Practical Issues in Geriatrics

Series Editor

Stefania Maggi
Ageing Branch
CNR-Neuroscience Institute
Padua
Italy

This practically oriented series presents state of the art knowledge on the principal diseases encountered in older persons and addresses all aspects of management, including current multidisciplinary diagnostic and therapeutic approaches. It is intended as an educational tool that will enhance the everyday clinical practice of both young geriatricians and residents and also assist other specialists who deal with aged patients. Each volume is designed to provide comprehensive information on the topic that it covers, and whenever appropriate the text is complemented by additional material of high educational and practical value, including informative video-clips, standardized diagnostic flow charts and descriptive clinical cases. Practical Issues in Geriatrics will be of value to the scientific and professional community worldwide, improving understanding of the many clinical and social issues in Geriatrics and assisting in the delivery of optimal clinical care.

More information about this series at http://www.springer.com/series/15090

Antonio Capurso • Gaetano Crepaldi
Cristiano Capurso

Benefits of the Mediterranean Diet in the Elderly Patient

FONDAZIONE
DIETA
MEDITERRANEA
ONLUS

Springer

Antonio Capurso
Department of Internal Medicine
School of Medicine
University of Bari
Bari
Italy

Gaetano Crepaldi
Department of Biomedical Science
CNR Neuroscience Institute
Padua
Italy

Cristiano Capurso
Department of Medical and
Surgical Sciences
School of Medicine, University of Foggia
Foggia
Italy

ISSN 2509-6060 ISSN 2509-6079 (electronic)
Practical Issues in Geriatrics
ISBN 978-3-030-08614-5 ISBN 978-3-319-78084-9 (eBook)
https://doi.org/10.1007/978-3-319-78084-9

Printed on acid-free paper

This Springer imprint is published by the registered company Springer International Publishing AG part of Springer Nature.
The registered company address is: Gewerbestrasse 11, 6330 Cham, Switzerland

Preface

This book illustrates the role of the Mediterranean diet in connection with well-being and particularly its impact on health and elderly care, as well as on the mechanisms of aging.

Aging is a natural process of human life. The knowledge that a healthy dietary regimen like the Mediterranean diet can effectively prevent or delay many diseases typically affecting aging people may help to better manage the aging process. From this point of view, knowledge of the numerous benefits of the Mediterranean-style diet may effectively reduce the burden of elderly care.

As early as the 1950s, Ancel Keys pointed out the effectiveness of the Mediterranean diet in helping to control, and possibly avoid, myocardial infarction and in improving cholesterol metabolism. Quite soon after the first studies were published, it became clear that the Mediterranean diet was beneficial in the prevention and management of not only cardiovascular disease but also many other diseases, from diabetes to hypertension, from cancer and thrombosis to neurodegenerative diseases, including dementia.

The biological effects of the Mediterranean diet appear to be due to the synergistic effects of its phytochemicals. This is why no single component can replace the combination of natural phytochemicals of the Mediterranean diet to achieve the observed health benefits. In this context, the Mediterranean diet with its main component virgin olive oil has been shown to exert a potent anti-inflammatory, anti-oxidant, and anti-cancer activity. The many components of Mediterranean diet, and particularly the polyphenols of virgin olive oil, promote these protective effects through epigenetic mechanisms, modifying the gene transcription activity toward a protective mode.

Examining those benefits in detail, this book offers a valuable educational tool for young professionals and caregivers, as well as for students and trainees in geriatrics and nutrition.

Bari, Italy	Antonio Capurso
Padua, Italy	Gaetano Crepaldi
Foggia, Italy	Cristiano Capurso

Acknowledgements

The authors would like to acknowledge the assistance of Ms. Linda Inverso in editing some of the book's chapters. This book has been endorsed by the "Fondazione Dieta Mediterranea, Ostuni, Italy" https://www.fondazionedietamediterranea.it/.

Contents

The Historical Origins and Composition of Mediterranean Diet

1

1.1 The Historical Scenario of Mediterranean Diet Around 1000 AD

Around the year 1000 AD, the eating habits of the European continent and of the Mediterranean area could be referred mainly to two well-defined models, which in turn derived from the two main European civilizations: the "classical" civilization and the "barbarian" civilization, which were very different one from the other and had been for a long time strongly pitted against each other.

The "classical" Greco-Roman civilization, which essentially had emerged and evolved in the Mediterranean basin, assigned a primary role to growing cereals (mostly grain) and arboriculture (mostly olive trees and grapes), alongside some livestock rearing, mainly of sheep and goats. This productive model was the main reference for a food culture mostly based on the "bread-olive oil-wine" triad, integrated, but only slightly, with meat and fish as well as sheep and goat cheeses.

The "barbarian" Celtic and Germanic civilization, which on the other hand had developed in the continental part of Europe, preferred a seminomadic lifestyle with an essentially silvo-pastoral economy based mainly on the exploitation of wild and forested areas through hunting, fishing, the gathering of wild fruits, and the rearing of free-range livestock, mostly of pigs. In this "barbarian" context, the growing of cereals played a marginal role as, instead of having the aim of producing flours, it was mostly destined to the production of beer, the beverage that in those lands replaced wine.

So, in that historical context, two main dietary models opposed each other, the European barbarian model, based on the "meat (from game), animal fats, and beer triad," and the Mediterranean *Greco-Roman* model based essentially on the "bread–olive oil–wine triad."

In 476 AD there was the fall of the *Roman Empire*. This date is historically considered as the end of the *Antiquity Era* and the passage to the *Middle Ages*. The subsequent centuries, from 400 to 800 AD, were characterized by huge human migrations in Europe, with northern and eastern European populations moving

A. Capurso et al., *Benefits of the Mediterranean Diet in the Elderly Patient*, Practical Issues in Geriatrics, https://doi.org/10.1007/978-3-319-78084-9_1

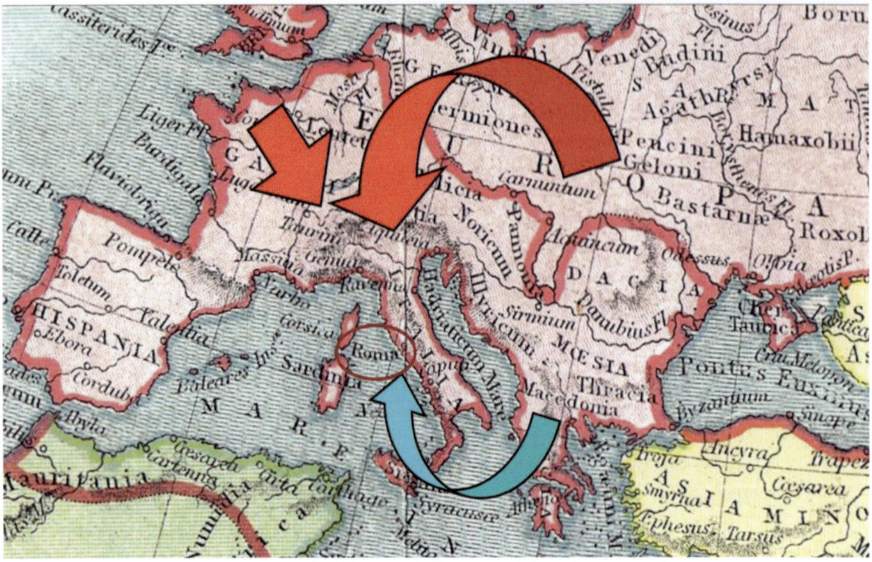

Fig. 1.1 The meeting/clash of the two civilizations, the Greek-Roman and the Barbarian

toward the south, toward the land of the Roman Empire. These "barbarian" migrations created an increasing pressure on the outer boundaries of the Roman territories, so greatly contributing to the collapse of the *Roman Empire*:

With the passage from *Antiquity* to the *Middle Ages*, the two "civilization" models, the *Greco-Roman* and the *Barbarian*, finally met and clashed with each other (Fig. 1.1).

It was a clash, because both civilizations tried to forcefully impose themselves on each other, and a meeting, because the two civilizations ended up blending into each other, growing richer with the most useful elements from the other. In this context, the food models also blended, with the growing of cereals, grapes, and olives typical of the Mediterranean spreading to Northern Europe. Bread, wine, and olive oil, the fundamental elements of the Mediterranean diet, became widespread in the northern countries, also because of their central role in the rituals and symbols of Christianity. With these elements regarded as liturgically indispensable, churches and monasteries became the means through which the food model of the "classical" civilization spread, with these products not remaining confined to the liturgical sphere but reaching also the daily food habits of the people.

At the same time, the Germanic production and dietary model was diffusing widely in the southern regions of Europe, concomitant with the political and social ascendancy of its propagator. So, in the southern regions, there began to spread a different attitude toward uncultivated areas—woods, pastures, and marshes—abundantly present in the south, left to grow wild and desolate during the premedieval transition ages. The novelty was that these uncultivated areas were to become used as places for breeding, hunting, fishing, and harvesting. The result was the diffusion of a mixed productive system—agro-silvo-pastoral—and, consequently, of a new feeding model in which animal products featured much more than before, along with products of vegetable origin. Regarding the vegetables, in particular, the *Greco-Roman* population learned from the barbarians to develop a localized horticultural production from small plots of land surrounded by uncultivated ground and the settlements, so introducing the consumption of vegetables in their Mediterranean diet.

Nevertheless, in the region of southern Italy, the peasant classes, less receptive to change, continued to produce and consume grain, olive oil, and wine, the typical products of the "classical" Roman and Mediterranean civilization, mostly because of the existing traditions and their dislike of innovations. The only innovation they accepted was that they learned to grow vegetables which entered their daily diet.

The northern regions, especially the Po river basin and Lombard Emilia, which had quickly become "Germanized," rapidly adopted the new "barbarian" models based on low-profile cereals, meat (especially pork), and animal fats.

To conclude, the roots of the Mediterranean diet are all derived from the classic *Greco-Roman* model of diet. It was therefore the southern peasants who, by resisting the penetration of the new "barbarian" food models imported by the Lombards, preserved the traditions of wheat bread, olive oil, wine, and of growing cereals. Several centuries had to pass before the "bread–oil–wine" triad was reconsidered from a new perspective, that is, an especially healthy diet that can prevent numerous diseases, particularly myocardial infarction and coronary heart diseases, cancer, and diabetes.

1.2 The Implementation of the Mediterranean Diet Along the Centuries

The basic elements of the basic Mediterranean diet, i.e., the "bread–olive oil–wine triad," progressively grew more diversified over the centuries (Fig. 1.2).

The first integration came from the "barbarian" invasions. The Germanic production and dietary model was rapidly and widely diffusing in the southern regions. In particular, the peasants learned from the *barbarians* to grow fresh vegetables in small plots of land near the house (the present backyard), and to harvest wild herbs and vegetables from the woods and uncultivated areas, to enrich their poor daily diet. Given the abundance of waters in the territory—marshes, ponds, rivers, streams, and lakes—freshwater fish consumption spread also extensively and took its place beside that of saltwater fish which, till then, had been the sole practice.

The second important integration of Mediterranean diet took place after the discovery of America by Christopher Columbus, August 3, 1492 AD. Spanish sailors imported to Europe new kinds of foods that Europeans had never heard of or seen: tomatoes, potatoes, corn, bell peppers, chili peppers, beans, pumpkins, pineapples, blueberries, sunflowers, peanuts, cocoa (chocolate), vanilla, tobacco, and unfortunately also syphilis.

So, the present Mediterranean diet is the result of a progressive enrichment along the centuries, starting from the basic *Greco-Roman* triad—bread, olive oil, and wine—with subsequent important contributions from "barbarian" invasions and from the discovery of America, the new continent.

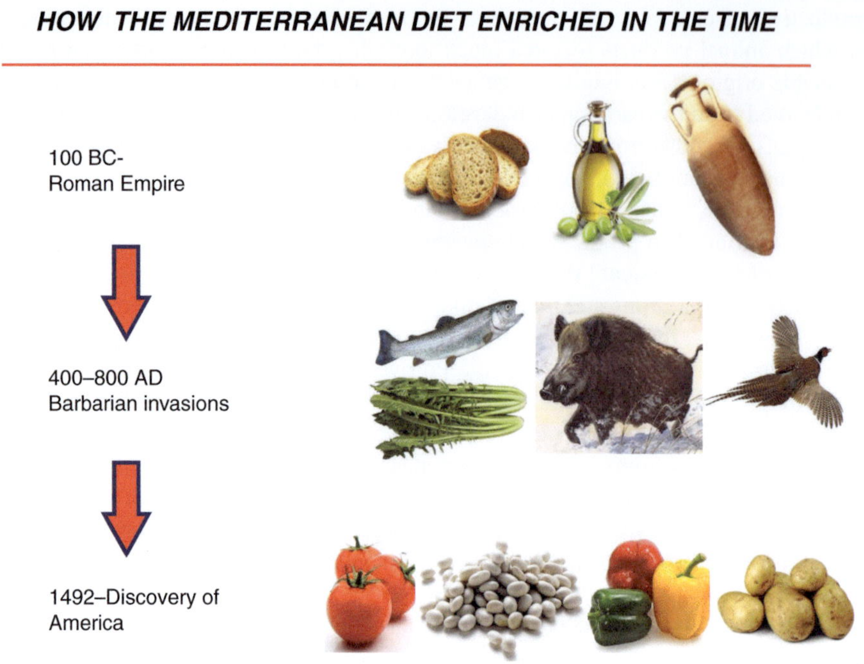

Fig. 1.2 How Mediterranean diet developed over the centuries

1.3 The Rediscovery of the Mediterranean Diet

The rediscovery of Mediterranean diet was essentially due to Ancel Keys, in the early 1950s.

Ancel Keys, professor of Human Physiology at the University of Minnesota and expert in nutrition and epidemiology, foresaw the benefits of this diet while visiting the isle of Crete in the 1940s, during the Second World War. Keys's attention was especially caught by how people in Crete never suffered from myocardial infarction, a disease that was almost unknown on the island, and he realized that their diet, based on oil, bread, and wine with vegetables, legumes, and fresh fruits, was the main reason for it.

Ancel Keys came to Italy for the first time in 1944, during the Second World War, landing at Paestum with the 5th US Army, and was so struck by the beauty of the place and the quality of the diet that he decided to come back in the future. In the early 1950s, traveling through several European countries together with Professor Paul White, Eisenhower's cardiologists, Ancel Keys noticed that wherever cholesterol levels were low, there were very few cases of myocardial infarction. A critical event in his trip was the 1st International Conference on Human Nutrition held in Rome in 1952, where Ancel Keys met professor Bergami, chair of Human Physiology at the University of Naples, who invited him to verify the cholesterol levels among different social classes of Naples and to meet with doctors who reported the rarity of myocardial infarction cases at their hospitals. The low cholesterol levels in southern Italy were immediately self-evident, leading to an early pilot study on cholesterol levels and diet in *Nicotera*, Calabria. Soon after, Ancel Keys embarked on the "Seven Countries Study," which conclusively demonstrated the effects of diet on human health and in particular the negative impact of animal fats, as opposed to the positive effects of unsaturated vegetable fats (extra-virgin olive oil) on the levels of cholesterol in the blood and on myocardial infarction incidence.

The "Seven Countries Study" [1], which could be considered the major breakthrough study on coronary risk factors, enrolled 12,520 subjects aged 40–59 from 7 countries (the United States, Italy, Finland, the Netherlands, Greece, Yugoslavia, and Japan), free of atherosclerosis and coronary artery disease. The subjects were monitored over an average period (*follow-up*) of 5 years. The number of fatal and nonfatal myocardial infarctions was much lower in southern European countries, the ones that had the lowest level of serum cholesterol and a diet rich in unsaturated fatty acids, derived essentially from olive oil (Greece, 20 cases of infarction per 10,000 people per year; Yugoslavia, 53 cases/10,000; Italy, 100 cases/10,000), compared to the northern Europe countries and the United States, whose level of serum cholesterol was much higher and the diet was very rich in saturated (animal) fats (Holland, 139/10,000; United States, 177/10,000; Finland, 198/10,000). The main data that emerged from the study was that the food habits of the populations living on the shores of the Mediterranean Sea protected the hearts of this population from infarctions, and the most important element of these food habits was the considerable daily consumption of extra-virgin olive oil, which supplied up to 40% of the daily caloric intake. In this study, Ancel Keys coined the term "Mediterranean diet" [2].

1.4 What Is the Mediterranean Diet?

The Mediterranean diet is a way of eating based on the traditional foods (and drinks) of the countries surrounding the Mediterranean Sea.

There are many Mediterranean diets. At least 16 countries border the Mediterranean Sea. Diets vary between these countries and also between regions within a country. Many differences in culture, ethnic background, religion, economy, and agricultural production result in different diets but with a common Mediterranean pattern, consisting of:

- High consumption of fruits, vegetables, bread and other cereals, potatoes, beans, nuts, and seeds
- Olive oil as an important monounsaturated fat source
- Dairy products, fish and poultry consumed in low to moderate amounts, and little red meat
- Eggs consumed zero to four times a week
- Wine consumed in low to moderate amounts, only during meals

Because olive oil was the principal source of fat in the Cretan diet (see section 1.5.1 this chapter), the model has been extended to include diets consumed in Mediterranean regions where olive oil is produced. In this manner, the generic term "Mediterranean diet" is used, in practice, to refer to dietary patterns similar to that of Crete in the early 1960s and other regions in the Mediterranean area where olive oil is a major fat source.

For Trichopoulou et al. [3], who studied older people in Greek villages, the eight characteristics of the traditional Greek Mediterranean diet are:

1. A high ratio of monounsaturated to saturated fat
2. Moderate alcohol consumption
3. High consumption of legumes
4. High consumption of cereals (including bread)
5. High consumption of fruits
6. High consumption of vegetables
7. Low consumption of meat and meat products
8. Low consumption of milk and dairy products

In a south Italy cohort (Bari-Casamassima) the dietary habits of the residents, 65–85 years old, were assessed by our group in the context of the large "Italian Longitudinal Study on Aging" (ILSA) [4], a prospective open study conducted in eight Italian areas to evaluate aging factors in a normal elderly population and the relationships between dietary macronutrient intakes and age-related changes, including cognitive functions. A semiquantitative food frequency questionnaire evaluating macronutrient energy intakes was administered to non-demented elderly subjects from the randomized cohort of 704 subjects. The daily diet of this elderly population resulted to be the typical Mediterranean diet (Fig. 1.3), with 47–50% of daily energy intakes derived from carbohydrates (bread and pasta), 12–14% from

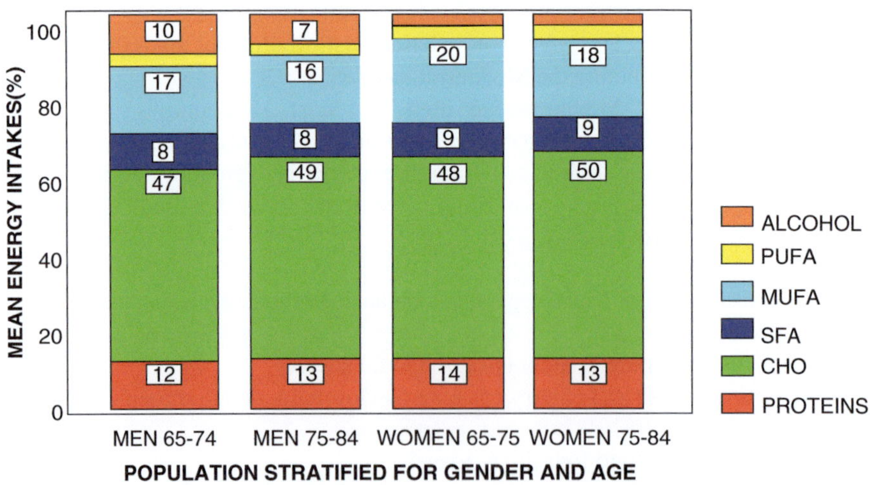

Fig. 1.3 The mean energy intakes stratified for gender and age by the ILSA study

proteins (mostly plant proteins coming from cereals and pulses), and 30% from fats, of which 7–8% from saturated fats, 20% from monounsaturated fats (extra-virgin olive oil), and 6–7% from polyunsaturated fats. Daily caloric intake from alcohol was 4–10% (Fig. 1.3). A significant inverse correlation between monounsaturated fatty acid (MUFA) energy intake and cognitive decline (MMSE <24) was found. The effect of education on the odds of having a MMSE score < 24 decreased exponentially with the increase of MUFA intakes, from an OR of 32 in the subjects of the lower percentile with a daily intake of 800 KJ of MUFA to an OR of 0.6 in the highest percentile with a daily intake of 2000–2400 KJ from MUFA. The conclusions were that in the elderly south Italy population with a typical Mediterranean diet, high daily MUFA intakes resulted in a strong protection against age-related cognitive decline (ARCD and MCI).

A good example of Mediterranean diet is the Mediterranean diet pyramid suggested by Willett, Trichopoulou et al. [5]. This pyramid reflects Mediterranean dietary traditions which historically have been associated with good health. This pyramid is based on food patterns typical of Crete, the rest of Greece, and of southern Italy in the early 1960s, where adult life expectancy was among the highest in the world and rates of coronary heart disease, cancers, and other diet-related chronic diseases were among the lowest.

1.5 The First Studies on the Mediterranean Diet

1.5.1 The Rockefeller Foundation Report: The Cretan Study

The first description of a Mediterranean-style diet is illustrated in a report of the Rockefeller Foundation of the 1950s. In 1948, the Greek government, concerned about the need to improve the postwar economic, social, and health conditions of the Greek population, invited the Rockefeller Foundation to undertake a major epidemiologic study on the island of Crete to determine how best to raise the population's standard of living. The Rockefeller Foundation appointed the epidemiologist Leland Albaugh. The survey was conducted in 1948–1949. The results were published in 1953 [6]. The data of the survey evidenced that 61% of daily caloric intake of the Cretan population was essentially derived from cereals, pulses, potatoes, vegetables, fresh fruit, and nuts, and another 30% of caloric intake was derived from extra-virgin olive oil as the unique alimentary fat. Contrary to this Mediterranean-style diet, the US diet in the same years had 65% of its daily caloric intake from meat, eggs, dairy products, fats, and sugar and 25% of calories from bread [6].

The Cretan cuisine was described as follows: "Olives, cereal grains, pulses, wild greens and herbs, and fruits, together with limited quantities of goat meat and milk, game, and fish have remained the basic Cretan foods for forty centuries… No meal was complete without bread… Olives and olive oil contributed heavily to the energy intake… Food seemed literally to be swimming in oil" [6].

However, despite the wealth of information provided by the Rockefeller Foundation report, the interest in the health implications of Mediterranean diet began with the work of Ancel Keys in the 1950s.

1.5.2 The Meeting of Ancel Keys with the Mediterranean Diet

Keys reported that his introduction to the Mediterranean diet began in the early 1950s when he was a visiting professor at Oxford. In 1951 he chaired the first conference of the Food and Agriculture Organization of the United Nations at their headquarters in Rome. Ancel Keys said: "The conference focused only on nutritional deficiencies. When I asked about the diet and the new epidemic of coronary heart disease, Gino Bergami, Professor of Physiology at the University of Naples, said coronary heart disease was not a problem in Naples."

In 1952, impressed by the low rates of heart disease in the Mediterranean region, Ancel Keys initiated a series of investigations on the diet in several populations.

Probably the best description of Mediterranean diet is that of Ancel Keys, when he came in Italy at the beginning of 1950s:

"Home made minestrone … pasta in endless variety … served with tomato sauce and a sprinkle of cheese, only occasionally enriched with some bits of meat or served with a little local seafood … a hearty dish of beans and short lengths of macaroni … lots of bread never more than a few hours from the oven and never served with any kind of spread; great quantities of fresh vegetables, a modest portion of meat or fish perhaps twice a week, wine of the type we used to call 'Dago red' … always fresh fruit for dessert" [7].

Later, Keys said "The heart of what we now consider the Mediterranean diet is mainly vegetarian: pasta in many forms, leaves sprinkled with olive oil, all kinds of vegetables in season and often cheese, all finished off with fruit and frequently washed down with wine … it is much lower in meat and dairy products and there are some differences in dessert. What we call pie is almost unknown, as are cornstarch and steamed puddings. Cakes are mostly special types for Christmas and Easter and fresh fruit is the standard dessert" [8].

In the book *Eat Well and Stay Well* [9], published in 1960 in collaboration with his wife Margaret, Keys said: "Years later, when called on to devise a diet for the possible prevention of coronary heart disease, we looked back and concluded it would be hard to do better than imitate the diet of the common folk of Naples in the early 1950s."

Having found that the typical dietary pattern of the Greek island of Crete and south Italy was associated with especially good health, this pattern has come to be viewed as the Mediterranean diet model.

As olive oil was the principal source of fat in the Cretan and south Italian diets, the model of Mediterranean diet was extended to include diets consumed in olive-producing Mediterranean regions. In this manner, the generic term "Mediterranean diet" was used in practice to refer to dietary patterns similar to those of Crete and south Italy in the early 1960s and in other regions in the Mediterranean area where olive oil is a major fat source.

Finally, it should be said that Mediterranean diet is not only a diet but rather a philosophy of life, which includes non-dietary lifestyle factors such as moderate physical activity (walking every day) and resting in the middle of the day (siesta) after an enjoyable family meal (Fig. 1.4).

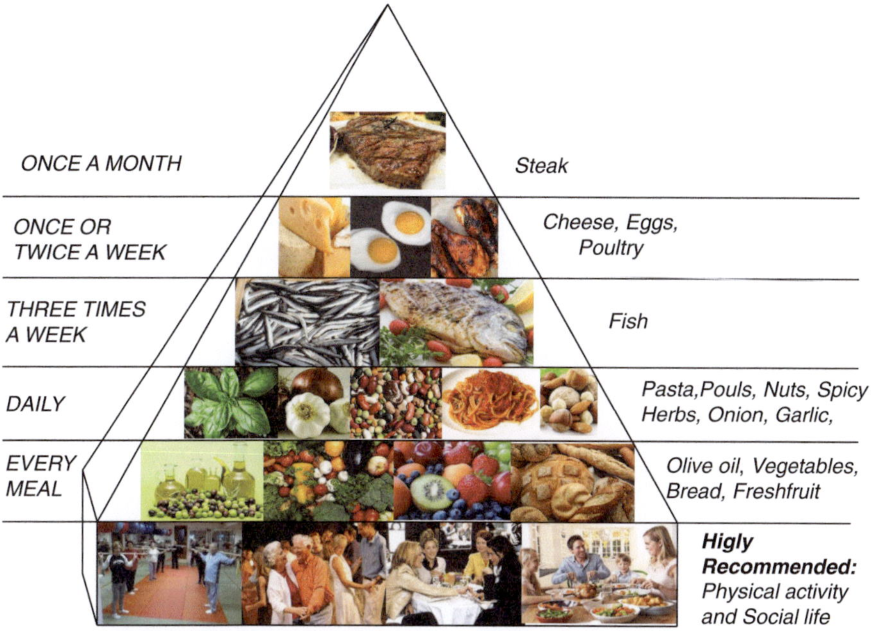

Fig. 1.4 A south Italy Mediterranean diet pyramid

References

1. Keys A, et al. Coronary heart disease in seven countries. Circulation. 1970;41:1–211.
2. Keys A, Keys M. How to eat well and stay well. The Mediterranean way. New York: Doubleday; 1975.
3. Trichopoulou A, Kouriros-Blazos A, Vassilakou T, Gnaudellis C, Polychronopoulos E, Venizelos M, Laggiou P, Wahlqvist ML, Trichopoulous D. Diet and survival of elderly Greek: a link to the past. Am J Clin Nutr. 1995;61:1346S–50S.
4. Solfrizzi V, Panza F, Torres F, Mastroianni F, Del Parigi A, Venezia A, Capurso A. High mono-unsaturated fatty acids intake protects against age-related cognitive decline. Neurology. 1999;52:1563–9.
5. Willett WC, Sachs F, Trichopoulou A, Dnescher G, Ferro-Luzzi A, Helsing E, Trichopoulos D. Mediterranean diet pyramid: a cultural model for healthy eating. Am J Clin Nutr. 1995;61:1402S–6S.
6. Albaugh LG, Soule G. Crete: a case study of an underdeveloped area. Princeton, NJ: Princeton University Press; 1953.
7. Nestle M. Mediterranean diets: historical and research overview. Am J Clin Nutr. 1995;61:1313S–20S.
8. Keys A. Mediterranean diet and public health: personal reflections. Am J Clin Nutr. 1995;61:1321S–3S.
9. Keys A, Keys M. Eat well and stay well: the Mediterranean way. New York: Doubleday & Co; 1959. p. 4.

Extra-Virgin Olive Oil (EVOO): History and Chemical Composition

2

2.1 The History of Olive Oil and Olive Trees

The historical scenario of olive oil begins during the Copper Age (sixth millennium BC), when humans began hunting, fishing, and agricultural activities: from a spiny bush with small fruits, big kernel, and a little pulp, a thick-oily-beneficial-tasty liquid could be obtained. The plant and its fruit were then improved over the centuries.

In that ancient time, along the Mediterranean coastline, from Syria to North Africa, from Greece to South Italy, there were bushy olive groves. The hills sloping down to the sea were covered with these evergreens with the silvery leaves.

A similar sight filled Abraham and his people with admiration when they arrived 2000 years before Christ at the east Mediterranean coast from the ancient Mesopotamian city of Ur, after a long journey across the desert.

Palestine must have seemed to be a happy land to the eyes of the ancient Hebrews. In Canaan, the new people soon learned to use the olive berries for their oil.

Two thousand years later, in the time of Jesus Christ, the olive groves still covered the hills of Palestine. In the Gospel according to St. Mark, it is recorded that Jesus, coming with his disciples from Galilee to Jerusalem, after having been to Jericho and restored sight to the blind man, stopped near the Mount of Olives, which was a hill covered with olive trees on the outskirt of Jerusalem. In David's city, there was another place, called Gethsemane, where one could rest in the shade of olive trees. Jesus went there with his disciples and prayed before his arrest. Today, in the garden of Gethsemane, there are eight centuries-old olive trees, certainly regenerated from shoots of earlier olive stumps.

The quotations from the Bible and the Gospels are surest documentation that the olive has a millenary presence in the Middle East.

It should be mentioned, however, that in the West, along the Mediterranean coast up to 40 miles from the sea, the olive was part of the spontaneous vegetation of 50 million years ago. Fossilized olive leaves of the Cenozoic Era have been found in Italy, around Senigallia and Mongardino Bolognese, and in Tuscany. Olive country,

A. Capurso et al., *Benefits of the Mediterranean Diet in the Elderly Patient*, Practical Issues in Geriatrics, https://doi.org/10.1007/978-3-319-78084-9_2

therefore, is not this or that land but all lands that look on the Mediterranean, whether plain or hill, and even with rocky soil.

In antiquity, the olive was a wild plant, with the features of a tree of little account: a trunk of limited height with compact foliage; long narrow, silvery green leaves; and black shiny drupes with little flesh and a bitter taste. Such is the portrait of the *oleaster* or wild olive tree *Olea europaea sylvestris et oleaster*. This plant has no claim to fame except for its having given life to the sweet-natured and better featured arboreal line of *Olea europaea sativa*. This is the domesticated or cultivated olive which combined in it the more rustic shapes of the *oleaster* and the more graceful shapes of our present olive trees.

To whom is the merit for first cultivating the olive? It is difficult to say: the ability to transform a spiny, bitter-berried plant into a docile tree in man's care has been acquired through the experience of many people through the centuries.

It is known for certain that, from very early times, the olive was cultivated and appreciated for its oil in Syria, Palestine, and Crete. The Phoenicians, considered the most expert navigators and capable merchants of 2000 BC, exported olives from southern Syria and Lebanon, their lands of origin, to the coastal countries of the Mediterranean and made known the good qualities of the "liquid gold" to the peoples with whom they had commercial contact.

In the twelfth century BC, the Phoenicians, oppressed at home by the invasion of the "People of the Sea," emigrated to those places which up till then had been simply their landings and transformed them into naval and trade colonies. Mozia (a small island off Marsala), Solunto, and Panormo (now, Palermo) thus became market based for mercantile activity in the West.

Large Phoenician sail- and oar-propelled ships navigated in the shelter of the Mediterranean coast, so they could better meet the dangers of both storms and attacks by sea robbers who, alas, made raids on everything. The mariner-merchants, when things went well, landed at the usual coastal villages where they knew by experience they could do good business. As soon as they arrived, they began unloading their wares, which were brought ashore, in large hemp baskets: They dealt in small, glass vases, kitchen utensils, weapons, ornaments and jewels, and woolen cloth of a reddish violet color tinted with purple. Large terra-cotta amphorae contained victuals: cereals, wine, and oil; there were black olives, too, picked, well-ripened, left to dry in the sun, and then preserved in amply-sized clay bowls.

When the merchants landed at the little centers of the African coast, the inhabitants ran to the shore, curious to see the new goods. With circumspection, they looked over the vases carefully before the bartering began. They were diffident, the natives, and they were not wrong: the Phoenician was notorious for his ability to cheat his neighbor.

Herodotus, the Greek historian of the fifth century BC, wrote of the Phoenicians: "… When they arrived, they unloaded their merchandise and laid it out orderly along the shore: then, returning to their ships, they sent up smoke signals, on seeing which the natives repaired to the sea, setting beside the goods the golden they offered in exchange and then withdrew. The Phoenicians came back to the shore, looked and, if they thought the amount of gold was adequate to the merchandise, they collected it up and went away, if not, they went aboard and waited for a satisfactory offer". This was the common method of trading and it lasted until Rome sacked Carthage, the cornerstone of Phoenician civilization.

In 1971, in the depths off the island of Mozia, a Carthaginian ship sunk during the first Punic War (264–241 BC) was found. On board were found various objects: wood, rope, spearheads, swords, and even small broom. Two hemp baskets, containing stalks of *Cannabis sativa* (cultivated cannabis) and some amphorae for wine, give one to imagine that the sailors were fond of stimulating and intoxicating drinks to boost their energy and bravery levels in battle. The stalks of cannabis sativa were infused to make an inebriating drink similar to tea. The crew ate meat rather than fish as proved by the ovine, deer, and domesticated animals' bones found in the hold. The small sizes of the earthenware pots and crockery on board suggest that probably only aromatic sauces for meat were prepared, but not soup, for meals. Olives, walnuts, almonds, and pistachios were consumed in great quantity, and perhaps they were used as comforting snacks during the short rest periods. A sprig of olive found on the ship suggests propitiatory rites in honor of the gods, frequently performed especially in time of war.

At the end of the Phoenician colonization, signs of that civilization remained long in Sicily. It is thought that the ability of cultivating the olive arrived at Rome from Sicily, through Campania. Pliny the Elder argued on the other hand that olive culture was introduced into Rome by the Etruscans, who were deeply involved in trade with the Phoenicians.

The other channel by which olive culture entered was by the Greeks. In the eighth century BC, a wave of Greek emigration gave rise to the nucleus of colonies along the south Italian Ionic coast, which came to be called *Magna Grecia*. The new Greek cities reached such economic and cultural power as to permit them to mint their own money. The monies of Messina and Crotone carried representations of olive foliage, which witness to a widespread presence in the fifth century BC of the olive tree in South Italy. Trade contacts between the Greeks of the colonies and the Romans must have fostered cultivation of the olive in the Roman territory, for then the Romans greatly admired everything coming from Greece.

It is certain that, in the Augustan Era, the stores of Rome held immense stocks of olive oil, much of it from Tunisia, Algeria, and Libya, territories conquered by the Romans.

Plutarch, in the *Parallel Lives*, records that when Julius Cesar returned to Rome after the war in Africa, he was welcomed with great festivities for having ensured Rome three million liters of oil per year. The province of Africa continued to supply Rome with olive oil. At the death of Septimius Severus (third century BC), stocks were enough to meet the needs of the entire Italian peninsula for 5 years.

Rome's fortune changed with the fall of the Roman Empire, and the olive, which was "the companion of the decadence of all virtue and social good," experienced similar change (Table 2.1).

Table 2.1 The olive oil over the centuries [1]

Period	Events
Copper Age (sixth millennium BC)	First extraction of thick oily liquid from olive fruit
Seventh millennium BC	Use of olive oil for cosmetic and basic medical purposes
Eighth–ninth century BC	Use for care (burned skin, dermatitis, intestinal pains)
Sixth century	Solone decreed a law for preservation of olive trees
Fifth century BC	In Panathenaean games, the winners of competitions were rewarded an olive twig and numerous amphorae (29–35 L) filled of olive oil
460–377 BC	For Hippocrates, father of medicine, olive oil was highly regarded
106–43 BC	Cicero wrote of the healthy aspect of "pinguis liquor olivae"
70–19 BC	Virgil mentioned the olive oil produced by "the sweet olive trees from the mild lake of Garda"
24–79 AD	Pliny the Elder in his *Historia Naturalis* listed 48 medicines made with olive oil
146–211 AD	Under the Roman emperor Settimio Severo free distribution of olive oil was given to the urban masses
Fourth century AD	Under Constantine: At least 250 bakeries and 2300 olive oil distributors
Middle age	The medical monks of the abbeys used preparation containing olive oil to treat burned skin and swellings, as well as numerous infections
Renaissance	The jars containing oil were present in all pharmacies
Nineteenth century	Olive oil is still used as a home remedy for several ailments

2.2 Olive Oil Composition

Olive oil is composed mainly of triglycerides (triacylglycerols) and contains small quantities of free fatty acids (FFA), glycerol, phosphatides, pigments, flavor compounds, sterols, and microscopic bits of olive. Different processing methods produce virgin, ordinary, or pomace olive oil. Virgin olive oil is produced by direct pressing or centrifugation of the olives. Virgin olive oils with an acidity greater than 3.0 degrees (presence in the oil of free fatty acids not linked to triacylglycerol) are submitted to a refining process in which some components, mainly phenolic compounds and to a lesser degree squalene, are lost. By mixing virgin and refined olive oil, an ordinary olive oil (UE 1991) is produced and marketed. After virgin olive oil production, the rest of the olive drupe and seed is processed and submitted to a refining process, resulting in pomace olive oil, to which a certain quantity of virgin olive oil is added before marketing.

From a chemical point of view, two olive oil fractions are identified, depending on the behavior in the presence of heating and strong alkaline solutions (concentrated solutions of KOH or NaOH):

- *The saponifiable fraction*, representing 98–99% of the total weight, is composed of substances that form soaps in the above conditions.
- *The unsaponifiable fraction*, representing the remaining 1–2% of the total weight, is composed of substances that fail to form soaps in the above conditions.

2.2.1 The Saponifiable Fraction

The saponifiable fraction of olive oil is composed of (1) unsaturated fatty acids (75–85% of the total fatty acids) and (2) saturated fatty acids (15–23%).

1. *Unsaturated fatty acids.* Oleic acid is the major fatty acid in olive oil. According to the rules laid down by the International Olive Oil Council (IOOC), its concentration must range from 55 to 83% of total fatty acids. Linoleic acid is the most abundant polyunsaturated fatty acid in olive oil. Its concentration must vary between 2.5 and 21% (IOOC). Because of its degree of unsaturation (two double bonds = n-6 fatty acid), it is more easily subject to oxidation; this means that an oil rich in linoleic acid becomes more easily rancid and therefore can be stored for a shorter time.

   Alpha-linolenic acid (three double bonds; n-3 fatty acid) is a very minor component of olive oil; it must be present in ≤1% according to IOOC standards. It is an omega-3 polyunsaturated fatty acid, which may have health benefits. However, because of its high degree of unsaturation (three double bonds), it is very susceptible to oxidation, and therefore it promotes rancidity of olive oil that contains it.
2. *Saturated fatty acids.* Palmitic (7.5–20%) and stearic acids (0.5–5%) are the main saturated fatty acid of olive oil. Myristic, heptadecanoic, arachidic, behenic, and lignoceric acids may be present in trace amounts.

Actually, the fatty acid composition of olive oil is not constant because it is influenced by several factors, i.e., the climate, the latitude, and the zone of production. Particularly important is the zone of production. In fact, Italian, Spanish, and Greek olive oils are high in oleic acid (56–83%) and low in palmitic and linoleic acids, while Tunisian olive oils are high in palmitic and linoleic acids but lower in oleic acid. Therefore, olive oils can be divided into two groups: (a) oils rich in oleic acid and low in palmitic and linoleic acids and (b) oils rich in palmitic and linoleic acids and low in oleic acid. The degree of olive ripeness at the time of extraction is important; in fact, oleic acid is formed first in the fruit, and data indicate a competitive relationship between oleic and palmitic acid and palmitoleic and linoleic acid.

Olive oil is essentially formed by *triglycerides* (three fatty acid molecules that esterify one glycerol molecule), with minimal amounts of diglycerides and monoglycerides that are normally present. The presence of mono- and diglycerides is due to incomplete synthesis and/or partial hydrolysis of triglycerides.

The content of *diglycerides* in virgin olive oil ranges from 1 to 2.8%. 1,2-diglycerides prevail in fresh olive oil, representing the majority of diglycerides (80%). During oil storage, isomerization occurs with a progressive increase of the more stable 1,3 isomers which, after about 10 months, become the major diglyceride.

Monoglycerides are present in a much lower amount than diglycerides, <0.25%, with 1-monoglycerides much higher than 2-monoglycerides.

2.2.2 The Unsaponifiable Fraction

The unsaponifiable fraction of olive oil represents the remaining 1–2% of the total weight and is composed of substances that fail to form soaps in the above conditions.

The unsaponifiable fraction is composed of a large number of different molecules which are very important from a nutritional point of view, as they contribute significantly to the health effect of olive oil. This fraction includes tocopherols, sterols, polyphenols, pigments, hydrocarbons, aromatic and aliphatic alcohol, triterpene acids, waxes, and other minor components.

The components of unsaponifiable fraction are responsible for the stability and the taste of olive oil. Their content is influenced by numerous factors, i.e., the cultivar, the degree of ripeness of the olives, the zone of production, the harvesting practices, the storage time of olives, the oil extraction process, and the storage conditions of the oil.

The unsaponifiable fraction can be subdivided into two types: (1) the "nonpolar" (non-water-soluble) fraction that could be extracted with solvents after the saponification of the oil; this fraction contains squalene and other triterpenes, sterols, tocopherol, and pigments and (2) the "polar," water-soluble fraction that includes the phenolic compounds.

2.2.2.1 Phenolic Compounds (Polyphenols)

Polyphenols are among the most important components of extra-virgin olive oil, for their beneficial impact on human health.

Extra-virgin olive oil contains approximately 36 phenolic compounds, and it is this minor phenolic fraction that is responsible for most of the health benefits associated with extra-virgin olive oil intake. Polyphenols make up 18–37% of the unsaponifiable fraction of olive oil. An average concentration of phenolic compounds of 230 mg/kg in extra-virgin olive oil has been reported [2]. The polyphenol concentration in extra-virgin olive oil actually varies from 50 to 800 mg/kg [3].

Polyphenols are an heterogeneous group of molecules with important organoleptic and nutritional properties (see also Chap. 10, Sect. 10.10.1., this book).

Olive oil polyphenols have been reported to be highly bioavailable compared to other plant polyphenols. Their absorption efficiency was evaluated about 55–66 mmol% in humans [4]. Tyrosol and hydroxytyrosol, two of the most important phenols of olive oil, are absorbed by humans in a dose-dependent manner in relation to the phenolic content of the olive oil administered [5].

Among polyphenols, there are molecules with simple structure, such as phenolic acids and alcohols, and molecules with complex structure, such as flavonoids, secoiridoids, and lignans.

Phenolic acids: They are aromatic acid compounds that include substances containing a phenolic ring and an organic carboxylic acid function. The main phenolic acids are (a) hydroxybenzoic acids (gallic, protocatechuic, and 4-hydroxybenzoic acids) and (b) hydroxycinnamic acids (caffeic, vanillin, syringic, p-coumaric, o-coumaric acids).

Phenolic alcohols: Among phenolic alcohols, the most abundant are hydroxytyrosol (3,4-dihydroxyphenyl ethanol) and tyrosol [2-(4-hydroxyhenyl)ethanol], which constitute around 90% of the total phenolic content of virgin olive oil [6]. The hydroxytyrosol derives from the hydrolysis of the secoiridoid oleuropein (Fig. 2.1). The hydroxytyrosol is by far the most potent antioxidant of virgin olive oil. It was recently reported to protect the blood lipids against oxidative damage as reported by the European Food Safety Authority (EFSA) panel on dietetic products, nutrition, and allergies. The panel considered that in order for olive oil to bear the "heart-health" claim, 5 mg of hydroxytyrosol and its derivatives (e.g., oleuropein complex and tyrosol) in olive oil should be consumed daily [7, 8].

Secoiridoids: Secoiridoids are the olive oil polyphenols with the more complex structure and are produced from the secondary metabolism of terpenes. They are glycosylated compounds and are characterized by the presence of elenolic acid in their structure. Oleuropein, demethyloleuropein, ligstroside, and nuzenide are the main secoiridoids. Oleuropein and demethyloleuropein are abundant in the pulp, while nuzenide is present only in the kernel.

Oleuropein, a bitter glycoside, is an important phenolic compound in the drupe and constitutes up to 14% of the fruit's dry weight. With the progression of blooming and maturation, oleuropein undergoes enzymatic and nonenzymatic hydrolysis and yields several simpler compounds (e.g., hydroxytyrosol, oleuropein

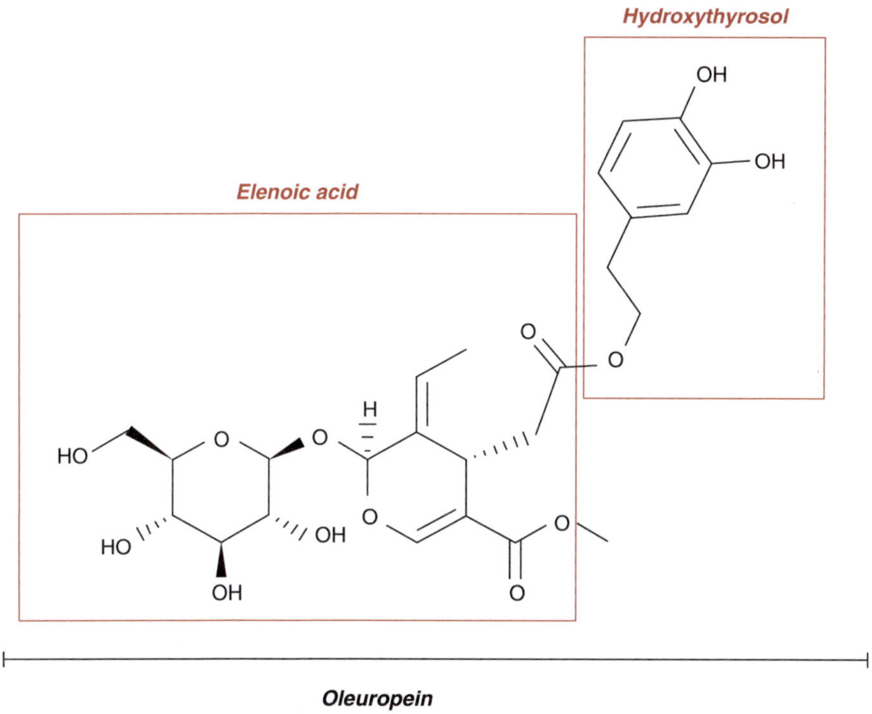

Fig. 2.1 Oleuropein, hydroxytyrosol and elenolic acid

aglycone, and ligstroside) that build up the full fruity taste that connoisseurs of olive oil search for.

Oleuropein aglycone, found in ripening olives and olive oil, is the phenolic secoiridoid liberated from the glucoside form, oleuropein, upon the action of a β-glucosidase. In olive oil, oleuropein is degraded into elenolic acid, the secoiridoid moiety, and hydroxytyrosol, the phenolic moiety (Fig. 2.1). Oleuropein aglycone and hydroxytyrosol are characterized by the orthodiphenolic structures, but in olive oil, there are also corresponding monophenolic structures of ligstroside aglycone and tyrosol. Tyrosol, hydroxytyrosol, and their corresponding secoiridoid derivatives constitute around 90% of the total phenolic content of virgin olive oil [9]. Hydroxyisochromans are formed by reaction between hydroxytyrosol and aromatic aldehydes (vanillin and benzaldehyde) under very mild conditions [9].

Oleuropein, the ester of hydroxytyrosol and elenolic acid (Fig. 2.1), is the most important secoiridoid of olive oil and the main olive oil polyphenol. It is present in very high quantities in olive leaves, as also in all the constituent parts of the olive, including peel, pulp, and kernel. Oleuropein accumulates in olives during the growth phase, up to 14% of the net weight; when the fruit turns greener, its quantity reduces. Finally, when the olives turn dark brown, color due to the presence of anthocyanins, the reduction in its concentration becomes more evident. During the reduction of oleuropein levels (and of the levels of other secoiridoids), an increase of compounds such as flavonoids, verbascosides, and simple phenols takes place.

Lignans: Lignans, in particular (+)-1-acetoxypinoresinol and (+)-pinoresinol, are another group of polyphenols in olive oil. It has been also found in the olive kernel. Lignans are not present in the pericarp of the olives nor in leaves and sprigs that may accidentally be pressed with the olives. Therefore, how they can pass into the olive oil becoming one of the main phenolic fractions is not yet known. (+)-1-Acetoxypinoresinol and (+)-pinoresinol are absent in seed oil and virtually absent in refined virgin olive oil, while they may reach a concentration of 100 mg/kg in extra-virgin olive oil. As seen for simple phenols and secoiridoids, there is considerable variation in their concentration among olive oils of various origins, variability probably related to differences between olive varieties, production areas, climate, and oil production techniques.

2.2.2.2 Hydrocarbons

They make up 30–50% of the unsaponifiable fraction. Squalene Hydrocarbons and beta-carotene are the main molecules.

Squalene, a hydrocarbon and a triterpene isolated for the first time from shark liver, is the major constituent of the unsaponifiable fraction and constitutes more than 90% of the hydrocarbons. Its concentration ranges from 136 to 708 mg/100 g in olive oil, compared to 19–36 mg for corn oil. It is an intermediate in the biosynthesis of the four-ring structure of steroids, and it seems to be responsible for several health effects of olive oil. In the hydrocarbon fraction of virgin olive oil, n-paraffins, diterpene and triterpene hydrocarbons, and isoprenoidal polyolefins are also found.

Beta-carotene, an organic, strongly colored red-orange pigment abundant in plant and fruits, is a nonpolar compound that acts both as antioxidant, protecting oil during storage, and as dye.

2.2.2.3 Sterols

Four classes of sterols are present in olive oil: common sterols, 4-methylsterols, triterpene alcohols, and triterpene dialcohols. Their content ranges from 1000 mg/kg, the minimum value required by the IOOC standard, to 2000 mg/kg. The lowest values are found in refined oils because the refining processes may cause losses up to 25%.

Common sterols or 4α-desmethylsterols: Common sterols are present mainly in the free and esterified form. The main molecules are beta-sitosterol, which makes up 75–90% of the total sterol; Δ5-avenasterol, 5–20%; and campesterol, 4%. Other components found in lower amounts or traces are, for example, stigmasterol, 2%, cholesterol, brassicasterol, and ergosterol.

4-Methylsterols: They are intermediates in the biosynthesis of sterols and are present both in the free and esterified form. They are present in small amounts, much lower than those of common sterols and triterpene alcohols, varying between 50 and 360 mg/kg. The main molecules are obtusifoliol, cycloeucalenol, citrostadienol, and gramisterol.

Triterpene alcohols or 4,4-dimethylsterols: They are a complex class of sterols, present both in the free and esterified form. They are found in amounts ranging from 350 to 1500 mg/kg. The main components are beta-amyrin, 24-methylenecycloartanol, cycloartenol, and butyrospermol; other molecules present in lower/trace amounts are, for example, cyclosadol, cyclobranol, germanicol, and dammaradienol.

Triterpene dialcohols: The main triterpene dialcohols found in olive oil are erythrodiol and uvaol. Erythrodiol is present both in the free and esterified form; in virgin olive oil, its level varies between 19 and 69 mg/kg, and the free form is generally lower than 50 mg/kg.

2.2.2.4 Tocopherols

The tocopherol content of olive oil is ~10 times lower than that of seed oils because of the lack of extraction of olive seeds, where most of the tocopherols are located.

Tocopherols make up 2–3% of the unsaponifiable fraction and include vitamin E. Of the eight E vitamins (alpha-, beta-, gamma-, and delta-tocopherol and alpha-, beta-, gamma-, and delta-tocotrienol), alpha-tocopherol represents about 90% of tocopherols in virgin olive oil. It is present in the free form and in very variable amount but on average higher than 100 mg/kg of olive oil. Thanks to its in vivo antioxidant properties, its presence is a protective factor for health. Alpha-tocopherol concentration seems to be related to the high levels of chlorophylls and to the concomitant requirement for deactivation of singlet oxygen. Beta-tocopherol, delta-tocopherol, and gamma-tocopherol are usually present in low amounts.

2.2.2.5 Pigments

This group includes chlorophylls and carotenoids. In olive oil, chlorophylls are present as pheophytins, mainly pheophytin a (i.e., a chlorophyll from which magnesium has been removed and substituted with two hydrogen ions), and confer the characteristic green color to olive oil. They are photosensitizer molecules that contribute to the photooxidation of olive oil itself. Beta-carotene and lutein are the main carotenoids in olive oil. Several xanthophylls are also present, such as antheraxanthin, beta-cryptoxanthin, luteoxanthin, mutatoxanthin, neoxanthin, and violaxanthin.

Olive oil's color is the result of the presence of chlorophylls and carotenoids and of their green and yellow hues. Their presence is closely related.

2.2.2.6 Triterpene Acids

They are present in trace amounts in the oil. Oleanolic and maslinic acids are the main triterpene acids in virgin olive oil: they are present in the olive husk, from which they are extracted in a small amount during processing.

2.2.2.7 Aliphatic and Aromatic Alcohols

Fatty alcohols and diterpene alcohols are the most important ones. Aliphatic alcohols have a number of carbon atoms between 20 and 30 and are located mostly inside the olive stones, from where they are partially extracted by milling.

Fatty Alcohols

Fatty alcohols are linear saturated alcohols with more than 16 carbon atoms. They are found in the free and esterified form and are present, in virgin olive oil, in an amount not generally higher than 250 mg/kg. Docosanol (C22), tetracosanol (C24), hexacosanol (C26), and octacosanol (C28) are the main fatty alcohols in olive oil, with tetracosanol and hexacosanol present in larger amounts. Waxes, which are minor constituents of olive oil, are esters of fatty alcohols with fatty acids, mainly of palmitic acid and oleic acid. They can be used as a criterion to discriminate between different types of oils; for example, they must be present in virgin and extra-virgin olive oil at levels <150 mg/kg, according to the IOOC standards.

Diterpene Alcohols

Geranylgeraniol and phytol are two acyclic diterpene alcohols present in the free and esterified form. Among esters present in the wax fraction of extra-virgin olive oil, oleate, eicosenoate, eicosanoate, docosanoate, and tetracosanoate have been found, mainly as phytyl derivatives.

2.2.2.8 Volatile Compounds

More than 280 volatile compounds have been identified in olive oil, such as hydrocarbons, the most abundant fraction, alcohols, aldehydes, ketones, esters, acids, ethers, and many others. However, only about 70 of them are present at levels higher than the perception threshold beyond which they may contribute to the aroma of virgin olive oil.

2.2.2.9 Minor Components

Among the minor components of olive oil, there are some phospholipids. The main phospholipids are phosphatidylserine, phosphatidylethanolamine, phosphatidylcholine, and phosphatidylinositol. In the unfiltered oils, trace amounts of proteins may be found.

2.2.2.10 Biological Activities of Olive Oil Phenolics

Thanks to the availability of pure compounds, the biological activities of the olive oil phenolics oleuropein and hydroxytyrosol have been thoroughly investigated in in vitro studies [10]. These studies included the antioxidant capacity of these phenolics. The results showed that olive oil phenolics are potent free radical scavengers, inhibit chemically induced LDL oxidation, inhibit platelet aggregation and eicosanoid production by activated human leukocytes, with a consequent antithrombotic activity [11], and potentiate the macrophagic response to endotoxin challenge by increasing their production of nitric oxide [12]. Finally, it was clearly demonstrated a dose-dependent absorption of olive oil phenolics by humans [5].

References

1. Caramia G, Gori A, Valli E, Cerretani L. Virgin olive oil in preventive medicine: from legend to epigenetics. Eur J Lipid Sci Technol. 2012;114:375–88.
2. Owen RW, Giacosa A, Hull WE, Haubner R, Spiegelhalder B, Bartsch H. The antioxidant/anticancer potential of phenolic compounds isolated from olive oil. Eur J Cancer. 2000;36:1235–47.
3. Perona JS, Cabello-Moruno R, Ruiz-Gutierrez V. The role of virgin olive oil components in the modulation of endothelial function. J Nutr Biochem. 2006;17:429–45.
4. Vissers MN, Zock PL, Katan MB. Bioavailability and antioxidant effects of olive oil phenols in humans: a review. Eur J Clin Nutr. 2004;58:955–65.
5. Visioli F, Galli C, Bornet F, Mattei A, Patelli R, Galli G, Caruso D. Olive oil phenolics are dose-dependently absorbed in humans. FEBS Lett. 2000;468:159–60.
6. de la Torre-Carbot K, Chavez-Servin JL, Jauregui O, Castellote AI, Lamuela-Raventós RM, Fitó M, Covas MI, Muñoz-Aguayo D, López-Sabater MC. Presence of virgin olive oil phenolic metabolites in human low density lipoprotein fraction: determination by high-performance liquid chromatography-electrospray ionization tandem mass spectrometry. Anal Chim Acta. 2007;583:402–10.
7. EFSA, NDA Panel. Scientific opinion on the substantiation of health claims related to polyphenols in olive and protection of LDL particles from oxidative damage. EFSA J. 2011;9:2033.
8. Martin-Pelaez S, Covas MI, Fito M, Kusar A, Pravst I. Health effects of olive oil polyphenols: recent advances and possibilities for the use of health claims. Mol Nutr Food Res. 2013;57:760–71.
9. Bendini A, Cerretani L, Carrasco-Pancorbo A, Gómez-Caravaca AM, Segura-Carretero A, Fernández-Gutiérrez A, Lercker G. Phenolic molecules in virgin olive oils: a survey of their sensory properties, health effects, antioxidant activity and analytical methods. An overview of the last decade. Molecules. 2007;12:1679–719.
10. Visioli F, Galli C. Olive oil: more than just oleic acid. Am J Clin Nutr. 2000;72:853.
11. Frost Larsen L, Jespersen J, Marckmann P. Are olive oil diets antithrombotic? Diets enriched with olive, rapeseed, or sunflower oil affect postprandial factor VII differently. Am J Clin Nutr. 1999;70:976–82.
12. Visioli F, Galli C. The effect of minor constituent of olive oil on cardiovascular disease: new findings. Nutr Rev. 1998;56:142–7.

Extra-Virgin Olive Oil and Cardiovascular Disease

3

3.1 Premises: Cardiovascular Disease

Cardiovascular disease (CVD) is the leading cause of death in the Western countries: more people die annually from CVDs than from any other cause. An estimated 17.7 million people died from CVDs in 2015, representing 31% of all global deaths. Of these deaths, an estimated 7.4 million are due to coronary heart disease and 6.7 million to stroke.

In the United States, CVD is the leading cause of death. About 610,000 people die from heart disease in every year. Coronary heart disease (CHD) is the most common type of heart disease killing 370,000 people annually in the United States. Every year about 735,000 Americans have a heart attack. Of these, 525,000 are a first attack, and 210,000 happen in people who have already had a heart attack [1, 2].

High blood pressure, high cholesterol, and smoking are the major risk factors that could lead to CVD and stroke. Other important risk factors are type 2 diabetes mellitus, obesity, and physical inactivity. A number of other, nonmajor, risk factors have been described.

3.2 The History of CHD Risk Factors

The research into the causes of atherosclerosis began in 1907, when Alexander Ignatowski (1875–1955) began his studies on atherosclerosis. Believing that a toxic metabolite of animal protein led to atherosclerosis, he fed meat to adult rabbits and milk and egg yolk to weanling rabbits and caused atherosclerosis. Rabbits fed with animal proteins soon developed pronounced atherosclerosis of the aorta. In 1908 Ignatowski published his pioneering work that first revealed a relationship between animal protein and experimental atherosclerosis [3]. This early experimental work paved a way to the metabolic study of the mechanism of atherosclerosis [4–8].

Subsequently, experimental efforts from many laboratories were directed at determining which, if any, animal protein was the most atherogenic. The subsequent

A. Capurso et al., *Benefits of the Mediterranean Diet in the Elderly Patient*, Practical Issues in Geriatrics, https://doi.org/10.1007/978-3-319-78084-9_3

discovery that dietary cholesterol per se was atherogenic turned attention to fat and cholesterol, eclipsing work on dietary protein. In 1912, using Ignatowski's experimental protocols, Theodor Fahr produced early atherosclerosis in 5–8 months and severe atherosclerotic damage to the aorta, with elevated blood pressure, in 9–10 months [9]. The same year, Nikolai Anichkov and Semen Chalatov reproduced Ignatowski's experiments and showed that atherosclerosis can be caused by cholesterol [10, 11]. Since 1912, extensive research has been conducted on the mechanism of atherosclerosis. Ignatowski's pioneering experiments became classic and were reproduced by many research scientists all over the world, which ultimately led to our current understanding of the atherosclerotic process.

In 1948, researchers under the direction of the National Heart Institute (now National Heart, Lung, and Blood Institute) initiated the Framingham Heart Study, the first major study to help understand heart disease. In 1949, the term "arteriosclerosis" (known as "atherosclerosis" today) was added to the International Classification of Diseases, which caused a sharp increase in reported deaths from heart disease.

The Framingham Study

The Framingham Heart Study is a long-term, ongoing cardiovascular cohort study on residents of the town of Framingham, Massachusetts. The study began in 1948 with 5209 adult subjects from Framingham and is now on its third generation of participants. Prior to it almost nothing was known about the "epidemiology of hypertensive or arteriosclerotic cardiovascular disease." Much of the now-common knowledge concerning heart disease, such as the effects of diet, exercise, and common medications such as aspirin, is based on this longitudinal study. It is a project of the National Heart, Lung, and Blood Institute, in collaboration with Boston University since 1971.

The initial population was 5209 healthy men and women aged 30–62, not the whole of the town population, as is sometimes assumed.

It was rightly assumed from the start of the Framingham Heart Study that cardiac health can be influenced by lifestyle and environmental factors and by inheritance. With the Framingham Heart Study, the term "risk factor" was introduced. Before the Framingham Heart Study, doctors had little sense of prevention. In the 1950s, it was believed that clogging of arteries and narrowing of arteries (atherosclerosis, arteriosclerosis) was a normal part of aging and occurred universally as people became older. High blood pressure (hypertension) and elevated serum cholesterol (hypercholesterolemia) were also seen as normal consequences of aging in the 1950s, and no treatment was initiated.

The Framingham Heart Study, along with other important large studies, e.g., the Seven Countries Study, Nurses' Health Study, and Women's Health Initiative, showed the importance of healthy diet, not being overweight or obese, and doing regular exercise in maintaining good health. It was observed that there were differences in cardiovascular risk between men and women. It was also confirmed that cigarette smoking is a highly significant factor in the development of heart disease, leading to angina pectoris, myocardial infarction (MI), and coronary death.

Major findings from the Framingham Heart Study, according to the researchers, were:

1960s: *Cigarette smoking increases risk of heart disease. Increased cholesterol and elevated blood pressure increase risk of heart disease. Exercise decreases risk of heart disease, and obesity increases it.*

1970s: *Elevated blood pressure increases risk of stroke. In women who are postmenopausal, risk of heart disease is increased, compared with women who are premenopausal. Psychosocial factors affect risk of heart disease.*

1980s: *High levels of HDL cholesterol are associated with a reduced risk of heart disease.*

1990s: *Having an enlarged left ventricle of the heart (left ventricular hypertrophy) increases risk of stroke. Elevated blood pressure can progress to heart failure. Framingham Risk Score is published and correctly predicts 10-year risk of future coronary heart disease (CHD) events. At 40 years of age, the lifetime risk for CHD is 50% for men and 33% for women.*

2000s: *So called "high-normal blood pressure" increases risk of cardiovascular disease (high-normal blood pressure is called pre-hypertension in medicine; it is defined as a systolic pressure of 120–139 mmHg and/or a diastolic pressure of 80–89 mmHg). Lifetime risk of developing elevated blood pressure is 90%. Obesity is a risk factor for heart failure. Serum aldosterone levels predict risk of elevated blood pressure. Lifetime risk for obesity is approximately 50%. The "SHARe" project (SHARe, SNP Health Association Resource), a genome-wide association study within the Framingham Heart Study, is announced. Social contacts of individuals are relevant to whether a person is obese and whether cigarette smokers decide to quit smoking. Four risk factors for a precursor of heart failure are described. Thirty-year risk for serious cardiac events can be calculated. American Heart Association considers certain genomic findings of the Framingham Heart Study as one of the top research achievements in cardiology. Some genes increase risk of atrial fibrillation. Risk of poor memory is increased in middle-aged men and women if the parents had suffered from dementia.*

In 1950, the University of California researcher John Gofman (1918–2007) and his associates identified today's two well-known cholesterol types: low-density lipoprotein (LDL) and high-density lipoprotein (HDL). He discovered that men who developed atherosclerosis had elevated levels of LDL and low levels of HDL.

Also in the 1950s, American scientist Ancel Keys (1904–2004) discovered in his travels to Southern Italy that heart disease was rare in those Mediterranean populations where people consumed a lower-fat diet. Keys' interest in diet and cardiovascular disease (CVD) was prompted, in part, by seemingly counterintuitive data: American business executives, presumably among the best-fed persons, had high rates of heart disease, while in postwar Europe CVD rates had decreased sharply in the wake of reduced food supplies. Keys postulated a correlation between cholesterol levels and CVD and initiated a study of Minnesota businessmen (the first prospective study of CVD) [12]. At a 1955 expert meeting at the World Health Organization in Geneva, Keys presented his diet-lipid-heart disease hypothesis with "his usual confidence and bluntness" [13]. Naples was the first case study that seemed to support his hypothesis [14].

After observing in Southern Italy the highest concentration of centenarians in the world, Keys hypothesized that a Mediterranean-style diet low in animal fat protected against heart disease and that a diet high in animal fats led to heart disease. The results of the *Seven Countries Study*, published on Circulation in 1970 [15], clearly showed that serum cholesterol was strongly related to coronary heart disease mortality both at the population and at the individual level [16]. As a result, representatives of the American Heart Association appeared on television to inform people that a diet which included large amounts of butter, lard, eggs, and beef would lead to coronary heart disease. This resulted in the American government recommending that people adopt a low-fat diet in order to prevent heart disease. Keys had concluded that saturated fats as found in milk and meat have adverse effects, while unsaturated fats found in vegetable oils had beneficial effects. This message was obscured for a 20-year period starting around 1985, when all dietary fats were considered unhealthy.

The Seven Country Study

The Seven Countries Study was formally started in fall 1958 in Yugoslavia. In total, 12,763 males, 40–59 years of age, were enrolled as 16 cohorts, in 7 countries, in 4 regions of the world (the United States, Northern Europe, Southern Europe, Japan). One cohort was in the United States, two cohorts in Finland, one in the Netherlands, three in Italy, five in Yugoslavia (two in Croatia and three in Serbia), two in Greece, and two in Japan. The entry examinations were performed between 1958 and 1964 with an average participation rate of 90%, lowest in the United States with 75% and highest in one of the Japanese cohorts, with 100%. The Seven Countries Study has continued for more than 50 years.

A 2015 systematic review and meta-analysis by the Cochrane Collaboration, an organization which promotes evidence-based medicine, found that reducing saturated fat intake reduced the risk of cardiovascular disease, concluding: "Lifestyle advice to all those at risk of cardiovascular disease and to lower-risk population groups should continue to include permanent reduction of dietary saturated fat and partial replacement by unsaturated fats" [17].

3.3 EVOO and CHD

CHD is largely preventable, as unhealthy lifestyles (smoking, lack of exercise, and poor dietary habits) contribute to nearly 80% of population-attributable risk [18, 19]. Among these lifestyle components, diet has been well studied. After decades of epidemiological, clinical, and experimental research, an impressive body of scientific evidence has been built on the profound influence that nutrients, foods, and dietary patterns have on health outcomes, including CHD [20, 21].

There are accumulating scientific evidences that, among widely followed dietary patterns, the Mediterranean diet might be the healthiest one. In this regard, a recent meta-analysis [22] of 18 prospective cohort studies showed that adherence to the Mediterranean diet confers a significant and consistent protection in relation to the occurrence of major chronic degenerative diseases, including CVD incidence and mortality [22]. Additionally, a systematic review of the effects of 32 candidate dietary factors on CHD risk ranked the Mediterranean diet first as the most likely dietary model to provide causal protection [21].

The Mediterranean diet is identified as the traditional dietary pattern found in Crete, Greece, Italy, and Spain in the early 1960s and is characterized by a high intake of cereals, vegetables, fruits, nuts, and olive oil; a moderate intake of fish and alcohol, mostly wine; and a low intake of dairy products, meat and meat products, and sweets [23] (see also Chap. 1, this book). However, different to other healthy diets, the Mediterranean diet has a high fat content as a distinguishing feature. This is because of the customarily high intake of olive oil, which is used abundantly as culinary fat and for dressing dishes, which facilitates intake of substantial quantities of vegetables.

Olive oil is a flavorsome, tasty, and nutritious edible fat that is usually obtained directly from pressing ripe olives; thus, it can be considered as an olive juice. When produced by mechanically pressing olives, olive oil is called "virgin" and contains both the fat, made up mostly of the MUFA oleic acid (cis-18: 1n-9), and minor components from the fruit, many of which are bioactive phytochemicals (see Chap. 2, Sect. 2.2.2., this book). While the virgin variety of olive oil has a unique composition of beneficial compounds, i.e., the antioxidant minor components contained in unsaponifiable fraction, ordinary or refined olive oil loses minor components, particularly the polyphenols, during the refining process. Nevertheless, whether virgin or refined, the high MUFA content still confers olive oil-specific characteristics that make this fat protective against numerous degenerative disease, including CVD.

3.4 EVOO and CHD: The Epidemiological Studies

Many randomized clinical trials have shown that consumption of olive oil, particularly virgin olive oil, is associated with beneficial effects on intermediate cardiovascular biomarkers, such as blood lipids, blood pressure, inflammation, and thrombosis. It is widely assumed that olive oil, particularly virgin olive oil, due to its antioxidant potential and MUFA content, is the main component of the Mediterranean diet that makes this diet cardioprotective [24]. An Italian study [25] showed that regular consumption of olive oil, compared with no or infrequent consumption, significantly reduced mortality risk by 24% in men and women with previous myocardial infarction; however, these results cannot be extrapolated to a healthy adult population.

However, given the consistent evidence on the cardiovascular benefit of the Mediterranean diet, there has been a surprising paucity of epidemiological data on olive oil consumption and CVD. One reason is the difficulty of disentangling olive oil from the other components of the Mediterranean diet. Probably this is the main reason for which epidemiological studies centered on olive oil consumption and CHD have often provided contradictory results.

The impact of olive oil and Mediterranean diet on overall mortality and several chronic degenerative disease, including CVD, was investigated in the European Prospective Investigation into Cancer and Nutrition (EPIC) study, a large, prospective observational, multicenter cohort study conducted in ten European countries and designed to investigate the relation between dietary, nutritional, metabolic, and lifestyle factors and the risk of cancer and other chronic diseases.

The sub-study EPICOR [26] was a study aimed to investigate the association between consumption of fruit, vegetables, and olive oil and the incidence of coronary heart disease (CHD) in 29,689 women enrolled between 1993 and 1998 in five EPIC cohorts in Northern (Turin and Varese), Central (Florence), and Southern (Naples and Ragusa) Italy. During a mean follow-up of 7.85 years, 144 major CHD events were identified. A strong CHD risk reduction was reported among participants in the highest quartile of olive oil consumption (>31.2 g/day), with a multivariate-adjusted hazard ratio (HR) of 0.56 (95% CI 0.31, 0.99; $P = 0.04$).

The EPIC Spain evaluated the association between olive oil and overall and cause-specific mortality in the Spanish population in the EPIC Spain [27]. A total of 40,622 participants (62% female) aged 29–69 years were recruited from five Spanish regions in 1992–1996. During the 13 years of follow-up, a total of 1915 deaths were reported, of which 4516 were CVD deaths. In comparison with non-consumers (15% of the sample), the highest quartile of olive oil consumers was associated with a 26% (95% CI: 13%, 36%) reduction in risk of overall mortality and a 44% (95% CI: 21%, 60%) reduction in CVD mortality. For each increase in olive oil of 10 g, there was a 7% decreased risk of overall mortality and a 13% decreased risk of CVD mortality. The authors concluded that olive oil was associated with a decreased risk of overall mortality with an important reduction in CVD mortality [27].

A further important report on olive oil consumption and CVD was the Three-City Study from France, whereby the association between olive oil consumption and incident stroke was evaluated in 7625 aged men and women after follow-up for 5–25 years [28]. Compared to subjects who never used olive oil (23% of the sample), those who used it for both cooking and dressing (37% of the sample) had a 41% (95% CI 6, 63) lower risk of stroke after adjustment for various confounders. No distinction between virgin and refined olive oil was made in this study.

The PREDIMED study [29] was a multicenter, parallel-group, randomized trial conducted in Spain on a population of 7447 persons at high cardiovascular risk but with no cardiovascular disease at enrolment. Participants were assigned to one of three diets: a Mediterranean diet supplemented with extra-virgin olive oil, a Mediterranean diet supplemented with mixed nuts, and a control diet (advice to reduce dietary fat). The primary end point was the rate of major cardiovascular events (myocardial infarction, stroke, or death from cardiovascular causes). After a median follow-up of 4.8 years, the multivariable-adjusted hazard ratios were 0.70 (95% CI, 0.54–0.92) and 0.72 (95% CI, 0.54–0.96) for the group assigned to a Mediterranean diet with extra-virgin olive oil (96 events) and the group assigned to a Mediterranean diet with nuts (83 events), respectively, versus the control group (109 events). The conclusions were that persons at high cardiovascular risk, a Mediterranean diet supplemented with extra-virgin olive oil or nuts reduced significantly (~30%) the incidence of major cardiovascular events.

The abovementioned studies made up a significant addition to the literature on olive oil consumption and CVD reduced rate, although some concerns were still represented by some confounding factors, i.e., subjects who consumed more olive oil were more educated, had less adiposity, and, when reported, had a healthier overall diet than low or no consumers. The data of PREDIMED study assessed with no further doubts the clear causal effect of high intake of extra-virgin olive oil and a substantial reduction in the risk of major cardiovascular events among high-risk persons.

Although the biological pathways by which olive oil reduces mortality per se are not completely clear, it is likely that various different mechanisms are involved and are linked to the protective effect that olive oil has on the risk of chronic diseases such as CVD, specific types of cancer, diabetes, and metabolic syndrome [24, 30]. Olive oil contains a high proportion of MUFAs, vitamin E, and diverse phenolic compounds that have been shown to have anti-inflammatory, antioxidant, antiatherogenic, and possibly anticarcinogenic effects. Extra-virgin olive oil has been shown to decrease a range of CVD risk factors by improving lipid profiles and platelet function homeostasis, lowering blood pressure, and reducing the atherogenic process [31–33] . Randomized controlled trials have also found that olive oil improves systemic inflammation and glycemic control [24].

However, the probably most important effect of virgin olive oil on risk reduction is its action on gene transcription through epigenetic mechanisms, which will be discussed in Chap. 7, this book.

3.5 EVOO and CHD: The Impact of EVOO at the Molecular and Clinical Level

The effects of EVOO in reducing the CVD and CHD death rate occur at molecular and clinical level.

3.5.1 Its Impact at the Molecular Level

The effects of EVOO at molecular level include anti-inflammatory, antioxidant, anti-angiogenic, and nutrigenomic effects.

3.5.1.1 Anti-inflammatory Effects

Major and minor olive oil components have been shown to be protective against inflammation and endothelial activation [34]. In this context, oleic acid and polyphenols antioxidants have been shown to have a leading role in anti-inflammatory activity.

In animal models, a diet rich in olive oil suppressed the natural killer cell activity [35] and the expression of receptors for interleukin (IL)-2 [36]. In human studies, LDL-induced monocyte adhesion to endothelial cells was lower after MUFA consumption than after that of SFA or PUFA in healthy individuals [37]. When exposed to oxidative stress, human LDL enriched in oleic acid promoted less monocyte chemotaxis (52% lower) and a reduced monocyte adhesion (77%) compared with linoleic-enriched LDL, [38]. Consumption of an oleic acid-rich diet for 2 months promoted a decrease in the expression of the intracellular adhesion molecule-1 (ICAM-1) in PBMC of healthy subjects [39]. Inflammatory markers, such as the high-sensibility C-reactive protein and IL-6, and cell adhesion molecules, such as ICAM-1, have been reported to decrease after both short-term (3 months) [40] and long-term (2 years) [30] consumption of olive oil-rich diets, such as the Mediterranean diet.

Although the protective mechanism of oleic acid-rich diets on inflammation has been attributed to a decrease in the LDL linoleic acid content and increase in oleic acid, oleic acid doesn't seem to be the single responsible factor for the anti-inflammatory properties of olive oil.

Olive oil minor components have been shown to have anti-inflammatory, antihypertensive, and anti-endothelial activation properties in experimental in vitro studies [41]. EVOO phenolic fraction has been shown to reduce the VEGF-induced angiogenic response and the NADPH oxidase activity in human cultured endothelial cells. The phenolic extracts, at concentration achievable nutritionally, significantly reduced, in a concentration-dependent manner, the VEGF-induced cell migration, invasiveness, and tubelike structure formation through the inhibition of MMP-2 and MMP-9. OOPE significantly ($P < 0.05$) reduced VEGF-induced intracellular reactive oxygen species by modulating NADPH oxidase activity, p47phox membrane translocation, and the expression of Nox2 and Nox4. Moreover, the treatment of endothelial cells with serum obtained 4 h after acute intake of extra-virgin olive oil, with high polyphenol content, decreased VEGF-induced NADPH oxidase activity and Nox4 expression, as well as MMP-9 expression.

Overall, native polyphenols and serum metabolites of extra-virgin olive oil rich in polyphenols are able to lower the VEGF-induced angiogenic responses by preventing endothelial NADPH oxidase activity and decreasing the expression of selective NADPH oxidase subunits [42].

The olive oil phenolics have been also shown to be effective in reducing the eicosanoid inflammatory mediators derived from arachidonic acid, such as thromboxane B_2 and 6-keto-prostaglandin $F_{1\alpha}$ [43–46] and other inflammatory markers, such as high-sensibility C-reactive protein or IL-6 [47]. The effect of phenolic compounds on cell adhesion molecules has shown contrasting results. A decrease of ICAM-1 and vascular cell adhesion molecule-1 serum levels at postprandial state after VOO when compared with refined olive oil ingestion has been reported [48]. However, no differences in ICAM-1 levels were reported after sustained virgin or refined olive oil consumption [47].

The anti-inflammatory effect of EVOO phenols has been shown to be associated with a modulation of the inflammatory and antioxidant gene expression [49] (see also Chap. 7). Treatment of human umbilical vein endothelial cells (HUVEC) with serum obtained 2 h after the intake of the high-phenol EVOO-based breakfast decreased p65 and MCP-1 gene expression and increased MT-CYB, SDHA, and SOD1 gene expression. In the same study, the treatment with serum obtained 4 h after the intake of the high-phenol EVOO-based breakfast decreased MCP-1 and CAT gene expression and increased MT-CYB gene expression, as compared to the treatment with serum obtained 4 h after the intake of the low-phenol VOO-based breakfast. These results suggested that the consumption of virgin olive oil rich in phenolic compounds reduces the risk of atherosclerosis development by decreasing inflammation and improving the antioxidant profile in the vascular endothelium [49].

Among the numerous polyphenols with anti-inflammatory effects, the oleocanthal has been described as having similar properties to that of the anti-inflammatory molecule ibuprofen (Fig. 3.1.) [50]. The bioavailability of oleocanthal in humans from olive oil ingestion remains, however, to be elucidated.

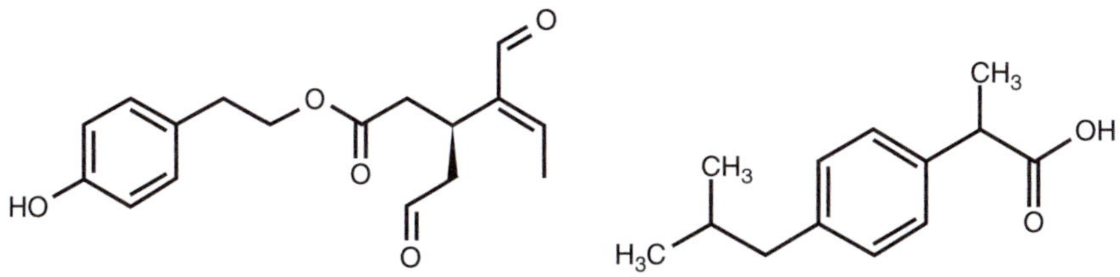

Fig. 3.1 Chemical formulas of oleocanthal (left) and ibuprofen (right)

3.5.1.2 Antioxidant Effects

Oxidized LDL is currently thought to be more damaging to the arterial wall than native LDL due to the ability of oxidized LDL to promote the atherosclerotic process.

Elevated concentrations of circulating oxidized LDL are predictors for coronary heart disease development [51].

The phenolic compounds of olive oil have shown to have antioxidant activity both in experimental models and in human studies [34]. It is important that phenolic compounds from olive oil are bioavailable in humans, even from low doses (25 mL) of olive oil, and this reinforces their protective role in vivo [52, 53]. Oleate-rich LDLs have been shown to be less susceptible to oxidation than linoleate-rich LDLs [54]. In a meta-analysis of 14 studies, the MUFA-rich diets have shown to promote a higher resistance of LDL to oxidation than the PUFA-rich ones [55].

A postprandial oxidative stress condition has been largely described. It appears that this oxidative condition is linked with postprandial lipemia and hyperglycemia [56]. With the intake of olive oil at adequate doses where oxidative stress occurs (equal to or greater than 40 mL) [57, 58], the in vivo lipid oxidative damage was inversely correlated in a dose-dependent manner with the phenolic content of the olive oil administered [59]. Oxidative stress associated with postprandial lipemia also contributes to endothelial dysfunction, which shifts hemostasis to a more thrombogenic state. In this sense, a VOO with a high content of phenolic compounds changes the postprandial hemostatic profile to a less thrombogenic state compared with a low phenolic content olive oil [60, 61] (see also Sect. 3.5.2.3 and Sect. 3.5.3, below).

Concerning sustained olive oil consumption, the results of EUROLIVE (*the effect of olive oil consumption on oxidative damage in European populations*) study have provided definitive evidence on the in vivo antioxidant role of phenolic compounds from olive oil in humans [50]. The EUROLIVE was a large, crossover, multicenter, clinical trial performed in 200 individuals from five European countries. Participants were randomly assigned to receive 25 mL/day of three similar olive oils, but with differences in their phenolic content, in intervention periods of 3 weeks preceded by 2-week washout periods in which olive oil and olives were avoided. Results of the study showed that all olive oils increased HDL cholesterol and the ratio between reduced and oxidized forms of glutathione and decreased triglycerides total to HDL cholesterol ratio and DNA oxidative damage [50, 62]. Consumption of medium and high phenolic content olive oil decreased the LDL/

HDL cholesterol ratio and the in vivo plasma-circulating oxidized LDL, serum uninduced conjugated dienes, and serum hydroxy fatty acids. The increase in HDL cholesterol and the decrease in lipid oxidative damage were observed in a dose-dependent manner of the phenolic content of the olive oil administered [50].

Concerning the possible protective effects on DNA oxidation, in the EUROLIVE study, no differences were observed in the protective effect of olive oil on DNA oxidation related to its phenolic content [62]. On the contrary, protective effects of olive oil phenols on in vivo DNA oxidation, measured as 8-oxodeoxyguanosine in peripheral blood mononuclear cells (PBMCs) and in urine, were found in healthy male subjects in a short-term study in which participants were previously submitted to a very low antioxidant diet [63].

In postmenopausal women, consumption of high-phenol extra-virgin oil reduced the DNA oxidation, measured by the comet assay in peripheral blood lymphocytes, compared with low-phenol olive oil [64].

Although the protective effects EVOO polyphenols on DNA oxidation are important, they don't appear to be the most important, due to the terrific epigenetic effects of polyphenols on DNA transcription activity (Chap. 7).

3.5.1.3 Nutrigenomic Effects

Besides their role as scavengers of reactive oxygen species and chain-breaking antioxidants, olive oil components can exert their health effects by acting at the genomic level, directly or through a decrease in reactive oxygen species, by modulating the expression of key genes for disease processes. Most of the data, however, come from in vitro or animal studies and only a few from studies in humans.

In endothelial cell models, oleic acid inhibited the expression of the vascular cell adhesion molecule-1 messenger RNA (mRNA) levels and the nuclear factor kB [65, 66]. Pomace olive oil upregulated the extracellular nitric oxide synthase expression in spontaneously hypertensive rat aortic rings [67]. Also, an olive oil enriched with the unsaponifiable fraction upregulated the expression of obesity- and insulin sensitivity-related genes in Apo E-deficient mice [68]. In agreement with the previously described cyclooxygenase-2 (COX-2) inhibitory activity of oleocanthal [50], a reduction in COX-2 expression in cell cultures, via inhibition of p38/cyclic adenosine monophosphate response element-binding protein phosphorylation, by olive oil phenolic compounds, has also been reported [69]. The COX-2-765C allele is associated with a low degree of inflammation in human studies. However, the polymorphism COX-2-765G.C has been reported as not modifying the anti-inflammatory effect of an olive oil-rich Mediterranean diet [70]. In experimental studies, the antioxidant scavenger enzyme transcriptome response has been shown to be upregulated by olive oil phenolic compounds. They activated the mRNA transcription of glutathione-related enzymes in murine J774 A.1 macrophage-like cells [71]. In agreement with this, olive oil feeding increased catalase and glutathione peroxidase expression in the islets of Langerhans in mice [72].

Few studies have analyzed the in vivo changes in gene expression associated with olive oil consumption in humans. In a study on normal volunteers [73], postprandial triglyceride-rich lipoproteins (TRL) were obtained after ingestion of meals enriched in refined olive oil (ROO), butter, or a mixture of vegetable and fish oil (VEFO). With the use of cDNA microarrays, the gene expression was evaluated in human coronary artery smooth muscle cells (HCASMC). TRL-butter, TRL-ROO, and TRL-VEFO provoked different transcriptional profiles in HCASMC. Sixty-six genes were regulated by TRL-butter, 55 by TRL-ROO, and 47 by TRL-VEFO. The data showed that TRL-butter predominantly activated genes involved in the regulation of cell proliferation and inflammation. Likewise, TRL-VEFO induced the expression of genes implicated in inflammation, while TRL-ROO promoted a less atherogenic gene profile. The authors concluded that the pathophysiological contribution of TRL to the development of atherosclerosis and the stability of atherosclerotic plaques may depend on the fatty acid composition of TRL [73].

In in vivo studies, the gene expression response in human peripheral blood mononuclear cells (PBMCs) after breakfasts rich in butter, walnuts, or olive oil has been compared [74, 75]. Butter elicited a higher increase in tumor necrosis factor-α (TNFα) mRNA than olive oil or walnuts [74]. Butter and walnuts, but not olive oil, elicited a nuclear factor kB postprandial activation in PBMCs of healthy volunteers [75].

In another study [76], the postprandial gene expression microarray analysis was performed on peripheral blood mononuclear cells during postprandial period. Two virgin olive oil-based breakfasts with high (398 ppm) and low (70 ppm) content of phenolic compounds were administered to 20 patients suffering from metabolic syndrome following a double-blinded, randomized, crossover design. Microarray analysis identified 98 differentially expressed genes (79 underexpressed and 19 overexpressed) when comparing the intake of phenol-rich olive oil with low-phenol olive oil. Many of these genes seem linked to obesity, dyslipemia, and type 2 diabetes mellitus. Among these, several genes appeared to be involved in inflammatory processes mediated by transcription factor NF-kB, activator protein-1 (AP-1) transcription factor complex, cytokines, mitogen-activated protein kinases (MAPKs) or arachidonic acid pathways, and COX-2. The conclusions were that intake of virgin olive oil-based breakfast rich in phenol compounds is able to repress in vivo expression of several pro-inflammatory genes, thereby switching activity of peripheral blood mononuclear cells to a less deleterious inflammatory profile.

A single dose of 50 mL of olive oil has been shown to elicit a rapid response of insulin sensitivity-related genes at postprandial time [77]. Insulin sensitivity after an olive oil-rich diet has been shown to be modulated by the polymorphism exon 1 variants of the scavenger receptor class B type 1 (SCARB1) [78]. In another study [79], the mononuclear transcriptome response in human PBMCs after sustained VOO consumption (3 weeks) has been reported. In agreement with the previous reports concerning the protective effects of sustained olive oil consumption on lipid and DNA oxidative damage [52, 62–64], some related genes such as lipoic acid synthase (LIAS), aldehyde dehydrogenase A1 (ALDH1A1), and genes corresponding to the DNA repairing proteins such as the excision repair cross-complementation group (ERCC5) and X-ray repair complementing defective repair in Chinese hamster cells 5 (XRCC5) were upregulated [79]. Although further studies are needed, nutrigenomic responses could be key mechanisms to explain the benefits associated with olive oil consumption.

3.5.2 Its Impact at the Clinical and Laboratory Level

3.5.2.1 Lipid Metabolism

Several studies have shown that vegetable oil, particularly olive oil, is able to reduce LDL cholesterol levels. However, it was also shown the superiority of olive oil, rich in MUFA, in modifying lipid parameters, in that seeds oils reduce HDL cholesterol while olive oil do not modify or increase HDL cholesterol levels.

In a randomized double-blind [80], five-period crossover study design, the effects of the different diets on serum lipids and lipoproteins were evaluated. The study compared the CVD risk profile of an average American diet (AAD) with those of four cholesterol-lowering diets: an American Heart Association/National Cholesterol Education Program Step II diet and three high-MUFA diets [olive oil (OO), peanut oil (PO), and peanuts and peanut butter (PPB)]. The high-MUFA diets lowered total cholesterol by 10% and LDL cholesterol by 14%. This response was comparable with that observed for the Step II diet. Triacylglycerol concentrations were 13% lower in subjects consuming the high-MUFA diets and were 11% higher with the Step II diet than with the AAD. The high-MUFA diets did not lower HDL cholesterol, whereas the Step II diet lowered it by 4% compared with the AAD. The OO, PO, and PPB diets decreased CVD risk by an estimated 25%, 16%, and 21%, respectively, whereas the Step II diet lowered CVD risk by 12%. The author concluded that a high-MUFA, cholesterol-lowering diet may be preferable to a low-fat diet because of more favorable effects on the CVD risk profile [80].

In another study on hypercholesterolemic patients [81], the effects on serum lipids and other intermediate markers of cardiovascular risk of replacing 40% of the fat in the background diet with virgin olive oil (VOO), walnuts, or almonds were evaluated. LDL cholesterol was reduced from baseline by 7.3%, 10.8%, and 13.4% after the VOO, walnut, and almond diets, respectively ($P = 0.001$). Total cholesterol and LDL/HDL ratios decreased in parallel. LDL cholesterol decreases were greater than predicted from dietary fatty acid and cholesterol exchanges among diets. The results of this study confirmed the cholesterol-lowering effects of olive and nut oils; the data also suggested that phenolic-rich VOO has a cholesterol-lowering effect independently of its fatty acid content.

Lipid profiles were improved in participants of the large crossover human study EUROLIVE, (previously mentioned) [58] which enrolled 200 European participants receiving olive oil for 3 weeks. Participants were randomly assigned to three groups of olive oil differing in their phenolic content (low, medium, and high). HDL-C linearly increased with the phenolic content, whereas TC/HDL-C ratio linearly decreased. LDL-C/HDL-C ratio and triglycerides decreased in those consuming medium and high phenolic olive oils.

The data of these studies have shown that, as far as the lipid metabolism is concerned:

1. The virgin olive oil is effective in reducing the level of lipid and LDL oxidation.
2. Oleic acid appears to be effective in reducing total and LDL cholesterol without reducing HDL cholesterol, which was also increased.
3. Besides oleic acid, the best activity of virgin olive oil comes from polyphenols, which have shown to increase HDL cholesterol and to work as antioxidant significantly reducing the LDL oxidability.

3.5.2.2 Blood Pressure and Hypertension

It has been reported that the adherence to a Mediterranean diet increases the likelihood of controlling arterial blood pressure (BP) [82, 83]. Although genetic factors appear to be responsible for as much as 20–40% of BP variations in the general population [84], epidemiologic data suggest that lifestyle factors, such as dietary habits, are a major contributor to the high prevalence of hypertension [41, 85]. Olive oil intake, per se, has been inversely associated with both systolic BP (SBP) and diastolic BP (DBP) [82].

Data from the literature have shown that (1) monounsaturated fatty acids (MUFA) and (2) polyphenols have the main impact on blood pressure and hypertension.

1. *MUFA*. Numerous epidemiological studies have assessed important relationships between dietary fat, particularly MUFA, and incidence of blood hypertension [86–93]. Most of these studies, however, have been conducted in the United States and Northern Europe, where overall MUFA consumption is only moderate and comes mainly from some types of meat and hence is highly correlated with the intake of saturated fat. In fact, most epidemiological studies conducted outside Mediterranean countries have not found relevant associations between MUFA intake and the risk of hypertension.

On the contrary, the few epidemiological studies conducted in Southern Europe show very different results, suggesting a protective role for MUFA or olive oil. Southern European countries, where a substantial proportion of the population still follows the traditional olive oil-rich Mediterranean diet, appear to be the ideal setting to ascertain this association, thus avoiding the association between MUFA and meat intake.

Investigators from the Italian Nine Communities Study [92] assessed the relationship between olive oil consumption and BP in almost 5000 middle-aged non-hypertensive individuals. Results showed a statistically significant inverse association, both for systolic and diastolic BP and for both men and women when analyzed separately [92]. In this same study, PUFA were associated with lower systolic BP but had no effect on diastolic BP.

A cross-sectional analysis of 20,343 participants in EPIC study [82] showed that the MUFA/SFA intake ratio was inversely associated with systolic and diastolic BP, after adjustment for potential confounders. Similarly, olive oil consumption was inversely associated with BP, even after adjustment for vegetable consumption [82]. For each 22 g increase in the daily consumption of olive oil, systolic and diastolic BP were 0.8 and 0.3 mmHg lower, on average, after adjustments were made for sex, age, education, body mass index, waist-to-hip ratio, energy intake, physical activity, and vegetable consumption.

Another study that has assessed the relationship between MUFA, olive oil, and BP is the SUN (Seguimiento Universidad de Navarra) study. This cohort study has been specifically designed to assess prospectively the effect of a Mediterranean dietary pattern on hypertension, diabetes, obesity, and cardiovascular disease [94]. In a baseline assessment of the first 8800 participants in this cohort, MUFA intake was associated with a lower prevalence of hypertension among those individuals with low fruit and vegetable consumption, while this effect was not apparent among those with higher fruit and vegetable consumption [95].

While the three previous studies had a cross-sectional design, with their problems in establishing causal relationships, the prospective analysis of the SUN study showed that olive oil consumption was inversely associated with the risk of developing blood hypertension among men [93], but no effect was observed among women. In this study, 5573 participants free of hypertension at baseline were followed up for a median of 28.5 months. Men in the highest quintile of olive oil consumption had a 50% reduction in the risk of incident hypertension compared with those in the lowest quintile of consumption, with a statistically significant linear trend. This association was independent of other known risk factors for hypertension including relevant dietary factors. Among women, there was not a clear relationship probably due to a low number of incident cases of hypertension observed in the women of this cohort during that period.

Since the late 1980, numerous feeding trials have been conducted to examine the effect of MUFA and olive oil on BP. These studies were conducted in very controlled environments, with tight monitoring of the diets to which participants were allocated, leading to a sharp contrast between the dietary profiles of compared groups. Additionally, none of them were funded by the olive oil industry.

One of the earliest studies was conducted in Italy on 57 normotensive volunteers aged 30–50 years. These individuals underwent a dietary intervention with a 70% increase in energy from SFA and a corresponding decrease in MUFA and carbohydrates. After 6 weeks, a significant increase in systolic and average BP was observed. BP reverted to baseline values when participants returned to their usual diet [96].

In a study conducted in Spain, 42 subjects were fed two different diets during 5-week periods. Diets differed in their fatty acid composition, while energy intake from carbohydrate, proteins, and fat was held constant. Compared with a diet rich in SFA (17% of total energy intake), an olive oil-enriched diet (21% of total energy intake from MUFA) was associated with lower levels of mean BP [97]. A similar study, conducted in 41 male young volunteers, showed that a diet rich in MUFA (22% of total energy intake), from olive oil, had a beneficial effect on glucose metabolism and BP compared with a diet rich in SFA or carbohydrate [98]. Similarly, in another study an olive oil-rich diet (30% of total energy intake from MUFA) administered during 3 weeks significantly reduced systolic and diastolic BP compared with a

PUFA-rich diet (27% of total energy intake) in a group of 16 normotensive type 2 diabetics [99]. This same group reported a beneficial effect of an olive oil-enriched diet compared with a high-carbohydrate diet [100]. Another study in 47 healthy normotensive volunteers showed a reduction of BP after a diet with a high amount of MUFA, from olive oil, compared with a diet rich in SFA. However, in this case, the MUFA diet did not perform better than a high-carbohydrate diet [101].

A diet rich in extra-virgin olive oil has been reported to be associated with a reduced need for antihypertensive medication compared with a diet enriched in sunflower oil [102]. In this randomized crossover trial, 23 hypertensive patients were assigned to each diet over periods of 6 months. Compared with the sunflower oil diet, the olive oil diet reduced significantly both systolic and diastolic BP (28 mmHg and 26 mmHg, respectively). Daily drug dosage was significantly reduced during the olive oil diet but not with the sunflower oil diet (approximately 50% vs. 4% reduction). This study suggests that olive oil can be used as a non-pharmacological approach in the treatment of hypertension.

The *OmniHeart* crossover randomized trial compared the effect of three different diets on BP, a carbohydrate (CHO)-rich DASH (Dietary Approaches to Stop Hypertension) diet, a protein-rich diet, and a MUFA-rich diet, in a group of 164 adults older than 30 years with prehypertension or stage 1 hypertension. After 6 weeks, the protein- and MUFA-rich diets produced higher reductions in BP than the CHO diet. However, there were no differences between the MUFA- and protein-rich diets [103].

Some studies have found that systolic blood pressure may be more responsive to extra-virgin olive oil (EVOO) compared to diastolic blood pressure, if the comparison is to an oil that is rich in polyunsaturated fats. For example, in a study on 62 elderly (mean age: 84 years) men and women in Spain, half of whom had hypertension, 4 weeks each of 60 g a day of EVOO or sunflower oil were compared [104]. Systolic blood pressure was decreased to what the authors considered "normalized" (136 ± 10 mmHg) in the hypertensive participants after the EVOO phase, compared to the sunflower oil (150 ± 8 mmHg), but neither oil had a significant impact on diastolic blood pressure. In another study on 41 overweight (BMI 29 ± 1 kg/m^2), but otherwise healthy adults, 3 months daily intake of EVOO compared to 49 g day of a corn and soybean oil combination (control) lowered systolic blood pressure, but there was no difference between the oils for diastolic blood pressure [105].

These studies, and several others, have documented the beneficial effect of MUFA and olive oil on blood pressure. However, it has been hypothesized that the effect of olive oil on BP could be not only mediated through its MUFA content. Other compounds, such as the polyphenols present in virgin olive oil, can have a favorable effect. Anyway, although some inconsistencies, MUFA from vegetable sources, especially from olive oil in the context of Mediterranean diets, can be beneficial in the management of hypertension, and it is very likely that it plays a role in the primary prevention of this disorder.

2. *Polyphenols*. Although a clear inverse correlation has been demonstrated between MUFA from olive oil and blood pressure, the rich polyphenol content of extra-virgin olive oil (EVOO) has been shown to play an important role in reducing the blood pressure.

EVOO is characterized by its high content in phenols (see also Chap. 2, this book). Due to minimal processing, EVOO is the only oil that retains important natural phenols. EVOO is processed in a manner similar to many fruit juices: the fruit is crushed and the juice is centrifuged. It is known that daily use of at least two tablespoon of EVOO can lower blood pressure. EVOO with higher phenol content generally provides more benefits that EVOO with lower phenol content.

The effects of a moderate consumption of olive oil on lipid profile, BMI, and blood pressure (BP) were evaluated in a group of 160 healthy men from non-Mediterranean and Mediterranean regions [106]. The study was a randomized, crossover trial with three intervention periods of 3 weeks and two washout periods of 2 weeks. At the intervention periods, three similar olive oils (25 mL/day), differing only in their phenolic concentration, were administered to the healthy volunteers. General linear models showed that the administration of the sequence of the three olive oils was responsible for a 3% decrease in systolic BP, but not in diastolic BP, in the non-Mediterranean subjects. The results of this study suggest that a moderate consumption of olive oil may be used as an effective tool to reduce SBP of healthy men who do not typically consume a Mediterranean diet.

Other studies specifically indicate phenols as determinants for blood pressure-lowering effect. For example, in 40 men (mean age = 67) with coronary heart disease, 19 of whom had hypertension, refined olive oil (ROO) containing very little phenols was compared to EVOO containing a medium total phenol content (161 mg/kg total phenols) for 3 weeks of daily consumption. The EVOO phase significantly decreased systolic blood pressure for the hypertensive participants compared to the ROO phase (mean difference for EVOO compared to ROO = −2.53 mmHg). However, neither of the oils had a significant impact on diastolic blood pressure [107].

In contrast, the EUROLIVE (*effect of olive oil consumption on oxidative damage in European populations*) study [108] found that total phenol content may have an impact on diastolic but not systolic blood pressure. The study compared ROO to EVOO with a moderately high total phenol content of 366 mg/kg at 25 mL/day for 3 weeks in 18 healthy men. The study found that compared to the ROO, the high total phenol EVOO reduced diastolic blood pressure, but neither oil had a significant impact on systolic blood pressure [108].

Another key study found that EVOO with a high total phenol content may reduce both systolic and diastolic blood pressure. In this study [109], 24 young women classified with high-normal blood pressure (120–139/80–89 mmHg) or stage 1 essential hypertension (140–159/90–99 mmHg) who consumed EVOO with 564 mg/kg total polyphenol or ROO for 8 weeks each were studied. When compared to baseline values, only the polyphenol-rich olive oil diet led to a significant ($P < 0.01$) decrease of 7.91 mmHg in systolic and 6.65 mmHg of diastolic BP. The polyphenol-rich olive oil diet also elicited an increase in plasma nitrites/nitrates (+4.7 ± 6.6 μmol/L, $P < 0.001$) and hyperemic area after ischemia (+345 ± 386 perfusion units (PU)/s, $P < 0.001$). It is noteworthy that this study showed that high-phenol EVOO was more effective in reducing blood pressure than the reductions reported from the DASH (Dietary Approaches to Stop Hypertension) study [110], which required consuming close to nine servings per day of fruits and vegetables to lower systolic blood pressure by 2.8 mmHg and diastolic blood pressure by 1.1 mmHg.

Also in the previously mentioned PREDIMED study, EVOO reduced blood pressure [111]. Briefly, the PREDIMED primary prevention trial was a randomized, single-blinded, controlled trial conducted in Spanish primary healthcare centers. Seven thousand four hundred forty-seven men (aged 55–80 years) and women (aged 60–80 years) who had high risk for cardiovascular disease were recruited. Participants were assigned to a control group or to one of two Mediterranean diets. The control group received education on how to follow a low-fat diet, while the groups on Mediterranean diets received nutritional education on either extra-virgin olive oil (50 mL/day) or nuts (30 g). The percentage of participants with controlled BP increased in all three intervention groups (P-value for within-group changes: $P < 0.001$). Participants allocated to either of the two Mediterranean diet groups had significantly lower diastolic BP than the participants in the control group (−1.53 mmHg (95% confidence interval (CI) −2.01 to −1.04) for the Mediterranean diet supplemented with extra-virgin olive oil and −0.65 mmHg (95% CI −1.15 to −0.15) mmHg for the Mediterranean diet supplemented with nuts). No between-group differences in changes of systolic BP were seen. The authors concluded that both the traditional Mediterranean diet and a low-fat diet exerted beneficial effects on BP and could be part of advice to patients for controlling BP. However, lower values of diastolic BP were found in the two groups promoting the Mediterranean diet with extra-virgin olive oil or with nuts than in the control group.

To conclude, the studies indicate that daily use of at least two tablespoons of EVOO can lower blood pressure, compared to oils rich in polyunsaturated fats or to refined olive oil. EVOO with a higher total phenolic content may be more effective than EVOO with a lower phenolic content in lowering blood pressure. It is not clear why EVOO with a higher total phenolic content has differing effects on systolic and diastolic blood pressure. One explanation is that specific phenols could have greater effects than others, an issue that the studies did not examine. Specific phenols and their amounts vary greatly depending on olive variety, growing conditions, and harvesting (see Chap. 2, this book).

Future research should seek to verify the level of total phenols needed for blood pressure improvements and to determine which specific phenols have a greater effect on blood pressure. The currently available research indicates that a trial of daily use of EVOO could be considered prior to prescribing medication for any person with hypertension.

3.5.2.3 Thrombosis

Numerous studies have demonstrated the significant impact of olive oil on thrombosis, in that olive oil and EVOO greatly attenuate the tendency toward thrombosis elicited by physiological and pathological conditions. Albeit an initial stage in which monounsaturated fatty acids (mainly oleic acid) were studied as the sole player of these effects, the knowledge about the micronutrients has evolved to a much more complex model in which the processing of the oil and the content in some minor components of the virgin olive oil play a fundamental role.

The role of EVOO in thrombosis is quite complex and involves the two processes of primary and secondary hemostasis (see Box 3.1).

Box 3.1: Primary and Secondary Hemostasis

The hemostasis is the normal physiological response that prevents significant blood loss after vascular injury, while thrombosis is the pathological intravascular phenomenon that leads to the formation of a clot along the wall of a blood vessel causing frequently the occlusion of the vessel.

The hemostasis depends on a complex series of events that involve platelets and activation of specific blood proteins, known as coagulation factors (Figs. 3.2, 3.3, and 3.4). These coagulation factors are generally serine proteases (enzymes), with the exception of factor V (FV) and FVIII which are glycoproteins and FXIII which is a transglutaminase. They circulate as inactive zymogen (inactive enzyme precursor) and act by cleaving downstream proteins, in a way that they become active enzymes.

The coagulation process begins almost instantly after an injury to the blood vessel has damaged the endothelium lining the vessel. The exposure of blood to the space under the endothelium initiates two processes: the primary and the secondary hemostasis.

1. The primary hemostasis is a phase in which the platelets change their status and adhere to the site of injury to form a primary cloth. When the

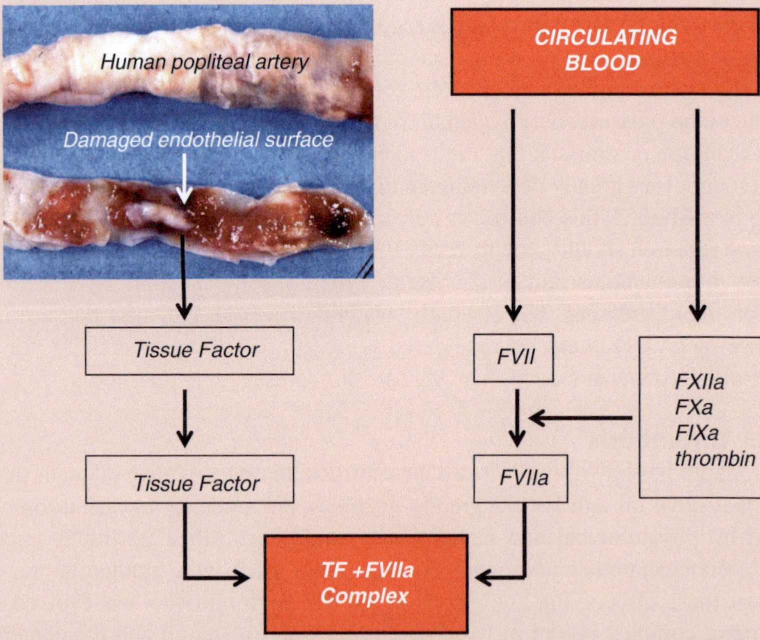

Fig. 3.2 The extrinsic, tissue factor-activated, coagulation pathway. When blood comes in contact with cell membranes with exposed TF, the monomer FVII is activated to the active dimer FVIIa, in the presence of FXIIa, FXa, FIXa, and thrombin and binds to TF forming the FVIIa-TF complex, which starts the cascade of the extrinsic coagulation pathway

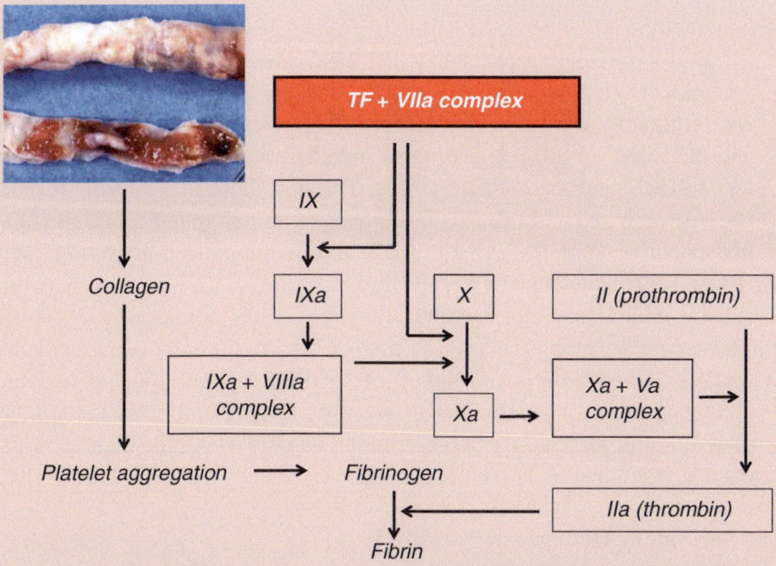

Fig. 3.3 The extrinsic coagulation pathway. Once the TF-FVIIa complex is formed, a cascade of several coagulation factors takes place leading to fibrin formation, in the context of the secondary hemostasis

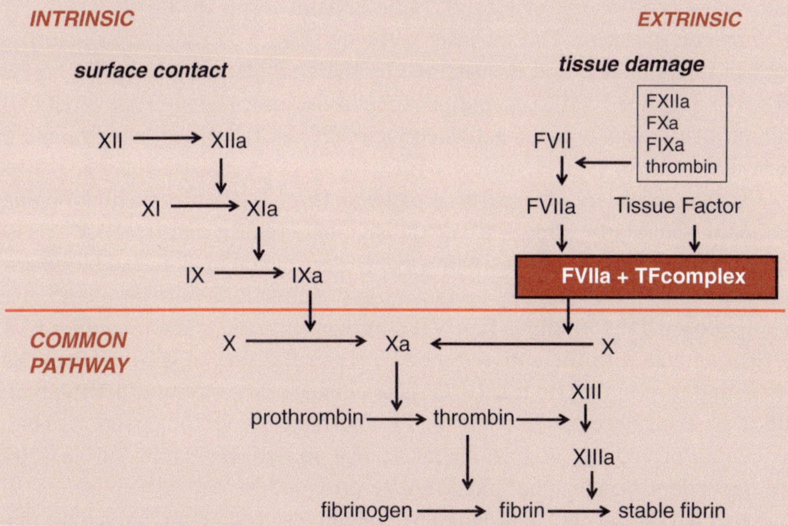

Fig. 3.4 Extrinsic and intrinsic coagulation pathways. Both extrinsic and intrinsic coagulation pathways converge on FX, which is activated into FXa. The FXa starts the last part of the coagulation process that intrinsic and extrinsic pathways have in common (the area under the red line), leading to the fibrin (clot) formation

endothelium is damaged, the normally isolated, underlying collagen becomes exposed to circulating platelets which bind directly to collagen with collagen-specific glycoprotein Ia/IIa surface receptors. This adhesion is strengthened further by von Willebrand factor (vWF) released from the endothelium and platelets; vWF forms additional links between the platelets' glycoprotein Ib/IX/V and the collagen fibrils. Through these mechanisms platelets become activated and release the contents of stored granules into the blood plasma. The granules include ADP, serotonin, platelet-activating factor (PAF), vWF, platelet factor IV, and thromboxane A2 (TXA2), which, in turn, activate additional platelets which adhere to the site of injury.

2. The secondary hemostasis is a complex phenomenon consisting in the formation of insoluble, cross-linked fibrin through the action of activated coagulation factors, particularly thrombin. Fibrin stabilizes the primary platelet plug, particularly in larger blood vessels where the platelet plug is insufficient alone to stop hemorrhage.

The Secondary Hemostasis Pathways

To stabilize the primary cloth, a secondary insoluble cloth, made of cross-linked fibrin, takes place. This phenomenon represents the core of "secondary hemostasis."

Traditionally, the secondary hemostasis has been divided into three distinct pathways: intrinsic, extrinsic, and common pathways (Fig. 3.4).

Intrinsic pathway: The intrinsic pathway (Fig. 3.4) starts after a surface contact phenomenon and is sustained by the coagulation factors FXII, FXI, FIX, the cofactor FVIII, Ca, and phosphatidylserine. The ultimate product of the intrinsic pathway is the activated factor IX (FIXa) which, with the aid of activated cofactor FVIIIa, activates FX.

Extrinsic pathway: The extrinsic pathway (Fig. 3.4) is the coagulation phenomenon that starts when a tissue damage takes place and is called "tissue factor (TF)-activated extrinsic pathway." It starts when in damaged blood vessels, circulating FVII comes in contact with subendothelial cell membranes with exposed TF, forming a TF-FVII complex (Fig. 3.2). The monomer FVII is then activated to the active dimer FVIIa in the presence of FXIIa, FXa, FIXa, and thrombin. The role of TF is to enhance the activity of FVIIa, making it an efficient catalyst of factor IX and factor X (FX) activation. These sequential proteolytic activations take place on cell membrane surfaces and are dependent on phospholipids, mostly provided by activated platelets but also by endothelial cells and leukocytes. Platelets, which are attracted to the vessel wall by collagen, become activated and release several of their constituents, including fibrinogen, causing thrombosis in concert with activated coagulation and fibrin formation (Figs. 3.3 and 3.4).

Common pathway: The extrinsic and intrinsic coagulation pathways converge on FX (Fig. 3.4), which is activated to FXa. The FXa starts the final part of the coagulation process shared by intrinsic and extrinsic pathways (Fig. 3.4, the area under the red line), leading to the fibrin (clot) formation.

3.5.3 Thrombosis: Factor VII

3.5.3.1 The Circulating Level of FVII Is Influenced by the Diet

Coagulation factor VII (FVII) is a 50 kDa single-chain vitamin K-dependent protease that plays an important role in the extrinsic pathway of blood coagulation. FVII is synthesized principally in the liver and is secreted as an inactive single-chain glycoprotein. In the presence of tissue factor, inactive FVII is converted by limited proteolysis to its fully activated two-chain form. Activation can be affected by a number of activated coagulation factors, including Xa, IXa, XIIa, and thrombin. After activation, FVIIa rapidly converts FIX and FX into their active forms, thus initiating the generation of thrombin and fibrin clot formation.

Numerous studies have demonstrated that (a) the levels of circulation FVII is influenced to some extent by the diet; (b) there is a substantial increase in FVII circulating levels in the postprandial phase; (c) the total intake of dietary fat appears to be the main determinant of the postprandial FVII plasma levels; and (d) the ratio of saturated/monounsaturated fatty acids in the diet is crucial to postprandial levels of FVII.

3.5.3.2 FVII Increases in the Postprandial Phase

FVIIc increases consistently in the postprandial phase. This FVII increase has been shown to be associated with postprandial triglyceride levels and takes place within 2–3 h after the intake of a fatty meal, persisting for several hours thereafter. The maximum activation of FVIIa takes place 8 h postprandially. Fat intake, rather than dietary energy intake, has been shown to be the primary determinant of the postprandial increase in FVIIc.

3.5.3.3 The Impact of EVOO and MUFA on Postprandial FVII Level

Alimentary fats are involved in the activity of FVII. Although the results on FVII and saturated-unsaturated fatty acids have given conflicting results, more recent data have shown that olive oil and its main fatty acid, the MUFA oleic acid, have a favorable impact on the activity of FVII, particularly in the postprandial phase.

It has been demonstrated that during the postprandial state, there exists a procoagulatory situation (an increase in thromboxanes and D-dimer and a decrease in tPA). It was found that the type of fat consumed, both in an acute meal and during the previous weeks, is the main determinant of these changes [112]. Also a sustained and remarkable increase in FVII antigen (FVIIag) and activity (FVIIa) takes place in the postprandial phase. Postprandial activation of FVIIa is mainly driven by a diet rich in long-chain saturated fatty acids. A single fat-rich meal, irrespective if rich in saturated fatty acids (SFAs) or polyunsaturated fatty acids (PUFAs), induces an increase in FVIIa only in individuals with a background diet rich in long-chain SFAs and not in those whose usual diet is rich in unsaturated fatty acids [113].

Of interest are the data on the different postprandial response to dietary fat in North Europe compared to the South Europe. FVIIc was shown to be significantly greater 8 h postprandially in Northern Europeans than in Southern Europeans, two populations that noteworthy follow different habitual diet, the northern rich in SFA and the southern rich in MUFA, particularly EVOO [114]. These data have been further confirmed in a comparative study where 40% of SFA was replaced with MUFA [115]: postprandial FVIIa and FVIIag were significantly lower after MUFA-rich diet than after SFA-rich diet. Also long-term dietary intervention studies [113] have confirmed the favorable effect of MUFA on FVII circulating levels. Compared with SFA-rich diet, consumption of a MUFA-rich diet for 16 weeks was associated with a significantly lower postprandial FVIIc and FVIIa levels. The beneficial effects of the MUFA-rich diet are sustained long term without any attenuation through adaptation.

Taken together, these data demonstrate that diets rich in MUFA, particularly from olive oil, are associated with a lower postprandial peak level of FVII and very likely explain the lower rates of CHD in countries whose diet is habitually rich in MUFA, such as the Southern European countries.

3.5.3.4 Mechanism of Action of MUFA on FVII: The Role of Triglycerides

The mechanism by which lipoproteins and fatty acids support the FVII increase/reduction is not completely clear. However, some studies have partially clarified these mechanisms.

The triglyceride-rich lipoprotein (TRLs: chylomicrons and VLDLs) particle size has been suggested to be a determinant of postprandial FVII activation.

It is known that a SFA-rich diet determines the postprandial formation of a high number of triglyceride-rich chylomicrons and activation of FVII. Different from SFA, a MUFA-rich diet results in the postprandial formation of a smaller number of larger chylomicron particles and in attenuation of the postprandial FVII activation.

It has been shown that chronic exposure to a MUFA-rich diet increases the capacity of large TRLs particles to transport lipids during the postprandial phase while reducing the absolute number of TRL particles [116]. Noteworthy FVII binds to the protein moiety of TRLs, thus prolonging the length of its stay in the bloodstream. By producing a smaller number of large TRL particles, the MUFA-rich diet makes that less FVII binds to TRL particles. This, in turn, determines less activation of FVII. Furthermore, the large TRL particles rich in MUFA or n-3 fatty acids are more easily cleared from the plasma than the particles rich in SFAs, thanks to their conformational structure [117]. In fact, the SFAs are located primarily in position s2 of the triacylglycerols, which interchange with greater difficulty from the surface of the chylomicrons than do the fatty acids located in position s1 and s3 of the acylglycerols, occupied preferentially by MUFA and n-3 fatty acids. This combination of factors, i.e., the smaller number of large TRL particles and the shorter stay in the bloodstream of MUFA-rich particles than SFA-rich particles, may explain the lower concentration of FVII after MUFA-rich diet as well as the differences between MUFA- and SFA-rich diets in postprandial changing from fasting.

Another suggested mechanism implicated in postprandial levels of FVII is the different affinity of fatty acids for peroxisome proliferator-activated receptor alpha (PPARα), a nuclear hormone receptor that plays a critical role in regulating lipid metabolism. The PPARα activity could be part of a more complex mechanism responsible of the FVII activation, at least in the acute test meal situation.

3.5.4 Platelets

3.5.4.1 Effects of EVOO, MUFA, and n-3 PUFA

Platelets are small cell fragments that are produced by the breakdown of megakaryocytes, the large precursor cells found in the bone marrow. On release into the circulation, they circulate for approximately 9–12 days. The normal platelet count varies from 140 to 400 × 10^9/L. As discussed above, platelets are involved in the primary hemostasis, with the formation of a "white" thrombus.

Dietary fats, which are expected to modify the composition of platelet membrane, would affect their function. In principle, diets high in saturated fat, particularly long-chain fatty acids, are associated with a greater incidence of thrombosis than when a diet high in monounsaturated or polyunsaturated fat is fed. Studies in vitro and in vivo have shown that long-chain saturated fatty acids increase the platelet aggregation, contrary to unsaturated fatty acids which inhibit it.

Studies in human have largely demonstrated the antiplatelet aggregation effect of EVOO and MUFA. In an 8-week study, a diet containing 17.5% energy as MUFA decreased significantly platelet aggregation in response to collagen and arachidonic acid [118]. In another study [119], a 21 g/day supplementation of olive oil for 8 weeks reduced platelet aggregation induced by ADP and collagen. In a population study on young adults, consumption of a MUFA-rich diet, compared to a SFA-rich diet, resulted in a significant decrease in platelet aggregation in response to ADP, collagen, and arachidonic acid at 8 weeks, and the reduced platelet aggregation was maintained at 16 weeks [120]. Despite the contrasting results of other studies, the weight of evidence suggests a significant beneficial effect of a MUFA-rich diet on platelet aggregation.

Studies in rabbits have also shown that oleic acid is a potent inhibitor of PAF (platelet-activating factor)-induced platelet aggregation. PAF is a platelet agonist, a powerful endogenous mediator of platelet aggregation, made of a mixture of unsaturated free fatty acids. The PAF effect on platelets is due to its interaction with a specific membrane receptor that induces the degradation of platelet plasma membrane phosphatidylinositol. Oleic acid has been demonstrated to induce an inhibition of phosphatidylinositol synthesis. To the effect of oleic acid on platelet activation has been attributed the beneficial effects of oleic acid and other unsaturated FFA in the thrombotic disease prevention [112].

The omega-3 (ω3 or n-3) polyunsaturated fatty acids (n-3 PUFA) eicosapentaenoic (EPA) and docosahexaenoic acid (DHA) extracted from fish oil have been demonstrated to actively reduce platelet aggregation. This effect is due to several mechanisms: (a) a competition with arachidonic acid, replacing the active thromboxane A_2 by thromboxane A_3, (b) an inhibition of cyclooxygenase, and (c) a direct antagonistic effect on the thromboxane A_2/prostaglandin H_2 receptor in human platelets.

The EPA and DHA metabolic activity, however, is not confined to the platelets anti-aggregation effects. Numerous studies and extensive reports have shown cardioprotective effects of dietary fish, fish oil, or a combination of EPA/DHA used in nutritional supplementation. Cardioprotection conferred by these PUFA species has been attributed to different mechanisms, including regulation of lipid metabolism and blood pressure, stabilization of atherosclerotic plaques, and antiarrhythmic and anti-inflammatory actions. Of importance, individual gene variations in apolipoprotein (apo) AI, apoA5, apoE, TNF alpha, PPAR alpha, NOS3, and ALOX5 interact with omega-3 PUFA intake modulating lipid metabolism and cardiovascular outcomes.

EPA and DHA have also lowering effect on triglyceride blood levels. The n-3 PUFA, in fact, interacts with triglyceride metabolism modulated by NOS and PPARα gene polymorphisms. Carriers of the minor allele for rs1799983 SNP of NOS3 gene have shown a negative correlation between plasma TG concentrations and plasma n-3 PUFA level. Following n-3 PUFA supplementation, subjects with the minor allele had a better response to the change in plasma n-3 PUFA in reducing serum TG concentration than major allele homozygous carriers.

Concerning the PPARα gene polymorphisms, the minor allele Leu162Val variant has been associated with higher triglycerides and apo C-III blood levels only in subjects consuming a low-PUFA diet. Conversely, high consumption of PUFA with diet modulates the effect of this SNP on lipid metabolism and triglyceride blood levels.

3.5.4.2 Polyphenols and Platelet Aggregation

As widely described elsewhere in this book (Chaps. 2 and 10), polyphenols are potent antioxidants present in several foods, particularly in fresh fruit, red wine, and extra-virgin olive oil (EVOO). As previously mentioned (Chap. 2), extra-virgin olive oil (EVOO) is particularly rich in phenolic compounds, and this richness depends on the mechanical procedures employed to obtain extra-virgin olive oil, without any use of chemical solvent. In fact, the common, or refined, olive oil, obtained with solvents by pomace, contains no polyphenols because solvents do not allow to recover any phenolic compound by the pomace. The refining process serves to remove color, odor, and flavor from low-quality olive oil and leaves behind a very pure form of olive oil that is tasteless, colorless, and odorless and without any bioactive compound. The EVOO, on the contrary, contains large amounts of polyphenols which, however, are only a tenth of the polyphenols contained in olives; in fact, the most part of these olives' bioactive compounds is lost during the various processing stages, particularly in the mill wastewater.

The major phenolic compounds in EVOO are oleuropein, tyrosol, hydroxytyrosol, and luteolin. These phenols, which represent almost 90% of the EVOO polyphenols, are only 4 of the almost 30 phenolic compounds present in EVOO.

The polyphenols have been mostly investigated in CHD where they have demonstrated to significantly reduce numerous cardiovascular risk factors. EVOO polyphenols possess antioxidant properties and influence many biological activities that may account, at least in part, for the observed effects of olive oil on the cardiovascular system. Some of these effects include (a) inhibition of LDL oxidation, (b) production of nitric oxide, and (c) downregulation of intercellular adhesion molecule-1(ICAM-1) and vascular cell adhesion molecule-1 (VCAM-1) expression in endothelial cells [121].

EVOO with a high phenolic compound content (400 mg/kg) has been demonstrated to significantly inhibit also PAI-1 and FVII.

As far as platelet aggregation is concerned, EVOO polyphenols have been demonstrated to reduce platelet aggregability. The EVOO phenol component [2-(3,4-dihydroxyphenyl)ethanol] decreases significantly platelet aggregation induced in vitro by ADP and collagen and the TxB_2 production by collagen and thrombin-stimulated platelet-rich plasma (PRP) [122]. Two isochroman polyphenols present in EVOO [1-(3′-cAMPmethoxy-4′-hydroxy-phenyl)-6,7dihydroxy-isochroman and 1-phenyl-6,7-dihydroxy-isochroman] inhibit in vitro platelet aggregation and thromboxane release induced by arachidonic acid and collagen [44]. In vivo beneficial effects of EVOO polyphenols on hemostasis have been also reported. In a study on volunteers, a significant reduction in plasma TxB_2 concentration after an EVOO-rich diet, compared to a high-oleic sunflower diet, was observed, and this effect was attributed to the greater amount of polyphenols in the EVOO-rich diet [123].

The molecular mechanisms of EVOO polyphenols antiplatelet activity have been studied.

Platelet activation is regulated by a number of physiological activators (thromboxane A_2, vasopressin, ADP, thrombin, serotonin) and inhibitors (endothelium-derived relaxing factor, prostaglandin inhibitor-2).

Platelet antagonists inhibit platelet function by increasing the intracellular levels of cyclic nucleotides cAMP and cGMP through the activation of the respective cyclases. Cyclic nucleotide levels are downregulated by degradation through phosphodiesterases (PDE). Platelets contain mainly PDE3, which preferentially hydrolyzes cAMP as substrate. EVOO phenols, particularly luteolin, have been demonstrated to act on cAMP-PDE complex, by inhibiting the PDE activity, so increasing the intracellular levels of cyclic nucleotides cAMP [124].

PMQ (3,3′,4′,5,7-pentamethylquercetin), a member of the polymethoxylated flavones family, is the methylated form of quercetin, a flavonol polyphenol found in many fruits, vegetables, teas, grains, and olive oil. PMQ is a potent antioxidant with anticarcinogenic activity and cardioprotective properties. In vitro studies have shown that PMQ exerts a potent inhibitory effect on platelet function and in vivo inhibits thrombus formation in acute animal model. PMQ has been shown to protect mice from death in the acute lung thromboembolism model and from carotid artery injury induced by ferric chloride. Moreover, PMQ inhibits platelet aggregation induced by several agonists and regulates functional responses of platelets, including the release of ATP and P-selectin. The molecular mechanisms of the inhibitory effects of PMQ on platelet function were shown to be the suppression of the PI3K/Akt-GSK3β and Syk-PLCγ2-Erk signaling cascades [123].

Finally, it should be pointed out that the very peculiar combination of biologically active compounds in EVOO produces a milder activation of the mechanisms of inflammation and coagulation during the postprandial phase, a situation that leads to reduced postprandial activation of NF-kB, an important cellular regulator that initiates the formation of procoagulant and pro-inflammatory signal peptides [112].

References

1. Miniño AM. Death in the United States, 2009. NCHS data brief, no 64. Hyattsville, MD: National Center for Health Statistics; 2011.
2. Mozaffarian D, Benjamin EJ, Go AS, et al. Heart disease and stroke statistics—2015 update: a report from the American Heart Association. Circulation. 2015;131:e29–322.
3. Ignatowski A. Changes in parenchymatous organs and in the aorta of rabbits under the influence of animal protein [in Russian]. Izvestia Imperatorskoi Voenno-Medicinskoi Akademii (St Petersburg). 1908;18:231–44.
4. Ignatowski A. Influence de la nourriture animale sur l'organisme des lapins. Arch Med Exp Anat Pathol. 1908;20:1–20.
5. Ignatowski A. Wirkung der tierischen nahrung auf den kaninchenorganismus. Ber Milit Med Akad. 1908;16:154–76.
6. Ignatowski A. Uber die wirkung des tierischen eiweisses auf die aorta und die parenchymatosen organe der kaninchen. Virchows Arch Pathol Anat Physiol Klin Med. 1909;198:248–70.
7. Kritchevsky D. Dietary protein, cholesterol and atherosclerosis: a review of the early history. J Nutr. 1995;125:589S–93S.
8. Konstantinov IE, Mejevoi N, Anichkov NM, Nikolai N. Anichkov and his theory of atherosclerosis. Tex Heart Inst J. 2006;33:417–23.
9. Fahr T. Beitrage zur experiemtellen atherosklerose unter besonderer beruchsichtgung der frage nach dem zusammenhang zwischen nebenierenveranderungen und atherosklerose. Verh Dtsch Ges Pathol. 1912;15:234–49.
10. Chalatow SS. Uber das verthalten der leber gegenuber den verschiedenen arten von speisefett. Virchows Arch Pathol Anat Physiol Klin Med. 1912;207:452–69.
11. Anichkow N, Chalatow S. Uber experimentelle cholesterin-steatose und ihre bedeuntung fur die entstehung einiger pathologischer prozess [in German]. Zentralbl Allg Pathol Anat. 1913;24:1–9.
12. Keys A, Taylor HL, Blackburn H, Brozek J, Anderson JT, Simonson E. Coronary heart disease among Minnesota business and professional men followed 15 years. Circulation. 1963;28:381–95.
13. Keys A. Seven countries: a multivariate analysis of death and coronary heart disease. Cambridge, MA: Harvard University Press; 1980.
14. da Silva AJM. La diète méditerranéenne, Discours et pratiques alimentaires en Méditerranée, vol. 2. Paris: L'Harmattan; 2015. p. 49–51.
15. Keys A. Coronary heart disease in seven countries. Circulation. 1970;41(4 Suppl):I 1–200.
16. Kromhout D. Serum cholesterol in cross-cultural perspective. The seven-countries study. Acta Cardiol. 1999;54:155–8.
17. Hooper L, Martin N, Abdelhamid A, Smith GD. Reduction in saturated fat intake for cardiovascular disease. Cochrane Database Syst Rev. 2015;6:CD011737.
18. Stampfer MJ, Hu FB, Manson JE, Rimm EB, Willett WC. Primary prevention of coronary heart disease in women through diet and lifestyle. N Engl J Med. 2000;343:16–22.
19. Yusuf S, Hawken S, Ounpuu S, Dans T, Avezum A, Lanas F, McQueen M, Budaj A, Pais P, Varigos J, Lisheng L, INTERHEART Study Investigators. Effect of potentially modifiable risk factors associated with myocardial infarction in 52 countries (the INTERHEART study): case–control study. Lancet. 2004;364:937–52.
20. Hu FB, Willett WC. Optimal diets for prevention of coronary heart disease. JAMA. 2002;288:2569–78.
21. Mente A, de Koning L, Shannon HS, Anand SS. A systematic review of the evidence supporting a causal link between dietary factors and coronary heart disease. Arch Intern Med. 2009;169:659–69.
22. Sofi F, Abbate R, Gensini GF, Casini A. Accruing evidence on benefits of adherence to the Mediterranean diet on health: an updated systematic review and meta-analysis. Am J Clin Nutr. 2010;92:1189–96.

23. Bach-Faig A, Berry EM, Lairon D, Reguant J, Trichopoulou A, Dernini S, Medina FX, Battino M, Belahsen R, Miranda G, Serra-Majem L, Mediterranean Diet Foundation Expert Group. Mediterranean diet pyramid today. Science and cultural updates. Public Health Nutr. 2011;14:2274–84.
24. Lòpez-Miranda J, Pérez-Jimenez F, Ros E, De Caterina R, Badimón L, Covas MI, Escrich E, Ordovás JM, Soriguer F, Abiá R, de la Lastra CA, Battino M, Corella D, Chamorro-Quirós J, Delgado-Lista J, Giugliano D, Esposito K, Estruch R, Fernandez-Real JM, Gaforio JJ, La Vecchia C, Lairon D, López-Segura F, Mata P, Menéndez JA, Muriana FJ, Osada J, Panagiotakos DB, Paniagua JA, Pérez-Martinez P, Perona J, Peinado MA, Pineda-Priego M, Poulsen HE, Quiles JL, Ramírez-Tortosa MC, Ruano J, Serra-Majem L, Solá R, Solanas M, Solfrizzi V, de la Torre-Fornell R, Trichopoulou A, Uceda M, Villalba-Montoro JM, Villar-Ortiz JR, Visioli F, Yiannakouris N. Olive oil and health: summary of the II international conference on olive oil and health consensus report, Jaen and Cordoba (Spain) 2008. Nutr Metab Cardiovasc Dis. 2010;20:284–94.
25. Barzi F, Woodward M, Marfisi RM, Tavazzi L, Valagussa F, Marchioli R. Mediterranean diet and all-causes mortality after myocardial infarction: results from the GISSI-Prevenzione trial. Eur J Clin Nutr. 2003;57:604–11.
26. Bendinelli B, Masala G, Saieva C, Salvini S, Calonico C, Sacerdote C, Agnoli C, Grioni S, Frasca G, Mattiello A, Chiodini P, Tumino R, Vineis P, Palli D, Panico S. Fruit, vegetables, and olive oil and risk of coronary heart disease in Italian women: the EPICOR Study. Am J Clin Nutr. 2011;93:275–83.
27. Buckland G, Mayén AL, Agudo A, Travier N, Navarro C, Huerta JM, Chirlaque MD, Barricarte A, Ardanaz E, Moreno-Iribas C, Marin P, Quirós JR, Redondo ML, Amiano P, Dorronsoro M, Arriola L, Molina E, Sanchez MJ, Gonzalez CA. Olive oil intake and mortality within the Spanish population (EPIC-Spain). Am J Clin Nutr. 2012;96:142–9.
28. Samieri C, Féart C, Proust-Lima C, Peuchant E, Tzourio C, Stapf C, Berr C, Barberger-Gateau P. Olive oil consumption, plasma oleic acid, and stroke incidence: the Three-City Study. Neurology. 2011;77:418–25.
29. Estruch R, Ros E, Salas-Salvadó J, Covas MI, Corella D, Arós F, Gómez-Gracia E, Ruiz-Gutiérrez V, Fiol M, Lapetra J, Lamuela-Raventos RM, Serra-Majem L, Pintó X, Basora J, Muñoz MA, Sorlí JV, Martínez JA, Martínez-González MA, PREDIMED Study Investigators. Primary prevention of cardiovascular disease with a Mediterranean diet. New Engl J Med. 2013;368:1279–90.
30. Esposito K, Marfella R, Ciotola M, Di Palo C, Giugliano F, Giugliano G, D'Armiento M, D'Andrea F, Giugliano D. Effect of a Mediterranean-style diet on endothelial dysfunction and markers of vascular inflammation in the metabolic syndrome: a randomized trial. JAMA. 2004;292:1440–6.
31. Covas MI, Konstantinidou V, Fito M. Olive oil and cardiovascular health. J Cardiovasc Pharmacol. 2009;54:477–82.
32. Estruch R. Anti-inflammatory effects of the Mediterranean diet: the experience of the PREDIMED study. Proc Nutr Soc. 2010;69:333–40.
33. Pérez-Lòpez FR, Chedraui P, Haya J, Cuadros JL. Effects of the Mediterranean diet on longevity and age-related morbid conditions. Maturitas. 2009;64:67–79.
34. Covas MI, Ruiz-Gutiérrez V, de la Torre R, Kafatos A, Lamuela-Raventòs RM, Osada J, Owen RW, Visioli F. Minor components of olive oil: evidence to date of health benefits in humans. Nutr Rev. 2006;64(Suppl 1):S20–30.
35. Yaqoob P, Newsholme EA, Calder PC. Inhibition of natural killer cell activity by dietary lipids. Immunol Lett. 1994;41:241–7.
36. Yaqoob P, Newsholme EA, Calder PC. The effect of dietary lipid manipulation on rat lymphocyte subsets and proliferation. Immunology. 1994;82:603–10.
37. Mata P, Alonso R, Lòpez-Farre A, Ordovas JM, Lahoz C, Garces C, Caramelo C, Codoceo R, Blazquez E, de Oya M. Effect of dietary fat saturation on LDL oxidation and monocyte adhesion to human endothelial cells in vitro. Arterioscler Thromb Vasc Biol. 1996;16:1347–55.

38. Tsimikas S, Philis-Tsimikas A, Alexopoulos S, Reaven PD. LDL isolated from Greek subjects on a typical diet or from American subjects on an oleate supplemented diet induces less monocyte chemotaxis and adhesion when exposed to oxidative stress. Arterioscler Thromb Vasc Biol. 1999;19:122–30.
39. Yaqoob P, Knapper JA, Webb DH, Williams CM, Newsholme EA, Calder PC. Effect of olive oil on immune function in middle-aged men. Am J Clin Nutr. 1998;67:129–35.
40. Estruch R, Martìnez-Gonzàlez MA, Corella D, Salas-Salvadó J, Ruiz-Gutiérrez V, Covas MI, Fiol M, Gómez-Gracia E, López-Sabater MC, Vinyoles E, Arós F, Conde M, Lahoz C, Lapetra J, Sáez G, Ros E, PREDIMED Study Investigators. Effects of a Mediterranean-style diet on cardiovascular risk factors: a randomized trial. Ann Intern Med. 2006;145:1–11.
41. Perona JS, Cabello-Moruno R, Ruìz-Gutìerrez V. The role of virgin olive oil components in the modulation of endothelial function. J Nutr Biochem. 2006;17:429–45.
42. Calabriso N, Massaro M, Scoditti E, D'Amore S, Gnoni A, Pellegrino M, Storelli C, De Caterina R, Palasciano G, Carluccio MA. Extra virgin olive oil rich in polyphenols modulates VEGF-induced angiogenic responses by preventing NADPH oxidase activity and expression. J Nutr Biochem. 2016;28:19–29.
43. Visioli F, Caruso D, Grande S, Bosisio R, Villa M, Galli G, Sirtori C, Galli C. Virgin olive oil study (VOLOS): vasoprotective potential of extra virgin olive oil in mildly dyslipidemic patients. Eur J Nutr. 2005;44:121–7.
44. Oubiña P, Sanchez-Muniz FJ, Rodenas S, Cuesta C. Eicosanoid production, thrombogenic ratio, and serum and LDL peroxides in normo- and hypercholesterolaemic post-menopausal women consuming two oleic acid-rich diets with different content of minor components. Br J Nutr. 2001;85:41–7.
45. Lèger CL, Carbonneau MA, Michel F, Mas E, Monnier L, Cristol JP, Descomps B. A thromboxane effect of a hydroxytyrosol-rich olive oil wastewater extract in patients with uncomplicated type I diabetes. Eur J Clin Nutr. 2005;59:727–30.
46. Bogani P, Galli C, Villa M, Visioli F. Postprandial anti-inflammatory and antioxidant effects of extra virgin olive oil. Atherosclerosis. 2007;190:181–6.
47. Fitò M, Cladellas M, de la Torre R, Martí J, Muñoz D, Schröder H, Alcántara M, Pujadas-Bastardes M, Marrugat J, López-Sabater MC, Bruguera J, Covas MI, SOLOS Investigators. Anti-inflammatory effect of virgin olive oil in stable coronary disease patients: a randomized, crossover, controlled trial. Eur J Clin Nutr. 2008;62:570–4.
48. Pacheco YM, Bermùdez B, Lopez S, Abia R, Villar J, Muriana FJ. Minor compounds of olive oil have postprandial anti-inflammatory effects. Br J Nutr. 2007;98:260–3.
49. Meza-Miranda ER, Rangel-Zúñiga OA, Marín C, Pérez-Martínez P, Delgado-Lista J, Haro C, Peña-Orihuela P, Jiménez-Morales AI, Malagón MM, Tinahones FJ, López-Miranda J, Pérez-Jiménez F, Camargo A. Virgin olive oil rich in phenolic compounds modulates the expression of atherosclerosis-related genes in vascular endothelium. Eur J Nutr. 2016;55:519–27.
50. Beauchamp GK, Keast RS, Morel D, Lin J, Pika J, Han Q, Lee CH, Smith AB, Breslin PA. Phytochemistry: ibuprofen-like activity in extra-virgin olive oil. Nature. 2005;437:45–6.
51. Meisinger C, Baumert J, Khuseyinova N, Loewel H, Koenig W. Plasma oxidized low density lipoprotein, a strong predictor for acute coronary heart disease events in apparently healthy, middle-aged men from the general population. Circulation. 2005;12:651–7.
52. Covas MI, Nyyssonen K, Poulsen HE, Kaikkonen J, Zunft HJ, Kiesewetter H, Gaddi A, de la Torre R, Mursu J, Bäumler H, Nascetti S, Salonen JT, Fitó M, Virtanen J, Marrugat J, EUROLIVE Study Group. The effect of polyphenols in olive oil on heart disease risk factors: a randomized trial. Ann Intern Med. 2006;145:333–41.
53. Weinbrenner T, Fitò M, Farré-Albaladejo M, Saez GT, Rijken P, Tormos C, Coolen S, De La Torre R, Covas MI. Bioavailability of phenolic compounds from olive oil and oxidative/antioxidant status at postprandial state in healthy humans. Drugs Exp Clin Res. 2004;30:207–14.
54. Parthasarathy S, Khoo JC, Miller E, Barnett J, Witztum JL, Steinberg D. Low density lipoprotein rich in oleic acid is protected against oxidative modification: implications for dietary prevention of atherosclerosis. Proc Natl Acad Sci U S A. 1990;87:3894–8.

55. Lapointe A, Couillard C, Lemieux S. Effects of dietary factors on oxidation of low-density lipoprotein particles. J Nutr Biochem. 2006;17:645–58.
56. Roche HM, Gibney MJ. The impact of postprandial lipemia in accelerating atherothrombosis. J Cardiovasc Risk. 2000;7:317–24.
57. Fitò M, Gimeno E, Covas MI, Miró E, López-Sabater Mdel C, Farré M, de LT, Marrugat J. Postprandial and short-term dietary intervention effects of virgin olive oil ingestion on the oxidative/antioxidative status. Lipids. 2002;37:245–51.
58. Covas MI, de la Torre K, Farré-Albaladejo M, Kaikkonen J, Fitó M, López-Sabater C, Pujadas-Bastardes MA, Joglar J, Weinbrenner T, Lamuela-Raventós RM, de la Torre R. Postprandial LDL phenolic content and LDL oxidation is modulated by olive oil phenolic compound in humans. Free Radic Biol Med. 2006;40:608–16.
59. Lòpez S, Bermùdez B, Pacheco YM, Villar J, Abia R, Muriana FJ. Distinctive postprandial modulation of beta cell function and insulin sensitivity by dietary fats: monounsaturated compared with saturated fatty acids. Am J Clin Nutr. 2008;88:638–44.
60. Pacheco YM, Lopez S, Bermudez B, Abia R, Muriana FJ. Extra-virgin vs. refined olive oil on postprandial hemostatic markers in healthy subjects. J Thromb Haemost. 2006;4:1421–2.
61. Ruano J, Lòpez-Miranda J, de la Torre R, Delgado-Lista J, Fernández J, Caballero J, Covas MI, Jiménez Y, Pérez-Martínez P, Marín C, Fuentes F, Pérez-Jiménez F. Intake of phenol-rich virgin olive oil improves the postprandial prothrombotic profile in hypercholesterolemic patients. Am J Clin Nutr. 2007;86:341–6.
62. Machowetz A, Poulsen HE, Gruendel S, Weimann A, Fitó M, Marrugat J, de la Torre R, Salonen JT, Nyyssönen K, Mursu J, Nascetti S, Gaddi A, Kiesewetter H, Bäumler H, Selmi H, Kaikkonen J, Zunft HJ, Covas MI, Koebnick C. Effect of olive oils on biomarkers of oxidative DNA stress in north and south Europeans. FASEB J. 2007;21:45–52.
63. Weinbrenner T, Fitò M, de la Torre R, Saez GT, Rijken P, Tormos C, Coolen S, Albaladejo MF, Abanades S, Schroder H, Marrugat J, Covas MI. Olive oils high in phenolic compounds modulate oxidative/antioxidative status in men. J Nutr. 2004;134:2314–21.
64. Salvini S, Sera F, Caruso D, Giovannelli L, Visioli F, Saieva C, Masala G, Ceroti M, Giovacchini V, Pitozzi V, Galli C, Romani A, Mulinacci N, Bortolomeazzi R, Dolara P, Palli D, et al. Daily consumption of a high-phenol extra-virgin olive oil reduces oxidative DNA damage in postmenopausal women. Br J Nutr. 2006;95:742–51.
65. Carluccio MA, Massaro M, Bonfrate C, Siculella L, Maffia M, Nicolardi G, Distante A, Storelli C, De Caterina R. Oleic acid inhibits endothelial activation: a direct vascular antiatherogenic mechanism of a nutritional component in the Mediterranean diet. Arterioscler Thromb Vasc Biol. 1999;19:220–8.
66. Massaro M, Carluccio MA, Paolicchi A, Bosetti F, Solaini G, De Caterina R. Mechanisms for reduction of endothelial activation by oleate: inhibition of nuclear factor-kappaB through antioxidant effects. Prostaglandins Leukot Essent Fatty Acids. 2002;67:175–81.
67. Rodrìguez-Rodrìguez R, Herrera MD, De Sotomayor MA, Ruiz-Gutierrez V. Pomace olive oil improves endothelial function in spontaneously hypertensive rats by increasing endothelial nitric oxide synthase expression. Am J Hypertens. 2007;20:728–34.
68. Acìn S, Navarro MA, Perona JS, Surra JC, Guillen N, Arnal C, Sarría AJ, Arbonés-Mainar JM, Carnicer R, Ruiz-Gutiérrez V, Osada J. Microarray analysis of hepatic genes differentially expressed in the presence of the unsaponifiable fraction of olive oil in apolipoprotein E-deficient mice. Br J Nutr. 2007;97:628–38.
69. Corona G, Deiana M, Incani A, Vauzour D, Dessì MA, Spencer JP. Inhibition of p38/CREB phosphorylation and COX-2 expression by olive oil polyphenols underlies their antiproliferative effects. Biochem Biophys Res Commun. 2007;362:606–11.
70. Corella D, Gonzàlez JI, Bullò M, Carrasco P, Portolés O, Díez-Espino J, Covas MI, Ruíz-Gutierrez V, Gómez-Gracia E, Arós F, Fiol M, Herrera MC, Santos JM, Sáez G, Lamuela R, Lahoz C, Vinyoles E, Ros E, Estruch R. Polymorphisms cyclooxygenase-2 2765G.C and interleukin-6 2174G.C are associated with serum inflammation markers in a high cardiovascular risk population and do not modify the response to a Mediterranean diet supplemented with virgin olive oil or nuts. J Nutr. 2009;139:128–34.

71. Masella R, Vari R, D'Archivio M, Di Benedetto R, Matarrese P, Malorni W, Scazzocchio B, Giovannini C. Extra virgin olive oil biophenols inhibit cell-mediated oxidation of LDL by increasing the mRNA transcription of glutathione-related enzymes. J Nutr. 2004;134:785–91.
72. Oliveras-Lòpez MJ, Bernà G, Carneiro EM, López-García de la Serrana H, Martín F, López MC. An extra-virgin olive oil rich in polyphenolic compounds has antioxidant effects in OF1 mice. J Nutr. 2008;138:1074–8.
73. Bermúdez B, López S, Pacheco YM, Villar J, Muriana FJ, Hoheisel JD, Bauer A, Abia R. Influence of postprandial triglyceride-rich lipoproteins on lipid-mediated gene expression in smooth muscle cells of the human coronary artery. Cardiovasc Res. 2008;79:294–303.
74. Jiménez-Gómez Y, López-Miranda J, Blanco-Colio LM, Marín C, Pérez-Martínez P, Ruano J, Paniagua JA, Rodríguez F, Egido J, Pérez-Jiménez F. Olive oil and walnut breakfasts reduce the postprandial inflammatory response in mononuclear cells compared with a butter breakfast in healthy men. Atherosclerosis. 2009;204:70–6.
75. Bellido C, López-Miranda J, Blanco-Colio LM, Pérez-Martínez P, Muriana FJ, Martín-Ventura JL, Marín C, Gómez P, Fuentes F, Egido J, Pérez-Jiménez F. Butter and walnuts, but not olive oil, elicit postprandial activation of nuclear transcription factor kappaB in peripheral blood mononuclear cells from healthy men. Am J Clin Nutr. 2004;80:1487–91.
76. Camargo A, Ruano J, Fernandez JM, Parnell LD, Jimenez A, Santos-Gonzalez M, Marin C, Perez-Martinez P, Uceda M, Lopez-Miranda J, Perez-Jimenez F. Gene expression changes in mononuclear cells in patients with metabolic syndrome after acute intake of phenol-rich virgin olive oil. BMC Genomics. 2010;11:253.
77. Konstantinidou V, Khymenets O, Covas MI, et al. Time course of changes in the expression of insulin sensitivity-related genes after an acute load of virgin olive oil. OMICS. 2009;13:431–8.
78. Peréz-Martìnez P, Pérez-Jimenez F, Bellido C, et al. A polymorphism exon 1 variant at the locus of scavenger receptor class B type 1 (SCARB1) gene is associated with differences in insulin sensitivity in healthy people during the consumption of an olive oil-rich diet. J Clin Endocrinol Metab. 2005;90:2297–300.
79. Khymenets O, Fitò M, Covas MI, et al. Mononuclear cell transcriptome response after sustained virgin olive oil consumption in humans: an exploratory nutrigenomics study. OMICS. 2009;13:7–19.
80. Kris-Etherton PM, Pearson TA, Wan Y, Hargrove RL, Moriarty K, Fishell V, Etherton TD. High-monounsaturated fatty acid diets lower both plasma cholesterol and triacylglycerol concentrations. Am J Clin Nutr. 1999;70:1009–15.
81. Damasceno NR, Pérez-Heras A, Serra M, Cofán M, Sala-Vila A, Salas-Salvadó J, Ros E. Crossover study of diets enriched with virgin olive oil, walnuts or almonds. Effects on lipids and other cardiovascular risk markers. Nutr Metab Cardiovasc Dis. 2011;21(Suppl 1):S14–20.
82. Psaltopoulou T, Naska A, Orfanos P, Trichopoulos D, Mountokalakis T, Trichopoulou A. Olive oil, the Mediterranean diet, and arterial blood pressure: the Greek European Prospective Investigation into Cancer and Nutrition (EPIC) study. Am J Clin Nutr. 2004;80:1012–8.
83. Panagiotakos DB, Pitsavos CH, Chrysohoou C. Status and management of hypertension in Greece: role of the adoption of a Mediterranean diet: the Attica study. J Hypertens. 2003;21:1483–9.
84. Ward R. Familial aggregation and genetic epidemiology of blood pressure. In: Laragh JH, Brenner BM, editors. Hypertension, pathophysiology, diagnosis and management. New York: Raven Press; 1990. p. 81–100.
85. Hermansen K. Diet, blood pressure and hypertension. Br J Nutr. 2000;83(Suppl 1):S113–9.
86. Witteman JCM, Willett WC, Stampfer MJ, Colditz GA, Sacks FM, Speizer FE, Rosner B, Hennekens CH. A prospective study of nutritional factors and hypertension among US women. Circulation. 1989;80:1320–7.
87. Ascherio A, Hennekens CH, Willett WC, Sacks F, Rosner B, Manson J, et al. Prospective study of nutritional factors, blood pressure, and hypertension among US women. Hypertension. 1996;27:1065–72.

88. Ascherio A, Rimm EB, Giovannucci EL, Colditz GA, Rosner B, Willett WC, Witteman J, Stampfer MJ. A prospective study of nutritional factors and hypertension among US men. Circulation. 1992;86:1475–84.
89. Stamler J, Liu K, Ruth KJ, Pryer J, Greenland P. Eight-year blood pressure change in middle-aged men: relationship to multiple nutrients. Hypertension. 2002;39:1000–6.
90. Stamler J, Caggiula A, Grandits GA, Kjelsberg M, Cutler JA. Relationship to blood pressure of combinations of dietary macronutrients: findings of the Multiple Risk Factor Intervention Trial (MRFIT). Circulation. 1996;94:2417–23.
91. Williams PT, Fortmann SP, Terry RB, Garay SC, Vranizan KM, Ellsworth N, Wood PD. Associations of dietary fat, regional adiposity, and blood pressure in men. J Am Med Ass. 1987;257:3251–6.
92. Trevisan M, Krogh V, Freudenheim J, Blake A, Muti P, Panico S, Farinaro E, Mancini M, Menotti A, Ricci G. Consumption of olive oil, butter, and vegetable oils and coronary heart disease risk factors. The Research Group ATS-RF2 of the Italian National Research Council. J Am Med Ass. 1990;263:688–92.
93. Alonso A, Martìnez-Gonzàlez MA. Olive oil consumption and reduced incidence of hypertension: the SUN Study. Lipids. 2004;39:1233–8.
94. Martìnez-Gonzàlez MA, Sànchez-Villegas A, de Irala-Estévez J, Martì A, Martìnez JA. Mediterranean diet and stroke: objectives and design of the SUN Project. Nutr Neurosc. 2002;5:65–73.
95. Alonso A, de la Fuente C, Martìn-Arnau AM, de Irala J, Martìnez JA, Martìnez-Gonzàlez MA. Fruit and vegetable consumption is inversely associated with blood pressure in a Mediterranean population with a high vegetable-fat intake: the Seguimiento Universidad de Navarra (SUN) Study. Br J Nutr. 2004;92:311–9.
96. Strazzullo P, Ferro-Luzzi A, Siani A, Scaccini C, Sette S, Catasta G, Mancini M. Changing the Mediterranean diet effects on blood pressure. J Hypertens. 1986;4:407–12.
97. Lahoz C, Alonso R, Ordovas JM, Lo'pez-Farre A, de Oya M, Mata P. Effects of dietary fat saturation on eicosanoid production, platelet aggregation and blood pressure. Eur J Clin Investig. 1997;27:780–7.
98. Salas J, López Miranda J, Jansen S, Zambrana JL, Castro P, Paniagua JA, Blanco A, López Segura F, Jiménez Perepérez JA, Pérez Jiménez F. La dieta rica en grasa monoinsaturada modifica de forma beneficiosa el metabolismo de los hidratos de carbono y la presiòn arterial. Med Clin (Barc). 1999;113:765–9.
99. Thomsen C, Rasmussen OW, Hansen KW, Vesterlund M, Hermansen K. Comparison of the effects on the diurnal blood pressure, glucose, and lipid levels of a diet rich in monounsaturated fatty acids with a diet rich in polyunsaturated fatty acids in type 2 diabetic subjects. Diabet Med. 1995;12:600–6.
100. Rasmussen OW, Thomsen C, Hansen KW, Vesterlund M, Winther E, Hermansen K. Effects on blood pressure, glucose, and lipid levels of a high-monounsaturated fat diet compared with a high-carbohydrate diet in NIDDM subjects. Diabetes Care. 1993;16:1565–71.
101. Mensink RP, Janssen MC, Katan MB. Effect on blood pressure of two diets differing in total fats but not in saturated and polyunsaturated fatty acids in healthy volunteers. Am J Clin Nutr. 1988;47:976–80.
102. Ferrara LA, Raimondi AS, d'Episcopo L, Guida L, Dello Russo A, Marotta T. Olive oil and reduced need for antihypertensive medications. Arch Intern Med. 2000;160:837–42.
103. Appel LJ, Sacks FM, Carey VJ, Obarzanek E, Swain JF, Miller ER 3rd, Conlin PR, Erlinger TP, Rosner BA, Laranjo NM, Charleston J, McCarron P, Bishop LM, OmniHeart Collaborative Research Group. Effects of protein, monounsaturated fat, and carbohydrate intake on blood pressure and serum lipids. Results of the OmniHeart Randomized Trial. J Am Med Ass. 2005;294:2455–64.
104. Perona JS, Canizares J, Montero E, Sanchez-Dominguez JM, Catala A, Ruiz-Gutierrez V. Virgin olive oil reduces blood pressure in hypertensive elderly subjects. Clin Nutr. 2004;23:1113–21.

105. Rozati M, Barnett J, Wu D, Hndelman G, Saltzman E, Wilson T, Li L, Wang J, Marcos A, Ordovàs JM, Lee JC, Meydani M, Meydani SN. Cardio-metabolic and immunological impacts of extra virgin olive oil consumption in overweight and obese older adults: a randomized controlled trial. Nutr Metab (Lond). 2015;12:28.
106. Bondia-Pons I, Schröder H, Covas MI, Castellote AI, Kaikkonen J, Poulsen HE, Gaddi AV, Machowetz A, Kiesewetter H, López-Sabater MC. Moderate consumption of olive oil by healthy European men reduces systolic blood pressure in non-Mediterranean participants. J Nutr. 2007;137:84–7.
107. Fito M, Cladellas M, de la Torre R, Martí J, Alcántara M, Pujadas-Bastardes M, Marrugat J, Bruguera J, López-Sabater MC, Vila J, Covas MI, Members of the SOLOS Investigators. Antioxidant effect of virgin olive oil in patients with stable coronary heart disease: a randomized, crossover, controlled, clinical trial. Atherosclerosis. 2005;181:149–58.
108. Castaner O, Fito M, Lopez-Sabater MC, Poulsen HE, Nyyssönen K, Schröder H, Salonen JT, De la Torre-Carbot K, Zunft HF, De la Torre R, Bäumler H, Gaddi AV, Saez GT, Tomás M, Covas MI, EUROLIVE Study Group. The effect of olive oil polyphenols on antibodies against oxidized LDL. A randomized clinical trial. Clin Nutr. 2011;30:490–3.
109. Moreno-Luna R, Munoz-Hernandez R, Miranda ML, Costa AF, Jimenez-Jimenez L, Vallejo-Vaz AJ, Muriana FJ, Villar J, Stiefel P. Olive oil polyphenols decrease blood pressure and improve endothelial function in young women with mild hypertension. Am J Hypertens. 2012;25:1299–304.
110. Appel LJ, Moore TJ, Obarzanek E, Vollmer WM, Svetkey LP, Sacks FM, Bray GA, Vogt TM, Cutler JA, Windhauser MM, Lin PH, Karanja N. A clinical trial of the effects of dietary patterns on blood pressure. DASH collaborative research group. N Engl J Med. 1997;336:1117–24.
111. Toledo E, Hu FB, Estruch R, Buil-Cosiales P, Corella D, Salas-Salvadó J, Covas MI, Arós F, Gómez-Gracia E, Fiol M, Lapetra J, Serra-Majem L, Pinto X, Lamuela-Raventós RM, Saez G, Bulló M, Ruiz-Gutiérrez V, Ros E, Sorli JV, Martinez-Gonzalez MA. Effect of the Mediterranean diet on blood pressure in the PREDIMED trial: results from a randomized controlled trial. BMC Med. 2013;11:207.
112. Delgado-Lista J, Lopez-Miranda J, Cortes B, Perez-Martinez P, Lozano A, Gomez-Luna R, Gomez P, Gomez MJ, Criado J, Fuentes F, Perez-Jimenez F. Chronic dietary fat intake modifies the postprandial response of hemostatic markers to a single fatty test meal. Am J Clin Nutr. 2008;87:317–22.
113. Roche HM, Zampelas A, Knapper JM, Webb D, Brooks C, Jackson KG, Wright JW, Gould BJ Kafatos A, Gibney MJ, Williams CM. Effect of long-term olive oil dietary intervention on postprandial triacylglycerol and factor VII metabolism. Am J Clin Nutr. 1998;68:552–60.
114. Zampelas A, Roche H, Knapper JM, Jackson KG, Tornaritis M, Hatzis C, Gibney MJ, Kafatos A, Gould BJ, Wright J, Williams CM. Differences in postprandial lipaemic response between Northern and Southern Europeans. Atherosclerosis. 1998;139:83–93.
115. Silva KD, Kelly CN, Jones AE, Smith RD, Wootton SA, Miller GJ, Williams CM. Chylomicron particle size and number, factor VII activation and dietary monounsaturated fatty acids. Atherosclerosis. 2003;166:73–84.
116. Duttaroy AK. Postprandial activation of hemostatic factors: role of dietary fatty acids. Prostaglandins Leukot Essent Fatty Acids. 2005;72:381–91.
117. Sirtori CR, Tremoli E, Gatti E, Montanari G, Sirtori M, Colli S, Gianfranceschi G, Maderna P, Dentone CZ, Testolin G. Controlled evaluation of fat intake in the Mediterranean diet: comparative activities of olive oil on plasma lipids and platelets in high-risk patients. Am J Clin Nutr. 1986;44:635–42.
118. Barradas MA, Chrirtofides JA, Jeremy JY, Mikhailidis DP, Fry DE, Dandona P. The effect of olive oil supplementation on human platelet function, serum cholesterol-related variables and plasma fibrinogen concentrations: a pilot study. Nutr Res. 1990;10:403–11.
119. Smith RD, Kelly CN, Fielding BA, Hauton D, Silva KD, Nydahl MC, Miller GJ, Williams CM. Long-term monounsaturated fatty acid diets reduce platelet aggregation in healthy young subjects. Br J Nutr. 2003;90:597–606.

120. Nunez D, Randon J, Gandh C, Siafaka-Kapadai A, Olson MS, Hanahan DJ. The inhibition of platelet-activating factor-induced platelet activation by oleic acid is associated with a decrease in polyphosphoinositide metabolism. J Biol Chem. 1990;265:18330–8.
121. Carluccio MA, Siculella L, Ancora MA, Massaro M, Scoditti E, Storelli C, Visioli F, Distante A, De Caterina R. Olive oil and red wine antioxidant polyphenols inhibit endothelial activation: antiatherogenic properties of Mediterranean diet phytochemicals. Arterioscler Thromb Vasc Biol. 2003;23:622–9.
122. Togna GI, Togna AR, Francon M, Marra C, Guiso M. Olive oil isochromans inhibit human platelet reactivity. J Nutr. 2003;133:2532–6.
123. Liang ML, Da XW, He AD, Yao GQ, Xie W, Liu G, Xiang JZ, Ming ZY. Pentamethylquercetin (PMQ) reduces thrombus formation by inhibiting platelet function. Sci Rep. 2015;5:11142.
124. Dell'Agli M, Maschi O, Galli GV, Fagnani R, Dal Cero E, Caruso D, Bosisio E. Inhibition of platelet aggregation by olive oil phenols via cAMP-phosphodiesterase. Br J Nutr. 2008;99:945–51.

Extra-Virgin Olive Oil and Type 2 Diabetes Mellitus

4

4.1 Premises: Insight Into Type 2 Diabetes Mellitus

Extra-virgin olive oil has been demonstrated to have a deep impact on type 2 diabetes mellitus and on several factors that predispose to diabetes.

The Type 2 diabetes mellitus (T2DM), also referred to as non-insulin-dependent diabetes mellitus (NIDDM) or adult-onset diabetes, maturity-onset diabetes, or ketosis-resistant diabetes, is a very complex disease and a long-term metabolic disorder characterized by high blood sugar, insulin resistance, and relative lack of insulin. Metabolically, T2DM is characterized by insulin resistance in appropriate hepatic glucose production and impaired insulin secretion. Long-term complications from high blood sugar include atherosclerosis and cardiovascular disease (CHD) including strokes, retinopathy which can result in blindness, kidney failure, and ischemic peripheral arteriopathy which can result in limb amputations.

T2DM makes up about 90% of cases of diabetes, with the other 10% due to type 1 diabetes mellitus and gestational diabetes.

4.2 Epidemiology

Rates of T2DM have increased markedly since 1960 in parallel with obesity [1]. This is important because obesity, particularly the abdominal obesity, appears to be the major determinant of the onset of T2DM.

As of 2015 there were approximately 392 million people diagnosed with diabetes compared to around 30 million in 1985, with T2DM making up about 90% of the cases [2]. This represents 8.3% of the adult population [3], with equal rates in both women and men [4]. As of 2014, trends suggested the rate would continue to rise. Diabetes at least doubles a person's risk of early death [5]. From 2012 to 2015, approximately 1.5 to 5.0 million deaths each year resulted from diabetes [5, 6]. The global economic cost of diabetes in 2014 was estimated to be US$ 612 billion [7]. In the United States, diabetes cost were $245 billion in 2012 [8].

A. Capurso et al., *Benefits of the Mediterranean Diet in the Elderly Patient*, Practical Issues in Geriatrics, https://doi.org/10.1007/978-3-319-78084-9_4

T2DM is primarily due to lifestyle factors and genetics [9]. A number of lifestyle factors are known to be important to the development of T2DM, including obesity (defined by a body mass index of greater than 30), lack of physical activity, poor diet, stress, and urbanization. Dietary factors influence the risk of developing T2DM. Consumption of sugar-sweetened drinks in excess is associated with an increased risk [10, 11]. The type of fats in the diet is also important, with saturated fat and trans fats increasing the risk and polyunsaturated and monounsaturated fat decreasing the risk [9]. A lack of physical activity is believed to cause 7% of cases [12].

4.3 Visceral Obesity, Metabolic Syndrome, and T2DM

T2DM is in most cases associated with a particular form of obesity, the abdominal-perivisceral adiposity, which is part of a complex syndrome, the metabolic syndrome (MetS), characterized by insulin resistance, impaired glucose metabolism, or overt T2DM, as well as atherogenic dyslipidemia, elevated blood pressure, and other comorbidities including a prothrombotic and pro-inflammatory state and non-alcoholic fatty liver disease [13–19]. All these conditions independently increase the risk of atherosclerotic disease, such as CHD and stroke.

Mediterranean diet and particularly MUFA and olive oil have a significant impact on these comorbidities, so influencing the fate of T2DM. We will consider first the role of these comorbidities, particularly visceral adiposity and the consequent insulin resistance, in the pathogenesis of T2DM and then the impact of Mediterranean diet and EVOO on the fate of T2DM.

At the origin of T2DM, insulin resistance induced by excess abdominal-perivisceral fat accumulation appears to be the starter of glucose metabolism impairment and T2DM onset.

4.3.1 Insulin Resistance

Insulin resistance (IR) is defined as an inadequate response by insulin target tissues—such as the skeletal muscle, liver, and adipose tissue—to the physiologic effects of circulating insulin. The hallmarks of impaired insulin sensitivity in these tissues are:

1. Decreased insulin-stimulated glucose uptake into the skeletal muscle
2. Impaired insulin-mediated inhibition of hepatic glucose production in the liver
3. A reduced ability of insulin to inhibit lipolysis in the adipose tissue

The primary cause of insulin resistance and T2DM appears to be the increase in fat mass and obesity, particularly the intra-abdominal fat accumulation [20]. We will discuss (a) the mechanisms of adipogenesis and fat accumulation and (b) the consequences of increased lipolysis of intra-abdominal adipose tissue and consequent excess of circulating free fatty acids (FFA) on insulin receptor (IR) activity.

4.3.2 Mechanisms of Adipogenesis and Fat Accumulation

Contrary to the previous belief that adipogenesis ceases early in the life, with a fixed number of adipocytes after birth, fat cells experience a dynamic turnover, by which mesenchymal cells undergo lineage commitment, preadipocyte proliferation, and terminal differentiation into mature adipocytes [21]. Approximately 10% of fat cells are renewed annually at the adult stage and at all levels of body mass index [22].

During a positive caloric balance, adipocytes normally undergo initial hypertrophy, which elicits cellular signaling for the recruitment, proliferation, and differentiation of new fat cells. If new adipogenesis from preadipocytes is impaired, as is the case in the MetS, the lack of excess energy storage may cause existing fat cells to undergo excessive hypertrophy, causing adipocyte dysfunction, the production of pathogenic adipocytes, and adipose tissue endocrine and immune responses [23]. Therefore, a failure of subcutaneous fat cell proliferation or differentiation results in excessive hypertrophy and dysfunction of fat cells and in a consequent ectopic fat storage, i.e., intra-abdominal, perimuscular, perivascular, pericardial, and periosteal fat accumulation [24–26]. Pericardial and perivascular adipose tissue may have direct pathogenic effects on the myocardium, coronary arteries, and peripheral vessels, via dysregulated local secretion of vasoactive and inflammatory factors that may contribute to atheroma instability and other cardiovascular diseases.

4.3.3 Visceral Fat: Role and Metabolism

The visceral adipose tissue (VAT) is localized primarily as intra-abdominal depots around the intestine, in the mesentery, omentum, and perirenal areas, and drains directly to the liver through the portal circulation.

Although the complex pathophysiology of VAT has not been completely elucidated, it is known that VAT adipocytes are more metabolically active, more sensitive to lipolysis, and more insulin-resistant than the subcutaneous adipose tissue (SCAT). Conversely, SCAT is more avid in the absorption of circulating free fatty acids (FFA), in triglyceride synthesis, and in the storage of lipids in fat cells [27, 28]. VAT metabolic activity is regulated by its peculiar physiochemical components, i.e., the presence of a greater number of glucocorticoid receptors and β-adrenoceptors and a lower number of insulin receptors (IR).

4.3.3.1 Glucocorticoid Receptors

Adipose tissue accumulation is controlled by steroid hormones. Glucocorticoids promote the accumulation of adipose tissue in the intra-abdominal depots [29]. Accordingly, VAT was demonstrated to undergo relative and absolute accumulation due to a fourfold increase in glucocorticoid receptors in VAT compared with SCAT [29]. Progesterone acts as a glucocorticoid receptor antagonist and blocks the effects of glucocorticoids in the adipose tissue. These data suggests that in premenopausal women progesterone might protect against cortisol-induced intra-abdominal fat accumulation. Thus, men and postmenopausal women, who normally have low progesterone level, might experience the full-blown cortisol effect on intra-abdominal fat accumulation and therefore tend to accumulate a larger proportion of their fat intra-abdominally. The increase in VAT is also attributable to the glucocorticoid-induced increase in appetite, as well as to a glucocorticoid-dependent increase in adipocyte differentiation and decrease in adipocyte proliferation, both of which promote adipocyte hypertrophy [30]. Due to these characteristics, VAT mass appears to be prone to very large increase, and VAT adipocytes to possibly become very hypertrophic [31].

4.3.3.2 Fat Mobilization: The Role of β_3 and α_2 Adrenoceptors

The process of fat mobilization from adipocytes consists of the hydrolysis of triacylglycerol stored in the adipocyte, to release nonesterified fatty acids (NEFA or FFA) into the circulation. The key enzyme is here an intracellular lipase, the hormone sensitive lipase (HSL), sensitive to catecholamines. Catecholamines have dual effects on the lipolysis rate, both accelerating (through β-adrenoceptors) and retarding lipolysis (through α_2-adrenoceptors). In men and women, the lipolytic response to noradrenaline, which acts through α_2- and β-adrenoceptors, is more marked in the visceral than in the gluteal or femoral fat [32]. It was also found [33] that the visceral fat cells from obese subjects were highly responsive to noradrenaline stimulation, which strongly enhances lipolytic response. The main finding was the markedly augmented β_3-adrenoceptor sensitivity and coupling efficiency in visceral adipocytes. It was suggested that this enhanced β_3-adrenoreceptor activity of VAT was due to an increased receptor number in obese subjects. Therefore, the elevated rate of lipolysis in visceral fat cells appears to be largely due to increased number and activity of β_3-adrenoceptors and, partly, to a reduced activity of α_2-adrenoceptors. As a consequence, more FFA are released into the portal system in obesity.

4.3.3.3 VAT Insulin Receptor Dysfunction

The density of insulin receptors (IR) in VAT is lower than in SCAT, and this makes the abdominal visceral adipose tissue more sensitive to lipolytic stimuli and less sensitive to the inhibitory action of insulin than SCAT [34]. Insulin inhibits lipolysis preferentially in the more insulin-sensitive subcutaneous adipocytes, thus leaving visceral fat more exposed to the action of catecholamines [35]. Other factors, however, intervene in the metabolic dysfunction of VAT IR, e.g., the chronic elevation of FFA and inflammatory adipocytokines, particularly TNF-α. An increase of FFA level in VAT, primarily due to excess of lipolysis promoted by the enhanced β_3-adrenoreceptor activity, appears to play a crucial role in the initial phases of insulin receptor dysfunction and insulin resistance primarily in VAT.

4.3.3.4 Adipose Tissue Chronic Inflammation

By definition, the obese adipose tissue is characterized by inflammation and progressive infiltration by macrophages as obesity develops. Besides its main function of lipid storage, the white adipose tissue has a major endocrine function, secreting several hormones, notably leptin, adiponectin, and monocyte chemoattractant protein-1(MCP-1), and a diverse range of other protein factors, which have been called adipocytokines or adipokines. The adipokinome includes proteins involved in lipid metabolism, insulin sensitivity, the complement system, blood pressure, and angiogenesis and a number of proteins involved in inflammation (TNFα, interleukin (IL)-1β, IL-6, IL-8, IL-10, transforming growth factor-β, nerve growth factor) and the acute phase response (plasminogen activator inhibitor (PAI)-1, haptoglobin, serum amyloid A) [21, 36]. The increased production and raised circulating levels of these proteins in obesity have led to the view that obese individuals are characterized by a state of chronic low-grade inflammation and that this is causally linked to insulin resistance, hyperlipidemia, and the MetS [36–41]. The unbalanced production of pro- and anti-inflammatory adipocytokines seen in visceral fat obesity critically contributes to the development of many aspects of the MetS [16, 18, 42].

A very interesting feature of this inflammatory profile is that it appears to be triggered, and reside predominantly, in the adipose tissue [43, 44]. While the role of adipocytes in metabolic pathways is clear, little is still understood about their role in inflammation. There is considerable evidence that the obese adipose tissue is markedly infiltrated by macrophages, which actively participate in the inflammatory pathways that are activated in the adipose tissue [45–47]. It is noteworthy that macrophage infiltration and inflammation-related gene expression in the adipose tissue precede the development of insulin resistance in animal models [45, 46], suggesting that infiltrated macrophages are an important source of inflammation in the adipose tissue. Most macrophages in adipose tissue are derived from the bone marrow and recruited by the adipose tissue [45].

4.3.3.5 The Timing of Adipose Tissue Inflammation (Fig. 4.1)

According to a proposed timing of adipose tissue inflammatory steps in obesity, hypertrophic adipocytes begin to secrete low levels of TNF-α, which stimulate preadipocytes to produce MCP-1 [46]. Endothelial cells also secrete MCP-1 in response to cytokines. Thus, preadipocytes, endothelial cells, or both appear to be responsible for attracting macrophages into the adipose tissue through the active secretion of MCP-1. Increased secretion of leptin (and/or decreased production of adiponectin) by adipocytes may also contribute to macrophage accumulation by stimulating transport of macrophages to the adipose tissue [48] and promoting the adhesion of macrophages to endothelial cells [49]. Also hyperinsulinemia promotes monocyte adhesion and recruitment by increasing the expression of vascular cell adhesion molecule (VCAM)-1 in endothelial cells [19, 50]. It is conceivable that physical damage to the endothelium, caused either by sheer size changes and crowding or by oxidative damage resulting from an increasingly lipolytic environment, can also play a role in macrophage recruitment, similar to what is seen in atherosclerosis. Additionally, the increased adipose tissue expression of chemotactic factors such as MCP-1 and its cognate receptor chemokine (C–C motif) receptor (CCR)-2 has been implicated in the control of monocyte recruitment to the adipose tissue [51]. Finally, recent evidence suggests that increased metabolic stresses such as endoplasmic reticulum (ER) stress, hypoxia, and oxidative stress, as well as the downregulation of mitogen-activated protein (MAP) kinase phosphatase (MKP)-1, are involved in

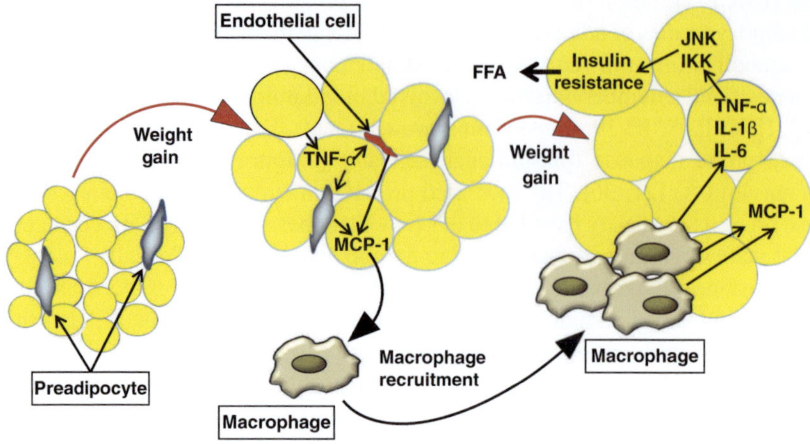

Fig. 4.1 The obese adipose tissue is characterized by inflammation and progressive infiltration by macrophages, as obesity develops. There is considerable evidence that the obese adipose tissue is markedly infiltrated by macrophages, which actively participate in the inflammatory pathways here activated. According to a proposed timing of adipose tissue inflammatory steps in obesity, hypertrophic adipocytes initially begin to secrete low levels of TNF-α, which stimulate preadipocytes to produce monocyte chemoattractant protein-1 (MCP-1) [46]. Endothelial cells also secrete MCP-1 in response to cytokines. Thus, preadipocytes, endothelial cells, or both appear to be responsible for attracting macrophages into the adipose tissue through the active secretion of MCP-1. Once macrophages are present and active in the adipose tissue, they, along with adipocytes and other cell types, perpetuate a vicious cycle of macrophage recruitment, production of inflammatory cytokines, and impairment of adipocyte function. The inflammatory cytokines IL-6, IL-1β, and TNF-α activate JNK and IKK serine kinases, which promote IRS-1 serine 307–312 phosphorylation. This serine phosphorylation is responsible for a reduction in IRS protein and a consequent inhibition of insulin receptor signaling by interrupting IRS/insulin receptor interaction. This molecular mechanism promotes insulin resistance in adipocytes and likely starts in the visceral adipose tissue (see also Figs. 4.2 and 4.3). Source: Capurso C, Capurso A. From excess adiposity to insulin resistance: the role of free fatty acids. Vasc Pharmacol 2012; 57: 91–97

the induction of inflammatory changes in adipocytes during the course of adipocyte hypertrophy [51]. Whatever the initial stimulus, once macrophages are present and active into the adipose tissue, they, along with adipocytes and other cell types, perpetuate a vicious cycle of macrophage recruitment, production of inflammatory cytokines, and impaired adipocyte function.

4.3.3.6 The Insulin Receptor Activity (Fig. 4.2)

To understand the role of excess FFA and other factors in the onset of insulin resistance, one has to consider the insulin receptor (IR) structure and metabolic activity (Fig. 4.2).

The IR, which belongs to the large class of tyrosine kinase receptors, is a transmembrane receptor that is activated by insulin [52]. The IR is a heterotetrameric protein consisting of two extracellular α-subunits and two transmembrane β-subunits, connected by disulfide bridges. Tyrosine kinase receptors, including the IR, mediate their activity by causing the addition of a phosphate group to particular

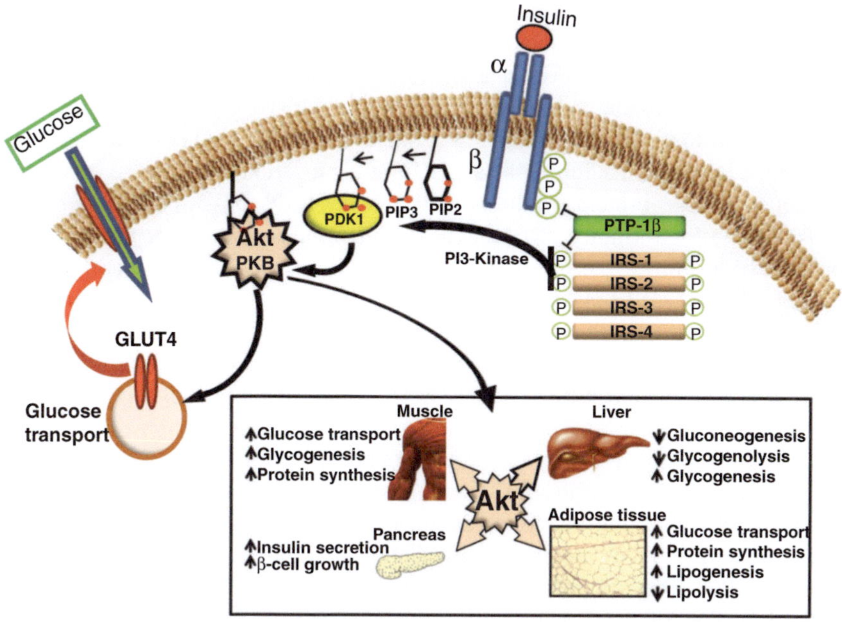

Fig. 4.2 The binding of insulin to the α-subunit of the insulin receptor activates autophosphorylation reactions whereby the intracellular part of the insulin receptor (β-subunit) becomes tyrosine-phosphorylated by the protein kinase activity of these same receptors. A phosphorylation cascade follows, initiating a protein phosphorylation cascade. The phosphorylation of IRS-1 and IRS-2 leads to binding and activation of phosphatidylinositol 3-kinase (PI3K), which converts phosphatidylinositol 3,4-bisphosphate [PI(3,4)P2] to phosphatidylinositol 3,4,5-trisphosphate [PI(3,4,5)P3]. These nucleotides act as anchors, binding protein kinases to the plasma membrane and activating them. [PI(3,4,5)P3] bound to the plasma membrane associates with phosphoinositol-dependent kinase-1 (PDK-1), and this leads to phosphorylation and activation of protein kinase B, otherwise known as Akt. Activated Akt is thought to initiate many of the metabolic actions of insulin in the adipose tissue, the muscle, the liver, and the pancreas. Source: Capurso C, Capurso A. From excess adiposity to insulin resistance: the role of free fatty acids. Vasc Pharmacol 2012; 57: 91–97

tyrosines on certain proteins within the cells. With the binding of insulin to the IR, a number of endogenous substrates are phosphorylated on tyrosine residue [53]. The first substrate to be tyrosine-phosphorylated by the insulin signaling is the transmembrane beta-subunit of the IR itself, with a mechanism of autophosphorylation. The preliminary tyrosine autophosphorylation of the IR tyrosine residues provides docking sites for the recruitment of a number of proteins, each capable of initiating a distinct signaling pathway, starting up a protein phosphorylation cascade. First among such proteins are a set of proteins known as IR substrates (IRS)1–4. The extracellular insulin binding induces the intracytoplasmic binding of IRS-1 to the receptor, through its src homology 2 (SH2) domains. Multiple tyrosine residues of IRS-1 itself are then phosphorylated by the receptor. Tyrosine-phosphorylated IRS-1 and IRS-2 serve as the major docking proteins for numerous proteins containing SH2 domain. This enables IRS-1 to activate several additional protein kinase signal systems. It has been suggested that the most dominant one is the signaling of phosphatidylinositol 3-kinase (PI3K) (Fig. 4.2), which converts phosphatidylinositol 3,4-bisphosphate [PI(3,4)P2] to phosphatidylinositol 3,4,5-trisphosphate [PI(3,4,5)P3]. These nucleotides act as anchors, binding downstream protein kinases to the plasma membrane and activating them, particularly the kinase Akt. It has been suggested that Akt (also known as protein kinase B, PKB) is the central element in the actions of insulin, such as GLUT4 translocation and glucose transport, glycogen synthesis, protein synthesis, and anti-lipolysis [54–58] (Fig. 4.2). The increase in the high-affinity glucose transporter GLUT4 molecules on the outer membrane of insulin-responsive tissues, including the muscular and the adipose tissue, leads to increased uptake of glucose from blood into these tissues. In other words, the glucose transporter GLUT4 is transported from cellular vesicles to the cell surface, where it can then mediate glucose transport into the cell [59]. IRS-1 plays a key role in transmitting signals from the IR to intracellular pathways of PI3K/Akt.

The degradation of IRS-1 by the proteasome degradation system acts as a feedback mechanism to turn off insulin signals. Insulin itself stimulates IRS-1 degradation, thus itself inhibiting insulin signaling [53]. After activation of IR signaling pathway, insulin induces membrane association of a protein kinase, the isoform theta (Θ) of PKC (PKC-Θ), which is known to be negatively associated with insulin sensitivity in the cells [60, 61]. Upon activation, PKC-Θ is phosphorylated by a mechanism of autophosphorylation. IRS-1 binds to activated (phosphorylated) PKC-Θ and becomes phosphorylated in IRS-1protein serine 307 in rodents and serine 312 in humans [62, 63]. Serine-phosphorylated IRS uncouples from the IR and is degraded by the proteasome system [53]. Other mechanisms of negative feedback have been described. Upon insulin stimulation, IRS-1 is tyrosine-phosphorylated by the IR, resulting in the activation of PI3-kinase, that mediates serine 307 phosphorylation of IRS-1, in turn inhibiting the ability of IRS-1 to be further tyrosine-phosphorylated by the IR and propagating insulin signaling [64]. Despite the complexity of insulin signaling, there is agreement that serine/threonine phosphorylation of IRS-1 inhibits IR-catalyzed IRS-1 tyrosine phosphorylation and the subsequent downstream signaling actions of insulin [53].

4.3.3.7 The Interruption of Insulin Receptor Signaling

As obesity develops, the fine and complex mechanisms that regulate insulin receptor activity become seriously perturbed by some factors that initiate "turnoff" reactions. Among the numerous factors described, excess of circulating FFA and TNF-α appears to be crucial in quenching IR function (Fig. 4.3).

4.3.3.8 FFA and Insulin Receptor Inactivation

It has been long known that FFA can induce insulin resistance [65, 66]. It was suggested that FFA cause insulin resistance through inhibition of insulin signaling, which occurs through activation of a serine kinase cascade [67].

Obesity results in an increased flux of FFA into the circulation and subsequent uptake by the myocyte, hepatocyte, or adipose tissue. Activated fatty acids (i.e., fatty acyl-CoA) are metabolized primarily via one of two pathways, oxidation and

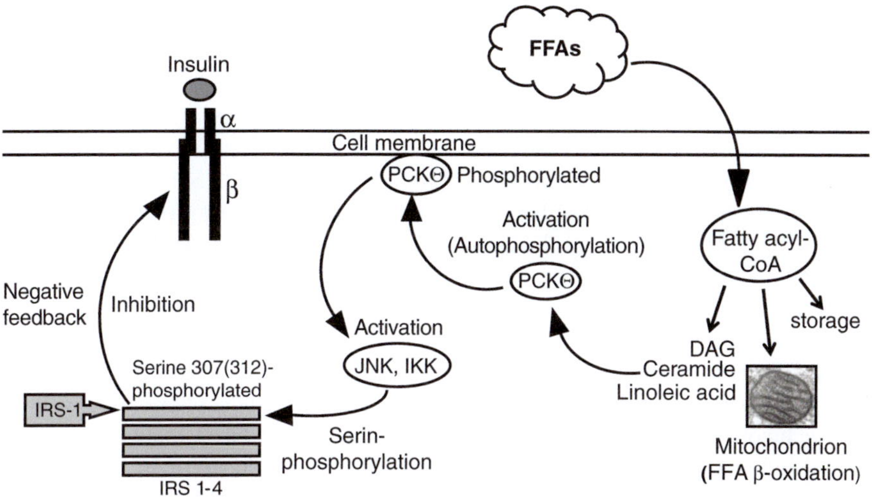

Fig. 4.3 Fatty acids, in their activated form (fatty acyl-CoAs), are metabolized primarily via one of two pathways, oxidation or storage. When fatty acid flux exceeds the capacity of these pathways, as it occurs in obesity, fatty acids and intermediates of fatty acid metabolism [linoleic acid, diacylglycerol (DAG), phosphatidic acid (PA), lysophosphatidic acid (LPA), ceramide] accumulate and activate phosphokinase C-theta (PKC-Θ), which becomes phosphorylated. Phosphorylated PKC-Θ starts a downstream activation of two serine kinases, the c-JUN NH2-terminal kinase (JNK) and the inhibitor kappaB kinase (IKK). JNK and IKK associate with IRS-1, promoting its serine phosphorylation (serine 312 in humans, serine 307 in rodents). The serine phosphorylation is responsible for IRS-1 blocking and the occurrence of insulin resistance by interrupting insulin receptor/IRS interaction and promoting IRS-1 protein degradation. Source: Capurso C, Capurso A. From excess adiposity to insulin resistance: the role of free fatty acids. Vasc Pharmacol 2012; 57: 91–97

storage (Fig. 4.3). When fatty acid flux exceeds the ability of these pathways to dispose of fatty acyl-CoA, fatty acids and intermediates of fatty acid metabolism (e.g., linoleic acid, diacylglycerol (DAG), phosphatidic acid (PA), lysophosphatidic acid (LPA), ceramide) accumulate. In turn, these fatty acid intermediates can activate a number of different serine kinases that negatively affect insulin action. Recently, some studies have better elucidated the role of FFA in the IR inactivation and degradation [18, 68]. FFA directly (e.g., linoleic acid) or through the intermediates DAG, PA, LPA, or ceramide activate the serine kinase PKC-Θ, which becomes phosphorylated at threonine 538 residue. Phosphorylated PKCΘ starts a downstream activation of other two serine kinases, the c-JUN NH2-terminal kinase (JNK) and the inhibitor kB kinase (IKK). JNK and IKK associate with IRS-1, promoting its serine phosphorylation on serine 312 in humans [53] and serine 307 in rodents [69] (Fig. 4.3). The serine phosphorylation is responsible for IRS-1 blocking and the occurrence of insulin resistance through interruption of IR/IRS interaction [70] and promotion of IRS-1 protein degradation [53]. The inactivated IR is then internalized into the cell and catabolized by lysosomes. This molecular pathway operates in many cell types including adipocytes, myocytes, and hepatocytes [68].

4.3.3.9 TNFα and Insulin Signaling

TNF-α, an inflammatory cytokine expressed mainly by macrophages of the adipose tissue (Fig. 4.1), inhibits insulin signaling and induces insulin resistance in human adipocytes by affecting IRS proteins [71, 72]. In adipocytes, TNF-α inhibits insulin-stimulated tyrosine phosphorylation of both IR and IRS-1 and downregulates the insulin-sensitive glucose transporter GLUT4. At the level of IRS-1, TNF-α acts by a double mechanism that involves (a) serine phosphorylation by IKK and by p38 MAP kinase (p38MAPK) at the serine 307 residue in rodents and serine 312 in humans and (b) tyrosine dephosphorylation by protein-tyrosine phosphatase 1B (PTP1B). Inhibition of IKK activation with salicylate restores insulin sensitivity also in the presence of TNF-α [73].

The mechanisms affecting IRS reduction involve proteasome-mediated degradation, phosphatase-mediated dephosphorylation, and serine phosphorylation of IRS-1, which converts IRS-1 to a form that inhibits IR tyrosine kinase activity [74, 75]. Obese individuals express 2.5-fold more TNF-α mRNA and protein in fat tissue relative to lean subjects, but circulating TNF-α levels are extremely low or undetectable. Therefore, rather than acting systemically, TNF-α seems to act locally at the site of the adipose tissue, through autocrine or paracrine mechanisms or both, having effects on insulin resistance and inducing IL-6 secretion [76]. In conclusion, the inhibitory effect of TNF-α on insulin signaling is mediated by a double mechanism of serine phosphorylation and tyrosine dephosphorylation of IRS-1, leading to IRS-1 inactivation and degradation [53].

4.3.3.10 Summarizing the Insulin Receptor Functioning

IRS proteins appear to be the keystone of insulin signaling, through a mechanism of phosphorylation. IRS-1 may be phosphorylated at the level of tyrosine or serine residues, with opposite effects. Tyrosine residue phosphorylation of IRS-1 and consequent docking of IRS-1 to the transmembrane β-subunits of insulin receptor activate the insulin signaling cascade in the muscle, the liver, and the adipose tissue. Serine residue phosphorylation of IRS-1, on the contrary, functions as a stop signal for insulin receptor, with detachment of IRS-1 from insulin receptor and degradation in the proteasome system. Insulin promotes first the autophosphorylation of tyrosine residues of the transmembrane β-subunits of IR and then the docking of IRS-1 to insulin receptor and the tyrosine phosphorylation of IRS-1. Excess of circulating FFA plays an opposite role to that of insulin, quenching insulin receptor activity through a mechanism of serine phosphorylation of IRS-1 induced by the FFA-activated serine kinase PKC-Θ. Serine-phosphorylated IRS-1, up-anchoring it to insulin receptor, stops insulin receptor activity and prompts insulin receptor and IRS-1 degradation by the proteasome. The serine kinase PKC-Θ results to be chronically activated in obese individuals, and this is probably one important cause of insulin resistance in such conditions [68]. As far as the serine kinase activation is concerned, salicylate has been demonstrated to prevent the FFA-induced activation of the serine kinase IKK-beta, preventing the serine phosphorylation and consequent inactivation of IRS-1 and insulin receptor [73]. This capacity of salicylate to prevent fat-induced defects in insulin signaling makes it the prototype of a potentially novel class of therapeutic agents for type 2 diabetes and insulin resistance. Finally, the inflammatory cytokine TNF-α, expressed mainly by macrophages resident in the "low-inflamed" adipose tissue of obese individuals, inhibits insulin signaling by a double mechanism that involves serine phosphorylation by IKK and tyrosine dephosphorylation by PTP1B of IRS-1. It is noteworthy that salicylate restores insulin sensitivity also in the presence of TNF-α [73]. Such mechanisms may explain the transition from excess adiposity to insulin resistance and—subsequently—type 2 diabetes.

4.4 The Impact of Extra-Virgin Olive Oil on Type 2 DM

4.4.1 EVOO Reduces the Risk of Type 2 DM

Comprehensive meta-analyses have shown significant inverse associations between high adherence to Mediterranean diet and risk of type 2 diabetes mellitus (T2DM) [77] and consistent improvements in glycemic control among T2DM patients following a Mediterranean diet [78].

A Spanish prospective cohort study [79] assessed the relation between level of adherence to a Mediterranean diet and incidence of T2DM. Participant in the study were 13,380 Spanish university graduates without diabetes at baseline followed up for a median of 4.4 years. Dietary habits were assessed at baseline with a validated 136-item food frequency questionnaire and scored on a nine-point index. Participants who adhered closely to a Mediterranean diet had a lower risk of diabetes. The incidence rate ratios adjusted for sex and age were 0.41 (95% confidence interval 0.19–0.87) for those with moderate adherence (score 3–6) and 0.17 (0.04–0.75) for those with the highest adherence (score 7–9) compared with those with low adherence (score < 3). A two-point increase in the score was associated with a 35% relative reduction in the risk of diabetes (incidence rate ratio 0.65, 0.44 to 0.95).

It should be considered that EVOO is the main source of dietary fat in the Mediterranean diet [80, 81]. With its high content in monounsaturated fatty acids (MUFAs) and polyphenols (tyrosol, secoiridoids, and lignans), consumption of extra-virgin olive oil has beneficial effects in the prevention, development, and progression of T2DM [82].

The MUFA oleic acid, the principal fatty acid of EVOO representing 70–75% of this oil, has been shown to have an important role in maintaining glycemic homeostasis and preventing metabolic risk factors. Meta-analyses of randomized controlled trials (RCTs) have shown that replacing carbohydrates (~5–10% of total energy intake) with MUFA as a specific dietary compound has beneficial effects on metabolic risk factors in T2DM patients [83–87], provided that MUFAs were derived from olive oil. In fact, in a meta-analysis of 32 cohort studies [88], MUFA of mixed animal and vegetable sources per se did not yield any significant effects on all-cause mortality and risk of cardiovascular disease, when the top and bottom thirds of baseline dietary fatty acid intake were compared. However, providing

MUFA via olive oil was associated with reduced risk of all-cause mortality, stroke, and cardiovascular events [88].

In a recent meta-analysis [89], 4 cohort studies, including 15,784 T2DM, and 29 RCTs have been analyzed to evaluate the relation of olive oil with the risk of T2DM. The study duration varied between 5.7 and 22 years for cohort studies enrolling 183,370 participants and between 2 weeks and 4.1 years for RCTs enrolling 3698 participants. The use of olive oil was inversely associated with the risk of T2DM. When the highest olive oil intake category was compared with the lowest intake category, an RR of 0.84 (95% CI, 0.77–0.92, $P < 0.01$) was found. The dose–response meta-analysis revealed that each 10 g daily increase in olive oil was associated with a 9% reduced risk of T2DM (RR, 0.91; 95% CI, 0.87–0.95; $P < 0.01$). A nonlinear relationship ($P < 0.01$) between olive oil intake and risk of T2DM was also found. The risk of T2DM was shown to decrease by 13% with increasing intake of olive oil up to ~15–20 g day^{-1}. No benefit for increasing intake was found above this value.

4.4.2 EVOO and MUFA Improve Glycemic Control

While in healthy individuals diets rich in olive oil, as the Mediterranean diet, reduce the incidence of T2DM, in people with T2DM a diet rich in monounsaturated fatty acids improves glycemic control, suggesting that a high intake of EVOO improves insulin sensitivity and insulin secretion [90–93].

The effect of EVOO in glycemic control has been shown in a sub-study of the PREDIMED study, a multicenter, randomized, primary prevention trial of cardiovascular disease. In this sub-study [94], 772 asymptomatic persons 55–80 years of age at high cardiovascular risk but free from T2DM were recruited and assigned to a low-fat diet or to 1 of 2 Mediterranean diets. Those allocated to Mediterranean diets received either free virgin olive oil, 1 L per week, or free nuts, 30 g/day. Compared with the low-fat diet, the mean changes (reductions) of plasma glucose levels in the Mediterranean diet with olive oil group or with nuts group were −0.39 mmol/L (95% CI, −0.70 to −0.07 mmol/L) and −0.30 mmol/L (CI, −0.58 to −0.01 mmol/L), respectively.

A MUFA-rich diet has been demonstrated to be better than a carbohydrate-rich diet in controlling fasting and postprandial serum glucose concentration. In a prospective study [93], 11 offsprings of obese and T2DM patients regarded as insulin-resistant after an OGTT were randomly divided into 3 groups and underwent 3 dietary periods each of 28 days in a crossover design: (a) diet high in saturated fat (SAT), (b) diet rich in monounsaturated fat (MUFA, from olive oil), and (c) diet rich in carbohydrate (CHO). Body weight and resting energy expenditure did not changed during the three dietary periods. Fasting serum glucose concentrations fell during MUFA-rich and CHO-rich diets compared with high-SAT diets (5.02 ± 0.1, 5.03 ± 0.1, 5.50 ± 0.2 mmol/L, respectively). However, the MUFA-rich diet improved insulin sensitivity, as indicated by lower homeostasis model analysis-insulin resistance (HOMA-IR), compared with CHO-rich and high-SAT diets

(2.32 ± 0.3, 2.52 ± 0.4, 2.72 ± 0.4, respectively). After a MUFA-rich and high-SAT breakfast (443 kcal), the postprandial integrated area under curve (AUC) of glucose and insulin was lower compared with isocaloric CHO-rich breakfast (7.8 ± 1.3, 5.84 ± 1.2, 11.9 ± 2.7 mmol, 180 min/L, and 1004 ± 147, 1253 ± 140, 2667 ± 329 pmol, 180 min/L, respectively), while the integrated glucagon-like peptide-1 response increased with MUFA and SAT breakfasts compared with isocaloric CHO-rich meals (4.22 ± 0.7, 4.34 ± 1.1, 1.85 ± 1.1, respectively). The conclusions were that weight maintenance with a MUFA-rich diet improves HOMA-IR and fasting proinsulin levels in insulin-resistant subjects. Ingestion of a virgin olive oil-based breakfast decreased postprandial glucose and insulin concentrations and increased HDL-C and GLP-1 concentrations as compared with CHO-rich diet.

In another study, a cross-sectional, population-based study undertaken in Pizarra, a small town in Spain, 538 normal subjects randomly chosen were given a prospective, 7-day nutritional questionnaire [95]. The intake of MUFA represented just over 50% of the total amount of dietary fat and about 18% of the energy consumed. 53.3% of the subjects usually consumed olive oil, 25.3% sunflower oil, and 21.4% both. The fatty acid composition of the serum phospholipids was used as a biological marker of the type of fat consumed. Beta-cell function and insulin resistance index were estimated. The results showed that insulin secretion was directly related with the intake of MUFA-rich fats, independently of the level of insulin resistance. Neither the saturated fatty acids nor the PUFA accounted for part of the variability of the β-cell function in a multiple regression analysis, confirming the favorable relationship of MUFA with β-cell insulin secretion. Studies both in healthy subjects and in persons with type 2 diabetes mellitus have demonstrated that levels of GLP-1 are increased more by dietary MUFA than by dietary saturated fatty acids [96] and that the greater postprandial clearance of an oral overload of MUFA-rich fats is associated with a greater increase in postprandial incretins such as GLP-1 or gastric inhibitory polypeptide. MUFAs from olive oil, therefore, appear to significantly increase the insulin and GPL-1 secretion.

It should be considered that a particular feature of Mediterranean diet is the large use of virgin olive oil for cooking, frying, spreading on bread, or dressing salads. This leads to a quite high daily intake of MUFA and to a high ratio of monounsaturated fatty acids to saturated fatty acids. Therefore, despite the relatively high total fat content, this food pattern is rich in monounsaturated fatty acids and poor in saturated fatty acids.

4.4.3 EVOO and the Pro-inflammatory State

Numerous studies have suggested that a pro-inflammatory state is one component of T2DM and metabolic syndrome [97–100]. The diabetic state per se confers an increased propensity to accelerated atherogenesis. Inflammation is pivotal in atherosclerosis; in addition to the established risk factors, inflammation appears to play an important role in diabetes and its complications. Evidence for increased inflammation includes increased levels of plasma C-reactive protein, the prototypic marker of inflammation, increased levels of plasminogen activator inhibitor, increased monocyte superoxide and pro-inflammatory cytokine release (IL-1, IL-6, and TNF-alpha), increased monocyte adhesion to the endothelium, increased NF-kappaB activity, and increased Toll-like receptor 2 and 4 expression and activity in diabetes. The low-grade inflammation is also associated with endothelial dysfunction [37, 101].

Mediterranean diet and EVOO have been demonstrated to favorably influence the pro-inflammatory state.

A randomized, single-blind study [102] conducted on 180 patients with metabolic syndrome was aimed to assess the effect of a Mediterranean-style diet rich in olive oil on endothelial functions and inflammatory markers. Patients in intervention group ($n = 90$) were instructed to follow a Mediterranean diet rich in olive oil, while patients in control group ($n = 90$) followed a prudent diet. Nutrient intake; endothelial function score as a measure of blood pressure and platelet aggregation response to L-arginine; lipid and glucose parameters; insulin sensitivity; and circulating levels of hs-CRP and IL-6, IL-7, and IL-18 were evaluated. After 2 years patients following the Mediterranean diet with olive oil, compared with patients consuming the control diet, had significantly reduced serum concentrations of hs-CRP ($P = 0.01$), IL-6 ($P = 0.04$), IL-7 ($P = 0.4$), and IL-18 ($P = 0.3$), as well as decreased insulin resistance ($P < 0.001$). Endothelial function score improved in the intervention group (mean [SD] change, +1.9 [0.6]; $P < 0.001$), while it remained stable in the control group (+0.2 [0.2]; $P = 0.33$). The conclusions were that olive oil and Mediterranean diet improve vascular inflammatory markers and endothelial function in subjects with DM and metabolic syndrome.

In a PREDIMED sub-study [94] conducted on 772 asymptomatic persons at high cardiovascular risk, Mediterranean diet enriched in EVOO (50 ml/week) reduced significantly C-reactive protein levels by 0.54 mg/L (CI, 1.04 to 0,03) compared with low-fat diet.

In a systematic review [103] aimed to synthesize data from randomized controlled trials investigating the effects of olive oil on markers of inflammation and endothelial function, 30 studies enrolling 3106 participants were included. Olive oil interventions (with daily consumption ranging approximately between 1 and 50 mL) resulted in a significantly more pronounced decrease in *C*-reactive protein (mean difference, −0.64 mg/L (95% confidence interval (CI) −0.96 to −0.31), $p < 0.0001$, $n = 15$ trials) and interleukin-6 (mean difference, −0.29 (95% CI −0.7 to −0.02), $p < 0.04$, $n = 7$ trials) as compared to controls, respectively. Values of flow-mediated dilatation (given as absolute percentage) were significantly more increased in individuals subjected to olive oil interventions (mean difference, 0.76% (95% CI 0.27 to 1.24), $p < 0.002$, $n = 8$ trials). These results confirm that olive oil exerts beneficial effects on markers of inflammation and endothelial function, thus representing a key ingredient contributing to the cardiovascular-protective effects of a Mediterranean diet.

4.4.4 Phenolic Compounds in EVOO

The minor components of EVOO, particularly polyphenols, have been demonstrated to favorably affect the blood glucose levels.

Polyphenols are well known to have antioxidant properties, chemopreventive activity, and capacity to improve endothelial functions by decreasing the expression of cell adhesion molecules, increasing nitric oxide disposability, and quenching intracellular free radicals [104]. They are also able to modify the hemostasis, inhibiting platelet-induced aggregation and showing antithrombotic properties both in experimental and human intervention trials [105].

As far as glucose metabolism is concerned, polyphenols have been demonstrated to interact with carbohydrate metabolism, improving plasma glucose levels and insulin secretion [106, 107].

*Polyphenols, or poly-hydroxy-phenol, are a group of plant metabolites thought to provide health benefits in humans through cell signaling pathways and antioxidant effects. They are considered as antioxidant phytochemicals that tend to prevent or neutralize the damaging effects of free radicals, the oxidative stress (see also Chap. 10, paragraph and Fig. 10.9.1; and Chap. 2, Sect. 2.2.2.1). It should be considered, however, that the bioactivity of these compounds is highly dependent on their intestinal absorption and generally they are ingested as nonabsorbable precursors that are transformed into bioactive forms by specific microorganisms in the intestine. Clostridium and Eubacterium genera, which are phylogenetically associated, have been shown to be involved in the metabolism of many phenolics. Through the action of gut microbiota, polyphenols are transformed to a much smaller number of metabolites. However, little is known about the impact of these ingested polyphenols upon the human gut microbiota, but a modulation of gut microbiota population by phenolics has been demonstrated. Therefore, the health benefits from phenolic consumption, in most cases, should be attributed to their bioactive metabolites and also to the modulation of the intestinal bacterial population [*108, 109*].*

*Virgin olive oil contains numerous phenolic compounds, i.e., phenolic acid, phenolic alcohols, secoiridoids, lignans, squalene, beta-carotene, sterols, and tocopherols. The most represented phenolic compounds of olive oil are tyrosol and hydroxytyrosol. These phenolics, derived by the hydrolysis of a precursor, the secoiridoid oleuropein, constitute around 90% of the total phenolic content of virgin olive oil [*110*]. It has been shown that, different from other diet polyphenols, coming essentially from vegetables and fresh fruit, tyrosol and hydroxytyrosol from virgin olive oil are dose-dependently absorbed in humans after ingestion and are excreted in the urine as glucuronide conjugates. Therefore, they are not degraded by gut microbiota but are just conjugated with glucuronic acid in the liver to increase their hydrophilicity that favors urinary secretion [*111–113*].*

Polyphenols affect glucose metabolism via an inhibition of carbohydrate digestion and absorption, a reduction of glucose release from the liver and a stimulation of glucose uptake in peripheral tissues [106]. The inhibition of carbohydrate digestion and absorption takes place through an inhibition of some digestive enzymes, especially the carbohydrate-hydrolyzing enzymes α-amylase and α-glucosidase. Inhibition of these enzymes retards carbohydrate digestion, thus causing a reduction in glucose absorption rate. This mechanism is particularly active with beans and wild fruits (blueberries, blackcurrants). Effective α-amylase and α-glucosidase polyphenol-type inhibitors from natural resources have been reported to be useful in reducing postprandial hyperglycemia [114]. Polyphenols from legumes, particularly several types of beans, have been demonstrated to actively inhibit α-amylase and α-glucosidase.

With their antioxidative properties, polyphenols diminish the production of advanced glycosylated end products such as HbA1c [115].

Polyphenols affect glucose metabolism also enhancing insulin secretion. The analysis of the results of a subgroup of participants of the PREDIMED trial revealed an inverse association between polyphenol excretion and fasting glucose [116], and the application of oleuropein and hydroxytyrosol as a supplement resulted in enhanced insulin secretion and sensitivity following oral glucose challenge [117].

These effects of polyphenol on glucose metabolism determine a reduced risk of T2DM. In fact, a high intake of total polyphenols, flavonoids (specifically flavanones and dihydroflavonols), and stilbenes has been found to be associated with a reduced risk of diabetes in elderly persons at high risk of cardiovascular disease. In a sub-study of PREDIMED [118], 3430 of the 7447 participants were selected because they were free of diabetes at baseline. Polyphenol intake was calculated by matching food consumption data from repeated food frequency questionnaires with the Phenol-Explorer database on the polyphenol content of each reported food. A 28% reduction in new-onset diabetes in the highest compared with the lowest tertile of total polyphenol intake was observed. The diabetes risk was inversely associated with the intake of subclasses of polyphenols, including total flavonoids (HR, 0.67; 95% CI, 0.48, 0.93; P-trend = 0.02), stilbenes (HR, 0.57; 95% CI, 0.38, 0.84; P-trend = 0.003), dihydroflavonols (HR, 0.59; 95% CI, 0.40, 0.88; P-trend = 0.003), and flavanones (HR, 0.69; 95% CI, 0.49, 0.97; P-trend = 0.03). The authors concluded that a high intake of total polyphenols, total flavonoids (specifically flavanones and dihydroflavonols), and stilbenes is associated with a reduced risk of diabetes in elderly persons at high risk of cardiovascular disease.

Another study showed that supplementation with olive leaf polyphenols (51.1 mg oleuropein and 9.7 mg hydroxytyrosol per day) for 12 weeks significantly improved insulin sensitivity and pancreatic β-cell secretory capacity after oral glucose challenge in overweight, middle-aged men at the risk of developing the metabolic syndrome [119]. Similarly, in a randomized, placebo-controlled trial in subjects with T2D, supplementation of a 500 mg olive leaf extract tablet once daily for 14 weeks was shown to significantly lower HbA1c and fasting insulin with no significant changes in postprandial insulin levels [119, 120].

Finally, polyphenols of olive oil have been demonstrated to inhibit the formation of advanced glycation products (AGEs). AGEs, which are readily formed and accumulated with sustained hyperglycemia, contribute to the development of diabetic complications. As a consequence, inhibition of AGE formation constitutes an attractive therapeutic/preventive target. AGEs are deeply involved in the aging and the development of common chronic diseases.

In a recent study [121], hydroxytyrosol (HT) and its acetate derivative (HTA) exert a significant inhibitory activity on the formation of fluorescent AGEs in bovine serum albumin glycation model systems induced by methylglyoxal and glucose. HT and HTA have also shown relevant carbonyl scavenging capacity toward methylglyoxal and glyoxal, which are the most potent promoters of the glycation in vivo. At equimolar concentrations, the ester linkage did not significantly affect the antiglycative activity and carbonyl trapping capacity of the orthodiphenolic ring structure. Results have been confirmed with the specific inhibition of the formation of the principal AGEs. Formation of carboxymethyllysine, argpyrimidine, and carboxyethyl-lysine has been shown to be significantly reduced by 61.9%, 71.4%, and 20.9%, respectively.

In another study [107], the methanolic olive leaf extract inhibited fluorescent AGE formation in a bovine serum albumin (BSA)-ribose system in vitro. Among the major phenolic components (luteolin, hydroxytyrosol, luteolin-4′-*O*-*β*-D-glucopyranoside, luteolin-7-*O*-*β*-D-glucopyranoside, and oleuropein), luteolin and luteolin-4′-*O*-*β*-D-glucopyranoside were assigned as potent inhibitors of AGE formation.

To conclude, the benefits of EVOO and dietary polyphenols on type 2 diabetes can be summarized as follows: improving of blood glucose levels, protection of pancreatic β-cells against glucose toxicity, improving insulin sensitivity and pancreatic β-cell secretory capacity, reduction of glucose release from the liver and stimulation of glucose uptake in peripheral tissues, anti-inflammatory and antioxidant effects, inhibition of α-amylases and α-glucosidases with consequent decrease of starch digestion, and inhibition of advanced glycation end product formation.

References

1. Moscou S. Getting the word out: advocacy, social marketing, and policy development and enforcement. In: Truglio-Londrigan M, Lewenson SB, editors. Public health nursing: practicing population-based care. 2nd ed. Burlington, MA: Jones & Bartlett Learning; 2013. p. 317.
2. Gardner DG, Shoback D. Chapter 17: pancreatic hormones & diabetes mellitus. In: Greenspan's basic & clinical endocrinology. 9th ed. New York: McGraw-Hill Medical; 2011.
3. Saenz A, Fernandez-Esteban I, Mataix A, Ausejo M, Roque M, Moher D. Metformin monotherapy for type 2 diabetes mellitus. Cochrane Database Syst Rev. 2005;20(3):CD002966.
4. Malanda UL, Welschen LM, Riphagen II, Dekker JM, Nijpels G, Bot SD. Self-monitoring of blood glucose in patients with type 2 diabetes mellitus who are not using insulin. Cochrane Database Syst Rev. 2012;1:CD005060.
5. World Health Organization. The top 10 causes of death. Fact sheet 310.
6. International Diabetes Federation. IDF Diabetes Atlas. 7th ed.
7. International Diabetes Federation. IDF Diabetes Atlas. 6th ed. 2013. p. 7.
8. American Diabetes, Association. Economic costs of diabetes in the U.S. in 2012. Diabetes Care. 2013;36:1033–46.
9. Risérus U, Willett WC, Hu FB. Dietary fats and prevention of type 2 diabetes. Progr Lipid Res. 2009;48:44–51.
10. Malik VS, Popkin BM, Bray GA, Després JP, Hu FB. Sugar sweetened beverages, obesity, type 2 diabetes and cardiovascular disease risk. Circulation. 2010;121:1356–64.
11. Malik VS, Popkin BM, Bray GA, Després JP, Willett WC, Hu FB. Sugar-sweetened beverages and risk of metabolic syndrome and type 2 diabetes: a meta-analysis. Diabetes Care. 2010;33:2477–83.
12. Lee IM, Shiroma EJ, Lobelo F, Puska P, Blair SN, Katzmarzyk PT. Effect of physical inactivity on major non-communicable diseases worldwide: an analysis of burden of disease and life expectancy. Lancet. 2012;380(9838):219–29.
13. DeFronzo RA, Ferrannini E, Koivisto V. New concepts in the pathogenesis and treatment of noninsulin-dependent diabetes mellitus. Am J Med. 1983;74:52–81.

14. Ferrannini E, Barrett EJ, Bevilacqua S, DeFronzo RA. Effect of fatty acids on glucose production and utilization in man. J Clin Invest. 1983;72:1737–47.
15. Kelley DE, Mokan M, Simoneau JA, Mandarino LJ. Interaction between glucose and free fatty acid metabolism in human skeletal muscle. J Clin Invest. 1993;92:91–8.
16. Berg AH, Scherer PE. Adipose tissue, inflammation, and cardiovascular disease. Circ Res. 2005;96:939–49.
17. Bays H, Ballantyne C. Adiposopathy: why do adiposopathy and obesity cause metabolic disease? Future Lipidol. 2006;1:389–420.
18. Schenk S, Saberi M, Olefsky JM. Insulin sensitivity: modulation by nutrients and inflammation. J Clin Invest. 2008;118:2992–3002.
19. Madonna R, De Caterina R. Atherogenesis and diabetes: focus on insulin resistance and hyperinsulinema. Rev Esp Cardiol. 2012;65:309–13.
20. Fujioka S, Matsuzawa Y, Tokunaga K, Tarui S. Contribution of intra-abdominal fat accumulation to the impairment of glucose and lipid metabolism in human obesity. Metabolism. 1987;36:54–9.
21. Bays HE. Adiposopathy is "sick fat" a cardiovascular disease? J Am Coll Cardiol. 2011;57:2461–73.
22. Spalding KL, Arner E, Westermark PO, Bernard S, Buchholz BA, Bergmann O, Blomqvist L, Hoffstedt J, Näslund E, Britton T, Concha H, Hassan M, Rydén M, Frisén J, Arner P. Dynamics of fat cell turnover in humans. Nature. 2008;453:783–7.
23. Bays HE, González-Campoy JM, Bray GA, Kitabchi AE, Bergman DA, Schorr AB, Rodbard HW, Henry RR. Pathogenic potential of adipose tissue and metabolic consequences of adipocyte hypertrophy and increased visceral adiposity. Expert Rev Cardiovasc Ther. 2008;6:343–68.
24. Danforth E Jr. Failure of adipocyte differentiation causes type II diabetes mellitus? Nat Genet. 2000;26:13.
25. Ravussin E, Smith SR. Increased fat intake, impaired fat oxidation, and failure of fat cell proliferation result in ectopic fat storage, insulin resistance, and type 2 diabetes mellitus. Ann N Y Acad Sci. 2002;967:363–78.
26. Pasarica M, Xie H, Hymel D, Bray G, Greenway F, Ravussin E, Smith SR. Lower total adipocyte number but no evidence for small adipocyte depletion in patients with type 2 diabetes. Diabetes Care. 2009;32:900–2.
27. Martin ML, Jensen MD. Effects of body fat distribution on regional lipolysis in obesity. J Clin Invest. 1991;88:609–13.
28. Ibrahim MM. Subcutaneous and visceral adipose tissue: structural and functional differences. Obes Rev. 2010;11:11–8.
29. Pedersen SB. Studies on receptors and actions of steroid hormones in adipose tissue. Dan Med Bull. 2005;52:258.
30. Tomlinson JW, Walker EA, Bujalska IJ, Draper N, Lavery GG, Cooper MS, Hewison M, Stewart PM. 11beta-hydroxysteroid dehydrogenase type 1: a tissue-specific regulator of glucocorticoid response. Endocr Rev. 2004;25:831–66.
31. Rebuffe-Scrive M, Krotkiewski M, Elfverson J, Bjorntorp P. Muscle and adipose tissue morphology and metabolism in Cushing's syndrome. J Clin Endocrinol Metab. 1988;W67:1122–8.
32. Krotkiewski M, Bjorntorp P, Sjostrom L, Smith U. Impact of obesity on metabolism in men and women: importance of regional adipose tissue distribution. J Clin Invest. 1983;72:1150–62.
33. Lonnqvist F, Thome A, Nilsell K, Hoffstedt J, Arner P. A pathogenic role of visceral fat beta 3-adrenoceptors in obesity. J Clin Invest. 1995;95:1109–16.
34. Kopelman PG, Albon L. Obesity, non-insulin-dependent diabetes mellitus and the metabolic syndrome. Br Med J. 1997;53:322–40.
35. Rebuffe-Scrive M, Andersson B, Olbe L, Bjorntorp P. Metabolism of adipose tissue in intraabdominal depots of non-obese men and women. Metabolism. 1989;38:453–61.
36. Trayhurn P, Wood IS. Adipokines: inflammation and the pleiotropic role of white adipose tissue. Br J Nutr. 2004;92:347–55.

37. Yudkin JS, Stehouwer CD, Emeis JJ, Coppack SW. C-reactive protein in healthy subjects: associations with obesity, insulin resistance, and endothelial dysfunction: a potential role for cytokines originating from adipose tissue? Arterioscler Thromb Vasc Biol. 1999;19:972–8.
38. Das UN. Is obesity an inflammatory condition? Nutrition. 2001;17:953–66.
39. Festa A, D'Agostino R Jr, Williams K, Karter AJ, Mayer-Davis EJ, Tracy RP, Haffner SM. The relation of body fat mass and distribution to markers of chronic inflammation. Int J Obes. 2001;25:1407–15.
40. Hotamisligil GS. Inflammatory pathways and insulin action. Int J Obes. 2003;27(Suppl. 3):S53–5.
41. Yudkin JS. Adipose tissue, insulin action and vascular disease: inflammatory signals. Int J Obes. 2003;27(Suppl. 3):S25–8.
42. Hotamisligil GS. Inflammation and metabolic disorders. Nature. 2006;444:860–7.
43. Wellen KE, Hotamisligil GS. Obesity-induced inflammatory changes in adipose tissue. J Clin Invest. 2003;112:1785–8.
44. Hirosumi J, Tuncman G, Chang L, Görgün CZ, Uysal KT, Maeda K, Karin M, Hotamisligil GS. A central role for JNK in obesity and insulin resistance. Nature. 2002;420:333–6.
45. Weisberg SP, McCann D, Desai M, Rosenbaum M, Leibel RL, Ferrante AW Jr. Obesity is associated with macrophage accumulation in adipose tissue. J Clin Invest. 2003;112:1796–808.
46. Xu H, Barnes GT, Yang Q, Tan G, Yang D, Chou CJ, Sole J, Nichols A, Ross JS, Tartaglia LA, Chen H. Chronic inflammation in fat plays a crucial role in the development of obesity-related insulin resistance. J Clin Invest. 2003;112:1821–30.
47. Clement K, Viguerie N, Poitou C, Carette C, Pelloux V, Curat CA, Sicard A, Rome S, Benis A, Zucker JD, Vidal H, Laville M, Barsh GS, Basdevant A, Stich V, Cancello R, Langin D. Weight loss regulates inflammation-related genes in white adipose tissue of obese subjects. FASEB J. 2004;18:1657–69.
48. Sierra-Honigmann MR, Nath AK, Murakami C, García-Cardeña G, Papapetropoulos A, Sessa WC, Madge LA, Schechner JS, Schwabb MB, Polverini PJ, FloresRiveros JR. Biological action of leptin as an angiogenic factor. Science. 1998;281:1683–6.
49. Maeda N, Shimomura I, Kishida K, Nishizawa H, Matsuda M, Nagaretani H, Furuyama N, Kondo H, Takahashi M, Arita Y, Komuro R, Ouch N, Kihara S, Tochino Y, Okutomi K, Horie M, Takeda S, Aoyama T, Funahashi T, Matsuzawa Y. Diet-induced insulin resistance in mice lacking adiponectin/ACRP30. Nat Med. 2002;8:731–7.
50. Madonna R, Pandolfi A, Massaro M, Consoli A, De Caterina R. Insulin enhances vascular cell adhesion molecule-1 expression in human cultured endothelial cells through a pro-atherogenic pathway mediated by p38 mitogen-activated protein-kinase. Diabetologia. 2004;47:532–6.
51. Suganami T, Ogawa Y. Adipose tissue macrophages: their role in adipose tissue remodeling. J Leukoc Biol. 2010;88:33–9.
52. Ward CW, Lawrence MC. Ligand-induced activation of the insulin receptor: a multi-step process involving structural changes in both the ligand and the receptor. BioEssays. 2009;31:422–34.
53. Greene MW, Sakaue H, Wang L, Alessi DR, Roth RA. Modulation of insulin-stimulated degradation of human insulin receptor substrate-1 by serine 312 phosphorylation. J Biol Chem. 2003;278:8199–211.
54. Cho H, Mu J, Kim JK, Thorvaldsen JL, Chu Q, Crenshaw EB III, Kaestner KH, Bartolomei MS, Shulman GI, Birnbaum MJ. Insulin resistance and a diabetes mellitus-like syndrome in mice lacking the protein kinase Akt2 (PKB beta). Science. 2001;292:1728–31.
55. Summers SA, Kao AW, Kohn AD, Backus GS, Roth RA, Pessin JE, Birnbaum MJ. The role of glycogen synthase kinase 3beta in insulin-stimulated glucose metabolism. J Biol Chem. 1999;274:17934–40.
56. Kitamura T, Kitamura Y, Kuroda S, Hino Y, Ando M, Kotani K, Konishi H, Matsuzaki H, Kikkawa U, Ogawa W, Kasuga M. Insulin-induced phosphorylation and activation of cyclic nucleotide phosphodiesterase 3B by the serine-threonine kinase Akt. Mol Cell Biol. 1999;19:6286–96.

57. Proud CG, Wang X, Patel JV, Campbell LE, Kleijn M, Li W, Browne GJ. Interplay between insulin and nutrients in the regulation of translation factors. Biochem Soc Trans. 2001;29:541–7.
58. Shepherd PR. Mechanisms regulating phosphoinositide 3-kinase signalling in insulin-sensitive tissues. Acta Physiol Scand. 2005;183:3–12.
59. Saltiel AR, Kahn CR. Insulin signalling and the regulation of glucose and lipid metabolism. Nature. 2001;414:799–806.
60. Standaert ML, Bandyopadhyay G, Galloway L, Soto J, Ono Y, Kikkawa U, Farese RV, Leitges M. Effects of knockout of the protein kinase C gene on glucose transport and glucose homeostasis. Endocrinology. 1999;140:4470–7.
61. Leitges M, Plomann M, Standaert ML, Bandyopadhyay G, Sajan MP, Kanoh Y, Farese RV. Knockout of PKC enhances insulin signaling through PI3K. Mol Endocrinol. 2002;16:847–58.
62. Stephens JM, Lee J, Pilch PF. Tumor necrosis factor-a-induced insulin resistance in 3T3-L1 adipocytes is accompanied by a loss of insulin receptor substrate-1 and GLUT4 expression without a loss of insulin receptor-mediated signal transduction. J Biol Chem. 1997;272:971–6.
63. Sun XJ, Goldberg JL, Qiao LY, Mitchell JJ. Insulin induced insulin receptor substrate-1 degradation is mediated by the proteasome degradation pathway. Diabetes. 1999;48:1359–64.
64. Rui L, Aguirre V, Kim JK, Shulman GI, Lee A, Corbould A, Dunaif A, White MF. Insulin/IGF-1 and TNF-α stimulate phosphorylation of IRS-1 at inhibitory Ser307 via distinct pathways. J Clin Invest. 2001;107:181–9.
65. Boden G, Jadali F, White J, Liang Y, Mozzoli M, Chen X, Coleman E, Smith C. Effects of fat on insulin stimulated carbohydrate metabolism in normal men. J Clin Invest. 1991;88:960–6.
66. Boden G. Role of fatty acids in the pathogenesis of insulin resistance and NIDDM. Diabetes. 1997;46:3–10.
67. Griffin ME, Marcucci MJ, Cline GW, Bell K, Barucci N, Lee D, Goodyear J, Kraegen EW, White MF, Shulman GI. Free fatty acid-induced insulin resistance is associated with activation of protein kinase C theta and alterations in the insulin signaling cascade. Diabetes. 1999;48:1270–4.
68. Gao Z, Zhang X, Zuberi A, Hwang D, Quon MJ, Lefevre M, Ye J. Inhibition of insulin sensitivity by free fatty acids requires activation of multiple serine kinases in 3T3–L1 adipocytes. Mol Endocrinol. 2004;18:2024–34.
69. Gual P, Le Marchand-Brustel Y, Tanti JF. Positive and negative regulation of insulin signaling through IRS-1 phosphorylation. Biochimie. 2005;87:99–109.
70. Aguirre V, Werner ED, Giraud J, Lee YH, Shoelson SE, White MF. Phosphorylation of ser307 in insulin receptor substrate-1 blocks interactions with the insulin receptor and inhibits insulin action. J Biol Chem. 2002;277:1531–7.
71. Hotamisligil GS, Arne P, Caro JF, Atkinson RL, Spiegelman BM. Increased adipose tissue expression of tumor necrosis factor-alpha in human obesity and insulin resistance. J Clin Invest. 1995;95:2409–15.
72. Skolnik EY, Marcusohn J. Inhibition of insulin receptor signaling by TNF: potential role in obesity and non-insulin-dependent diabetes mellitus. Cytokine Growth Factor Rev. 1996;7:161–73.
73. Kim JK, Kim YJ, Fillmore JJ, Chen Y, Moore I, Lee J, Yuan M, Li ZW, Karin M, Perret P, Shoelson SE, Shulman GI. Prevention of fat-induced insulin resistance by salicylate. J Clin Invest. 2001;108:437–46.
74. White MF. Insulin signaling in health and disease. Science. 2003;302:1710–1.
75. Pirola L, Johnston AM, Van Obberghen E. Modulation of insulin action. Diabetologia. 2004;47:170–84.
76. Arner P. The adipocyte in insulin resistance: key molecules and the impact of the thiazolidinediones. Trends Endocrinol Metab. 2003;14:137–45.
77. Schwingshackl L, Missbach B, Konig J, Hoffmann G. Adherence to a Mediterranean diet and risk of diabetes: a systematic review and meta-analysis. Public Health Nutr. 2015;18:1292–9.

78. Huo R, Du T, Xu Y, Xu W, Chen X, Sun K, et al. Effects of Mediterranean-style diet on glycemic control, weight loss and cardiovascular risk factors among type 2 diabetes individuals: a meta-analysis. Eur J Clin Nutr. 2015;69:1200–8.
79. Martînez-Gonzàlez MA, Nunez-Cordoba JM, Basterra-Gortari FJ, Beunza JJ, Vazquez Z, Benito S, Tortosa A, Bes-Rastrollo M. Adherence to Mediterranean diet and risk of developing diabetes: prospective cohort study. Br Med J. 2008;336:1348–51.
80. Trichopoulou A, Martinez-Gonzalez MA, Tong TY, Forouhi NG, Khandelwal S, Prabhakaran D, et al. Definitions and potential health benefits of the Mediterranean diet: views from experts around the world. BMC Med. 2014;12:112.
81. Schwingshackl L, Hoffmann G. Does a Mediterranean-type diet reduce cancer risk? Curr Nutr Rep. 2016;5:9–17.
82. Lopez-Miranda J, Perez-Jimenez F, Ros E, De Caterina R, Badimon L, Covas MI, et al. Olive oil and health: summary of the II international conference on olive oil and health consensus report, Jaen and Cordoba (Spain) 2008. Nutr Metab Cardiovasc Dis. 2010;20:284–94.
83. Qian F, Korat AA, Malik V, Hu FB. Metabolic effects of monounsaturated fatty acid–enriched diets compared with carbohydrate or polyunsaturated fatty acid–enriched diets in patients with type 2 diabetes: a systematic review and meta-analysis of randomized controlled trials. Diabetes Care. 2016;39:1448–57.
84. Schwingshackl L, Hoffmann G. Monounsaturated fatty acids and risk of cardiovascular disease: synopsis of the evidence available from systematic reviews and eta-analyses. Forum Nutr. 2012;4:1989–2007.
85. Schwingshackl L, Strasser B, Hoffmann G. Effects of monounsaturated fatty acids on glycaemic control in patients with abnormal glucose metabolism: a systematic review and meta-analysis. Ann Nutr Metab. 2011;58:290–6.
86. Schwingshackl L, Strasser B. High-MUFA diets reduce fasting glucose in patients with type 2 diabetes. Ann Nutr Metab. 2012;60:33–4.
87. Schwingshackl L, Strasser B, Hoffmann G. Effects of monounsaturated fatty acids on cardiovascular risk factors: a systematic review and meta-analysis. Ann Nutr Metab. 2011;59:176–86.
88. Schwingshackl L, Hoffmann G. Monounsaturated fatty acids, olive oil and health status: a systematic review and meta-analysis of cohort studies. Lipids Health Dis. 2014;13:154.
89. Schwingshackl L, Lampousi AM, Portillo MP, Romaguera D, Hoffmann G, Boeing H. Olive oil in the prevention and management of type 2 diabetes mellitus: a systematic review and meta-analysis of cohort studies and intervention trials. Nutr Diabetes. 2017;7:e262.
90. Garg A. High monounsaturated-fat diets for patients with diabetes mellitus: a meta-analysis. Am J Clin Nutr. 1998;67(Suppl 3):577–82S.
91. Rocca AS, LaGreca J, Kalitsky J, Brubaker PL. Monounsaturated fatty acid diets improve glycemic tolerance through increased secretion of glucagon-like peptide-1. Endocrinology. 2001;142:1148–55.
92. Ros E. Dietary cis-monounsaturated fatty acids and metabolic control in type 2 diabetes. Am J Clin Nutr. 2003;78(Suppl 3):617–25S.
93. Paniagua JA, de la Sacristana AG, Sánchez E, Romero I, Vidal-Puig A, Berral FJ, et al. MUFA-rich diet improves postprandial glucose, lipid and GLP-1 responses in insulin-resistant subjects. J Am Coll Nutr. 2007;26:434–44.
94. Estruch R, Martínez-González MA, Corella D, Salas-Salvadó J, Ruiz-Gutiérrez V, Covas MI, Fiol M, Gómez-Gracia E, López-Sabater MC, Vinyoles E, Arós F, Conde M, Lahoz C, Lapetra J, Sáez G, Ros E. PREDIMED Study Investigators effects of a Mediterranean-style diet on cardiovascular risk factors: a randomized trial. Ann Inter Med. 2006;145:1–11.
95. Rojo-Martínez G, Esteva I, Ruiz de Adana MS, García-Almeida JM, Tinahones F, Cardona F, Morcillo S, García-Escobar E, García-Fuentes E, Soriguer F. Dietary fatty acids and insulin secretion: a population-based study. Eur J Clin Nutr. 2006;60:1195–2000.
96. Thomsen C, Storm H, Holst JJ, Hermansen K. Differential effects of saturated and monounsaturated fats on posprandial lipemia and glucagon-like peptide 1 response in patients with type 2 diabetes. Am J Clin Nutr. 2003;77:605–11.

97. Han TS, Sattar N, Williams K, Gonzalez-Villalpando C, Lean ME, Haffner SM. Prospective study of C-reactive protein in relation to the development of diabetes and metabolic syndrome in the Mexico City Diabetes study. Diabetes Care. 2002;25:2016–21.
98. Esposito K, Pontillo A, Giugliano F, Marfella R, Nicoletti G, Giugliano D. Association of low interleukin-10 levels with the metabolic syndrome in obese women. J Clin Endocrinol Metab. 2003;88:1055–8.
99. Tamakoshi K, Yatsuya H, Kondo T, Hori Y, Ishikawa M, Zhang H, Murata C, Otsuka R, Zhu S, Toyoshima H. The metabolic syndrome is associated with elevated circulating C-reactive protein in healthy reference range, a systemic low-grade inflammatory state. Int J Obes Relat Metab Disord. 2003;27:443–9.
100. Ridker PM, Buring JE, Cook NR, Rifai N. C-reactive protein, the metabolic syndrome, and risk of incident cardiovascular events: an 8-year follow-up of 14719 initially healthy American women. Circulation. 2003;107:391–7.
101. Ziccardi P, Nappo F, Giugliano G, Esposito K, Marfella R, Cioffi M, D'Andrea F, Molinari AM, Giugliano D. Reduction of inflammatory cytokine concentrations and improvement of endothelial functions in obese women after weight loss over one year. Circulation. 2002;105:804–9.
102. Esposito K, Marfella R, Ciotola M, Di Palo C, Giugliano F, Giugliano G, D'Armiento M, D'Andrea F, Giugliano D. Effect of a Mediterranean-style diet on endothelial dysfunction and markers of vascular inflammation in the metabolic syndrome: a randomized trial. JAMA. 2004;292:1440–6.
103. Schwingshackl L, Christoph M, Hoffmann G. Effects of olive oil on markers of inflammation and endothelial function. A systematic review and meta-analysis. Forum Nutr. 2015;7:7651–75.
104. Carluccio MA, Siculella L, Ancora MA, Massaro M, Scoditti E, Storelli C, Visioli F, Distante A, De Caterina R. Olive oil and red wine antioxidant polyphenols inhibit endothelial activation: antiatherogenic properties of Mediterranean diet phytochemicals. Arterioscler Thromb Vasc Biol. 2003;23:622–9.
105. Visioli F, Caruso D, Grande S, Bosisio R, Villa M, Galli G, Sirtori C, Galli C. Virgin olive oil study (VOLOS): vasoprotective potential of extra virgin olive oil in mildly dyslipidemic patients. Eur J Nutr. 2005;44:121–7.
106. Hanhineva K, Törrönen R, Bondia-Pons I, Pekkinen J, Kolehmainen M, Mykkänen H, Poutanen K. Impact of dietary polyphenols on carbohydrate metabolism. Int J Mol Sci. 2010;11:1365–402.
107. Kim Y, Keogh JB, Clifton PM. Polyphenols and glycemic control. Nutrients. 2016;8:E17.
108. Valdés L, Cuervo A, Salazar N, Ruas-Madiedo P, Gueimonde M, González S. The relationship between phenolic compounds from diet and microbiota: impact on human health. Food Funct. 2015;6(8):2424–39.
109. Selma MV, Espín JC, Tomás-Barberán FA. Interaction between phenolics and gut microbiota: role in human health. J Agric Food Chem. 2009;57:6485–501.
110. Bendini A, Cerretani L, Carrasco-Pancorbo A, Gómez-Caravaca AM, Segura-Carretero A, Fernández-Gutiérrez A, Lercker G. Phenolic molecules in virgin olive oils: a survey of their sensory properties, health effects, antioxidant activity and analytical methods. An overview of the last decade. Molecules. 2007;12:1679–719.
111. Visioli F, Galli C, Bornet F, Mattei A, Patelli R, Galli G, Caruso D. Olive oil phenolics are dose-dependently absorbed in humans. FEBS Lett. 2000;468(2–3):159–60.
112. Tuck KL, Freeman MP, Hayball PJ, Stretch GL, Stupans I. The in vivo fate of hydroxytyrosol and tyrosol, antioxidant phenolic constituents of olive oil, after intravenous and oral dosing of labeled compounds to rats. J Nutr. 2001;131:1993–6.
113. Miró-Casas E, Covas MI, Fitó M, Farré-Albadalejo M, Marrugat J, de la Torre R. Tyrosol and hydroxytyrosol are absorbed from moderate and sustained doses of virgin olive oil in humans. Eur J Clin Nutr. 2003;57:186–90.
114. Gao H, Huang YN, Gao B, Xu PY, Inagaki C, Kawabata J. α-glucosidase inhibitory effect by the flower buds of *Tussilago farfara* L. Food Chem. 2008;106:1195–201.

115. Xiao JB, Högger P. Dietary polyphenols and type 2 diabetes: current insights and future perspectives. Curr Med Chem. 2015;22:23–38.
116. Medina-Remón A, Tresserra-Rimbau A, Pons A, Tur JA, Martorell M, Ros E, et al. Effects of total dietary polyphenols on plasma nitric oxide and blood pressure in a high cardiovascular risk cohort. The PREDIMED randomized trial. Nutr Metab Cardiovasc Dis. 2015;25:60–7.
117. de Bock M, Derraik JG, Brennan CM, Biggs JB, Morgan PE, Hodgkinson SC, et al. Olive (Olea Europaea L.) leaf polyphenols improve insulin sensitivity in middleaged overweight men: a randomized, placebo-controlled, crossover trial. PLoS One. 2013;8:e57622.
118. Tresserra-Rimbau A, Guasch-Ferré M, Salas-Salvadó J, Toledo E, Corella D, Castañer O, Guo X, Gómez-Gracia E, Lapetra J, Arós F, Fiol M, Ros E, Serra-Majem L, Pintó X, Fitó M, Babio N, Martínez-González MA, Sorli JV, López-Sabater MC, Estruch R, Lamuela-Raventós RM, PREDIMED study investigators. Intake of total polyphenols and some classes of polyphenols is inversely associated with diabetes in elderly people at high cardiovascular disease risk. J Nutr. 2016;146:767–77.
119. De Bock M, Derraik JG, Brennan CM, Biggs JB, Morgan PE, Hodgkinson SC, Hofman PL, Cutfield WS. Olive (olea europaea l.) leaf polyphenols improve insulin sensitivity in middle-aged overweight men: a randomized, placebo-controlled, crossover trial. PLoS One. 2013;8:e57622.
120. Wainstein J, Ganz T, Boaz M, Bar Dayan Y, Dolev E, Kerem Z, Madar Z. Olive leaf extract as a hypoglycemic agent in both human diabetic subjects and in rats. J Med Food. 2012;15:605–10.
121. Navarro M, Morales FJ. In vitro investigation on the antiglycative and carbonyl trapping activities of hydroxythyrosol. Eur Food Res Technol. 2016;242:1101–10.

Extra-virgin Olive Oil, the Mediterranean Diet, and Neurodegenerative Diseases

5

5.1 Premises

Among its numerous beneficial effects, Mediterranean diet has been also demonstrated to reduce the risk of neurodegenerative diseases.

In a recent umbrella review [1] which included 13 meta-analyses of observational studies and 16 meta-analyses of randomized controlled trials (RCTs) investigating the association between the adherence to the Mediterranean diet and 37 different health outcomes, for a total population of over 12,800,000 subjects, a robust evidence for a greater adherence to the Mediterranean diet and a reduced risk of overall mortality, cardiovascular disease, coronary heart disease, myocardial infarction, overall cancer incidence, diabetes, and neurodegenerative diseases was found. It was reported that a two-point increase of adherence to the Mediterranean diet determined a significant 8% reduction of death from any causes, a 10% reduction from death and/or incidence of cardio- and cerebrovascular diseases, a 6% reduction from death and/or the incidence of neoplastic diseases, and a 13% reduction of the incidence of neurodegenerative diseases, including Parkinson's disease and Alzheimer's disease. Mild cognitive impairment (MCI), generally considered a pre-dementia syndrome, has been also found to have an incidence risk reduction by high adherence to Mediterranean diet [2–6].

In this chapter, mild cognitive impairment (MCI), Alzheimer's disease (AD), and Parkinson's disease (PD) will be treated, in the order.

5.2 Mild Cognitive Impairment (MCI) and the Mediterranean Diet

Mild cognitive impairment (MCI), also known as age-related cognitive decline (ARCD), age-associated cognitive decline (AACD), or age-associated memory impairment (AAMI), is an intermediate stage between the expected cognitive decline of normal aging and the more serious decline of dementia. According to

A. Capurso et al., *Benefits of the Mediterranean Diet in the Elderly Patient*, Practical Issues in Geriatrics, https://doi.org/10.1007/978-3-319-78084-9_5

DSM-IV, MCI could be defined as an objective decline in cognitive functioning associated with the aging process but within normal limits given the person's age. The cognitive decline may be self-reported or referred by a reliable informant and can involve one of the cognitive areas, i.e., memory and learning, attention and concentration, thinking, language, and visuospatial functioning.

Whether MCI and cognates are expression of a normal aging process or represent distinct clinical entities or, eventually, a continuum with dementia is still unclear [7, 8]. The causes of mild cognitive decline are unknown, but some studies have suggested that it may be prevented [9]. Cardiovascular and other chronic diseases [10, 11], hypertension [12], diabetes mellitus [13], depression [14], and low levels of physical activity have been identified as risk factors for MCI [15]. On the contrary, high socioeconomic status, a flexible personality in middle age, and the maintenance of vision and hearing have been identified as protective factors against MCI [16]. The diet seems to have a role in the cognitive decline. Deficiencies of micronutrients (vitamins B1, B2, B6, B12, and C and folate) have been described quite frequently in elderly people and found to be significantly associated with cognitive impairment [17, 18].

As far as the impact of diet on MCI is concerned, in a study of our group, the relationships between dietary macronutrient intakes and age-related changes in cognitive functions in Southern Italy, a region with the typical Mediterranean dietary pattern [2, 19, 20], were evaluated. Actually, it was a sub-study of the larger *Italian Longitudinal Study on Aging (ILSA),* promoted by the Italian National Research Council-Targeted Project on Aging, with a sample of 5632 subjects aged 65–84 years, free living or institutionalized [2]. In this sub-study, a standardized test battery assessing global cognitive functions (Mini-Mental State Examination, MMSE), selective attention (Digit Cancellation Test, DCT), and episodic memory (Babcock Story Recall Test), and a semi-quantitative food frequency questionnaire evaluating macronutrient energy intakes, was performed on 278 non-demented elderly subjects from the randomized cohort of Casamassima, Bari (n = 704). Results showed an inverse relationship between energy intake from monounsaturated fatty acids (MUFAs) and cognitive decline. We demonstrated that the odds of having a compromised cognitive function (MMSE score < 24) was very high (OR 33; CI 8.2–133) in the lowest percentile of daily MUFA intake (<800 kJ day^{-1}), but it decreased exponentially with the increase of daily MUFA intake, reaching an odds ratio of 0.69 in the highest percentile of MUFA intake, i.e., population with a daily MUFA intake of ≥2400 kJ day^{-1}. Moreover, a significant inverse association between MUFA intakes and DCT score (odds ratio, 0.99) was observed, while no association was found between nutritional variables and episodic memory (Table 5.1).

In this study, high MUFA intake was associated with the preservation of cognitive functions in healthy elderly people. We hypothesized that this protective effect of MUFA could be related to the role of fatty acids in maintaining the structural integrity of neuronal membranes. Dietary fatty acids, in fact, can modify neuronal membrane fluidity. Polyunsaturated fatty acids (PUFAs) regulate the fluidity of synaptosomal membranes and thereby regulate neuronal transmission [21]. Moreover,

Table 5.1 Change in the odds ratio (OR) and 95% confidence interval (CI) for cognitive decline, as assessed by Mini-Mental State Examination (MMSE) score, with the increase of energy daily intake from monounsaturated fatty acids (MUFAs)

	Adjusted for education		Adjusted for education and age	
MUFA intake (kJ day^{-1})	OR	95% CI	OR	95% CI
<800	33.0	8.2–133	37.5	9–156
801–1200	14.9	6.2–35.8	16.9	6.7–42.7
1201–1600	6.7	3.7–12	7.6	3.9–14.6
1601–2000	3.0	1.3–6.7	3.4	1.4–8
2001–2400	1.3	0.4–4.9	1.5	0.4–5.9
2401–2800	0.6	0.1–4.5	0.7	0.1–4.5

essential fatty acids can modify the function of the neurotransmitters' receptors such as cholinergic receptors, nicotinic receptors, adrenergic receptors, dopaminergic receptors, muscarinic receptors,and N-methyl-D-aspartate receptors. Finally, free fatty acids, lipid metabolites, and phospholipids modify the function of membrane proteins, including ion channels. In fact, some studies have examined the effects of essential fatty acids on membrane function as they can affect the calcium, chloride, and potassium ion channels [22]. In a study on the fatty acid composition of neuronal membranes, an increase in MUFA content and a decrease in PUFA content with advancing age were found [23], suggesting that in the aging process, there is an increasing demand of MUFA. Moreover, unsaturated fatty acids have been shown to be essential for the proliferation of cells, particularly hematopoietic cells. In fact, an increase of D^9 desaturase activity, which converts stearic acid to oleic acid and increases the degree of differentiation of cells, has been found in a study on lymphocytic and macrophage-like cells [24]. High PUFA intake, on the contrary, has been found to be positively associated with cognitive impairment, while high fish consumption tended to be inversely associated with cognitive impairment [25].

Another study confirmed the protective effect of high adherence to Mediterranean diet toward MCI [4]. The study, conducted in a multiethnic community in New York, investigated the association between adherence to the Mediterranean diet (0–9 scale, higher scores indicate higher adherence) and the incidence of MCI. There were 1393 cognitively normal participants, 275 of whom developed MCI during a mean follow-up of 4.5 years. Compared with subjects in the lowest Mediterranean diet adherence tertile, subjects in the middle tertile had a nonsignificant 17% less risk of developing MCI, and those in the highest tertile had a significant 28% less risk (HR = 0.72; 95% CI, 0.52–1.00; $P = 0.05$) of developing MCI.

A recent systematic review and meta-analysis [6] evaluated the association between Mediterranean diet and cognitive impairment. A total of five papers (six cohorts) were included, of which three were from the United States and one each from Australia and France. A total of 3636 participants from 2 studies and 3901 participants from 3 studies were included in the analysis of incident MCI. The Mediterranean diet score, as a continuous variable, was not associated with incident MCI (HR = 0.95; 95% CI, 0.84–1.08, $p = 0.45$). When examining the tertiles, the highest Mediterranean diet tertile was associated with a reduced risk of MCI (adjusted HR = 0.73; 95% CI, 0.56–0.96, $p = 0.02$), and there was also a trend for the middle tertile (HR = 0.82; 95% CI, 0.64–1.05, $p = 0.11$), compared to the lowest.

To summarize, cross-sectional and prospective studies have provided evidence that higher adherence to a Mediterranean-type diet is associated with slower cognitive decline and a reduced risk of progression from MCI to AD. These findings suggest that adherence to the Mediterranean diet may affect pre-dementia syndromes and their progression to overt dementia. At present, epidemiological evidence suggests a possible association between some Mediterranean diet components (fish consumption, MUFA, PUFA, particularly, n-3 PUFA, antioxidant polyphenols) and reduced risk of cognitive decline and dementia. Fruit and vegetable consumption, although the limited epidemiological evidence available, is also acknowledged to have a protective role against cognitive decline, dementia, and AD.

5.3 The Incidence of MCI and the Rate of Progression to Dementia

An important question is to what extent MCI progresses to dementia. In a study of our group [26], we evaluated the prevalence, incidence, and rate of progression of MCI to dementia and correlated vascular risk factors with incident MCI and its progression to dementia. 2963 individuals from a population-based sample of 5632 subjects 65 to 84 years old, of the Italian Longitudinal Study on Aging (ILSA), were evaluated, with a 3.5-year follow-up. In this population sample, 139 MCI patients were diagnosed at the baseline survey. During the 3.5-year follow-up, 113 new events of MCI were diagnosed with an estimated incidence rate of 21.5 per 1000 person-years. We found a progression rate of MCI to dementia (all causes) of 3.8/100 person-years. Specific progression rates for AD, vascular dementia (VaD), and other types of dementia were 2.3, 1.3, and 0.3/100 person-years, respectively. Furthermore, age was a risk factor for incident MCI (RR, 5.93; 95% CI, 3.17–11.10), while high education was protective (RR, 0.06; 95% CI, 0.03–0.10), and serum total cholesterol evidenced a borderline nonsignificant trend for a protective effect. There was a nonsignificant trend for stroke as a risk factor of progression of MCI to dementia. Among those who progressed to dementia, 60% progressed to AD and 33% to VaD. Vascular risk factors influenced incident mild cognitive impairment and the rate of progression to dementia.

In another study [27] on subtypes of MCI and progression to dementia, 52 elderly outpatients with a diagnosis of MCI and a mean follow up of 1.21 ± 0.61 years were evaluated. Mean age was 72.8 ± 6.6 years, and males were 61.5%. Mean baseline Mini-Mental State Examination (MMSE) score was 27.1 ± 1.5. There were 15 incident cases of dementia (28.8%), with Alzheimer's disease (AD) accounting for 53.3% of all cases, AD with cerebrovascular disease for 33.4%, and frontotemporal dementia for 13.3%. Overall rate of conversion was 23.8 per 100 person-years. During the same follow-up period, 53.8% of participants remained stable and 17.3% reverted to normal. Rates of conversion for the specific MCI subtypes were 38 per 100 person-years for amnestic MCI, 20 per 100 person-years for non-amnestic

MCI, and 16 per 100 person-years for memory plus other cognitive domains of MCI. With respect to non-converters, converters were generally older (76.1 ± 4.2 vs. 71.5 ± 7.0 years, $p = 0.021$) and had a lower MMSE score (26.4 ± 1.66 vs. 27.4 ± 1.4, $p = 0.035$) and a higher prevalence of atrophy at neuroimaging (73.7% vs. 42.4%, $p = 0.047$). Moreover, with respect to non-converters, converters tended to have higher serum high-density lipoprotein (HDL) levels and lower serum folate levels. No difference was observed for the other study variables, including MCI subtype.

To investigate the risk factors associated with the conversion of MCI to dementia of Alzheimer type (AD), 119 subjects affected by amnestic MCI (aMCI) were studied with a multidimensional assessment and a neuropsychological battery, with a follow-up of 1 year [28]. Demented MCI ($N = 40$; 33.6%) were older (mean age 73.5 ± 8.5 vs. 69.2 ± 7.0; $p = 0.006$) when compared to stable MCI ($N = 79$; 66.4). The demented MCI global cognitive performances, at baseline, were more compromised when assessed by ADAS-Cog (mean score 10.7 ± 3.9 vs. 6.7 ± 3.4; $p = 0.000$) and by MMSE (mean score 26.1 ± 1.9 vs. 27.3 ± 1.8; $p = 0.002$). Demented were similarly compromised in basic activities of daily living (BADL mean 0.2 ± 0.4 vs. 0.1 ± 0.3 functions lost; $p =$ NS) but more compromised on instrumental daily functions (IADL mean 0.7 ± 0.8 vs. 0.1 ± 0.5 functions lost; $p = 0.001$). The presence of white matter lesions (WML) on CT or MRI was more pronounced in demented group ($p = 0.02$). After 1 year, demented worsened on phonemic verbal fluency (PFL) ($p = 0.009$), Raven's colored matrices ($p = 0.003$), and Trail Making Tests A and B ($p = 0.008$ and $p = 0.007$, respectively) and in instrumental activities of daily living (IADL) ($p = 0.000$) with respect to stable. Logistic regression analysis revealed that ADAS-Cog basal score, Trail Making B, and IADL but not memory deterioration were significantly associated with the conversion to AD. The authors concluded that in subjects with aMCI, poor global cognitive performance at baseline and the worsening on executive functions and on functional status but not the worsening on memory functions are independently associated with the conversion to dementia of Alzheimer type at 1-year follow-up [28].

Summarizing, the mild decline in cognitive functioning associated with the aging (MCI), generally affecting the memory domain, progresses to dementia in nearly 30% of cases, becoming Alzheimer's dementia in 60%, vascular dementia 30%, and frontotemporal dementia 10%. Risk factors are low education, folate deficiency, low intake on micronutrients, depression, vascular risk factors, and stroke. Mediterranean diet reduces the risk of progression of MCI to dementia by 28%; some Mediterranean diet components (fish consumption, MUFA, PUFA, particularly, n-3 PUFA) and fruit and vegetable consumption are acknowledged to have a protective role against progression of MCI to dementia.

5.4 The Mediterranean Diet and the Incidence of Dementia

Numerous studies have shown that a higher adherence to the Mediterranean diet is associated with a reduced risk of cognitive impairment, MCI, and Alzheimer's disease (AD), as well as with a reduced progression of MCI to AD. The associations have been shown to be significant even for the sensitivity analysis. The studies in particular have shown that Mediterranean diet may be protective for AD particularly in subjects with high adherence to this diet.

In a meta-analysis [6] on association of Mediterranean diet and Alzheimer's disease (5 studies, 6 cohorts, for a total of 7537 subjects), each one-point increase in the Mediterranean diet score in cognitively normal individuals was associated with an 8% reduced risk of developing AD (adjusted HR, 0.92; 95% CI, 0.85–0.99. $p = 0.03$). Examining the Mediterranean diet in tertiles, subjects in the middle tertile of Mediterranean diet had a 13% not significant reduced risk (adjusted HR = 0.87; 95% CI, 0.66–1.14, $P = 0.31$), while the subjects in the higher tertile had a significant 36% risk reduction (adjusted HR = 0.64; 95% CI, 0.46–0.89, $P = 0.007$) as compared to the lowest tertile.

The role and the mechanisms of the Mediterranean diet in the pathogenesis of cognitive decline and dementia appears quite complex. Several mechanisms have been suggested. Higher adherence to Mediterranean diet has been found to be associated with low level of C-reactive protein and lower interleukin levels [29–31]. Therefore a possible underlying mechanism for the neuroprotective effects of the Mediterranean diet could be its vascular protective properties and its ability to reduce inflammation and oxidative stress, which are associated with the pathophysiology of degenerative disease in general [32–34]. Another protective effect of Mediterranean diet could derive through the action of individual components, i.e., vegetables [35], high ratio of monounsaturated fatty acids to saturated fatty acids [36], alcohol [35], and fish [37]. Another important pathway for the protective effects of Mediterranean diet could be due to the proposed cardioprotective role of Mediterranean diet, by lowering the risk of cardiovascular comorbidities, such as hypertension, dyslipidemia, and coronary artery disease [34, 38, 39]. It should be noted that Mediterranean diet is also associated with a significant reduction in plasma glucose level, serum insulin levels, and insulin resistance, so improving the features of metabolic syndrome and obesity [34, 40, 41].

The role of the diet in the pathogenesis of cognitive decline has been confirmed by some findings showing that elderly African-Americans [42] and Japanese living in the United States [43, 44] have a much higher prevalence of Alzheimer's disease (AD) (6.24% and 4.1%, respectively) than those still living in their ethnic homelands (<2%), suggesting that the prevalence of AD is strongly influenced by diet and nutrition, environment, and/or lifestyle than by genetics.

Recent papers linking clinical expression of AD to oxidative stress [45, 46] and cerebral infarct indicate that the clinical expression of AD is facilitated by cerebral infarction or stroke and confirmed the diet as a key factor in the development of AD [47, 48].

Regression analyses have been performed on the prevalence of AD in the population aged 65+ of 11 countries, obtained from 18 community-wide studies versus components of the national diets [49]. The primary findings have been that the contributions of fat and total calories have the highest correlations with AD prevalence rates. Fish consumption has been found to reduce the prevalence of AD in European and North American countries.

Some dietary components and supplements have been found effective in delaying the onset of AD, including antioxidants, fish, and nonsteroidal anti-inflammatory drugs [50]. In the Rotterdam Study, where total dietary fat was found to be a high risk factor for the development of AD, fish consumption was confirmed to reduce AD risk, and linoleic acid was inversely correlated with AD [51]. A significant inverse correlation was found between the fraction of calories derived from cereals and AD prevalence [50].

Red wine – another component of the Mediterranean diet – was also investigated in relation to AD. In the PAQUID study, the relative risk of dementia was 0.21 and of AD 0.25 among the 318 subjects of this cohort who drank 3 or 4 glasses of wine each day, compared with a relative risk of 1 glass in the 971 total abstainers. Among the 922 older subjects who drank no more than 1 or 2 glasses of wine each day, the relative risk for AD was significantly reduced (RR, 0.55) [52]. Other studies confirmed these protective effects of red wine against AD [53, 54]. In a study of our group [55], the protective effects of red wine on cognition and AD were confirmed: subjects with mild cognitive impairment who were moderate drinkers (less than one drink/day, approximately 15 g of alcohol) had a lower rate of progression to dementia than abstainers (hazard ratio [HR] 0.15; 95% CI 0.03–0.78). Higher levels of drinking (> or =1 drink/day) were not associated with the rate of progression to dementia in subjects with MCI compared to abstainers. The conclusions of this study were that in subjects with mild cognitive impairment, up to one drink/day of alcohol or wine may decrease the rate of progression to dementia [55].

Concerning the mechanisms by which red wine protects from AD, several hypotheses have been made. Some studies have suggested that many kinds of natural polyphenols may have neuroprotective effects both in vivo and in vitro, possibly due to their abilities to scavenge reactive oxygen species [56–61]. The green tea polyphenol epigallocatechin gallate was shown to attenuate b-amyloid-induced neurotoxicity in cultured hippocampal neurons through scavenging reactive oxygen species [60]. In another in vitro study [62], the effects of wine-related polyphenols (myricetin, morin, quercetin, kaempferol (+)-catechin and (−)-epicatechin) on the formation, extension, and destabilization of β-amyloid fibrils (fAβ) at pH 7.5 at 37C were examined. All examined polyphenols dose-dependently inhibited formation of fAβ from fresh Aβ (1-40) and Aβ (1-42), as well as their extension. Moreover, these polyphenols dose-dependently destabilized preformed fAβs. The overall activity of the molecules examined was in the order of myricetin ¼ morin ¼ quercetin > kaempferol > (+)-catechin ¼ (−)-epicatechin. It was suggested that polyphenols and other organic compounds with antioxidant motifs (melatonin, NDGA, nicotine) could bind specifically to Aβ and/or to fAβ, inhibit fAβ formation, and/or destabilize pre-formed fAβ. The authors concluded that although the mechanisms by which polyphenols inhibit fAβ formation from Aβ and destabilize pre-formed fAβ in vitro are still unclear, polyphenols could be a key molecule for the development of preventives and therapeutics for AD.

An interesting recent approach to dementia is the nutrigenomic approach, with the microRNAs' (miRNAs) impact on silencing brain genes.

A microRNA (miRNA) is a small noncoding RNA molecule containing about 22 nucleotides, found in plants, animals, and some viruses, that functions in RNA silencing and post-transcriptional regulation of gene expression. While the majority of miRNAs are located within the cell, some miRNAs, commonly known as circulating miRNAs or extracellular miRNAs, have been found in extracellular environment, including various biological fluids and cell culture media. Encoded by eukaryotic nuclear DNA in plants and animals and by viral DNA in certain viruses whose genome is based on DNA, miRNAs function via *base pairing with complementary sequences within mRNA molecules. As a result, the mRNA molecules are silenced, by one or more of the following processes:*

- *Cleavage of the mRNA strand into two pieces*
- *Destabilization of the mRNA through shortening of its poly(A) tail*
- *Less efficient translation of the mRNA into proteins by ribosomes*

In a recent study in mice treated from age 10 to 16 months with an EVOO naturally rich in phenols (H-EVOO), both the gene and miRNA expression profiles of the brain were changed after the intervention, and these changes were associated with reduced age-related decline of motor coordination and contextual memory [64]. At the end of the treatment, most of the aging-dependent genes were downregulated and restricted to the cerebral cortex. Compared to L-EVOO (the same oil deprived of phenols), the treatment with H-EVOO stimulated a significant upregulation of genes associated with synaptic plasticity and with motor and cognitive behavior, such as Notch1, BMPs, NGFR, GLP1R, and CRTC3. miRNAs were mostly upregulated in old L-EVOO animals compared to young. Moreover, H-EVOO-fed mice cortex displayed miRNA expression profiles similar to those observed in young mice. Sixty-three miRNAs, out of 1203 analyzed, were significantly downregulated compared to the L-EVOO group; among them, miRNAs whose predicted target genes were upregulated by the treatment, such as miR-484, miR-27, miR-137, miR-30, miR-34, and miR-124, were found. Further, some of the H-EVOO-modulated miRNAs were found to target genes associated with synaptic plasticity and neuronal function protection, whose expression was also modified by the treatment. A computational analysis on miRNAs allowed to identify a restricted list of 14 age-modulated miRNAs and a partially overlapped list of 6 treatment-modulated miRNAs. Among the age-modulated miRNAs, those with top scores were miR-681, miR-2709, and miR-2706, all reduced in aging, and miR-230a-5p, which was upregulated in older mice. Of the six treatment-modulated miRNAs, all downregulated in the H-EVOO group, five were also upregulated in aging: miR-30a-5p, miR-2434-5p, miR-2369-5p, miR-2451, and miR-2126-3p. At the top ranking score was miR-30a-5p, predicted to control a large number of genes involved in pathways, such as axon guidance, ubiquitin-mediated proteolysis, regulation of actin cytoskeleton, and long-term potentiation. miR-126, a well-studied miRNA in vascular biology, was already described to respond to phenolics. Its levels were increased in colon-derived myofibroblast cells upon treatment with wine-derived polyphenols, and that response was associated with a reduced expression of inflammatory genes (NF-kB, ICAM-1, VCAM-1, and PECAM-1) [65].

These data clearly show that a dietary intervention starting from middle age with food rich in phenols can actively modulate, at the cerebral level, the expression of genes and miRNAs involved in neuronal function and synaptic plasticity, along with cognitive, motor, and emotional behavior, towards a more protective mode [64].

5.5 The Mediterranean Diet and Parkinson's Disease

Parkinson's disease (PD) is the second most common neurodegenerative disorder after Alzheimer's disease (AD) affecting roughly 1% of individuals over age 60 in North America and Europe [66].

As a prototypic neurodegenerative disorder, Parkinson's disease (PD) is characterized by the progressive loss of specific neuronal subpopulations leading to a late-onset movement disorder. Based on familial forms of PD, to date a significant number of genes were identified that allowed first insight into the molecular pathogenesis of this common movement disorder. The pathways involved include impaired protein degradation and subsequent aggregation within neuronal cells and impaired mitochondrial function followed by energy depletion due to oxidative stress leading to cell death.

Genetic and epidemiological studies hint to a complex interplay of genetic susceptibility factors and environmental risk factors to converge to processes of pathological protein accumulation and mitochondrial damage that trigger neurodegeneration in PD. Therefore large-scale genetic–epidemiological studies combining genetic whole-genome approaches with a detailed ascertainment of environmental exposures are expected to provide important clues to decipher the complexity of neurodegeneration of this most frequent neurodegenerative movement disorder.

The role of environmental exposures in the pathogenesis of PD has been studied [67, 68]. However, most studies that have investigated associations between PD risk and intake of individual foods and nutrients have reported inconsistent results. The most consistent data are those who support the association between higher consumption of dairy products and increased PD risk [69–71].

Numerous cohort studies and meta-analyses have evaluated the impact of environmental factors, particularly the diet, on the incidence of PD.

In a prospective analysis of two large cohorts, the Health Professionals Follow-Up Study (HPFS) (1986-2002) and the Nurses' Health Study (NHS) (1984-2000), the associations between dietary patterns and risk of PD have been examined [72]. 49,692 men and 81,676 women free of PD at baseline were included. After a follow-up of 16 years, 508 new PD cases were documented. The principal components analysis identified two dietary patterns: prudent and Western. The prudent dietary pattern, characterized by high intakes of fruit, vegetables, and fish, was inversely associated with PD risk, while the Western pattern was not. The pooled multivariate-adjusted RR for the top compared with the bottom quintiles of the prudent score was 0.78 (95% CI, 0.56, 1.07; *P* for trend 0.04). For the AHEI (*Alternate Healthy Eating Index*), the pooled multivariate-adjusted RR for the top compared with the bottom quintile was 0.70 (95% CI, 0.51, 0.94; *P* for trend 0.01) and for aMED (*alternate Mediterranean Diet Score*) was 0.75 (95% CI, 0.57, 1.00; *P* for trend 0.07). The authors concluded that dietary patterns with a high intake of fruit, vegetables, legumes, whole grains, nuts, fish, and poultry and a low intake of saturated fat and a moderate intake of alcohol may protect against PD. To note, the prudent diet characteristics appear to be very similar to the characteristics of the Mediterranean diet.

A meta-analysis [63] conducted to systematically review all the prospective cohort studies that have analyzed the relation between adherence to a Mediterranean diet, mortality, and incidence of chronic diseases in a primary prevention setting was performed. The cumulative analysis among 8 cohorts (514,816 subjects and 33,576 deaths) showed a beneficial role for greater adherence to a Mediterranean diet on cardiovascular mortality (pooled relative risk 0.91, 0.87 to 0.95), incidence of or mortality from cancer (0.94, 0.92–0.96), and incidence of Parkinson's disease and Alzheimer's disease (0.87, 0.80–0.96). The data of this meta-analysis confirmed that a greater adherence to a Mediterranean diet is associated with a significant improvement in health status, as seen by a significant reduction in overall mortality (9%), mortality from cardiovascular diseases (9%), incidence of or mortality from cancer (6%), and incidence of Parkinson's disease and Alzheimer's disease (13%).

In a recent case–control study [73] aimed to determine to what extent the Mediterranean diet adherence was somewhat associated with Parkinson's disease (PD), 257 PD participants and 198 controls were studied. The Willett semiquantitative food frequency questionnaire was used to collect dietary data regarding average food consumption in the past year before the assessment, and the Mediterranean diet score was obtained applying the method described by Trichopoulou and colleagues [74]. The results were that higher Mediterranean-type diet adherence was associated with reduced odds for PD after adjustment for all covariates (OR, 0.86; 95% CI, 0.77–0.97; $P = 0.010$). Lower Mediterranean-type diet score was associated with earlier PD age at onset.

Recently [75] it was shown the primary role of the oxidant stress in the pathogenesis of PD in an in vitro study on human dopaminergic neurons derived from patients with idiopathic and familial PD. A time-dependent pathological cascade was identified, beginning with mitochondrial oxidant stress leading to oxidized dopamine accumulation, ultimately resulting in reduced glucocerebrosidase enzymatic activity, lysosomal dysfunction, and α-synuclein accumulation. Thus, dopamine oxidation has shown to be an important link between mitochondrial and lysosomal dysfunction in PD pathogenesis.

To summarize, environmental and genetic pathways converge in the pathogenesis of Parkinson's disease. High adherence to a Mediterranean-style diet is associated with a reduced risk of PD. Dietary patterns with a high intake of fruit, vegetables, legumes, whole grains, nuts, fish, and poultry and a low intake of saturated fat and a moderate intake of alcohol appear to be protective toward PD. Among the components of Mediterranean diet, antioxidants contained in vegetables and fresh fruit appear to have a pivotal role in preventing the oxidative damage of dopaminergic neurons leading to the onset of PD.

Conclusions

Numerous studies and meta-analyses have shown that Mediterranean diet or a Mediterranean-style diet may reduce the risk of neurological and cognitive diseases. In particular, MCI incidence, transition of MCI to dementia, incidence of AD, and incidence of Parkinson's disease are significantly prevented by a diet rich in whole grains, vegetables, legumes, fresh fruit, nuts, fish, and poultry, a low intake of saturated fat, and a high intake of MUFA particularly from olive oil. Extra-virgin olive oil appears to have an additional protective effect due to its high content of polyphenols, which have not only antioxidant effects but also nutrigenomic effects, by which they modulate, at cerebral level, the expression of genes and miRNAs involved in neuronal function and synaptic plasticity, along with cognitive, motor, and emotional behavior.

References

1. Dinu M, Pagliai G, Casini A, Sofi F. Mediterranean diet and multiple health outcomes: an umbrella review of meta-analyses of observational studies and randomised trials. Eur J Clin Nutr. 2017;72:30. https://doi.org/10.1038/ejcn.2017.58.
2. Solfrizzi V, Panza F, Torres F, Mastroianni F, Del Parigi A, Venezia A, Capurso A. High monounsaturated fatty acids intake protects against age-related cognitive decline. Neurology. 1999;52:1563–9.
3. Panza F, Solfrizzi V, Colacicco AM, D'Introno A, Capurso C, Torres F, Del Parigi A, Capurso S, Capurso A. Mediterranean diet and cognitive decline. Public Health Nutr. 2004;7:959–63.
4. Scarmeas N, Stern Y, Mayeux R, Manly JJ, Schupf N, Luchsinger JA. Mediterranean diet and mild cognitive impairment. Arch Neurol. 2009;66:216–25.
5. Solfrizzi V, Frisardi V, Seripa D, Logroscino G, Imbimbo BP, D'Onofrio G, Addante F, Sancarlo D, Cascavilla L, Pilotto A, Panza F. Mediterranean diet in predementia and dementia syndromes. Curr Alzheimer Res. 2011;8:520–42.
6. Singh B, Parsaik AK, Mielke MM, Erwin PJ, Knopman DS, Petersen RC, Roberts RO. Association of Mediterranean diet with mild cognitive impairment and Alzheimer's disease: a systematic review and meta-analysis. J Alzheimers Dis. 2014;39:271–82.
7. Hanninen T, Hallikainen M, Koivisto K, Helkala EL, Reinikainen KJ, Soininen H, et al. A follow-up study of age-associated memory impairment: neuropsychological predictors of dementia. J Am Geriatr Soc. 1995;43:1007–15.
8. Brayne C, Calloway P. Normal ageing, impaired cognitive function and senile dementia of Alzheimer type: a continuum? Lancet. 1988;1:1265–7.
9. Nolan KA, Blass JP. Preventing cognitive decline. Clin Geriatr Med. 1992;8:19–34.
10. Fillit HM. The clinical significance of normal cognitive decline in late life. In: Fillit HM, Butler RN, editors. Cognitive decline. Strategies for prevention. Oxford: Oxford University Press; 1997. p. 1–7.
11. Breteler MM, Claus JJ, Grobbee DE, Hofman A. Cardiovascular disease and distribution of cognitive function in elderly people: the Rotterdam study. Br Med J. 1994;308:1604–8.

12. Launer LJ, Masaki K, Petrovich H, Foley D, Havlik RJ. The association between midlife blood pressure levels and latelife cognitive function. J Am Med Assoc. 1995;274:1846–51.
13. Richardson JT. Cognitive function in diabetes mellitus. Neurosci Biobehav Rev. 1990;14:385–8.
14. Blazer D, Burchett B, Service C, George LK. The association of age and depression among the elderly: an epidemiologic exploration. J Gerontol. 1991;46:M210–5.
15. Rogers RL, Meyer JS, Mortal KF. After reaching retirement age, physical activity sustains cerebral perfusion and cognition. J Am Geriatr Soc. 1990;38:123–8.
16. White LR, Foley DJ, Havlik RJ. Lifestyle risk factors for cognitive impairment. In: Fillit HM, Butler RN, editors. Cognitive decline. Strategies for prevention. Oxford: Oxford University Press; 1997. p. 23–32.
17. Sahyoun NR, Otradovec CL, Hartz SC, Jacob RA, Peters H, Russell RM, et al. Dietary intakes and biochemical indicators of nutritional status in an elderly, institutionalized population. Am J Clin Nutr. 1988;47:524–33.
18. Goodwin J, Goodwin J, Garry P. Association between nutritional status and cognitive functioning in a healthy elderly population. JAMA. 1983;249(21):2917.
19. Capurso A, Solfrizzi V, Panza F, Tores F, Mastroianni F, Grassi A, Del Parigi A, Capurso C, Pirozzi MR, Centonze S, Misciagna G. Dietary patterns and cognitive functions in elderly subjects. Aging Clin Exp Res. 1997;9(Suppl. 4):45–7.
20. Solfrizzi V, Panza F, Capurso A. The role of diet in cognitive decline. J Neural Transm. 2003;110:95–110.
21. Jones CB, Arai T, Rapoport SI. Evidence for the involvement of docosahexanoic acid in cholinergic stimulated signal transduction at the synapse. Neurochem Res. 1997;22:663–70.
22. Yehuda S, Rabinovitz S, Mostofsky DI. Essential fatty acids are mediators of brain biochemistry and cognitive functions. J Neurosci Res. 1999;56:565–70.
23. Lopez GH, Ilincheta de Boschero MG, Castagnet PI, Giusto NM. Age-associated changes in the content and fatty acids composition of brain glycerophospholipids. Comparative Biochemistry and Physiology. Part B. Biochem Mol Biol. 1995;112:331–43.
24. Marzo I, Martinez-Lorenzo MJ, Anel A, Desportes P, Alava MA, Naval J, et al. Biosynthesis of unsaturated fatty acids in the main cell lineages of human leukemia and lymphoma. Biochim Biophys Acta. 1995;1257:140–8.
25. Kalmijn S, Feskens EJ, Launer LJ, Kromhout D. Polyunsaturated fatty acids, antioxidants, and cognitive functions in very old men. Am J Epidemiol. 1997;145:33–41.
26. Solfrizzi V, Panza F, Colacicco AM, D'Introno A, Capurso C, Torres F, Grigoletto F, Maggi S, Del Parigi A, Reiman EM, Caselli RJ, Scafato E, Farchi G, Capurso A, Italian Longitudinal Study on Aging Working Group. Vascular risk factors, incidence of MCI, and rates of progression to dementia. Neurology. 2004;63:1882–91.
27. Maioli F, Coveri M, Pagni P, Chiandetti C, Marchetti C, Ciarrocchi R, Ruggero C, Nativio V, Onesti A, D'Anastasio C, Pedone V. Conversion of mild cognitive impairment to dementia in elderly subjects: a preliminary study in a memory and cognitive disorder unit. Arch Gerontol Geriatr. 2007;44(Suppl 1):233–41.
28. Rozzini L, Chilovi BV, Conti M, Bertoletti E, Delrio I, Trabucchi M, Padovani A. Conversion of amnestic mild cognitive impairment to dementia of Alzheimer type is independent to memory deterioration. Int J Geriatr Psychiatry. 2007;22:1217–22.
29. Fung TT, McCullough ML, Newby PK, Manson JE, Meigs JB, Rifai N, Willett WC, Hu FB. Diet-quality scores and plasma concentrations of markers of inflammation and endothelial dysfunction. Am J Clin Nutr. 2005;82:163–73.
30. Esposito K, Giugliano F, Di Palo C, Giugliano G, Marfella R, D'Andrea F, D'Armiento M, Giugliano D. Effect of lifestyle changes on erectile dysfunction in obese men: a randomized controlled trial. JAMA. 2004;291:2978–84.
31. Chrysohoou C, Panagiotakos DB, Pitsavos C, Das UN, Stefanadis C. Adherence to the Mediterranean diet attenuates inflammation and coagulation process in healthy adults: The ATTICA Study. J Am Coll Cardiol. 2004;44:152–8.
32. Steele M, Stuchbury G, Munch G. The molecular basis of the prevention of Alzheimer's disease through healthy nutrition. Exp Gerontol. 2007;42:28–36.

33. Cummings JL. Alzheimer's disease. N Engl J Med. 2004;351:56–67.
34. Frisardi V, Panza F, Seripa D, Imbimbo BP, Vendemiale G, Pilotto A, Solfrizzi V. Nutraceutical properties of Mediterranean diet and cognitive decline: possible underlying mechanisms. J Alzheimers Dis. 2010;22:715–40.
35. Roberts RO, Geda YE, Cerhan JR, Knopman DS, Cha RH, Christianson TJ, Pankratz VS, Ivnik RJ, Boeve BF, O'Connor HM, Petersen RC. Vegetables, unsaturated fats, moderate alcohol intake, and mild cognitive impairment. Dement Geriatr Cogn Disord. 2010;29:413–23.
36. Panza F, Capurso C, D'Introno A, Colacicco AM, Del Parigi A, Gagliardi G, Breglia G, Capurso A, Solfrizzi V. Mediterranean diet, mild cognitive impairment, and Alzheimer's disease. Exp Gerontol. 2007;42:6–7. author reply 8–9
37. Eskelinen MH, Ngandu T, Helkala EL, Tuomilehto J, Nissinen A, Soininen H, Kivipelto M. Fat intake at midlife and cognitive impairment later in life: a population-based CAIDE study. Int J Geriatr Psychiatry. 2008;23:741–7.
38. Singh RB, Dubnov G, Niaz MA, Ghosh S, Singh R, Rastogi SS, Manor O, Pella D, Berry EM. Effect of an indo-Mediterranean diet on progression of coronary artery disease in high risk patients (indo-Mediterranean diet heart study): a randomised single-blind trial. Lancet. 2002;360:1455–61.
39. Psaltopoulou T, Kyrozis A, Stathopoulos P, Trichopoulos D, Vassilopoulos D, Trichopoulou A. Diet, physical activity and cognitive impairment among elders: the EPIC-Greece cohort (European prospective investigation into cancer and nutrition). Public Health Nutr. 2008;11:1054–62.
40. Esposito K, Marfella R, Ciotola M, Di Palo C, Giugliano F, Giugliano G, D'Armiento M, D'Andrea F, Giugliano D. Effect of a Mediterranean-style diet on endothelial dysfunction and markers of vascular inflammation in the metabolic syndrome: a randomized trial. JAMA. 2004;292:1440–6.
41. Jula A, Marniemi J, Huupponen R, Virtanen A, Rastas M, Ronnemaa T. Effects of diet and simvastatin on serum lipids, insulin, and antioxidants in hypercholesterolemic men: a randomized controlled trial. JAMA. 2002;287:598–605.
42. Hendrie HC, Osuntokun BO, Hall KS, Ogunniyi AO, Hui SL, Unverzagt FW, Gureje O, Rodenberg CA, Baiyewu O, Musick BS. Prevalence of Alzheimer's disease and dementia in two communities: Nigerian Africans and African Americans. Am J Psychiatr. 1995;152:1485–92.
43. Graves AB, Larson EB, Edland SD, Bowen JD, McCormick WC, McCurry SM, Rice MM, Wenzlow A, Uomoto JM. Prevalence of dementia and its subtypes in the Japanese American population of King County, Washington state. The kame project. Am J Epidemiol. 1996;144:760–71.
44. White L, Petrovitch H, Ross GW, Masaki KH, Abbott RD, Teng EL, Rodriguez BL, Blanchette PL, Havlik RJ, Wergowske G, Chiu D, Foley DJ, Murdaugh C, Curb JD. Prevalence of dementia in older Japanese American men in Hawaii: the Honolulu–Asia aging study. J Am Med Assoc. 1996;276:955–60.
45. Harman D. Free radical theory of aging: Alzheimer's disease pathogenesis. Age. 1995;18:97–119.
46. Smith MA, Sayre L, Perry G. Morphological aspects of oxidative damage in Alzheimer's disease. In: Beal MF, Howell H, Bodis-Wollner I, editors. Mitochondria and free radicals in neurodegenerative diseases. New York: WileyLiss Inc.; 1997. p. 50.
47. Hulette C, Nochlin D, McKeel D, Morris JC, Mirra SS, Sumi SM, Heyman A. Clinical–neuropathologic findings in multi-infarct dementia: a report of six autopsied cases. Neurology. 1997;48:668–72.
48. Snowdon DA, Greiner LH, Mortimer JA, Riley KP, Greiner PA, Markesbery WR. Brain infarction and the clinical expression of Alzheimer's disease. The Nun study. J Am Med Assoc. 1977;277:811–7.
49. Grant B. Dietary links to Alzheimer's disease. Alzheimer's Dis Rev. 1997;2:42–55.
50. Grant B. Dietary links to Alzheimer's disease: 1999 update. J Alzheimers Dis. 1999;1:197–201.
51. Kalmijn S, Lauher LJ, Ott A, Witteman JC, Hofman A, Breteler MM. Dietary fat intake and the risk of incident dementia in the Rotterdam study. Ann Neurol. 1997;42:776–82.

52. Orgogozo JM, Dartigues JF, Lafont S, Letenneur L, Commenges D, Salamon R. Wine consumption and the elderly: a prospective community study in the Bordeaux area. Rev Neurol. 1997;153:185–92.
53. Dorozynski A. Wine may prevent dementia. Br Med J. 1997;314:997.
54. Truelsen T, Thudium D, Gronbaek M. Amount and type of alcohol and risk of dementia: the Copenhagen City heart study. Neurology. 2002;59:1313–9.
55. Solfrizzi V, D'Introno A, Colacicco AM, Capurso C, Del Parigi A, Baldassarre G, Scapicchio P, Scafato E, Amodio M, Capurso A, Panza F, Italian Longitudinal Study on Aging Working Group. Alcohol consumption, mild cognitive impairment, and progression to dementia. Neurology. 2007;68:1790–9.
56. Inanami O, Watanabe Y, Syuto B, Nakano M, Tsuji M, Kuwabara M. Oral administration of (−) catechin protects against ischemia-reperfusion-induced neuronal death in the gerbil. Free Radic Res. 1998;29:359–65.
57. Shutenko Z, Henry Y, Pinard E, Seylaz J, Potier P, Berthet F, Girard P, Sercombe R. Influence of the antioxidant quercetin in vivo on the level of nitric oxide determined by electron paramagnetic resonance in rat brain during global ischemia and reperfusion. Biochem Pharmacol. 1999;57:199–208.
58. Bastianetto S, Zheng WH, Quirion R. Neuroprotective abilities of resveratrol and other red wine constituents against nitric oxide-related toxicity in cultured hippocampal neurons. Br J Pharmacol. 2000;131:711–20.
59. Virgili M, Contestabile A. Partial neuroprotection of in vivo excitotoxic brain damage by chronic administration of the red wine antioxidant agent, trans-resveratrol in rats. Neurosci Lett. 2000;281:123–6.
60. Choi YT, Jung CH, Lee SR, Bae JH, Baek WK, Suh MH, Park J, Park CW, Suh SI. The green tea polyphenol (−)-epigallocatechin gallate attenuates beta-amyloid-induced neurotoxicity in cultured hippocampal neurons. Life Sci. 2001;70:603–14.
61. Levites Y, Weinreb O, Maor G, Youdim MB, Mandel S. Green tea polyphenol (−)-epigallocatechin-3-gallate prevents Nmethyl-4-phenyl-1,2,3,6-tetrahydropyridine-induced dopaminergic neurodegeneration. J Neurochem. 2001;78:1073–82.
62. Ono K, Yoshiike Y, Takashima A, Hasegawa K, Naiki H, Yamada M. Potent anti-amyloidogenic and fibril-destabilizing effects of polyphenols in vitro: implications for the prevention and therapeutics of Alzheimer's disease. J Neurochem. 2003;87:172–81.
63. Sofi F, Cesari F, Abbate R, Gensini GF, Casini A. Adherence to Mediterranean diet and health status: meta-analysis. BMJ. 2008;337:a1344.
64. Luceri C, Bigagli E, Pitozzi V, Giovannelli LA. Nutrigenomics approach for the study of anti-aging interventions: olive oil phenols and the modulation of gene and microRNA expression profiles in mouse brain. Eur J Nutr. 2017;56:865–77.
65. Angel-Morales G, Noratto G, Mertens-Talcott S. Red wine polyphenolics reduce the expression of inflammation markers in human colon-derived CCD-18Co myofibroblast cells: potential role of microRNA-126. Food Funct. 2012;3:745–52.
66. Nussbaum RL, Ellis CE. Alzheimer's disease and Parkinson's disease. N Engl J Med. 2003;348:1356–64.
67. Tanner CM. Advances in environmental epidemiology. Mov Disord. 2010;25(Suppl 1):S58–62.
68. Tanner CM, Ottman R, Goldman SM, et al. Parkinson disease in twins: an etiologic study. JAMA. 1999;281:341–6.
69. Chen H, Zhang SM, Hernan MA, Willett WC, Ascherio A. Diet and Parkinson's disease: a potential role of dairy products in men. Ann Neurol. 2002;52:793–801.
70. Chen H, O'Reilly E, McCullough ML, et al. Consumption of dairy products and risk of Parkinson's disease. Am J Epidemiol. 2007;165:998–1006.
71. Park M, Ross GW, Petrovitch H, et al. Consumption of milk and calcium in midlife and the future risk of Parkinson disease. Neurology. 2005;64:1047–51.
72. Gao X, Chen H, Fung TT, Logroscino G, Schwarzschild MA, Hu FB, Ascherio A. Prospective study of dietary pattern and risk of Parkinson disease. Am J Clin Nutr. 2007;86:1486–94.

73. Alcalay RN, Gu Y, Mejia-Santana H, Cote L, Marder KS, Scarmeas N. The association between Mediterranean diet adherence and Parkinson's disease. Mov Disord. 2012;27:771–4.
74. Trichopoulou A, Costacou T, Bamia C, Trichopoulos D. Adherence to a Mediterranean diet and survival in a Greek population. N Engl J Med. 2003;348:2599–608.
75. Burbulla LF, Song P, Mazzulli JR, Zampese E, Wong YC, Jeon S, Santos DP, Blanz J, Obermaier CD, Strojny C, Savas JN, Kiskinis E, Zhuang X, Krüger R, Surmeier DJ, Krainc D. Dopamine oxidation mediates mitochondrial and lysosomal dysfunction in Parkinson's disease. Science. 2017;357(6357):1255–61. https://doi.org/10.1126/science.aam9080.

Extra-virgin Olive Oil and Cancer

6

6.1 Premises

“Contrary to what many believe, cancer is not a natural event. Adopting a healthy diet and lifestyle can prevent the majority of cancers. Old age should be graceful and peaceful” [1].

“Cancer growth can be turned on and off by nutrition, despite very strong predisposition” [1].

It is estimated that almost 1.5 million people in the United States are diagnosed with cancer every year [2]. There is also evidence that lifestyle factors increase cancer risk and, if modified, could significantly reduce the cancer burden [3].

Mortality rate due to cancer has been decreasing since the 1990s, most likely due to improved measures of preventive examinations as well as therapeutic interventions. This heterogeneous complex of diseases, however, still remains one of the major causes of premature death worldwide as it is ranked second to cardiovascular diseases in current statistics [4]. Cancer incidence is estimated to be 18% by the year 2030 [5].

Due to the substantial effect of modifiable lifestyle factors on the most prevalent cancers, it has been estimated that 50% of cancer is preventable [6]. Current recommendations for the major risk factors that can be modified to decrease risk for cancers include reducing tobacco use, increasing physical activity, controlling weight, improving diet, and limiting alcohol consumption [7].

The rapidly growing number of cancer survivors in Europe and the United States [8, 9] has led to investigate the causes of this survival improvement through observational and prospective cohort studies.

A. Capurso et al., *Benefits of the Mediterranean Diet in the Elderly Patient*, Practical Issues in Geriatrics, https://doi.org/10.1007/978-3-319-78084-9_6

6.2 Adherence to the Mediterranean Diet and Cancer

It was shown that overall cancer incidence is lower in Mediterranean countries compared to that in Northern countries, such as the United Kingdom and the United States. There is increasing evidence that adherence to a Mediterranean dietary pattern correlates with reduced risk of several types of cancer. Adherence to a Mediterranean-style diet has shown to improve the overall cancer mortality, incidence of different types of cancer, and cancer mortality risk in cancer survivors [10, 11].

Data on adherence to Mediterranean diet and cancer risk are actually very numerous, but not infrequently they appear incomplete. For example, cancer risk reduction in subjects with high adherence to Mediterranean diet has been shown in cohort studies but not in case–control or randomized studies and vice versa. We will consider the data of some important studies, particularly those coming from large meta-analysis or cohort studies.

In a large meta-analysis [11] including 83 studies and an overall population of 2,130,753 subjects, the highest adherence to a Mediterranean diet has been found to be significantly associated with a lower risk of cancer, both in cohort studies (RR 0.86; CI 0.81–0.91) and (although not significantly) in randomized controlled studies (RR 0.75; CI 0.17–3.33). In this large meta-analysis, colorectal and breast cancers were the only tumors which were concordantly inversely associated with high adherence to Mediterranean diet in all types of studies, i.e., observational, cohort, and case–control studies.

Concerning colorectal cancer, the highest adherence to a Mediterranean dietary pattern was found to be inversely associated with the incidence of this cancer in observational studies (RR 0.82; CI 0.75–0.88), cohort studies (RR 0.86; CI 0.80–0.92), and case–control studies (RR 0.71; CI 0.57–0.88).

Also breast cancer risk was significantly inversely associated with a high adherence to Mediterranean diet in all types of studies: randomized controlled studies (RR 0.43; CI 0.21–0.88), cohort studies (RR 0.94; CI 0.90–0.99), and case–control studies (RR 0.89; CI 0.85–0.94).

Concerning other cancers, liver cancer risk was found to be reduced in cohort and case–control studies (RR 0.62; CI 0.47–0.82 and 0.51; CI 0.34–0.77, respectively), but there are no randomized controlled studies. Biliary tract cancer risk was found significantly reduced, but data are derived only from cohort studies (RR 0.44; CI 0.25–0.67). Gallbladder cancer risk was significantly reduced in cohort studies (RR 0.42; CI 0.23–0.57).

Other cancers were reduced in some type of studies, but not in others. Prostate cancer risk was significantly reduced in cohort studies (RR 0.96; CI 0.92–1.00), but not in case–control studies (RR 0.90; CI 0.64–1.26). Gastric cancer risk was reduced in case–control studies (RR 0.65; CI 0.53–0.79), but not in cohort studies (RR 0.82; CI 0.61–1.10). Esophageal cancer risk was reduced in case–control studies (RR 0.26; CI 0.13–0.52), but not in cohort studies (RR 0.68; CI 0.34–1.36). Head and neck cancer incidence was significantly reduced only in case–control studies (RR 0.46; CI 0.32–0.67), not in cohort studies (RR 0.61; CI 0.33–1.14). Pancreatic cancer risk was reduced only in case–control studies (RR 0.48; CI 0.35–0.66), not in cohort studies (RR 0.99; CI 0.77–1.27). Other types of cancer were not reduced in high-adherence Mediterranean diet subjects: respiratory, bladder, endometrial, and ovarian cancer and lymphoma.

Also the report from a large cohort such as the European Prospective Investigation Into Cancer and Nutrition (EPIC study) [12] including 335,873 individuals found a lower overall cancer risk among individuals with greater adherence to Mediterranean diet (HR 0.96, 95% CI 0.95–0.98) for a two-point increment of the Mediterranean diet score. It was calculated that 4.7% of cancers among men and 2.4% in women would be avoided in that population if study subjects had a greater adherence to Mediterranean dietary pattern.

In a sub-study of EPIC, conducted on 45,275 participants of the Italian section of the EPIC study followed for a mean of 11.28 years, the Italian Mediterranean Index (*an index score calculated from intake of 11 items: high intakes of seven typical Mediterranean food and low intake of four "non-Mediterranean" foods*) was inversely associated with cancer risk (HR 0.50; 95% CI, 0.35, 0.71 for the highest category compared to the lowest; P-trend, 0.043). Results did not differ by sex. The highest Italian Mediterranean Index score (*meaning high adherence to Mediterranean diet*) was also significantly associated with reduced risks of any colon cancer (HR 0.54; 95% CI, 0.36, 0.81), distal colon cancer (HR 0.44; 95% CI, 0.26, 0.75), and rectal cancer (HR 0.41; 95% CI, 0.20, 0.81), but not of proximal colon cancer [13].

An investigation conducted among the women included in the EPIC cohort showed that adherence to a Mediterranean diet excluding alcohol was related to a modest reduced risk of breast cancer in postmenopausal women (HR 0.94; CI 0.88–1.00), and this association was stronger in receptor-negative tumors [14]. Similar findings have been reported in 33,731 women from the UK Women's Cohort Study with a nonsignificant inverse association with increasing adherence to the Mediterranean diet pattern in premenopausal but not postmenopausal women [15], whereas a marginally significant inverse association (HR 0.78 for every two points; 95% CI, 0.62, 0.98) among postmenopausal women in the Greek arm of the EPIC study was found [16].

Concluding, numerous studies have demonstrated that the Mediterranean diet is beneficial for cancer, in that it appears to be inversely associated with incidence and mortality. Mediterranean diet has been shown to be particularly beneficial in some types of cancer, i.e., breast and colorectal cancer. The beneficial effects are due to various components of Mediterranean diet, among which extra-virgin olive oil (EVOO) appears to play a pivotal role in the prevention and evolution of cancer disease.

6.3 Olive Oil and Cancer

Extra-virgin olive oil (EVOO), a vegetable oil very rich in antioxidants, particularly polyphenols (see Chap. 2, this book), has been demonstrated to be beneficial particularly to cardiovascular diseases but also to other diseases including cancer.

The effect of olive oil on human health has, till now, mainly been analyzed by studies deriving from Mediterranean populations, where it is consumed in large quantities. These studies frequently do not distinguish between "plain" olive oil, which is the most used in the world market, and extra-virgin olive oil, the oil obtained with mechanical procedures and very rich in polyphenols (see Chap. 2, this book). Moreover, as it has been already stated, before causally interpreting the usually observed inverse association of olive oil to certain malignancies, residual confounding is an issue arising from the fact that associations are reported mainly from case–control studies [17].

In the present chapter, we will consider data coming from some systematic review and meta-analysis on the effect of olive oil consumption on cancer occurrence, to highlight the deep impact of olive oil intake in various types of cancer.

In a systematic review and meta-analysis [18] conducted on 19 case–control studies, for a total of 13,800 cancer patients and 23,340 controls, it was found that compared to the lowest, the highest category of olive oil consumption was associated with lower odds of having any type of cancer (log odds ratio = −0.41, 95% CI −0.53, −0.29), irrespective of the country of origin (Mediterranean or non-Mediterranean). The combined effect of the highest percentile of olive oil intake compared to the lowest was highly significant ($p < 0.001$). Therefore, people in the highest group of olive oil consumption have shown to have a 0.66 times lower odds, or 34% lower likelihood, of having any type of cancer.

The level of association of olive oil consumption with single cancers will be now considered.

6.3.1 Breast Cancer

Several case–control studies conducted in Greece, Spain, Italy, and France have suggested that olive oil is significantly associated with decreased breast cancer. All these studies coming from different Mediterranean countries have shown a significant inverse association between high daily intake of olive oil and breast cancer occurrence.

In a Greek hospital-based case–control study of 820 women with breast cancer and 1548 controls, more frequent consumption of olive oil (more than once a day compared with once a day) was associated with a significantly reduced breast cancer risk (odds ratio, OR = 0.75). This protective association was concentrated in postmenopausal women [19].

In another study [16], 14,800 women of the Greek cohort of the EPIC study were followed for an average of 9.8 years to evaluate the relation of conformity to the Mediterranean diet with breast cancer. In this cohort, 240 incident breast cancer cases were identified. Results showed that although increasing conformity to the Mediterranean diet was not associated with lower breast cancer risk in the entire cohort, there was a significant inverse association among postmenopausal women (HR = 0.78 for every two points; 95% CI 0.62–0.98). However, when the analysis of association was pinpointed to olive oil only, extrapolated from Mediterranean diet, the results showed that an increased consumption of olive oil was associated with lower breast cancer risk in the entire cohort (HR = 0.93, 95% CI 0.80–1.08) and in the postmenopausal women (HR = 0.85, 95% CI 0.69–1.06), respectively, though not statistically significant.

Three case–control studies from Spain showed the following results: in the first one [20] (762 cases – 988 controls), the odds ratio for the highest versus the lowest quartile of consumption of olive oil was 0.66, with a significant dose–response trend; in the second study [21] (100 breast cancer cases – 100 controls), women in the highest tertile of monounsaturated fat consumption were at lower risk compared with women in the lowest tertile (RR = 0.30; 95% CI 0.1–1.08); in the third study, the Canary Islands study [22], the odds ratio for women in the three upper quintiles of olive oil consumption (≥8.8 g/day) was 0.27.

In a multicenter case–control study from Italy [23], 2564 cases and 2588 controls were studied. The odds ratio per unit (30 g) increase of olive oil consumption was 0.89 (95% CI 0.81–0.99); when the population study was stratified in quintiles of olive oil intake, compared with the lowest quintile, the odds ratios (ORs) were 1.05, 0.99, 0.93, and 0.87 for increasing quintiles of intake; in a model postulating linear logit increase, the OR per unit (30 g) was 0.89 (95% confidence interval [CI] = 0.81–0.99, $P = 0.03$).

In another study from Italy [24], a prospective study that used nutritional data from 8984 women in a follow-up of 9.5 years (ORDET cohort), there were 207 incident cases of breast cancer; the "salad vegetables" pattern, principally consisting of raw vegetables and olive oil, was associated with significantly lower (34–35%) breast cancer incidence (RR = 0.66, 95% CI 0.47–0.95), comparing the highest to lowest tertile.

In the south of France, a case–control study of 437 breast cancer cases and 922 controls showed an inverse association of olive oil intake with breast cancer risk [25]. In another study from France [26], a prospective study, the association between dietary patterns and breast cancer risk was evaluated; the analyses included 2381 postmenopausal invasive breast cancer cases diagnosed during a median 9.7-year follow-up period among 65,374 women from the E3N-EPIC cohort. Results showed that the "healthy/Mediterranean" pattern was negatively associated with breast cancer risk (HR = 0.85, 95% CI 0.75–0.95; $P = 0.003$ for linear trend), especially when tumors were estrogen receptor-positive/progesterone receptor-negative. Authors concluded that adherence to a dietary pattern including mostly fruits, vegetables, fish, and olive/sunflower oil, along with avoidance of Western-type foods, results in a substantial reduction in postmenopausal breast cancer risk.

The EURAMIC study [27], from five European centers including Malaga (Spain), used adipose biopsies with diverse fat intake patterns to see if oleic acid or other monounsaturates are associated with breast cancer. In 291 postmenopausal incident breast cancer patients and 351 controls, the OR (75th to 25th percentiles) was 0.40 in Malaga and 1.27 (not statistically significant) in all the other European centers pooled. Thus, the strong inverse association between oleic acid concentrations and breast cancer in the Spanish study population was not observed in the study's non-Spanish populations. This difference of association between Spain and other European countries could actually be explained by the fact that in Spain oleic acid is derived almost exclusively from extra-virgin olive oil (which contains numerous other active compounds as polyphenols), while in other European countries, oleic acid is derived from multiple sources, including pig's and cattle's meat. The authors concluded that the strong protective associations reported for olive oil intake in dietary studies may be due to other protective components of the extra-virgin olive oil and not to the direct effect of oleic acid uptake.

To conclude, several studies on the effect of olive oil and Mediterranean diet on breast cancer have convincingly shown that olive oil reduces significantly the risk of breast cancer, particularly in postmenopausal women and particularly in estrogen receptor-positive/progesterone receptor-negative tumors. This effect does not seem to be related to the intake of monounsaturated oleic acid but probably to the convergent and synergic action of the various components of extra-virgin olive oil, including the antioxidant polyphenols.

6.3.2 Colorectal Cancer

Colorectal carcinoma rates have been shown to be relatively low in Mediterranean countries compared with most other Western countries, but the components of the Mediterranean diet responsible for this favorable pattern are unclear. The association between colorectal cancer and olive oil doesn't appear so strong as for breast cancer. In case–control studies conducted in Mediterranean populations with colorectal cancer, olive oil has been found to have a slight protective effect, while monounsaturated fat intake appeared uninfluential.

In a case–control study conducted in 6 Italian areas [28], 1953 patients with incident, histologically confirmed colorectal carcinoma (1225 of the colon and 728 of the rectum) and 4154 control subjects with no history of cancer were studied. The odds ratios (ORs) for successive tertiles of olive oil intake, compared with the lowest one, were 0.87 (95% CI, 0.75–1.01) and 0.83 (95% CI, 0.70–0.99; P = 0.03) when colorectal carcinoma was analyzed as a whole, 0.82 (95% CI, 0.68–0.98) and 0.81 (95% CI, 0.66–0.99; *P* = 0.04) for colon carcinoma, and 0.96 (95% CI, 0.77–1.19) and 0.88 (95% CI, 0.66–1.12) for rectal carcinoma. Allowance for vegetable intake attenuated the apparent protection from olive oil consumption (OR, 0.94 for colon and 0.97 for rectum for the highest tertile), which still was apparent in younger subjects (OR, 0.82 for colon and 0.69 for rectum). The conclusions of this study were that there was some evidence for a differential effect of different fats on colorectal cancer, with a little protective effect for olive oil [28].

In a large, multicenter case–control study [29] conducted in Italy and Switzerland between 1992 and 2000, with 1394 cases of colon cancer, 886 cases of rectal cancer, and 4765 controls, the multivariate odds ratios (ORs) for an increment of one portion per week of fried foods were 0.97 (95% CI = 0.93–1.01) for colon cancer and 1.04 (95% CI = 1.00–1.09) for rectal cancer. When the type of fats mainly used for frying was analyzed, olive oil, but not other types of oils, appeared to protect from colon cancer risk (OR = 0.89, 95% CI = 0.82–0.98). The authors concluded that these results do not indicate a relevant role of fried foods on colorectal cancer, with a possible favorable effect of (fried) olive oil on colon cancer risk, but not on rectal cancer risk [29].

In a case–control study on 1953 individuals with colorectal cancer and 4154 controls, the role of monounsaturated fats appeared uninfluential in colon cancer occurrence, while saturated fat intake showed a modest direct association with rectal cancer [30].

Concluding, the available data do not show an appreciable role of olive oil in colon cancer incidence, although some protective effect has been found. The lower incidence of colon cancer in Mediterranean countries appears to be mostly due to the Mediterranean diet as a whole, with a prominent role played by high intake of vegetable and fresh fruit and low intake of meat and saturated fats.

6.3.3 Pancreatic Cancer

Studies on relationships between olive oil and pancreatic cancer are very few, and results are contrasting. Only one study showed a significant inverse association of pancreatic cancer with olive oil intake. In northern Italy, in a case–control study conducted between 1983 and 1992 (362 cases with histologically confirmed, pancreatic cancer risk and 1502 controls), cancer risk was inversely associated with consumption of olive oil (OR = 0.58 for subsequent tertiles of intake) after allowance for sociodemographic factors and tobacco smoking (ORs were 0.76 for intermediate and 0.60 for highest score of intake and the risk was significant) [31, 32].

6.3.4 Stomach Cancer

Also for stomach cancer, studies on the impact of olive oil are quite few. In an Italian study [33], 126 gastric patients were typed for MSI status (a distinctive molecular pathway of carcinogenesis). A MSI+ phenotype was detected in 43 of 126 cases (34.1%), whereas 83 cases were classified as MSI-. The risk of MSI+ tumors was positively associated with high consumption of red meat and meat sauce and negatively associated with consumption of white meat (OR 25.7; CI 6.4–102.8) and olive oil. A positive association was also seen with total protein and nitrite intake. For MSI- tumors, a significant protective effect was associated with frequent consumption of citrus and other fresh fruits, garlic, legumes, vegetables, and olive oil and with high intake of beta-carotene and other antioxidants. Olive oil showed a protective effect on gastric cancer in both MSI- (OR 0.6; CI 0.3–1.00) and MSI+ (OR 0.5; CI 0.2–1.1) phenotypes.

In another case–control study [34] on 1016 gastric cancer patients and 1159 population-based controls, the risk of gastric cancer was found to vary significantly with estimated nutrient intake. The risk rose with increasing consumption of nitrites and proteins and decreased in proportion to intake of olive oil, ascorbic acid, beta-carotene, and alpha-tocopherol. Ascorbic acid showed the strongest geographic gradient, with highest consumption in southern low-risk areas. The authors suggested that the protective effects reported for consumption of fresh fruit, fresh vegetables, and olive oil could be linked to the vitamins C and E contained in these foods.

The findings were consistent with the hypothesis that N-nitroso compounds are involved in gastric cancer risk, since elevated risk was apparent for agents (nitrites, protein) that promote nitrosation, while decreased risk was found for nutrients (ascorbic acid and alpha-tocopherol) which inhibit the process.

To conclude, the few studies on gastric cancer and olive oil appear to share the conclusion that the protective effect of olive on gastric cancer oil seems to operate in synergy with antioxidants contained in Mediterranean diet components, particularly fresh fruit and vegetable.

6.3.5 Esophageal Cancer

Olive oil has shown to protect from esophageal cancer. In a study conducted in northern Italy [35], 304 histologically confirmed squamous esophageal carcinoma cases and 743 controls were interviewed. After correction for multiple confounders, olive oil intake showed a significant reduction of cancer risk in the highest quintile versus lowest (OR 0.26; CI 0.13–0.51). Also after adjustment for total vegetable consumption, olive oil showed a significant reduction of cancer risk, with no monotonic exposure association, that is, even consumers of a minimal quantity of olive oil (the second quintile) appeared to be at a reduced risk for the disease (OR 0.30; CI 0.17–0.56), as consumers of a maximal quantity (the fifth quintile)(OR = 0.36, 95% CI = 0.18–0.73), compared to the lowest quintile of olive oil intake [35], and the same significant reduction was also found for monounsaturated fatty acids [36].

In another case–control study in France (208 cases and 399 controls) for olive oil, the OR for consumers versus nonconsumers was 0.70 (95% CI 0.54–0.90) [37].

6.3.6 Cancer of the Larynx

Some cross-sectional studies have shown a protective effect of olive oil on laryngeal cancer.

In a population-based, case–control study conducted in northern Italy [38], 220 incident male laryngeal cancer cases were studied. After an 8-year follow-up, new primaries occurred among 36 subjects. The occurrence of new primaries was influenced by dietary habits, in that those who had a high intake of olive oil had a one-third lower risk of developing a new primary at the eighth year of observation. The authors concluded that a healthy diet, and particularly olive oil, is protective among those who experience a laryngeal neoplasm and suggests that diet could be a potential preventive agent against the occurrence of new primaries among these patients.

In another study of the same authors [39], in a series of 215 incident cases of laryngeal cancer who were interviewed 10 years earlier in the framework of a population-based case–control study, multiple new primaries occurred in 36 subjects. Although the cancer seemed to be related to tobacco and alcohol intake, the statistical analysis showed a dose-dependent association with tobacco, whereas alcohol was not statistically related to outcomes. Survival resulted to be significantly improved by the intake of vegetables, citrus fruit, orange juice, bread, and olive oil, all of them typical components of Mediterranean diet. A differentiation between dietary patterns showed a 36% advantage in survival for those with higher intake of monounsaturated fatty acids.

In another study [40] conducted in northern Italy and Switzerland with 527 histologically confirmed laryngeal cancer cases and 1297 controls, an inverse association of the risk was observed with olive oil (OR = 0.4 for the highest compared to the lowest quintile of intake, $p = 0.003$), not statistically significant when controlling for total vegetable consumption (OR = 0.66, $p = 0.45$).

Finally, in an analysis where cancers of the oral cavity, pharynx other than nasopharynx, larynx, and esophagus were collectively assessed [41], olive oil used in salads and/or in cooking was significantly inversely associated with cancer (OR contrasting frequency of consumption above vs. below median = 0.78 with 95% CI 0.67–0.90).

To conclude, in the few studies on olive oil and laryngeal cancer, olive oil was associated with a lower risk of the occurrence of a new primary cancer and a 36% advantage in survival for those with higher intake of olive oil.

6.3.7 Oral and Pharyngeal Cancer

In the few case–control studies available, monounsaturated fats (and olive oil) appear to be inversely related to oral and pharyngeal cancer risk.

In a case–control analysis conducted in Italy with 598 cases and 1491 controls, the risk of oropharyngeal cancer was approximately halved in the highest compared to the lowest quintile of olive oil (OR = 0.4, 95% CI 0.3–0.7), which was slightly attenuated by allowance for vegetable intake [42].

In another case–control study conducted in Serbia which included 45 cases with histopathological diagnosis of undifferentiated carcinoma of nasopharyngeal type and 90 controls, frequent/moderate consumption of olive oil was significantly negatively associated with cancer compared with rare or never consumption of olive oil (OR = 0.42, 95% CI 0.19–0.91, $p = 0.03$) [43].

In a case–control study conducted in Greece on the oral cancer with 106 patients with oral carcinoma and an equal number of controls, added lipids, which in Greece are represented overwhelmingly by olive oil, were found inversely and significantly associated with oral carcinoma risk ($p = 0.04$) [44].

In another case–control study conducted in Greece, in the context of the European alcohol-related cancers and genetic susceptibility in Europe project [239 incident upper aerodigestive tract (UADT) cases and 194 hospital controls], authors concluded that stricter adherence to the Mediterranean diet was associated with a substantial and significant decrease in UADT cancer risk (30% for a two-unit increase in score), whereas after mutual adjustment, no individual dietary component of this diet was significantly associated with this risk [45].

In conclusion, also oropharyngeal cancer appears to be associated with Mediterranean diet and a high intake of olive oil, and the strength of this statistical association is only slightly reduced when vegetables are included in the analysis.

Therefore, Mediterranean diet, its vegetable components, and olive oil appear to reduce the risk of oropharyngeal cancer occurrence.

6.3.8 Lung Cancer

There is little evidence for an association of olive oil with lung cancer. In a hospital-based, case–control study of lung cancer in Italy (342 with primary lung cancer and 292 controls), use of olive oil was found to offer a protection toward lung cancer (OR = 0.67, 95% CI 0.45–0.99) [53]. Prospective studies on the association of lung cancer with dietary fat cannot be considered in countries, such as the United States and Norway, where monounsaturated fat intake is mainly derived from sources other than olive oil [46–48].

6.3.9 Ovarian Cancer

Data on impact of olive oil on ovarian cancer are quite few. In a case–control study conducted in Greece on189 epithelial ovarian cancer cases and 200 controls, an inverse relation of monounsaturated fat intake and risk for ovarian cancer was found (OR = 0.80, 95% CI 0.65–0.99 for 1SD increase in consumption on a daily basis) [49].

In a case–control study in Italy, 1031 cases and 2411 controls were included. After correction for multiple confounders, a reduced risk of ovarian cancer was observed for high intake of olive oil (OR = 0.68, 95% CI 0.50–0.93, for the highest quintile, compared with the lowest one), as well for higher intake of monounsaturated fat and oleic acid [50, 51].

6.3.10 Endometrial Cancer

Also for this cancer, data on impact of olive oil are very scarce. In a case–control study conducted in Switzerland and northern Italy (274 endometrial cancer cases and 572 controls), after correction for energy intake, more frequent consumption of olive oil was associated with a decreased risk for endometrial cancer, though results were not statistically significant (OR = 0.82 for highest vs. lowest tertile) [52].

In a case–control study from Greece, with 145 cases and 298 controls, the only statistically suggestive association was the inverse one with monounsaturated fats (OR = 0.74, 95% CI 0.54–1.03) [53]. In another Greek study (84 cases and 84 controls), a protective effect of added lipids, which in the Greek diet are primarily represented by olive oil, was highly suggestive [54].

6.3.11 Bladder Cancer

The few data available are contrasting. In a case–control study in Belgium (200 cases and 386 controls), results showed that there was a statistically significant inverse association between olive oil intake and bladder cancer, consistent with a linear dose–response relationship: middle versus the lowest tertile (OR = 0.62, 95% CI 0.39–0.99) and the highest versus the lowest tertile (OR = 0.47, 95% CI 0.28–0.78; p-trend = 0.002) [55]. However, findings from another study [56] showed that in a Spanish population with an average dietary pattern typical of Mediterranean populations, monounsaturated fat intake was associated with a moderate increase of risk, which disappeared after correction for saturated fat intake.

6.3.12 Prostate Cancer

Studies on association of Mediterranean diet and prostate cancer have shown contrasting results. However, some meta-analysis and follow-up studies have shown a positive impact of Mediterranean diet on prostate cancer. It should be noted that countries following the traditional Mediterranean diet, particularly Southern European countries, have lower prostate cancer incidence and mortality compared to other European regions. The beneficial effect has been attributed to the specific eating pattern.

In a recent review [57] examining the evidence of the effect of adherence to a Mediterranean diet as a whole and its single components on prostate cancer risk, a strong evidence supporting the associations between foods that are typical of a Mediterranean eating pattern and reduced prostate cancer risk was found.

In a prospective study, 47,867 men enrolled in the Health Professionals Follow-up Study were followed from 1986 to 2010. During the follow-up period, 6220 prostate cancer cases were confirmed. Although no association between Mediterranean diet (after diagnosis) and risk of lethal or fatal prostate cancer was evidenced, a 22% lower risk of overall mortality (hazard ratio, 0.78; CI 0.67–0.90) was found among men with greater adherence to the Mediterranean diet after prostate cancer diagnosis [58].

Concerning the correlation between olive oil intake and prostate cancer risk, the very few studies available have shown contrasting results.

A case–control study from Greece [59] included 320 patients with histologically confirmed incident prostate cancer and 246 controls without prostate cancer. Among major food groups, milk and dairy products as well as added lipids were marginally positively associated with risk for prostate cancer. Among added lipids, seed oils were significantly and butter and margarine nonsignificantly positively associated with prostate cancer risk, whereas olive oil was unrelated to this risk. Cooked tomatoes and to a lesser extent raw tomatoes were inversely associated with the risk for prostate cancer. Also vitamin E was inversely associated with prostate cancer.

In another study [60], a population-based case–control study on 858 men aged <70 years with histologically confirmed prostate cancer and 906 age-frequency-matched men, an inverse association with prostate cancer was observed (OR, 95% CI for tertile III compared with tertile I) for allium vegetables 0.7, 0.5–0.9, p trend 0.01; tomato-based foods 0.8, 0.6–1.0, p trend 0.03; and total vegetables 0.7, 0.5–1.0, p trend 0.04. Margarine intake was positively associated with prostate cancer (1.3, 1.0–1.7; p trend 0.04). The only statistically significant associations observed with nutrients were weak inverse associations for palmitoleic acid (p trend 0.04), fatty acid 17:1 (p trend 0.04), and 20:5 n-6 (p trend 0.05) and a nonsignificant trend for oleic acid (p trend 0.09). The authors concluded that, based on these findings, diets rich in olive oil (a source of oleic acid), tomatoes and *allium* vegetables might reduce the risk of prostate cancer.

Although data on the impact of dietary factors on prostate cancer risk are contrasting, those concerning the increased risk are more convincing than those associated with a reduced risk. In fact, numerous studies and large meta-analysis have convincingly shown the significant positive association of red and processed meat with increased risk of prostate cancer [61] as well as of other types of cancer as colorectal cancer. Also high daily intakes of dairy products have shown to be positively associated with increased risk of prostate cancer [62].

Concerning the protective effects of the diet, in addition to vegetables and *allium* products, tomatoes and its major carotenoid *lycopene* have been shown to reduce the prostate cancer risk (see Chap. 9, this book). A large meta-analysis [63] summarizing the results of 11 case–control studies and 10 cohort studies or nested case–control studies showed that for a high intake of cooked tomato products, the corresponding RR was 0.81 (95% CI 0.71–0.92). The RR of prostate cancer related to an intake of one serving/day of raw tomato (200 g) was 0.97 (95% CI 0.85–1.10) for the case–control studies and 0.78 (95% CI 0.66–0.92) for cohort studies. For serum- or plasma-based studies, the corresponding RRs were 0.74 (95% CI 0.59–0.92) for all studies, 0.55 (95% CI 0.32–0.94) for case–control studies, and 0.78 (95% CI 0.61–1.00) for cohort studies. This meta-analysis indicates that results from cohort studies and serum- or plasma-based studies support about a 25–30% reduction in the risk of prostate cancer. However, the association between tomato products and lycopene and lower prostate cancer risk, while suggestive, remains controversial, because not all the studies are supportive [64].

Conclusion

A large number of studies have demonstrated that nutritional factors play a major role in cancer initiation and development. In a meta-analysis already mentioned [18] that evaluated solely olive oil intake, data from 13,800 cancer patients and 23,340 controls showed that the combined effect of the highest percentile of olive oil intake with the lowest was highly significant, in that people in the highest group of olive oil consumption had 0.66 times lower odds of having any type of cancer (logOR = −0.41 95% CI −0.53 to −0.29) or 34% lower likelihood of having any type of cancer. The applied effect-equality test revealed that although the study-specific effect size measures were heterogeneous, all of them were to the same protective direction [18].

Ecologic comparisons and meta-analysis of prospective cohort studies suggest that cancer morbidity and mortality are lower in Mediterranean countries, where olive oil represents a substantial fraction of dietary fat [65]. Prospective studies have shown evidence that higher degree of adherence to the Mediterranean diet is associated with a reduced mortality for cancer of all types [66]. According to a large review, in Western countries, approximately 25% of the incidence of colorectal cancer, 15% of breast cancer, and 10% of prostate, pancreas, and endometrial cancer could be prevented if traditional Mediterranean dietary patterns were followed [67].

In a study conducted in 28 countries, 76% of the intercountry variation in colorectal cancer incidence rates could be attributed to three dietary factors, meat, fish, and olive oil, in combination; meat and fish were found positively associated, whereas olive oil was negatively associated. The authors suggested that olive oil could influence secondary bile acid patterns in the colon that, in turn, might influence polyamine metabolism in colonic cells reducing possibility to progression from normal mucosa to adenoma and, eventually, carcinoma [68].

Evidence to support that olive oil conveys protection against occurrence of different types of cancer, although already demonstrated by numerous observational, case–control and cohort studies, necessitates more epidemiological studies, especially prospective ones, specifically designed to address these issues. Well-designed cohort studies will help to further examine the association and questions arising, such as, firstly, if olive oil intake facilitates more vegetable intake, thus maximizing its beneficial effects to cancer prevention, and, secondly, if the possible beneficial effects of olive oil are attributed to its monounsaturated content or to its other components. Actually, olive oil in Mediterranean diet is frequently associated with vegetables, herbs (*allium*), and tomatoes, all of which have been significantly associated with a reduced risk of numerous diseases, including cancer.

References

1. Campbell CT, Campbell TM. The China study. Dallas, TX: Benbella Books Inc; 2006.
2. Cancer Facts and Figures 2007. Atlanta, GA: National Home Office, American Cancer Society, Inc.; 2007. p. 30239–4251.
3. Stein CJ, Colditz GA. Modifiable risk factors for cancer. Brit J Cancer. 2004;90:299–303.
4. Stewart BW, Bray F, Forman D, Ohgaki H, Straif K, Ullrich A, Wild CP. Cancer prevention as part of precision medicine: 'plenty to be done'. Carcinogenesis. 2016;37:2–9.
5. Tyrovolas S, Panagiotakos DB. The role of Mediterranean type of diet on the development of cancer and cardiovascular disease, in the elderly: a systematic review. Maturitas. 2010;65:122–30.
6. Colditz GA, DeJong W, Hunter DJ, Trichopoulos D, Willet WC, editors. Harvard report on cancer prevention. Cancer Causes Control. 1996;7(Suppl):S1–S55.
7. Curry SJ, Byers T, Hewitt M. Fulfilling the potential of cancer prevention and early detection. Washington, DC: The National Academies Press; 2003.
8. Rowland JH, Kent EE, Forsythe LP, Loge JH, Hjorth L, Glaser A, Mattioli V, Fosså SD. Cancer survivorship research in Europe and the United States: where have we been, where are we going, and what can we learn from each other? Cancer. 2013;119(Suppl. 11):2094–108.
9. DeSantis CE, Lin CC, Mariotto AB, Siegel RL, Stein KD, Kramer JL, Alteri R, Robbins AS, Jemal A. Cancer treatment and survivorship statistics, 2014. CA Cancer J Clin. 2014;64:252–71.
10. Schwingshackl L, Hoffmann G. Adherence to Mediterranean diet and risk of cancer: an updated systematic review and meta-analysis of observational studies. Cancer Med. 2015;4:1933–47.
11. Schwingshackl L, Schwedhelm C, Galbete C, Hoffmann G. Adherence to Mediterranean diet and risk of cancer: an updated systematic review and meta-analysis. Nutrients. 2017;9:E1063.

12. Couto E, Boffetta P, Lagiou P, Ferrari P, Buckland G, Overvad K, Dahm CC, Tjonneland A, Olsen A, Clavel-Chapelon F, Boutron-Ruault MC, Cottet V, Trichopoulos D, Naska A, Benetou V, Kaaks R, Rohrmann S, Boeing H, von Ruesten A, Panico S, Pala V, Vineis P, Palli D, Tumino R, May A, Peeters PH, Bueno-de-Mesquita HB, Büchner FL, Lund E, Skeie G, Engeset D, Gonzalez CA, Navarro C, Rodríguez L, Sánchez MJ, Amiano P, Barricarte A, Hallmans G, Johansson I, Manjer J, Wirfärt E, Allen NE, Crowe F, Khaw KT, Wareham N, Moskal A, Slimani N, Jenab M, Romaguera D, Mouw T, Norat T, Riboli E, Trichopoulou A. Mediterranean dietary pattern and cancer risk in the EPIC cohort. Br J Cancer. 2011;104:1493–9.
13. Agnoli C, Grioni S, Sieri S, Palli D, Masala G, Sacerdote C, Vineis P, Tumino R, Giurdanella MC, Pala V, Berrino F, Mattiello A, Panico S, Krogh V. Italian Mediterranean index and risk of colorectal cancer in the Italian section of the EPIC cohort. Int J Cancer. 2013;132(6):1404–11.
14. Buckland G, Travier N, Cottet V, Gonzalez CA, Lujan-Barroso L, Agudo A, Trichopoulou A, Lagiou P, Trichopoulos D, Peeters PH, May A, Bueno-de-Mesquita HB, Bvan Duijnhoven FJ, Key TJ, Allen N, Khaw KT, Wareham N, Romieu I, McCormack V, Boutron-Ruault M, Clavel-Chapelon F, Panico S, Agnoli C, Palli D, Tumino R, Vineis P, Amiano P, Barricarte A, Rodríguez L, Sanchez MJ, Chirlaque MD, Kaaks R, Teucher B, Boeing H, Bergmann MM, Overvad K, Dahm CC, Tjønneland A, Olsen A, Manjer J, Wirfält E, Hallmans G, Johansson I, Lund E, Hjartåker A, Skeie G, Vergnaud AC, Norat T, Romaguera D, Riboli E. Adherence to the Mediterranean diet and risk of breast cancer in the European prospective investigation into cancer and nutrition cohort study. Int J Cancer. 2013;132:2918–27.
15. Cade JE, Taylor EF, Burley VJ, Greenwood DC. Does the Mediterranean dietary pattern or the Healthy Diet Index influence the risk of breast cancer in a large British cohort of women? Eur J Clin Nutr. 2011;65:920–8.
16. Trichopoulou A, Bamia C, Lagiou P, Trichopoulos D. Conformity to traditional Mediterranean diet and breast cancer risk in the Greek EPIC (European Prospective Investigation into Cancer and Nutrition) cohort. Am J Clin Nutr. 2010;92:620–5.
17. Martin-Moreno JM. The role of olive oil in lowering cancer risk: is this real gold or simply pinchbeck? J Epidemiol Community Health. 2000;54:726–7.
18. Psaltopoulou T, Kosti RI, Haidopoulos D, Dimopoulos M, Panagiotakos DB. Olive oil intake is inversely related to cancer prevalence: a systematic review and a meta-analysis of 13,800 patients and 23,340 controls in 19 observational studies. Lipids Health Dis. 2011;10:127.
19. Trichopoulou A, Katsouyanni K, Stuver S, Tzala L, Gnardellis C, Rimm E, Trichopoulos D. Consumption of olive oil and specific food groups in relation to breast cancer risk in Greece. J Natl Cancer Inst. 1995;87:110–6.
20. Martin-Moreno JM, Willett WC, Gorgojo L, Banegas JR, Rodriguez-Artalejo F, Fernandez-Rodriguez JC, Maisonneuve P, Boyle P. Dietary fat, olive oil intake and breast cancer risk. Int J Cancer. 1994;58:74–80.
21. Landa MC, Frago N, Tres A. Diet and the risk of breast cancer in Spain. Eur J Cancer Prev. 1994;3:313–20.
22. García-Segovia P, Sánchez-Villegas A, Doreste J, Santana F, Serra-Majem L. Olive oil consumption and risk of breast cancer in the Canary Islands: a population-based case-control study. Public Health Nutr. 2006;9:163–7.
23. La Vecchia C, Negri E, Franceschi S, Decarli A, Giacosa A, Lipworth L. Olive oil, other dietary fats and the risk of breast cancer (Italy). Cancer Causes Control. 1995;6:545–50.
24. Sieri S, Krogh V, Pala V, Muti P, Micheli A, Evangelista A, Tagliabue G, Berrino F. Dietary patterns and risk of breast cancer in the ORDET cohort. Cancer Epidemiol Biomark Prev. 2004;13:567–72.
25. Bessaoud F, Daurès JP, Gerber M. Dietary factors and breast cancer risk: a case control study among a population in Southern France. Nutr Cancer. 2008;60:177–87.
26. Cottet V, Touvier M, Fournier A, Touillaud MS, Lafay L, Clavel-Chapelon F, Boutron-Ruault MC. Postmenopausal breast cancer risk and dietary patterns in the E3N-EPIC prospective cohort study. Am J Epidemiol. 2009;170:1257–67.
27. Simonsen NR, Fernandez-Crehuet Navajas J, Martin-Moreno JM, Strain JJ, Huttunen JK, Martin BC, Thamm M, Kardinaal AF, van't Veer P, Kok FJ, Kohlmeier L. Tissue stores of

individual monounsaturated fatty acids and breast cancer: the EURAMIC study. Am J Clin Nutr. 1998;68:134–41.
28. Braga C, La Vecchia C, Franceschi S, Negri E, Parpinel M, Decarli A, Giacosa A, Trichopoulos D. Olive oil, other seasoning fats and the risk of colorectal carcinoma. Cancer. 1998;82:448–53.
29. Galeone C, Talamini R, Levi F, Pelucchi C, Negri E, Giacosa A, Montella M, Franceschi S, La Vecchia C. Fried foods, olive oil and colorectal cancer. Ann Oncol. 2007;18:36–9.
30. Franceschi S, La Vecchia C, Russo A, Favero A, Negri E, Conti E, Montella M, Filiberti R, Amadori D, Decarli A. Macronutrient intake and risk of colorectal cancer in Italy. Int J Cancer. 1998;76:321–4.
31. Soler M, Chatenoud L, La Vecchia C, Francheschi S, Negri E. Diet, alcohol, coffee and pancreatic cancer: final results from an Italian study. Eur J Cancer Prev. 1998;7:455–60.
32. La Vecchia C, Negri E. Fats in seasoning and the relationship to pancreatic cancer. Eur J Cancer Prev. 1997;6:370–3.
33. Palli D, Russo A, Ottini L, Masala G, Saieva C, Amorosi A, Cama A, D'Amico C, Falchetti M, Palmirotta R, Decarli A, Mariani Costantini R, Fraumeni JF Jr. Red meat, family history, and increased risk of gastric cancer with microsatellite instability. Cancer Res. 2001;61:5415–9.
34. Buiatti E, Palli D, Decarli A, Amadori D, Avellini C, Bianchi S, Bonaguri C, Cipriani F, Cocco P, Giacosa A, Marubini E, Minacci C, Puntoni R, Russo A, Vindigni C, Fraumeni JF Jr, Blot WJ. A case-control study of gastric cancer and diet in Italy: II. Association with nutrients. Int J Cancer. 1990;45:896–901.
35. Bosetti C, La Vecchia C, Talamini R, Negri E, Levi F, Dal Maso L, Franceschi S. Food groups and risk of squamous cell esophageal cancer in northern Italy. Int J Cancer. 2000;87:289–94.
36. Franceschi S, Bidoli E, Negri E, Zambon P, Talamini R, Ruol A, Parpinel M, Levi F, Simonato L, La Vecchia C. Role of macronutrients, vitamins and minerals in the aetiology of squamous-cell carcinoma of the oesophagus. Int J Cancer. 2000;86:626–31.
37. Launoy G, Milan C, Day NE, Pienkowski MP, Gignoux M, Faivre J. Diet and squamous-cell cancer of the oesophagus: a French multicenter case-control study. Int J Cancer. 1998;76:7–12.
38. Russo A, Crosignani P, Berrino F. Tobacco smoking, alcohol drinking and dietary factors as determinants of new primaries among male laryngeal cancer patients: a case-cohort study. Tumori. 1996;82:519–25.
39. Crosignani P, Russo A, Tagliabue G, Berrino F. Tobacco and diet as determinants of survival in male laryngeal cancer patients. Int J Cancer. 1996;65:308–13.
40. Bosetti C, La Vecchia C, Talamini R, Negri E, Levi F, Dal Maso L, Franceschi S. Food groups and laryngeal cancer risk: a case-control study from Italy and Switzerland. Int J Cancer. 2002;100:355–60.
41. Lagiou P, Talamini R, Samoli E, Lagiou A, Ahrens W, Pohlabeln H, Benhamou S, Bouchardy C, Slamova A, Schejbalova M, Merletti F, Richiardi L, Kjaerheim K, Agudo A, Castellsague X, Macfarlane TV, Macfarlane GJ, Biggs AM, Barzan L, Canova C, Simonato L, Lowry RJ, Conway DI, McKinney PA, Znaor A, McCartan BE, Healy CM, Marron M, Hashibe M, Brennan P. Diet and upper-aerodigestive tract cancer in Europe: the ARCAGE study. Int J Cancer. 2009;124:2671–6.
42. Franceschi S, Favero A, Conti E, Talamini R, Volpe R, Negri E, Barzan L, La Vecchia C. Food groups, oils and butter, and cancer of the oral cavity and pharynx. Br J Cancer. 1999;80:614–20.
43. Nesić V, Sipetić S, Vlajinac H, Stosić-Divjak S, Jesić S. Risk factors for the occurrence of undifferentiated carcinoma of nasopharyngeal type: a case-control study. Srp Arh Celok Lek. 2010;138:6–10.
44. Petridou E, Zavras A, Lefatzis D, Conti E, Talamini R, Volpe R, Negri E, Barzan L, La Vecchia C. The role of diet and specific micronutrients in the etiology of oral carcinoma. Cancer. 2002;94:2981–8.
45. Samoli E, Lagiou A, Nikolopoulos E, Lagogiannis G, Barbouni A, Lefantzis D, Trichopoulos D, Brennan P, Lagiou P. Mediterranean diet and upper aerodigestive tract cancer: the Greek segment of the alcohol-related cancers and genetic susceptibility in Europe study. Br J Nutr. 2010;101:369–74.

46. Smith-Warner SA, Ritz J, Hunter DJ, Albanes D, Beeson WL, van den Brandt PA, Colditz G, Folsom AR, Fraser GE, Freudenheim JL, Giovannucci E, Goldbohm RA, Graham S, Kushi LH, Miller AB, Rohan TE, Speizer FE, Virtamo J, Willett WC. Dietary fat and risk of lung cancer in a pooled analysis of prospective studies. Cancer Epidemiol Biomark Prev. 2002;11(10 Pt 1):987–92.
47. Bandera EV, Freudenheim JL, Marshall JR, Zielezny M, Priore RL, Brasure J, Baptiste M, Graham S. Diet and alcohol consumption and lung cancer risk in the New York State Cohort (United States). Cancer Causes Control. 1997;8:828–40.
48. Veierød MB, Laake P, Thelle DS. Dietary fat intake and risk of lung cancer a prospective study of 51452 Norwegian men and women. Eur J Cancer Prev. 1997;6:540–9.
49. Tzonou A, Hsieh CC, Polychronopoulou A, Kaprinis G, Toupadaki N, Trichopoulou A, Karakatsani A, Trichopoulos D. Diet and ovarian cancer: a case-control study in Greece. Int J Cancer. 1993;55:411–4.
50. Bosetti C, Negri E, Franceschi S, Talamini R, Montella M, Conti E, Lagiou P, Parazzini F, La Vecchia C. Olive oil, seed oils and other added fats in relation to ovarian cancer (Italy). Cancer Causes Control. 2002;13:465–70.
51. Bidoli E, La Vecchia C, Montella M, Maso LD, Conti E, Negri E, Scarabelli C, Carbone A, Decarli A, Franceschi S. Nutrient intake and ovarian cancer: an Italian case-control study. Cancer Causes Control. 2002;13:255–61.
52. Levi F, Franceschi S, Negri E, La Vecchia C. Dietary factors and the risk of endometrial cancer. Cancer. 1993;71:3575–81.
53. Tzonou A, Lipworth L, Kalandidi A, Trichopoulou A, Gamatsi I, Hsieh CC, Notara V, Trichopoulos D. Dietary factors and the risk of endometrial cancer: a case-control study in Greece. Br J Cancer. 1996;73:1284–90.
54. Petridou E, Kedikoglou S, Koukoulomatis P, Dessypris N, Trichopoulos D. Diet in relation to endometrial cancer risk: a case-control study in Greece. Nutr Cancer. 2002;44:16–22.
55. Brinkman MT, Buntinx F, Kellen E, Van Dongen MC, Dagnelie PC, Muls E, Zeegers MP. Consumption of animal products, olive oil and dietary fat and results from the Belgian case-control study on bladder cancer risk. Eur J Cancer. 2011;47:436–42.
56. Riboli E, González CA, López-Abente G, Errezola M, Izarzugaza I, Escolar A, Nebot M, Hémon B, Agudo A. Diet and bladder cancer in Spain: a multicentre case-control study. Int J Cancer. 1991;49:214–9.
57. López-Guarnido O, Álvarez-Cubero MJ, Saiz M, Lozano D, Rodrigo L, Cozar JM, Rivas A. Mediterranean diet adherence and prostate cancer risk. Nutr Hosp. 2014;31:1012–9.
58. Kenfield SA, DuPre N, Richman EL, Stampfer MJ, Chan JM, Giovannucci EL. Mediterranean diet and prostate cancer risk and mortality in the health professionals follow-up study. Eur Urol. 2014;65:887–94.
59. Tzonou A, Signorello LB, Lagiou P, Wuu J, Trichopoulos D, Trichopoulou A. Diet and cancer of the prostate: a case-control study in Greece. Int J Cancer. 1999;80:704–8.
60. Hodge AM, English DR, McCredie MR, Severi G, Boyle P, Hopper JL, Giles GG. Foods, nutrients and prostate cancer. Cancer Causes Control. 2004;15:11–20.
61. Sinha R, Park Y, Graubard BI, Leitzmann MF, Hollenbeck A, Schatzkin A, Cross AJ. Meat and meat-related compounds and risk of prostate cancer in a large prospective cohort study in the United States. Am J Epidemiol. 2009;170:1165–77.
62. Aune D, Navarro Rosenblatt DA, Chan DS, Vieira AR, Vieira R, Greenwood DC, Vatten LJ, Norat T. Dairy products, calcium, and prostate cancer risk: a systematic review and meta-analysis of cohort studies. Am J Clin Nutr. 2015;101:87–117.
63. Etminan M, Takkouche B, Caamano-Isorna F. The role of tomato products and lycopene in the prevention of prostate cancer: a meta-analysis of observational studies. Cancer Epidemiol Biomark Prev. 2004;13:340–5.
64. Giovannucci E. Tomato products, lycopene, and prostate cancer: a review of the epidemiological literature. J Nutr. 2005;135:2030S–1S.
65. Sofi F, Cesari F, Abbate R, Gensini GF, Casini A. Adherence to Mediterranean diet and health status: meta-analysis. BMJ. 2008;337:1136–44.

66. Trichopoulou A, Costacou T, Bamia C, Trichopoulos D. Adherence to a Mediterranean diet and survival in a Greek population. N Engl J Med. 2003;348:2599–608.
67. Trichopoulou A, Lagiou P, Kuper H, Trichopoulos D. Cancer and Mediterranean dietary traditions. Cancer Epidemiol Biomark Prev. 2000;9:869–73.
68. Stoneham M, Goldacre M, Seagroatt V, Gill L. Olive oil, diet and colorectal cancer: an ecological study and a hypothesis. J Epidemiol Community Health. 2000;54:756–60.

7 Epigenetics/Epigenomics of Olive Oil and the Mediterranean Diet

7.1 Premises

"Mediterranean diet and olive oil modify gene transcription towards a protective mode."

Epigenetics/epigenomics are terms used to describe a variety of modifications to the genome that do not involve changes in DNA sequence and result in alteration of gene transcription allowing for differential expression of common genetic information. In a sense it constitutes the missing link between genetics, the environment, and disease [1].

Nutrigenomics, tightly connected with epigenetics/epigenomics, is a multidisciplinary science that comes after the human genome has been characterized and put the genomic techniques besides the biochemical and epidemiological aspects, with the aim to understand the etiologic aspects of chronic diseases such as cancer, type 2 diabetes mellitus (T2DM), obesity, cardiovascular diseases (CVD), metabolic syndrome, etc.

Nutrigenomics is linked to nutrigenetics, which studies the genetic basis of the different individual response to the same nutritional stimulus. This phenomenon arises from gene polymorphism. As a consequence, genes are important in determining a function, but nutrition is able to modify the degree of gene expression [2].

Among the mechanisms by which Mediterranean diet and its main fat component, olive oil, exert its beneficial effects on human health, gene–diet interactions have probably the most important role in the development of and in the protection against chronic degenerative diseases. From a nutrigenomic point of view, nutrients act as dietary signals, are detected by the cellular sensor, and modulate gene and protein expression and, subsequently, metabolite production [3].

A. Capurso et al., *Benefits of the Mediterranean Diet in the Elderly Patient*, Practical Issues in Geriatrics, https://doi.org/10.1007/978-3-319-78084-9_7

7.2 An Example of Gene–Diet Interaction

An example of gene–diet interaction is given by the PREDIMED study [4]. This was a parallel-group, multicenter, randomized prospective, primary prevention trial that included 7447 persons aged 55–80 years. The primary end point was the rate of major cardiovascular events (myocardial infarction, stroke, or death from cardiovascular causes). The subjects were randomly assigned to one of three diets: a Mediterranean diet supplemented with extra-virgin olive oil, a Mediterranean diet supplemented with mixed nuts, or a control diet (advice to reduce dietary fat). After a median follow-up of 4.8 years, a significant risk reduction of the primary end points was observed in the two groups assigned to Mediterranean diet, compared to control group, with a hazard ratio (HR) of 0.70 (CI, 0.54 to 0.92) and 0.72 (CI, 0.54 to 0.96) for the group assigned to a Mediterranean diet with extra-virgin olive oil and the group assigned to a Mediterranean diet with nuts, respectively, versus the control group. These findings provided evidence supporting the notion that Mediterranean diet reduces cardiovascular risk to a level (30%) within the range observed for pharmacological interventions.

Subsequently, a sub-study [5] on 7018 participants to the PREDIMED study, whose DNA was isolated, was undertaken, and the TCF7L2-rs7903146 polymorphism was determined to see whether the polymorphism (C > T) associations with type 2 diabetes, glucose, lipids, and cardiovascular disease incidence were modulated by Mediterranean diet. The TCF7L2 is a relevant transcription factor in the Wnt signaling pathway, located on chromosome 10q25.3, and consists of 17 exons (boxes). The rs7903146 (C > T) single nucleotide polymorphism (SNP) in intron 4 has been demonstrated to be the most important polymorphism associated with type 2 diabetes. The 7903146 T allele is significantly associated with higher type 2 diabetes risk. The results of the study showed that the TCF7L2-rs7903146 polymorphism was associated with type 2 diabetes (odds ratio 1.87; CI, 1.62–2.17) for TT compared with CC. When adherence to the Mediterranean diet was low, TT subjects had higher fasting glucose concentrations (132.3 mg/dL) than CC + CT (127.3 mg/dL) individuals ($P = 0.001$). Nevertheless, when adherence was high, this plasma glucose increase was not observed ($P = 0.605$). This modulation was also detected for total cholesterol, LDL cholesterol, and triglycerides (P interaction, 0.05 for all). Likewise, TT subjects had a higher stroke incidence in the control group (adjusted HR 2.91; $P = 0.006$ compared with CC), whereas dietary intervention with Mediterranean diet reduced significantly stroke incidence in TT homozygotes (adjusted HR 0.96; $P = 0.892$ for TT compared with CC) [5].

These results convincingly showed that Mediterranean diet can modulate gene expression via epigenetic mechanisms in fine-tuning gene expression.

7.3 The Activation/Inactivation of Gene Transcription

As we have said before, the term "epigenetics" is used to refer to the complex interactions between the genome and the environment involved in development and differentiation in higher organisms. Among environmental factors, diet is probably the most important element that can transiently change the transcription activity of genes through epigenetic modifications. Epigenetic modifications alter DNA accessibility and chromatin structure, thereby regulating patterns of gene expression. The major mechanisms in epigenetic regulation are (1) the long-term epigenetic modifications that involve DNA methylation and (2) the more flexible (short-term) modifications that involve histone modifications, such as methylation and acetylation.

A third mechanism in epigenetic regulation comes from microRNAs. These are small, noncoding RNA molecules that function in RNA silencing and posttranscriptional regulation of gene expression.

7.3.1 DNA Methylation

DNA methylation is a process by which methyl groups are added to the DNA molecule (Fig. 7.1). Methylation changes the activity of a DNA segment without changing the sequence. When located in a gene promoter, DNA methylation typically acts to repress gene transcription. DNA methylation is essential for normal development and is associated with a number of key processes including aging and carcinogenesis.

Most DNA methylation in humans occurs at cytosine–phosphate–guanine (CpG) dinucleotides and consists of the addition of a methyl group on position 5 of cytosine residues of the CpG island (Fig. 7.1). DNA methylation of CpG islands is unambiguously linked with transcriptional repression.

CpG-dense promoters of actively transcribed genes are never methylated, but transcriptionally silent genes do not necessarily carry a methylated promoter. Whereas DNA methylation is not necessary per se for transcriptional silencing, it is thought nonetheless to represent a "locked" state that definitely inactivates gene transcription.

In mouse and human, around 60–70% of genes have a CpG island in their promoter region and most of these CpG islands remain unmethylated independently of the transcriptional activity of the gene. DNA methylation may affect the transcription of genes in two ways. First, the methylation of DNA itself may physically impede the binding of transcriptional proteins to the gene, and second, and likely more important, methylated DNA may be bound by proteins known as methyl-CpG-binding domain proteins (MBDs). MBD proteins then recruit additional proteins to the locus, such as histone deacetylases and other chromatin remodeling

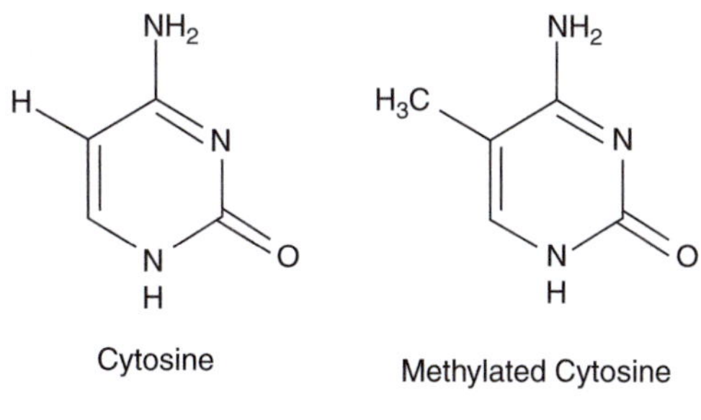

Fig. 7.1 Methylation of DNA.
The methyl group binds to nucleotide, at level of cytosine

proteins that can modify histones, thereby forming compact, inactive chromatin, termed heterochromatin.

At CpG sites there are single nucleotide polymorphisms (SNPs) that either create or disrupt a CpG with effects on methylation levels, not only in the site, but also in the surrounding region, hence linking genetic variation to epigenetic changes and increasing the number of regulatory factors.

DNA methylation in cancer. In many disease processes, DNA methylation appears of crucial importance. Alterations of DNA methylation have been recognized as an important component of cancer development. In cancer, gene promoter CpG islands acquire abnormal hypermethylation, which results in transcriptional silencing that can be inherited by daughter cells following cell division. Hypomethylation has also been implicated in the development and progression of cancer through different mechanisms. Typically, there is hypermethylation of tumor suppressor genes and hypomethylation of oncogenes [6]. Hypomethylation, in general, arises earlier and is linked to chromosomal instability and loss of imprinting, whereas hypermethylation is associated with promoters and can arise secondary to gene silencing (oncogene suppressor) and might be a target for epigenetic therapy [7].

Generally, in progression to cancer, hundreds of genes are silenced or activated. Although silencing of some genes in cancers occurs by mutation, a large proportion of carcinogenic gene silencing is a result of altered DNA methylation. DNA methylation causing silencing in cancer typically occurs at multiple CpG sites in the CpG islands that are present in the promoters of protein-coding genes. Silencing of DNA repair genes through methylation of CpG islands in their promoters appears to be especially important in progression to cancer.

Altered expressions of microRNAs (see miRNA paragraph, below) also silence or activate many genes in progression to cancer. Altered microRNA expression occurs through hyper-/hypomethylation of CpG sites in CpG islands in promoters controlling transcription of the microRNAs.

DNA methylation in atherosclerosis. DNA methylation is implicated also in atherosclerosis. Two of the cell types targeted for DNA methylation polymorphisms are monocytes and lymphocytes, which experience an overall hypomethylation. One proposed mechanism behind this global hypomethylation is elevated homocysteine level causing hyperhomocysteinemia, a known risk factor for cardiovascular disease. High plasma level of homocysteine inhibits DNA methyltransferases, which causes hypomethylation. Hypomethylation of DNA affects gene that alters smooth muscle cell proliferation, causes endothelial cell dysfunction, and increases inflammatory mediators, all of which are critical in forming atherosclerotic lesions [8]. High levels of homocysteine also result in hypermethylation of CpG islands in the promoter region of the estrogen receptor alpha (ERα) gene, causing its down-regulation [9]. ERα protects against atherosclerosis due to its action as a growth suppressor, causing the smooth muscle cells to remain in a quiescent state [10]. The ERα promoter does not appear to be methylated in situ (normal aorta), but becomes methylated in proliferating aortic smooth muscle cells. Hypermethylation of the ERα promoter thus allows intimal smooth muscle cells to proliferate excessively and contribute to the development of the atherosclerotic lesion [11].

DNA methylation in aging. In humans and other mammals, DNA methylation levels can be used to accurately estimate the age of tissues and cell types, forming an accurate epigenetic clock. In a study that analyzed the complete DNA methylomes of $CD4^+$ T cells in a newborn, in a 26-year-old individual, and in a 103-year-old individual, it was observed that the loss of methylation is proportional to age. Hypomethylated CpGs observed in the centenarian DNAs compared with the neonates covered all genomic compartments (promoters, intergenic, intronic, and exonic regions) [12]. However, some genes become hypermethylated with age, including genes for the *estrogen receptor*, *p16*, and *insulin-like growth factor 2* [6].

7.3.2 Histone Modification

In analogy to DNA methylation, the histone modifications are important mechanisms by which environmental factors, including the diet, modify the transcriptional activity of genes.

Chromatin is the complex of chromosomal DNA associated with proteins in the nucleus. DNA in chromatin is packaged around histone proteins, in units referred to as nucleosomes. A nucleosome has 147 bp of DNA associated with an octomeric core of histone proteins, consisting of two H3–H4 histone dimers surrounded by two H2A–H2B dimers. N-terminal histone tails protrude from nucleosomes into the nuclear lumen. It has been suggested that different combinations of histone modifications may regulate chromatin structure and transcriptional status [13, 14].

Of the many described histone modifications, histone acetylation at the ε-amino group of lysine residues in H3 and H4 tails is most consistently associated with promoting transcription. However, this description oversimplifies a complex process, as acetylated, open-chromatin structure may also allow access of transcriptional repressors.

Histone tail acetylation has received much attention over the last several years as a key mediator of chromatin structure and transcriptional regulation. Acetylation is targeted to regions of chromatin by the recognition and binding of DNA sequence-specific transcription factors that recruit one of a growing family of histone acetyltransferase (HAT) cofactors such as CREB-binding protein (CBP) and p300, MYST, and GNAT [15].

Deacetylation of histones correlates with CpG methylation and the inactive state of chromatin. There are four classes of histone deacetylase enzymes (HDACs), with members capable of deacetylation of histones and/or other protein targets [16].

DNA methyltransferase and histone deacetylase are believed to operate along the same mechanistic pathway to silence gene expression.

The histone tails can also be methylated on selected residues, such as lysine and arginine, and, depending on the amino acid and the histone modified, may exert a stimulatory or inhibitory effect on transcription. However, histone lysine methylation patterns and their effects on transcription are more complex than acetylation, in that some methylation sites are associated with transcriptionally permissive chromatin (euchromatin) and some are repressive, fostering heterochromatin formation.

In addition, ε-amino groups of lysine residues can be mono-, di-, or tri-methylated. Overall, the H3K27me3 and H3K9me states are associated with silencing, whereas the H3K4me3 and H3K36me3 states are transcriptionally permissive modifications.

7.3.3 MicroRNA (miRNA, MiRNA)

MicroRNAs (miRNAs) are very important factors that modify the gene transcription activity. Small-RNA-guided gene regulation has emerged as one of the fundamental principles in cell function.

A miRNA (Fig. 7.2) is a small noncoding RNA molecule containing 20–22 nucleotides found in plants, animals, and some viruses that functions in RNA silencing and posttranscriptional regulation of gene expression. While the majority of miRNAs are located within the cell, some miRNAs, commonly known as circulating miRNAs or extracellular miRNAs, have also been found in extracellular environment, including various biological fluids and cell culture media. Plant miRNAs usually have near-perfect pairing with their mRNA targets, which induces gene repression through cleavage of the target transcripts. In contrast, animal miRNAs are able to recognize their target mRNAs by using as little as 6–8 nucleotides (the seed region) at the 5′ end of the miRNA, which is not enough pairing to induce cleavage of the target mRNAs. A given miRNA may have hundreds of different mRNA targets, and a given target might be regulated by multiple miRNAs.

The mature miRNA is part of an active *RNA-induced silencing complex* (RISC) containing *Dicer* and many associated proteins. (*Dicer, also known as endoribonuclease Dicer, is an enzyme of the RNase III family that cleaves double-stranded RNA and pre-microRNA (pre-miRNA) into short double-stranded RNA fragments calle.3d small interfering RNA and microRNA, respectively.*) (Fig. 7.2)

miRNA genes are transcribed by the RNA polymerase II, which encodes a nucleotide sequence called *hairpin loop*. This hairpin loop structure, called also primary miRNA (pri-miRNA) composed of about 70 nucleotides, undergoes a first modification in the nucleus becoming a pre-miRNA. The hairpin double-stranded RNA in the pri-miRNA is recognized by a nuclear protein known as DGCR8 (*DiGeorge syndrome critical region 8*), which is associated with the enzyme *Drosha*, a protein that cuts RNA; this protein complex cuts about 11 nucleotides from the hairpin base, transforming the pri-miRNA in a pre-miRNA (precursor miRNA). The pre-miRNA is then exported from the nucleus into the cytoplasm where it is further processed and pre-miRNA is cleaved by the RNase III enzyme "Dicer," yielding a miRNA–miRNA duplex of about 22 nucleotides in length. Although either strand of the duplex may act as a functional miRNA, only one strand is usually incorporated into a silencing complex, the *RNA-induced silencing complex* (RISC), that interacts with its mRNA target. In fact, to become active, miRNAs have to bind to a protein complex, the Argonaute proteins, so becoming part of an active RISC containing *Dicer* and many associated proteins [17]. Therefore, miRNAs serve as a guide to direct Argonaute proteins to specific target messenger RNAs to repress protein

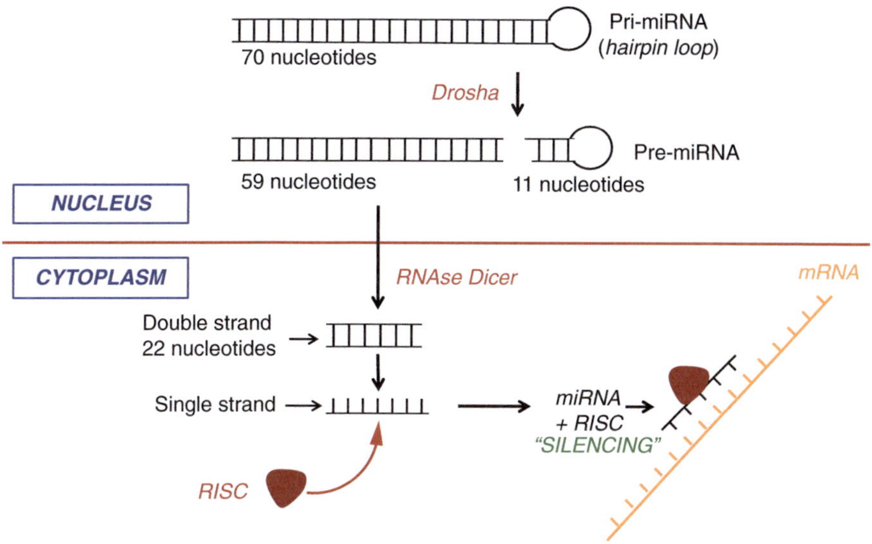

Fig. 7.2 microRNA (miRNA) transcription, modifications and binding to target site

expression. Argonaute proteins therefore are highly specialized binding modules that accommodate the small RNA component – the miRNAs – and coordinate downstream gene-silencing events by interacting with other protein factors. Argonaute protein family, therefore, is actually the key player in gene-silencing pathways guided by miRNAs.

Gene silencing may occur either via mRNA degradation or preventing mRNA from being translated. miRNAs function via base pairing with complementary sequences within mRNA molecules. As a result, these mRNA molecules are silenced, by one or more of the following processes: (a) cleavage of the mRNA strand into two pieces, (b) destabilization of the mRNA through shortening of its poly(A) tail, and (c) less efficient translation of mRNA into proteins by ribosomes [18, 19].

The human genome may encode over 2000 miRNAs [20], which are abundant in many mammalian cell types and appear to target about 60% of the genes of humans and other mammals [21, 22]. Therefore, 60% of human protein-coding genes are regulated by miRNAs [22]. Each miRNA expressed in a cell may target about 100–200 messenger RNAs that it downregulates.

miRNAs are well conserved in both plants and animals and are thought to be a vital and evolutionarily ancient component of gene regulation. A given miRNA may have hundreds of different mRNA targets, and a given target might be regulated by multiple miRNA [22].

Many miRNAs are epigenetically regulated, meaning that the diet can significantly modulate the activity of many miRNA. About 50% of miRNA genes are associated with CpG islands [23] that may be repressed by epigenetic methylation. Transcription from methylated CpG islands is strongly and heritably repressed [24].

Other miRNAs are epigenetically regulated by either histone modifications or by combined DNA methylation and histone modification [23].

Turnover of mature miRNA is needed for rapid changes in miRNA expression profiles. During miRNA maturation in the cytoplasm, uptake by the Argonaute protein is thought to stabilize the guide strand, while the opposite (or "passenger") strand is preferentially destroyed. In what has been called a "use it or lose it" strategy, Argonaute may preferentially retain miRNAs with many targets over miRNAs with few or no targets, leading to degradation of the nontargeting molecules [25].

7.4 MicroRNA Dysregulation and Diseases

Just as miRNA is involved in the normal functioning of eukaryotic cells, so has dysregulation of miRNA been associated with disease. For example, a mutation in the seed region of microRNA-96 (miR-96) has been shown to cause hereditary progressive hearing loss [26]; a mutation in the seed region of miR-184 causes hereditary keratoconus with anterior polar cataract [27]; deletion of the miR-17~92 cluster causes skeletal and growth defects [28].

7.4.1 MicroRNA Dysregulation and Cancer

Chronic lymphocytic leukemia was the first human disease demonstrated to be associated with miRNA dysregulation [29]. Many other miRNAs also have links with cancer and accordingly are sometimes referred to as "oncomirs." In malignant B cells, miRNAs participate in pathways fundamental to B-cell development like B-cell receptor (BCR) signaling, B-cell migration/adhesion, cell–cell interactions in immune niches, and the production and class switching of immunoglobulins. MiRNAs influence B-cell maturation and generation of pre-, marginal zone, follicular, B1, plasma, and memory B cells [29].

Leukemia can be caused by the insertion of a viral genome next to the 17–92 array of microRNAs, leading to increased expression of this microRNA [29]. Two types of miRNA inhibit the E2F1 protein, a protein that regulates cell proliferation. miRNA appears to bind to messenger RNA before it can be translated to proteins that switch genes on and off [29]. By measuring activity among 217 genes encoding miRNAs, patterns of gene activity that can distinguish types of cancers were identified. MiRNA profiling can determine whether patients with chronic lymphocytic leukemia had slow-growing or aggressive forms of the cancer [29].

Another role for miRNA in cancers is to use their expression level for prognosis. For example, one study on non-small-cell lung carcinoma found that low miR-324a levels could serve as an indicator of poor survival [30]. Either high miR-185 or low miR-133b levels correlate with metastasis and poor survival in colorectal cancer [31].

Furthermore, specific miRNAs may be associated with certain histological subtypes of colorectal cancer. For instance, expression levels of miR-205 and miR-373 have been shown to be increased in mucinous colorectal cancers and mucin-producing ulcerative colitis-associated colon cancers, but not in sporadic colonic adenocarcinoma that lacks mucinous components [32]. In vitro studies suggested that miR-205 and miR-373 may functionally induce different features of mucinous-associated neoplastic progression in intestinal epithelial cells [32].

In classical Hodgkin lymphoma, plasma miR-21, miR-494, and miR-1973 are promising disease response biomarkers [33].

miR-205 is significantly underexpressed in breast tumors compared with matched normal breast tissue. Moreover, breast cancer cell lines, including MCF-7 and MDA-MB-231, express a lower level of miR-205 than the nonmalignant MCF-10A cells. Ectopic expression of miR-205 significantly inhibits cell proliferation and anchorage-independent growth as well as cell invasion. These findings establish the tumor-suppressive role of miR-205, which probably is a direct targeting of oncogenes such as ErbB3 and Zeb1. Therefore, miR-205 may serve as a unique therapeutic target for breast cancer [34].

Five members of the microRNA-200 family (miR-200a, miR-200b, miR-200c, miR-141, and miR-429) are downregulated in tumor progression of breast cancer [35].

miR-506 has been found to work as a tumor antagonist. In fact, ectopic overexpression of miR-506 in ovarian cancer cells was sufficient to inhibit proliferation and to promote senescence by directly targeting the CDK4/6-FOXM1 axis in ovarian cancer [36]. A significant number of cervical cancer samples were found to have downregulated expression of miR-506. Additionally, studies found that miR-506 works to promote apoptosis of cervical cancer cells, through its direct target the hedgehog pathway transcription factor, Gli3 [37].

7.4.2 MicroRNA, DNA Repair, and Cancer

DNA damage is considered to be the primary underlying cause of cancer [38]. In fact, a number of measurable epigenetic alterations have been detected very early in normal appearing tissue undergoing histologically invisible tumorigenesis [38]. If DNA repair is deficient, damage can accumulate. Such damage can cause mutational errors during DNA replication due to error-prone translesion synthesis. It has been shown the central role of epigenetic deficiencies in DNA repair gene expression that arise during progression to cancer. Accumulated damage can cause epigenetic alterations due to errors during DNA repair. Such mutations and epigenetic alterations can give rise to cancer [39, 40].

In 29–66% of glioblastomas [41, 42], DNA repair is deficient due to epigenetic methylation of the O-6-methylguanine-DNA methyltransferase (MGMT) gene, which reduces protein expression of MGMT. However, for 28% of glioblastomas, the MGMT protein is deficient, but the MGMT promoter is not methylated [41]. In glioblastomas without methylated MGMT promoters, the level of microRNA miR-181d is inversely correlated with protein expression of MGMT, and the direct target of miR-181d is the MGMT mRNA 3'UTR [41]. Thus, in 28% of glioblastomas, increased expression of miR-181d and reduced expression of DNA repair enzyme MGMT may represent a causal factor.

HMGA proteins (HMGA1a, HMGA1b, and HMGA2) are implicated in cancer, and expression of these proteins is regulated by microRNAs. HMGA expression is almost undetectable in differentiated adult tissues but is elevated in many cancers. HMGA proteins are polypeptides of ~100 amino acid residues characterized by a modular sequence organization. These proteins have three highly positively charged regions, termed AT hooks, that bind the minor groove of AT-rich DNA stretches in specific regions of DNA. Human cancers, including thyroid, prostatic, cervical, colorectal, pancreatic, and ovarian carcinomas, show a strong increase of HMGA1a and HMGA1b proteins [43].

A 2003 study [44] showed that HMGA1 protein binds to the promoter region of DNA repair gene BRCA1 (involved in breast cancer) and inhibits BRCA1 promoter activity. They also showed that while only 11% of breast tumors had hypermethylation of the BRCA1 gene, 82% of aggressive breast cancers have low BRCA1 protein expression, and most of these reductions were due to chromatin remodeling by high levels of HMGA1 protein.

ERCC-1 (DNA excision repair protein) is a protein that in humans together with ERCC4 forms the ERCC1-XPF enzyme complex that participates in DNA repair and DNA recombination. HMGA2 protein specifically targets the promoter of ERCC1 gene, thus reducing the expression of this DNA repair gene [45]. ERCC-1 protein expression was deficient in 100% of 47 evaluated colon cancers [46]. In normal tissues, HGMA1 and HMGA2 genes are targeted (and thus strongly reduced in expression) by miR-15, miR-16, miR-26a, miR-196a2, and Let-7a [47]. Three of these microRNAs (miR-16, miR-196a and Let-7a) [48, 49] have methylated promoters and therefore low expression in colon cancer. For two of these, miR-15 and miR-16, the coding regions are epigenetically silenced in cancer due to histone deacetylase activity [50]. When these microRNAs are expressed at a low level, then HMGA1 and HMGA2 proteins are expressed at a high level. HMGA1 and HMGA2 target (reduced expression of) BRCA1 and ERCC1 DNA repair genes [51]. Thus DNA repair can be reduced, likely contributing to cancer progression [38].

In contrast to the previous example, where under-expression of miRNAs indirectly caused reduced expression of DNA repair genes, in some cases overexpression of certain miRNAs may directly reduce expression of specific DNA repair proteins. A study [52] referred to six DNA repair genes that are directly targeted by the miRNAs indicated *ATM* (miR-421), *RAD52* (miR-210, miR-373), *RAD23B* (miR-373), *MSH2* (miR-21), *BRCA1* (miR-182), and *P53* (miR-504, miR-125b). More recently, a study [53] listed multiple DNA repair genes directly targeted by these additional miRNAs: *ATM* (miR-100, miR-18a, miR-101), *DNA-PK* (miR-101), *ATR* (miR-185), *Wip1* (miR-16), *MLH1*, *MSH2*, *MSH6* (miR-155), *ERCC3*, *ERCC4* (miR-192), and *UNG2* (miR-16, miR-34c). Among these miRNAs, miR-16, miR-18a, miR-21, miR-34c, miR-101, miR-125b, miR-155, miR-182, miR-185, miR-192, and miR-373 were identified as overexpressed in colon cancer through epigenetic hypomethylation [49]. Overexpression of any one of these miRNAs can cause reduced expression of its target DNA repair gene.

To this purpose, we should recall that high red meat (HRM) intake is associated with increased colon cancer, while resistant starch is probably protective. Resistant starch fermentation produces butyrate, which can alter microRNA (miRNA) levels in colorectal cancer cells in vitro. In a randomized crossover study, 23 volunteers undertook 4-week dietary interventions: an HRM diet (300 g/day lean red meat) and an HRM + HAMSB diet (HRM with 40 g/day butyrylated high-amylose maize starch). Levels of oncogenic mature miRNAs, including miR-17–92 cluster miRNAs and miR-21, increased in the rectal mucosa with the HRM diet, whereas the HRM + HAMSB diet restored miR-17–92 miRNAs, but not miR-21, to baseline levels. Elevated miR-17–92 and miR-21 in the HRM diet corresponded with increased cell proliferation and a decrease in miR-17–92 target gene transcript levels, including the cell cycle inhibitor *CDKN1A (target of miR-17 and miR-20a)*. The oncogenic miR-17–92 cluster is differentially regulated by dietary factors that increase or decrease risk for colorectal cancer, and this may explain, at least in part, the respective risk profiles of HRM and resistant starch. These findings support the carcinogenic activity of a HRM (red meat) diet and the increased resistant starch consumption as a means of reducing risk associated with an HRM diet [54].

7.4.3 MicroRNA and Obesity

The most frequent disease associated with obesity and particularly with visceral obesity is the "metabolic syndrome," a constellation of symptoms, signs, and pathophysiological conditions including visceral obesity, insulin resistance, impaired glucose metabolism, and type 2 diabetes mellitus (DM), as well as atherogenic dyslipidemia, elevated blood pressure, and other comorbidities including a prothrombotic and pro-inflammatory state and nonalcoholic fatty liver disease. All these conditions independently increase the risk of atherosclerotic diseases, such as ischemic heart disease and stroke. Among metabolic derangements induced by excess fat accumulation, insulin resistance appears to be the most important metabolic consequence of abdominal fat accumulation, leading in most cases to insulin resistance and type 2 diabetes mellitus.

miRNAs play an important role in the regulation of stem cell progenitors differentiating into adipocytes. In immortalized human bone marrow-derived stromal cell line hMSC-Tert20, a decreased expression of miR-155, miR-221, and miR-222 has been found during the adipogenic programming of both immortalized and primary hMSCs, suggesting that they act as negative regulators of differentiation [55]. Conversely, ectopic expression of the miRNAs 155, 221, and 222 significantly inhibited adipogenesis and repressed induction of the master regulators PPARγ and CCAAT/enhancer-binding protein alpha (CEBPA) [56]. This paves the way for possible genetic obesity treatments.

7.4.4 MicroRNA and Atherosclerosis

MicroRNAs are also involved in atherosclerosis. miR-712 has been identified as a potential biomarker (i.e., predictor) for atherosclerosis, the well-known pathological condition of the arterial wall associated with lipid retention and inflammation.

The non-laminar blood flow is one among the numerous factors that influence the onset of atherosclerosis; it correlates with development of atherosclerosis as mechanosensors of endothelial cells respond to the shear force of disturbed flow (d-flow). A number of pro-atherogenic genes including matrix metalloproteinases (MMPs) are upregulated by d-flow, mediating pro-inflammatory and pro-angiogenic signals. These findings were observed in ligated carotid arteries of mice to mimic the effects of d-flow. Within 24 h, pre-existing immature miR-712 formed mature miR-712 suggesting that miR-712 is flow-sensitive [51]. Coinciding with these results, miR-712 is also upregulated in endothelial cells exposed to naturally occurring d-flow in the greater curvature of the aortic arch [51].

Concerning the mode of action of miR-712, this microRNA targets tissue inhibitor of metalloproteinases 3 (TIMP3) [51]. TIMPs normally regulate activity of matrix metalloproteinases (MMPs) which degrade the extracellular matrix (ECM). Arterial ECM is mainly composed of collagen and elastin fibers, providing the structural support and recoil properties of arteries [57]. These fibers play a critical role in regulation of vascular inflammation and permeability, which are important in the development of atherosclerosis [58]. Expressed by endothelial cells, TIMP3 is the only ECM-bound TIMP [57]. A decrease in TIMP3 expression results in an increase of ECM degradation in the presence of d-flow. Consistent with these findings, inhibition of pre-miR-712 increases expression of TIMP3 in cells, even when exposed to turbulent flow [51].

TIMP3 also decreases the expression of TNFα (a pro-inflammatory cytokine) during turbulent flow [51]. Activity of TNFα in turbulent flow was measured by the expression of TNFα-converting enzyme (TACE) in blood. TNFα decreased if miR-712 was inhibited or TIMP3 overexpressed [51], suggesting that miR-712 and TIMP3 regulate TACE activity in turbulent flow conditions.

Anti-miR-712 effectively suppresses d-flow-induced miR-712 expression and increases TIMP3 expression [51]. Anti-miR-712 also inhibits vascular hyperpermeability, thereby significantly reducing atherosclerosis lesion development and immune cell infiltration [51].

7.4.5 miRNA and Dementia

As previously described (Chap. 5, Sect. 5.4), miRNAs have been shown to have important protective role also on aging cognitive decline, with a significant impact on silencing numerous brain genes. This protective effect was mainly observed with olive oil polyphenols. Mice fed with high-polyphenol-content olive oil displayed a cortex miRNA expression profile similar to that observed in young mice. Numerous miRNAs have been shown to be actively modulated. At the top ranking score was miR-30a-5p, predicted to control a large number of genes involved in pathways, such as axon guidance, ubiquitin-mediated proteolysis, regulation of actin cytoskeleton, and long-term potentiation. For further details, see Chap. 5, Sect. 5.4.

7.5 EVOO, Oleic Acid, Polyphenols, and Gene Transcription

As described in previous chapters, intake of extra-virgin olive oil (EVOO), rich in polyphenols, is effective in lowering blood pressure in hypertensive patients, reducing lipid and DNA oxidation, ameliorating lipid profile and insulin resistance, inflammation, and endothelial dysfunction, thus leading to protection against cardiovascular disease (CVD). EVOO has been also shown to have a favorable effect on the tumorigenesis and cancer progression due to its ability to modify structure and function of cell membrane, the modulation of cell signal transduction pathways, the regulation of gene expression, and the oncogenes.

7.5.1 "In Vitro" Studies: The Effect of Oleic Acid

In "in vitro" studies on tumor-derived cell lines naturally exhibiting HER2 gene amplification and p185 (Her-2/neu) oncoprotein overexpression, the exogenous supplementation of oleic acid significantly downregulated HER2-coded p185 oncoprotein in cancer cells harboring amplification of HER gene. The exposure to oleic acid specifically repressed the transcriptional activity of the human HER gene promoter [59]. In fact, physiological concentrations of oleic acid were found to suppress the overexpression of HER2 (Her-2/neu, erbB-2), the well-characterized oncogene playing a key role in the etiology, progression, and response to chemotherapy and endocrine therapy in approximately 20% of breast carcinomas. Oleic acid treatment was also found to synergistically enhance the efficacy of trastuzumab, a humanized monoclonal antibody binding with high affinity to the ectodomain of the Her2-coded p185 (HER2) oncoprotein. Moreover, oleic acid exposure significantly diminished the proteolytic cleavage of the ectodomain of HER2 and, consequently, its activation status, a crucial molecular event that determines both the aggressive behavior and the response to trastuzumab of HER2-overexpressing breast carcinomas. Oleic acid suppressed HER2 at the transcriptional level, by upregulating expression of Ets protein PEA3-aDNA-binding protein that specifically blocks HER2 promoter activity in breast, ovarian, and stomach cancer cell lines.

This anti-HER2 property of oleic acid offered a previously unrecognized molecular mechanism by which olive oil may regulate the malignant behavior of cancer cell [59, 60].

7.5.2 "In Vivo" Studies: Single Dose Studies of EVOO

In a recent study [61] conducted on peripheral blood mononuclear cells (PBMCs), the intake of a single dose of olive oil rich in polyphenols modulated the transcription of genes and miRNAs involved in metabolism, inflammation, and cancer, switching PBMCs to a less deleterious inflammatory phenotype.

Twelve healthy subjects and 12 patients at the first diagnosis of metabolic syndrome were recruited for this study. After a 1-week washout period during which no olive oil consumption was allowed, the subjects underwent EVOO intake in a single dose. They received 50 mL of either high- or low-polyphenol EVOO. Samples for serum biochemistry and whole blood for PBMC isolation were collected 4 h after EVOO administration. Gene expression microarrays were performed in both healthy controls and patients with metabolic syndrome.

At the paired analysis (T0, baseline values, vs. T1, 4 h after EVOO administration), high-polyphenol EVOO induced the modulation of 2438 annotated genes (1376 upregulated and 1062 downregulated, out of total 2447 differentially modulated; $p < 0.05$) in the PBMCs of healthy subjects and of 954 annotated genes (403 upregulated and 551 downregulated, out of total 963 differentially modulated; $p < 0.05$) in the PBMCs of patients with metabolic syndrome. Of these hits, 389 annotated genes (195 overexpressed and 194 under-expressed) were consistently changed in both control and metabolic syndrome groups. High-polyphenol EVOO intake induced dramatic changes in the mRNA abundance of a number of genes, with important modulation of the immune response (e.g., *upregulation of CD28 signaling in T helper cells and Fcγ receptor-mediated phagocytosis in macrophages and monocytes; suppression of the NFAT in the regulation of the immune response and of PI3K signaling in B lymphocytes*) and of different inflammatory signals (*suppression of both B-cell and T-cell receptors, NF-κB, IL1/3/8, RANK, and thrombin signaling cascades as well as of the LPS-stimulated MAPK activation and of the NRF2-mediated oxidative stress responses*).

Also pathways involved in metabolism and cardio-metabolic risk appeared to be modulated by high-polyphenol EVOO intake, with suppression of protein kinase A, PI3K/AKT signaling, CREB, mTOR, and cholesterol biosynthesis, as well as of mechanisms involved in cardiac hypertrophy, adipogenesis, and circadian rhythms.

A negative modulation of cell proliferation pathways and cancer was also observed, with upregulation of the DNA damage response systems and suppression of different pathways involved in cell and cancer proliferation such as ERK/MAPK, CXCR4, HGF/EGF, and HIF1α signaling cascades.

Also glucose metabolism (both gluconeogenesis and glycolysis as well as the biosynthesis of acetyl-CoA by the pyruvate dehydrogenase complex) and pathways involved in the metabolism of different amino acids (aspartate, cysteine, isoleucine, leucine, methionine, valine, tryptophan) appeared upregulated.

High-polyphenol EVOO modulated also a set of transcripts coding for proteins participating to the transcriptional machinery of different nuclear receptors (e.g., both androgen and estrogen receptors, glucocorticoid receptor, and retinoid acid receptors).

Using RTqPCR to confirm the most important hits modulated by high-polyphenol EVOO, numerous genes were considered "biologically relevant" and defined "statistically significant" for $p < 0.05$ and "significantly modulated" for $p < 0.01$. Using these criteria, numerous genes were confirmed as upregulated, including the Argonaute RISC catalytic component 2 (AGO2), involved in miRNA biogenesis, and central modulator of RNA posttranscriptional modification and protein synthesis.

To confirm that also miRNAs were modulated by EVOO, miRNA expression profile was studied with microarrays. Six genes were confirmed as downregulated and two genes upregulated. The six downregulated genes were:

1. miR-146b-5p, overexpressed in human atherosclerotic plaques and upregulated in human monocytes/macrophages stimulated with oxidized LDL
2. miR-19a-3p, involved in oncogenesis
3. miR-181b-5p, involved in modulation on inflammation and cancer
4. miR-107, known to be suppressed by fatty acids and associated with obesity, insulin resistance and fatty liver, and acute myocardial infarction
5. miR-769-5p, overexpressed in melanoma cells; promotes cell proliferation
6. miR-192-5p, associated with impaired glucose metabolism, fatty liver, and acute myocardial infarction

The two upregulated genes were:

1. miR-23b-3p, known as anti-inflammatory
2. miR-519b-3p, known as tumor suppressor

The majority of these miRNAs were significantly modulated mainly in normal individuals, while in subjects affected by metabolic syndrome, they were much less modulated, so confirming that EVOO intake expresses the best of its effectiveness in healthy individuals, i.e., in primary prevention, than in secondary prevention, i.e., individual already affected by metabolic syndrome.

The results of this study [61] have shown that the intake of EVOO with high concentration of polyphenols (~400 ppm) exerts transcriptional effects potentially beneficial in insulin resistance (i.e., miR-107), inflammation (i.e., miR-181b-5p), and cancer (i.e., miR-19a-3p, miR-519-3p). As far as cancer is concerned, EVOO intake also showed to modulate protective mechanisms of tumorigenesis, i.e., upregulation of the DNA damage response system (protective for cancer) and suppression of different pathways involved in cell proliferation (e.g., ERK/MAPK, CXR4, HGF/EGF, and HIF1α signaling cascade). Finally, EVOO also downregulated AGO2, a key player in miRNA processing (pre-miRNA cleavage and mature miRNA release) [62], thus pointing to miRNA as possible targets modulated by EVOO.

In another study [63], the human in vivo gene expression changes were assessed in the postprandial period after intake of a single 50 mL dose of EVOO, by analyzing microarray data. The aim was to assess gene expression changes in PBMCs of healthy volunteers 6 h after the VOO dose. This time point was selected because it reflected the end of the postprandial state. At baseline (0 h) and at post-ingestion (6 h), total RNA was isolated and gene expression (29,082 genes) was evaluated by microarray. From microarray data, nutrient–gene interactions were observed in genes related to metabolism, cellular processes, cancer, and atherosclerosis (e.g., USP48 by 2.16; OGT by 1.68-fold change) and associated processes such as inflammation (e.g., AKAP13 by 2.30; IL-10 by 1.66-fold change) and DNA damage (e.g.,

DCLRE1C by 1.47; POLK by 1.44-fold change). The highest downregulation appeared in genes related to environmental information processing pathways. Microarray results were verified by qRT-PCR in all five upregulated genes (*ADAM17, IL10, OGT, USP48*, and *AKAP13*). When results obtained by microarray were verified by qRT-PCR in nine genes, full concordance was achieved only in the case of upregulated genes (*ADAM17, ADRB2, ALOX5AP, CD36, LIAS, OGT, PPARBP*). This acute 50 mL VOO dose also promoted in vivo time course changes, as measured by qRT-PCR, in the expression of genes related to insulin resistance, oxidative stress, and inflammation in healthy volunteers [64]. These results supported the hypothesis that postprandial protective changes related to olive oil consumption are mediated through gene expression changes.

In another study [65] on human PBMCs, a breakfast based on virgin olive oil, high in polyphenols (398 ppm), showed to postprandially repress the expression of pro-inflammatory genes when compared with a common olive oil-based breakfast (low in polyphenols, 70 ppm). Twenty adults (9 men, 11 women), fulfilling at least 3 criteria for metabolic syndrome, participated in this randomized crossover trial. 45,220 probe sets were tested to interrogate the expression of 30,886 unique human genes. Inflammatory disorder was the most highly represented disorder (39 genes). From these, 35 genes (PTGS2, IL1B, IL6, OSM, CCL3, CXCL1, CXCL2, CXCL3, CXCR4, NAMPT, DUSP1, DUSP2, EGR1, EGR2, EGR3, EREG, FOSB, G0S2, JUN, JUNB, NFKBIA, NFKBIZ, NR4A1, NR4A2, PER1, SOCS3, SOD2, TAGAP, TNFAIP3, ZFP36, AREG, CA2, CD69, CD83, CDKN2A) were under-expressed, and after intake of virgin olive oil with high content in phenolic compounds, 4 genes were overexpressed (CCR2, CA1, CPVL, FN1). Cellular functions most strongly associated with the differentially expressed genes were cell death (41 genes), cell migration (24 genes), cell division (23 genes), cell proliferation (32 genes), and transcription (25 genes). These data demonstrated that in vivo the phenol fraction of EVOO is able to repress the expression of several genes related to inflammation pathways in patients with metabolic syndrome during postprandial period. This finding draws interest since pro-inflammatory state remains one component of metabolic syndrome in which low-grade inflammation is often associated with endothelial dysfunction and by itself is associated with the development of atherosclerosis. The conclusions were that intake of breakfast based in virgin olive oil rich in phenol compounds is able to repress expression of several pro-inflammatory genes in vivo, thereby switching activity of PBMCs to a less deleterious inflammatory profile. These results provided at least a partial molecular basis for risk reduction of cardiovascular disease observed in Mediterranean countries, where EVOO represents a main source of dietary fat.

7.5.3 "In Vivo" Studies: Sustained EVOO Consumption

Ten healthy individuals, six men and four women, participated in a linear study with an intervention period of 3 weeks and a daily EVOO consumption of 25 mL/day, a common intake of EVOO in Mediterranean diet [66]. The objective of the study was to identify the PBMC genes that respond to EVOO consumption in order to ascertain the molecular mechanisms underlying the beneficial action of EVOO in the prevention of atherosclerosis. The response to EVOO consumption was confirmed for individual samples (n = 10) by qPCR for ten upregulated genes (ADAM17, ALDH1A1, BIRC1, ERCC5, LIAS, OGT, PPARBP, TNFSF10, USP48, and XRCC5). These results showed that 3 weeks of nutritional intervention with EVOO supplementation, at doses common in the Mediterranean diet, can alter the expression of genes related to atherosclerosis development and progression [66].

In another study [67], a randomized, parallel, double-blind trial, the effect of diets supplemented with a mixture of conjugated linoleic acids (CLAs) versus olive oil (control group) on adipocyte gene expression changes was examined. Eighty-one healthy postmenopausal women participated in this study. After a 16-week consumption, the CLA group had less total fat mass (4%) and lower-body fat mass (7%) than the control ($P = 0.02$ and <0.001, respectively). Post hoc analyses showed that serum insulin concentrations were greater in the CLA-mix group (34%) than the control group ($P = 0.02$) in the highest waist circumference tertile only. Adipose tissue mRNA expression of glucose transporter 4, leptin, and lipoprotein lipase was lower, whereas expression of TNFα was higher in the CLA-mix group than in the control group ($P < 0.04$). In conclusion, a 50:50 mixture of conjugated linoleic acids isomers resulted in less total and lower-body fat mass in postmenopausal women and greater serum insulin concentrations in the highest waist circumference tertile.

The specific effect of the MUFA-rich diet, mainly in the form of refined olive oil (OO), versus SFA-rich diets on gene expression has been reported [68]. In a parallel controlled-feeding trial conducted in 20 abdominally overweight subjects at risk of metabolic syndrome, who followed for 8 weeks a diet rich in saturated (SFA) or monounsaturated fat (MUFA), the insulin sensitivity, serum lipids, and gene expression profiles of adipose tissue were studied. Adipose tissue samples underwent whole-genome microarray and histologic analysis. Consumption of the SFA diet resulted in an increased expression of genes involved in inflammation processes in adipose tissue, determining a pro-inflammatory "obesity-linked" profile: upregulation of immune function and inflammation-related processes and downregulation of amino acid metabolism and fatty acid metabolism. The MUFA diet led to a more anti-inflammatory gene expression profile, which was accompanied by a decrease in serum LDL-cholesterol concentrations and an increase in plasma and adipose tissue oleic acid content. Microarray results were validated by q-PCR analysis in a set of genes involved in inflammatory processes. The *ADIPOQ* gene was downregulated, and *CCL5/RANTES*, *CD14*, and *RAC2* genes were upregulated both in microarrays and qPCR results, after SFA-rich diet. After MUFA-rich diet, the *CD163* gene was downregulated. For the other four genes tested (*C1QB*, *CTSS*, *ITGB2*, *PPAR*), qPCR changes did not reach statistical significance. The conclusions were that consumption of an SFA diet resulted in a pro-inflammatory "obesity-linked" gene expression profile, whereas consumption of a MUFA diet caused a more anti-inflammatory profile. These data suggested that replacement of dietary SFA with MUFA could prevent adipose tissue inflammation and may reduce the risk of inflammation-related diseases such as metabolic syndrome.

The first study proposing a possible molecular scheme of action after polyphenol-rich olive oil consumption in a human intervention study was a sub-study [69] of the EUROLIVE study. In this randomized, crossover, controlled trial, 18 healthy European volunteers received daily 25 mL olive oil with a low polyphenol content (LPC, 2.7 mg/kg) or a high polyphenol content (HPC, 366 mg/kg) in intervention periods of 3 weeks separated by 2-week washout periods. Results showed a decrease of systemic LDL oxidation and monocyte chemoattractant protein 1 and the expression of pro-atherogenic genes in peripheral blood mononuclear cells [i.e., CD40 ligand (CD40L), IL-23α subunit p19 (IL23A), adrenergic β-2 receptor (ADRB2), oxidized LDL (lectin-like) receptor 1 (OLR1), and IL-8 receptor-α (IL8RA)] after the HPC intervention compared with after the LPC intervention. Random-effect linear regression analyses showed (1) a significant decrease in CD40, ADRB2, and IL8RA gene expression with the decrease of LDL oxidation and (2) a significant decrease in intercellular adhesion molecule 1 and OLR1 gene expression with increasing concentrations of tyrosol and hydroxytyrosol in urine. On the basis of these results, an integrated scheme for the in vivo downregulation of the CD40/CD40L system and its downstream products promoted by olive oil polyphenol consumption was proposed. CD40 and sCD40L belong to the tumor necrosis factor (TNF) superfamily, and they are molecules with a dual prothrombotic and pro-inflammatory role [70]. The CD40L triggers inflammatory signals in cells of the vascular wall, representing a major pathogenetic pathway of atherosclerosis [71]. Systemic LDL oxidation, total cholesterol, and plasma MCP1 decreased after the high-polyphenol intervention compared with after the low-polyphenol intervention. The reduction in LDL oxidation and the increase in antioxidant polyphenols, promoted by the regular dietary intake of polyphenol-rich OO, were associated with a downregulation in the expression of genes related to the CD40/CD40L pathway.

7.5.4 The Combined Transcriptomic Effect of the Mediterranean Diet and the Polyphenols of Olive Oil

The numerous results on Mediterranean diet and EVOO polyphenols make plausible the hypothesis that changes in the expression of genes could be mediated by both the traditional Mediterranean diet and EVOO polyphenols, in association.

About this, a randomized, parallel, controlled clinical trial in healthy volunteers (n=90) aged 20–50 years was performed, aimed to assess whether benefits associated with the traditional Mediterranean diet (TMD) and virgin olive oil (VOO) consumption could be mediated through changes in the expression of atherosclerosis-related genes [72, 73]. Three-month intervention groups were as follows: (1) TMD with VOO (TMD + VOO), (2) TMD with washed virgin olive oil (TMD + WOO), and (3) control with participants' habitual diet. WOO was similar to VOO but with a lower polyphenol content (55 vs. 328 mg/kg, respectively). TMD consumption decreased plasma oxidative and inflammatory status and decreased gene expression related to both inflammation (interferon gamma, INFɣ), Rho GTPase-activating protein15 (ARHGAP15), and interleukin-7 receptor (IL7R) and

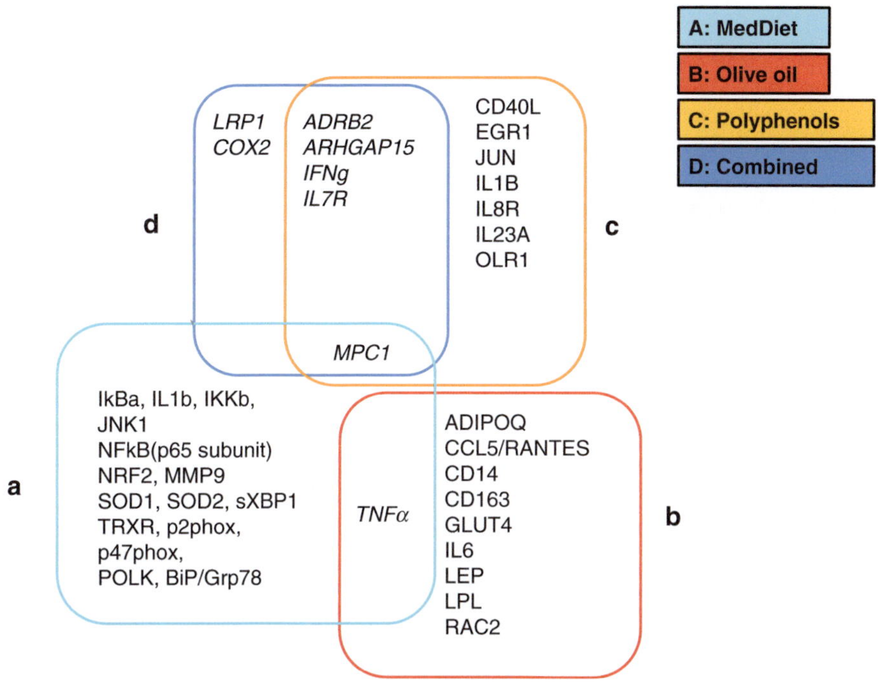

Fig. 7.3 Genes differentially expressed, as verified by qRT-PCR, in transcriptomic studies in humans after (**a**) Mediterranean diet intervention, (**b**) olive oil intervention, (**c**) olive oil phenolic compounds intervention, and (**d**) Mediterranean diet and olive oil combined intervention (From [71], modified)

oxidative stress [adrenergic beta(2)-receptor (ADRB2) and polymerase (DNA-directed) kappa (POLK)] in peripheral blood mononuclear cells. All effects, with the exception of the decrease in POLK expression, were particularly observed when VOO, rich in polyphenols, was present in the TMD dietary pattern. These results confirmed a significant role of olive oil polyphenols in the downregulation of pro-atherogenic genes in the context of a TMD. The benefits associated with a TMD and olive oil polyphenol consumption on cardiovascular risk clearly appear to be mediated through nutrigenomic effects (Fig. 7.3).

7.6 Conclusive Remarks

Mediterranean diet, its main fat component olive oil, and olive oil antioxidant polyphenols have been shown to exert a modulatory effect toward a protective mode on genes related to chronic degenerative diseases, particularly atherosclerotic processes (such as oxidation and inflammation), and cancer (Fig. 7.3).

There are convincing evidences that phenolic compounds present in the olive oil are responsible for the transcriptomic effect, as shown from randomized, controlled, human studies in which similar olive oils but with differences in their phenolic content have been tested in the trials. The benefits associated with olive oil and Mediterranean diet consumption result to be mediated through changes in the expression of genes related to chronic degenerative diseases, particularly inflammation and oxidative stress (i.e., *IFN*, *IL7R*, *ADRB2*, *MCP1*, *TNF*). Despite some heterogeneity of the studies, it is widely accepted that olive oil, the main source of fat in the Mediterranean diet, is more than a MUFA-rich source and its polyphenols account for a greater nutrigenomic, protective effect.

EVOO and polyphenols have been shown to modulate also cancer-related genes toward a protective mode.

Oleic acid from olive oil, with its blocking effect of the HER2 promoter, offered for the first time a previously unrecognized mechanism by which olive oil may regulate the malignant behavior of cancer cells. Indeed, the olive oil-induced transcriptional repression of HER2 oncogene has represented a first genomic explanation linking Mediterranean diet, olive oil, and cancer, also considering that HER2 oncogene operates equally in various types of Her-2/neu-related carcinomas.

Another effect of olive oil on cancer, probably the most important, is the modulation of a number of microRNAs. miR-19a-3p (oncogenesis), miR-181b-5p (inflammation and cancer), and miR-769-5p 8 (melanoma cells) are downregulated, while miR-519b-3p (tumor suppressor) is upregulated. The active role of these miRNA has been confirmed by RTqPCR.

The gene modulatory effect of oleic acid and polyphenol-rich EVOO takes place with three main mechanisms: DNA methylation, histone modification, and microRNA blocking action. Through these effects, gene transcription activity is blocked, and this effect is called *epigenetic*. The epigenetic effect coming from nutrients (mostly from polyphenol-rich olive oil) is defined as *nutrigenetic or nutrigenomic*, being *nutrigenetic* the effect of genetic variation on dietary response, while *nutrigenomic* the role of nutrients and bioactive food compounds on gene expression.

References

1. Miggiano GA, De Sanctis R. Nutritional genomics: toward a personalized diet. Clin Ter. 2006;157:355–61.
2. Muller M, Kersten S. Nutrigenomics: goals and strategies. Nat Rev Genet. 2003;4:315–22.
3. Corella D, Ordovás JM. How does the Mediterranean diet promote cardiovascular health? Current progress toward molecular mechanisms: gene-diet interactions at the genomic, transcriptomic, and epigenomic levels provide novel insights into new mechanisms. BioEssays. 2014;36:526–37.
4. Estruch R, Ros E, Salas-Salvadó J, Covas MI, Corella D, Arós F, Gómez-Gracia E, Ruiz-Gutiérrez V, Fiol M, Lapetra J, Lamuela-Raventos RM, Serra-Majem L, Pintó X, Basora J, Muñoz MA, Sorlí JV, Martínez JA, Martínez-González MA. PREDIMED study investigators. Primary prevention of cardiovascular disease with a Mediterranean diet. New Engl J Med. 2013;368:1279–90.
5. Corella D, Carrasco P, Sorlí JV, Estruch R, Rico-Sanz J, Martínez-González MÁ, Salas-Salvadó J, Covas MI, Coltell O, Arós F, Lapetra J, Serra-Majem L, Ruiz-Gutiérrez V, Warnberg J, Fiol M, Pintó X, Ortega-Azorín C, Muñoz MÁ, Martínez JA, Gómez-Gracia E, González JI,

Ros E, Ordovás JM. Mediterranean diet reduces the adverse effect of the TCF7L2-rs7903146 polymorphism on cardiovascular risk factors and stroke incidence: a randomized controlled trial in a high-cardiovascular-risk population. Diabetes Care. 2013;36(11):3803–11.
6. Gonzalo S. Epigenetic alterations in aging. J Appl Physiol. 2010;109:586–97.
7. Daura-Oller E, Cabre M, Montero MA, Paternain JL, Romeu A. Specific gene hypomethylation and cancer: new insights into coding region feature trends. Bioinformation. 2009;3:340–3.
8. Castro R, Rivera I, Struys EA, Jansen EE, Ravasco P, Camilo ME, Blom HJ, Jakobs C, Tavares de Almeida T. Increased homocysteine concentrations and S-adenosylhomocysteine concentrations and DNA hypomethylation in vascular disease. Clin Chem. 2003;49:1292–6.
9. Huang YS, Zhi Y, Wang SR. Hypermethylation of estrogen receptor-α gene in atheromatosis patients and its correlation with homocysteine. Pathophysiology. 2009;16:259–65.
10. Dong CD, Yoon W, Goldschmidt-Clermont PJ. DNA methylation and atherosclerosis. J Nutr. 2002;132:2406S–9S.
11. Ying AK, Hassanain HH, Roos CM, Smiraglia DJ, Issa JJ, Michler RE, Caligiuri M, Plass C, Goldschmidt-Clermont PJ. Methylation of the estrogen receptor- α gene promoter is selectively increased in proliferating human aortic smooth muscle cells. Cardiovasc Res. 2000;46:172–9.
12. Heyn H, Li N, Ferreira HJ, Moran S, Pisano DG, Gomez A, Diez J, Sanchez-Mut JV, Setien F, Carmona FJ, Puca AA, Sayols S, Pujana MA, Serra-Musach J, Iglesias-Platas I, Formiga F, Fernandez AF, Fraga MF, Heath SC, Valencia A, Gut IG, Wang J, Esteller M. Distinct DNA methylomes of newborns and centenarians. Proc Natl Acad Sci U S A. 2012;109:10522–7.
13. Jenuwein T, Allis CD. Translating the histone code. Science. 2001;293:1074–80.
14. Strahl BD, Allis CD. The language of covalent histone modifications. Nature. 2000;403:41–5.
15. Berndsen CE, Denu JM. Catalysis and substrate selection by histone/protein lysine acetyltransferases. Curr Opin Struct Biol. 2008;18:682–9.
16. Michan S, Sinclair D. Sirtuins in mammals: insights into their biological function. Biochem J. 2007;404:1–13.
17. Rana TM. Illuminating the silence: understanding the structure and function of small RNAs. Nat Rev Mol Cell Biol. 2007;8:23–36.
18. Bartel DP. MicroRNAs: target recognition and regulatory functions. Cell. 2009;136:215–33.
19. Fabian MR, Sonenberg N, Filipowicz W. Regulation of mRNA translation and stability by microRNAs. Ann Review Biochem. 2010;79:351–79.
20. Bentwich I, Avniel A, Karov Y, Aharonov R, Gilad S, Barad O, Barzilai A, Einat P, Einav U, Meiri E, Sharon E, Spector Y, Bentwich Z. Identification of hundreds of conserved and nonconserved human microRNAs. Nat Genet. 2005;37:766–70.
21. Lewis BP, Burge CB, Bartel DP. Conserved seed pairing, often flanked by adenosines, indicates that thousands of human genes are microRNA targets. Cell. 2005;120:15–20.
22. Friedman RC, Farh KK, Burge CB, Bartel DP. Most mammalian mRNAs are conserved targets of microRNAs. Genome Res. 2009;19:92–105.
23. Bernal JE, Duran C, Papiha SS. Transcriptional and epigenetic regulation of human microRNAs. Cancer Lett. 2012;331:1–10.
24. Goll MG, Bestor TH. Eukaryotic cytosine methyltransferases. Annu Rev Biochem. 2005;74:481–514.
25. Kai ZS, Pasquinelli AE. MicroRNA assassins: factors that regulate the disappearance of miRNAs. Nat Struct Mol Biol. 2010;17:5–10.
26. Mencía A, Modamio-Høybjør S, Redshaw N, Morín M, Mayo-Merino F, Olavarrieta L, Aguirre LA, del Castillo I, Steel KP, Dalmay T, Moreno F, Moreno-Pelayo MA. Mutations in the seed region of human miR-96 are responsible for nonsyndromic progressive hearing loss. Nat Genet. 2009;41:609–13.
27. Hughes AE, Bradley DT, Campbell M, Lechner J, Dash DP, Simpson DA, Willoughby CE. Mutation altering the miR-184 seed region causes familial keratoconus with cataract. Am J Human Genet. 2011;89:628–33.
28. de Pontual L, Yao E, Callier P, Faivre L, Drouin V, Cariou S, Van Haeringen A, Geneviève D, Goldenberg A, Oufadem M, Manouvrier S, Munnich A, Vidigal JA, Vekemans M, Lyonnet S, Henrion-Caude A, Ventura A, Amiel J. Germline deletion of the miR-17~92 cluster causes skeletal and growth defects in humans. Nat Genet. 2011;43:1026–30.

29. Musilova K, Mraz M. MicroRNAs in B cell lymphomas: how a complex biology gets more complex. Leukemia. 2014;29:1004–17.
30. Võsa U, Vooder T, Kolde R, Fischer K, Välk K, Tõnisson N, Roosipuu R, Vilo J, Metspalu A, Annilo T. Identification of miR-374a as a prognostic marker for survival in patients with early-stage nonsmall cell lung cancer. Genes Chromosomes Cancer. 2011;50:812–22.
31. Akçakaya P, Ekelund S, Kolosenko I, Caramuta S, Ozata DM, Xie H, Lindforss U, Olivecrona H, Lui WO. miR-185 and miR-133b deregulation is associated with overall survival and metastasis in colorectal cancer. Int J Oncol. 2011;39:311–8.
32. Eyking A, Reis H, Frank M, Gerken G, Schmid KW, Cario E. MiR-205 and MiR-373 are associated with aggressive human mucinous colorectal cancer. PLoS One. 2016;11:e0156871.
33. Jones K, Nourse JP, Keane C, Bhatnagar A, Gandhi MK. Plasma MicroRNA are disease response biomarkers in classical Hodgkin lymphoma. Clin Cancer Res. 2014;20:253–64.
34. Wu H, Mo YY. Targeting miR-205 in breast cancer. Expert Opin Ther Targets. 2009;13:1439–48.
35. Gregory PA, Bert AG, Paterson EL, Barry SC, Tsykin A, Farshid G, Vadas MA, Khew-Goodall Y, Goodall GJ. The miR-200 family and miR-205 regulate epithelial to mesenchymal transition by targeting ZEB1 and SIP1. Nat Cell Biol. 2008;10:593–601.
36. Liu G, Sun Y, Ji P, Li X, Cogdell D, Yang D, Zhang W. MiR-506 suppresses proliferation and induces senescence by directly targeting the CDK4/6-FOXM1 Axis in ovarian cancer. J Pathol. 2014;233:308–18.
37. Wen SY, Lin Y, Yu YQ, Cao SJ, Zhang R, Yang XM, Zhang ZG. miR-506 acts as a tumor suppressor by directly targeting the hedgehog pathway transcription factor Gli3 in human cervical cancer. Oncogene. 2015;34:717–25.
38. Bernstein C, Prasad AR, Nfonsam V, Bernstein H. DNA damage, DNA repair and cancer. New Res Dir DNA Repair. 2013:413–65.
39. O'Hagan HM, Mohammad HP, Baylin SB. Double strand breaks can initiate gene silencing and SIRT1-dependent onset of DNA methylation in an exogenous promoter CpG island. PLoS Genet. 2008;4:e1000155.
40. Cuozzo C, Porcellini A, Angrisano T, Morano A, Lee B, Di Pardo A, Messina S, Iuliano R, Fusco A, Santillo MR, Muller MT, Chiariotti L, Gottesman ME, Avvedimento EV. DNA damage, homology-directed repair, and DNA methylation. PLoS Genet. 2007;3:e110.
41. Zhang J, Hoadley K, Kushwaha D, Ramakrishnan V, Li S, Kang C, You Y, Jiang C, Song SW, Jiang T, Chen CC. miR-181d: a predictive glioblastoma biomarker that downregulates MGMT expression. Neuro-Oncology. 2012;14:712–9.
42. Spiegl-Kreinecker S, Pirker C, Filipits M, Lötsch D, Buchroithner J, Pichler J, Silye R, Weis S, Micksche M, Fischer J, Berger W. O6-Methylguanine DNA methyltransferase protein expression in tumor cells predicts outcome of temozolomide therapy in glioblastoma patients. Neuro-Oncology. 2010;12:28–36.
43. Sgarra R, Rustighi A, Tessari MA, Di Bernardo J, Altamura S, Fusco A, Manfioletti G, Giancotti V. Nuclear phosphoproteins HMGA and their relationship with chromatin structure and cancer. FEBS Lett. 2004;574:1–8.
44. Baldassarre G, Battista S, Belletti B, Thakur S, Pentimalli F, Trapasso F, Fedele M, Pierantoni G, Croce CM, Fusco A. Negative regulation of BRCA1 gene expression by HMGA1 proteins accounts for the reduced BRCA1 protein levels in sporadic breast carcinoma. Mol Cell Biol. 2003;23:2225–38.
45. Borman L, Schwanbeck R, Heyduk T, Seebeck B, Rogalla P, Bullerdiek J, Wisniewski JR. High mobility group A2 protein and its derivatives bind a specific region of the promoter of DNA repair gene ERCC1 and modulate its activity. Nucleic Acids Res. 2003;3:6841–51.
46. Facista A, Nguyen H, Lewis C, Prasad AR, Ramsey L, Zaitlin B, Nfonsam V, Krouse RS, Bernstein H, Payne CM, Stern S, Oatman N, Banerjee B, Bernstein C. Deficient expression of DNA repair enzymes in early progression to sporadic colon cancer. Genome Integr. 2012;3:3.
47. Palmieri D, D'Angelo D, Valentino T, De Martino I, Ferraro A, Wierinckx A, Fedele M, Trouillas J, Fusco A. Downregulation of HMGA-targeting microRNAs has a critical role in human pituitary tumorigenesis. Oncogene. 2012;31:3857–65.
48. Malumbres M. miRNAs and cancer: an epigenetics view. Mol Asp Med. 2013;34:863–74.

49. Schnekenburger M, Diederich M. Epigenetics offer new horizons for colorectal cancer prevention. Curr Colorectal Cancer Rep. 2012;8:66–81.
50. Sampath D, Liu C, Vasan K, Sulda M, Puduvalli VK, Wierda WG, Keating MJ. Histone deacetylases mediate the silencing of miR-15a, miR-16, and miR-29b in chronic lymphocytic leukemia. Blood. 2012;119:1162–1172.r.
51. Son DJ, Kumar S, Takabe W, Kim CW, Ni CW, Alberts-Grill N, Jang IH, Kim S, Kim W, Won Kang S, Baker AH, Woong Seo J, Ferrara KW, Jo H. The atypical mechanosensitive microRNA-712 derived from pre-ribosomal RNA induces endothelial inflammation and atherosclerosis. Nat Commun. 2013;4:3000.
52. Wan G, Mathur R, Hu X, Zhang X, Lu X. miRNA response to DNA damage. Trends Biochem Sci. 2011;36:478–84.
53. Tessitore A, Cicciarelli G, Del Vecchio F, Gaggiano A, Verzella D, Fischietti M, Vecchiotti D, Capece D, Zazzeroni F, Alesse E. MicroRNAs in the DNA damage/repair network and cancer. Int J Genomics. 2014;2014:820248.
54. Humphreys KJ, Conlon MA, Young GP, Topping DL, Hu Y, Winter JM, Bird AR, Cobiac L, Kennedy NA, Michael MZ, Le Leu RK. Dietary manipulation of oncogenic microRNA expression in human rectal mucosa: a randomized trial. Cancer Prev Res (Phila). 2014;7:786–95.
55. Skårn M, Namløs HM, Noordhuis P, Wang MY, Meza-Zepeda LA, Myklebost O. Adipocyte differentiation of human bone marrow-derived stromal cells is modulated by microRNA-155, microRNA-221, and microRNA-222. Stem Cells Dev. 2012;21:873–83.
56. Zuo Y, Qiang L, Farmer SR. Activation of CCAAT/enhancer-binding protein (C/EBP) alpha expression by C/EBP beta during adipogenesis requires a peroxisome proliferator-activated receptor-gamma-associated repression of HDAC1 at the C/ebp alpha gene promoter. J Biol Chem. 2006;281:7960–7.
57. Basu R, Fan D, Kandalam V, Lee J, Das SK, Wang X, Baldwin TA, Oudit GY, Kassiri Z. Loss of Timp3 gene leads to abdominal aortic aneurysm formation in response to angiotensin II. J Biol Chem. 2012;287:44083–96.
58. Libby P. Inflammation in atherosclerosis. Nature. 2002;420:868–74.
59. Menendez JA, Lupu R. Mediterranean dietary traditions for the molecular treatment of human cancer: anti-oncogenic actions of the main olive oil's monounsaturated fatty acid oleic acid (18,1 n-9). Curr Pharm Biotechnol. 2006;7:495–502.
60. Colomer R, Menéndez JA. Mediterranean diet, olive oil and cancer. Clin Transl Oncol. 2006;8:15–21.
61. D'Amore S, Vacca M, Cariello M, Graziano G, D'Orazio A, Salvia R, Sasso RC, Sabbà C, Palasciano G, Moschetta A. Genes and miRNA expression signatures in peripheral blood mononuclear cells in healthy subjects and patients with metabolic syndrome after acute intake of extra virgin olive oil. Biochim Biophys Acta. 1861;2016:1671–80.
62. Macfarlane LA, Murphy PR. MicroRNA: biogenesis, function and role in cancer. Curr Genomics. 2010;11:537–61.
63. Konstantinidou V, Khymenets O, Fito M, De La Torre R, Anglada R, Dopazo A, Covas MI. Characterization of human gene expression changes after olive oil ingestion: an exploratory approach. Folia Biol (Praha). 2009;55:85–91.
64. Konstantinidou V, Khymenets O, Covas MI, de la Torre R, Muñoz-Aguayo D, Anglada R, Farré M, Fito M. Time course of changes in the expression of insulin sensitivity-related genes after an acute load of virgin olive oil. OMICS. 2009;13:431–8.
65. Camargo A, Ruano J, Fernandez JM, Parnell LD, Jimenez A, Santos-Gonzalez M, Marin C, Perez-Martinez P, Uceda M, Lopez-Miranda J, Perez-Jimenez F. Gene expression changes in mononuclear cells in patients with metabolic syndrome after acute intake of phenol-rich virgin olive oil. BMC Genomics. 2010;11:253.
66. Khymenets O, Fitó M, Covas MI, Farré M, Pujadas MA, Muñoz D, Konstantinidou V, de la Torre R. Mononuclear cell transcriptome response after sustained virgin olive oil consumption in humans: an exploratory nutrigenomics study. OMICS. 2009;13:7–19.
67. Raff M, Tholstrup T, Toubro S, Bruun JM, Lund P, Straarup EM, Christensen R, Sandberg MB, Mandrup S. Conjugated linoleic acids reduce body fat in healthy postmenopausal women. J Nutr. 2009;139:1347–52.

68. van Dijk SJ, Feskens EJ, Bos MB, Hoelen DW, Heijligenberg R, Bromhaar MG, de Groot LC, de Vries JH, Müller M, Afman LA. A saturated fatty acid-rich diet induces an obesity-linked proinflammatory gene expression profile in adipose tissue of subjects at risk of metabolic syndrome. Am J Clin Nutr. 2009;90:1656–64.
69. Castañer O, Covas MI, Khymenets O, Nyyssonen K, Konstantinidou V, Zunft HF, de la Torre R, Muñoz-Aguayo D, Vila J, Fitó M. Protection of LDL from oxidation by olive oil polyphenols is associated with a downregulation of CD40-ligand expression and its downstream products in vivo in humans. Am J Clin Nutr. 2012;95:1238–44.
70. Antoniades C, Bakogiannis C, Tousoulis D, Antonopoulos AS. The CD40/CD40 ligand system: linking inflammation with atherothrombosis. J Am Coll Cardiol. 2009;54:669–77.
71. Prontera C, Martelli N, Evangelista V, D'Urbano E, Manarini S, Recchiuti A, Dragani A, Passeri C, Davì G, Romano M. Homocysteine modulates the CD40/CD40L system. J Am Coll Cardiol. 2007;49:2182–90.
72. Konstantinidou V, Covas MI, Muñoz-Aguayo D, Khymenets O, de la Torre R, Saez G, Tormos Mdel C, Toledo E, Marti A, Ruiz-Gutiérrez V, Ruiz Mendez MV, Fito M. In vivo nutrigenomic effects of virgin olive oil polyphenols within the frame of the Mediterranean diet: a randomized controlled trial. FASEB J. 2010;24:2546–57.
73. Konstantinidou V, Covas MI, Sola R, Fitò M. Up-to date knowledge on the in vivo transcriptomic effect of the Mediterranean diet in humans. Mol Nutr Food Res. 2013;57:772–83.

Cereals

8

8.1 Premises

Cereals have been the staple food in most population worldwide from time immemorial. In Mediterranean diet, cereals represent the main source of daily caloric intake. In a study conducted in eight Italian cities [1] where dietary habits of an elderly population (65–84 years) were investigated with a 7-day questionnaire, 47–50% of daily caloric intake resulted to be derived from cereals (bread and pasta), 30% from extra virgin olive oil, and 15% from proteins, mainly vegetal proteins (see Chap. 1, Figs. 1.3 and 1.4, this book).

Etymologically, the word cereal derives from *Cerealia*, a celebration that was offered in Ancient Rome to Ceres, goddess of agriculture, harvest, and fertility. In Ancient Greece, she was known as Demeter, nurturing mother of blond hair, representing the heads of wheat. Its name means "grow" and refers to the importance of grains for the survival and expansion of people throughout history.

The consumption of bread is still deeply rooted in the culture of the Mediterranean countries. Currently, cereals provide about 50% of daily energy in the Mediterranean diet.

From nutritional point of view, cereals are rich in carbohydrates but contain also proteins and vitamins, important for energy functions.

8.2 Wheat

Wheat (*Triticum*, most commonly *T. aestivum*) is a cereal grain originally from the Levant region but now cultivated worldwide. Globally, wheat is the leading source of vegetal protein in human food, having a protein content of about 13–14%, which is relatively high compared to other major cereals and staple foods. The major cultivated species of wheat are:

– (Hexaploid species) = common wheat or bread wheat (*Triticum aestivum*); spelt (*Triticum spelta*)

A. Capurso et al., *Benefits of the Mediterranean Diet in the Elderly Patient*, Practical Issues in Geriatrics, https://doi.org/10.1007/978-3-319-78084-9_8

- (Tetraploid species) = durum (*Triticum durum*); emmer (*Triticum dicoccon*), khorasan (*Triticum turgidum or turanicum*)
- (Diploid species) = einkorn (*Triticum monococcum*)

In the United States, the wheat types more frequently used are:

- *Durum*: a very hard grain used to make semolina flour for pasta.
- *Hard red winter*: hard, brownish, high-protein wheat used for bread, hard baked goods and as an adjunct in other flours to increase protein in pastry flour for pie crusts.
- *Hard white*: hard, light-colored, medium-protein wheat, used for bread and brewing.
- *Soft red winter*: soft, low-protein wheat used for cakes, pie crusts, biscuits, and muffins.
- *Soft white*: soft, light-colored, very low-protein wheat grown in temperate moist areas. Used for pie crusts and pastry. Pastry flour, for example, is sometimes made from soft white winter wheat.

8.2.1 History

The archaeological record suggests that wheat was first cultivated in the regions of the Fertile Crescent around 9600 BCE. Greeks and Romans collected wisdom of the Egyptians to make bread a staple in Rome. Then, agricultural grain was controlled by the state, and the loaves were baked in public ovens. Over the years, along with wine and olive oil, bread was a food of great religious importance.

The Fertile Crescent (also known as the cradle of civilization) is a crescent-shaped region containing the comparatively moist and fertile land of otherwise arid and semiarid Western Asia, the Nile Valley, and Nile Delta. In current usage, all definitions of the Fertile Crescent include Mesopotamia, the land in and around the Tigris and Euphrates rivers, and the Levant, the eastern coast of the Mediterranean Sea. The modern-day countries with significant territory within the Fertile Crescent are Iraq, Syria, Lebanon, Cyprus, Jordan, Israel, the State of Palestine, Egypt, as well as the southeastern fringe of Turkey and the western fringes of Iran.

8.2.2 Nutrients

100 grams wheat provides 327 calories and is a rich source of multiple essential nutrients, such as protein, dietary fiber, manganese, phosphorus, and niacin (see table "**Wheat, Hard, Red Winter**"). Several B vitamins and other dietary minerals are in significant content. Wheat is 13% water, 71% carbohydrates, and 1.5% fat. Its 13–14% protein content is comprised mostly of gluten as 75–80% of total wheat protein, which, upon digestion, contributes amino acids for human nutrition.

Wheat, Hard, Red Winter

Table of nutritional values per 100 g of wheat (variety Hard, Red Winter)

Energy	1368 kJ	(327 kcal)
Protein	12.61 g	
Total fat	1.54 g	
Carbohydrates	71.18 g	
Sugars	0.41 g	
Dietary fiber	12.2 g	
Thiamine (B_1)	0.383 mg	(33% DV)
Riboflavin (B_2)	0.115 mg	(10% DV)
Niacin (B_3)	5.464 mg	(36% DV)
Pantothenic acid (B_5)	0.954 mg	(19% DV)
Vitamin B_6	0.3 mg	(23% DV)
Folate (B_9)	38 μg	(10% DV)
Vitamin B_{12}	0 μg	(0% DV)
Choline	31.2 mg	(6% DV)
Vitamin E	1.01 mg	(7% DV)
Vitamin K	1.9 μg	(2% DV)
Calcium	29 mg	(3% DV)
Iron	3.19 mg	(25% DV)
Magnesium	126 mg	(35% DV)
Manganese	3.985 mg	(190% DV)
Phosphorus	288 mg	(41% DV)
Potassium	363 mg	(8% DV)
Selenium	70.7 μg	
Sodium	2 mg	(0% DV)
Zinc	2.65 mg	(28% DV)

Source: USDA National Nutrient Database

8.2.3 Gluten

The main protein of the wheat is represented by the gluten. Gluten is a protein complex that accounts for 75–85% of the total protein in wheat. Gluten, the main family of proteins in wheat, can be divided into glutenins and gliadins, which are present in varying amounts in all types of wheat. Gluten forms when glutenin molecules cross-link to form a submicroscopic network attached to gliadin, which contributes viscosity (thickness) and extensibility to the mix. If this dough is leavened with yeast, fermentation produces carbon dioxide bubbles, which, trapped by the gluten network, cause the dough to rise. Baking coagulates the gluten, which, along with starch, stabilizes the shape of the final product.

The development of gluten (i.e., enhancing its elasticity) affects the texture of the baked goods. Gluten's attainable elasticity is proportional to its content of glutenins with low molecular weights as this portion contains the preponderance of the sulfur atoms responsible for the cross-linking in the network. More refining (of the gluten) leads to chewier products such as pizza and bagels, while less refining yields tender baked goods such as pastry products. Generally, bread flours are high in gluten (hard wheat); pastry flours have a lower gluten content. Kneading promotes the formation of gluten strands and cross-links, creating baked products that are chewier (in contrast to crumbly).

Gluten, especially wheat gluten, is often the basis for imitation meats resembling beef, chicken, duck (see mock duck), fish, and pork. When cooked in broth, gluten absorbs some of the surrounding liquid (including the flavor) and becomes firm to the bite.

8.2.4 Health Effects

Consumed worldwide by billions of people, wheat is a significant food for human nutrition, particularly in the least developed countries where wheat products are primary foods. When eaten as the whole grain, wheat is a healthy food source of multiple nutrients and dietary fiber recommended for children and adults in several daily servings amounting to about one third of total food intake.

As a common component of breakfast cereals, whole wheat is associated with improved micronutrient intake and lower risk of several diseases. By supplying high dietary insoluble fiber content, whole wheat in the diet contributes toward lowering the risk of multiple diseases, including coronary heart disease, stroke, cancer, and type 2 diabetes, with lower all-cause mortality [2, 3].

Manufacturers of foods containing wheat as a whole grain in specified amounts are allowed a health claim for marketing purposes in the United States, stating: "low fat diets rich in fiber-containing grain products, fruits, and vegetables may reduce the risk of some types of cancer, a disease associated with many factors" and "diets low in saturated fat and cholesterol and rich in fruits, vegetables, and grain products that contain some types of dietary fiber, particularly soluble fiber, may reduce the risk of heart disease, a disease associated with many factors" [4]. Dietary fiber may also help people feel full and therefore help with a healthy weight [3]. Further, wheat is a major source for natural and biofortified nutrient supplementation, including dietary fiber, protein, and dietary minerals.

8.2.5 Celiac Disease

In genetically susceptible people, gluten can trigger celiac disease. Celiac disease affects about 1% of the general population in developed countries. There is evidence that most cases remain undiagnosed and untreated. The gliadins are considered to be the main cause of celiac disease. Celiac disease causes damage to the small intestine, resulting in impaired absorption of nutrients. Associated symptoms may be weight loss, bloating flatulence, diarrhea, constipation, stomach pain, and fatigue. The only known effective treatment is a strict lifelong gluten-free diet. Other diseases triggered by eating gluten are non-celiac gluten sensitivity.

8.2.6 Non-celiac Gluten Sensitivity

Non-celiac gluten sensitivity (NCGS) or gluten sensitivity is defined as a clinical entity induced by the ingestion of gluten leading to intestinal and/or extraintestinal symptoms that improve once the gluten-containing foodstuff is removed from the diet, and celiac disease and wheat allergy have been excluded. NCGS is included in the spectrum of gluten-free disorders. The pathogenesis of NCGS is not yet well understood. There is evidence that not only gliadin (main cytotoxic antigen of gluten) but also other proteins present in gluten and gluten-containing cereals (wheat, rye, barley, and their derivatives) may have a role in the development of symptoms. FODMAPs (short-chain carbohydrates that are poorly absorbed in the small intestine) present in gluten-containing grains have recently been identified as a possible cause of gastrointestinal symptoms in NCGS patients. Recently, a team of researchers published a study confirming that wheat exposure in this group is, in fact, triggering a systemic immune reaction and accompanying intestinal cell damage. It is estimated that the impacted population is equal to or even exceeds the number of individuals with celiac disease (the vast majority of whom remain undiagnosed).

8.2.7 Wheat Fiber

Whole wheat is high in fiber, but refined wheat contains virtually no fiber. The fiber content of whole-grain wheat ranges from 12 to 15% of the dry weight. Concentrated in the bran, most of the fibers are removed in the milling process and largely absent in refined flour. The most common fiber in wheat bran is arabinoxylan (70%), which is a type of hemicellulose. The rest is mostly made up of cellulose and beta-glucan [5]. These fibers are all insoluble. They pass through the digestive system almost intact, leading to increased fecal weight. Some of them also feed the friendly bacteria in the gut [6, 7].

In a double-blind, randomized, crossover study [8] carried out in 31 volunteers who were randomized into two groups and consumed daily 48 g breakfast cereals, either whole-grain cereals (WG) or wheat bran (WB) in two 3-week study periods, the numbers of fecal bifidobacteria and lactobacilli (the target genera for prebiotic intake) were significantly higher upon WG ingestion compared with WB. Ingestion of both breakfast cereals resulted also in a significant increase in ferulic acid concentrations in blood. Moreover, a significant reduction in total cholesterol was observed in volunteers in the top quartile of total cholesterol concentrations upon ingestion of either cereal. The authors concluded that daily consumption of WG wheat exerted a pronounced prebiotic effect on the human gut microbiota composition. This prebiotic activity may contribute toward the beneficial physiological effects of WG wheat.

Wheat also contains small amounts of soluble fibers (fructans) that may cause digestive symptoms in people with irritable bowel syndrome. However, in those who tolerate it, wheat bran have beneficial effects on gut health.

8.2.8 Antioxidants of Wheat and Protection Against Colon Cancer

Wheat contains numerous antioxidants. Most of the antioxidants in wheat are concentrated in the bran and the germ, parts of the grain that are absent from refined white wheat.

Wheat bran [9] contains phenolic acids, which can be divided into derivatives of either hydroxycinnamic acid or hydroxybenzoic acid. Hydroxybenzoic acid derivatives include *p*-hydroxybenzoic, vanillic, syringic, and gallic acids. However, the most abundant phenolic acids in wheat are derivatives of hydroxycinnamic acids, specifically ferulic acid, dehydrodimers and dehydrotrimers of ferulic acid, and sinapic and *p*-coumaric acids. The bran layers contain the majority of phenolic acids that are mostly linked with cell wall structural components through ester bonds.

The highest levels of antioxidants are found in the aleurone layer, a component of the bran. Therefore, the antioxidant potency of wheat grain fractions is predominantly determined by aleurone content, which can be attributed to the presence of relatively large amounts of phenolic compounds, primarily ferulic acid [10]. Ferulic acid, in fact, is the predominant antioxidant polyphenol found in wheat and other grains.

Wheat bran contains also other classes of antioxidants, namely, flavonoids, carotenoids (mostly lutein), and lignans [11, 12].

Wheat bran was shown to provide protection against colorectal cancer in human intervention and animal studies. Lignans in particular have been shown to be involved in the antitumor activity of wheat bran in colon cancer. The cancer preventive mechanisms have been attributed to the two prominent lignan metabolites, *enterolactone* and *enterodiol*. In a study on human colon cancer SW480 cells [12], these lignans metabolites have been shown to greatly contribute to the cancer prevention by wheat bran observed in APC-Min mice. The inhibition of cancer cells growth by lignan metabolites appeared to be mediated by cytostatic and apoptotic mechanisms.

Among the flavonoids of wheat bran, the flavonol quercetin has been shown to inhibit human SW480 colon cancer growth, similarly to lignans [13]. The molecular mechanism underlying the antitumor effect of quercetin in SW480 colon cancer cells appeared to be related to the inhibition of expression of cyclin D1 and survivin as well as the Wnt/beta-catenin signaling pathway. Due to these results, the Wnt/beta-catenin signaling pathway was qualified as one of the promising targets for innovative treatment strategies of colorectal cancer.

8.3 Spelt (*Triticum spelta*)

Spelt (*Triticum spelta*), also known as "dinkel wheat" or "hulled wheat," is a species of wheat cultivated since very ancient times. It is a wheat species known from genetic evidence to have originated as a naturally occurring hybrid of a domesticated tetraploid wheat such as *emmer wheat* and the wild goat grass *Aegilops tauschii*. This hybridization must have taken place in the Near East because this is where *Aegilops tauschii* grows, and it must have taken place before the appearance of common or bread wheat (*Triticum aestivum*, a hexaploid free-threshing derivative of spelt) in the archaeological record about 8000 years ago. The much later appearance of spelt in Europe might thus be the result of a later, second, hybridization between *emmer* and *bread wheat*. Recent DNA evidence supports an independent origin for European spelt through this hybridization. Whether spelt has two separate origins in Asia and Europe, or single origin in the Near East, is currently unresolved.

8.3.1 History

In Greek mythology spelt was a gift to the Greeks from the goddess Demeter and was first used by the Greeks. Being a sailing people, the Greeks taught the rest of the world how to use and cultivate.

Spelt is mentioned in the Bible. The seventh plague in Egypt in Exodus did not damage the harvest of wheat and spelt, as these were "late crops." Ezekiel 4:9 says: "Take thou also unto thee wheat, and barley, and beans, and lentils, and millet, and spelt, and put them in one vessel, and make thee bread thereof …". In Horace's *Satire* 2.6 (late 31–30 BC), which ends with the story of the country mouse and the city mouse, the country mouse eats spelt at dinner while serving his city guest finer foods. In the *Divine Comedy* of Dante Alighieri, Pietro della Vigna appears as a suicide in Circle VII, ring ii, Canto XIII of the Inferno. Pietro describes the fate awaiting souls guilty of suicide to Dante the Pilgrim and Virgil. According to Pietro, the soul of the suicide grows into a wild tree and is tormented by harpies that feast upon its leaves. Pietro likens the initial growth and transformation of the soul of the suicide to the germination of a grain of spelt (*Inferno* XIII, 94–102).

The earliest archaeological evidence of spelt is from the fifth millennium BC in Transcaucasia, northeast of the Black Sea, though the most abundant and best-documented archaeological evidence of spelt is in Europe. Remains of spelt have been found in some later Neolithic sites (2500–1700 BC) in Central Europe. During the Bronze Age, spelt spread widely in Central Europe. In the Iron Age (750–15 BC), spelt became a principal wheat species in southern Germany and Switzerland, and by 500 BC, it was in common use in southern Britain.

In the Middle Ages, spelt was cultivated in parts of Switzerland, Tyrol, and Germany. Spelt was introduced to the United States in the 1890s. In the twentieth century, spelt was replaced by bread wheat in almost all areas where it was still grown. The organic farming movement revived its popularity somewhat toward the end of the century, as spelt requires less fertilizer.

8.3.2 Nutrients

In a 100 g serving, uncooked spelt provides 338 calories and is an excellent source of protein, dietary fiber, several B vitamins, and numerous dietary minerals (see table "**Spelt, Uncooked**"). Richest nutrient contents include manganese (143% DV), phosphorus (57% DV), and niacin (46% DV). Cooking substantially reduces many nutrient contents. Spelt contains about 70% total carbohydrates, including 11% as dietary fiber, and is low in fat (see table "**Spelt, Uncooked**").

Spelt contains a moderate amount of gluten and is therefore suitable for baking, but this component also makes it unsuitable for people with gluten-related disorders, such as celiac disease, non-celiac gluten sensitivity, and wheat allergy. The spelt gluten is not as strong as wheat gluten. In comparison to hard red winter wheat, spelt has a more soluble protein matrix characterized by a higher gliadin:glutenin ratio [14]. For this reason, spelt gluten tends to be more extensible and less elastic than gluten from modern wheat, resulting in the typical, weaker spelt doughs. As a consequence, for bread, rolls or two-layer flat bread have been proposed high doses of ascorbic acid, shorter mixing times, reduced water addition, or longer dough rest times, and for pasta, high-temperature drying has been recommended [14].

Spelt: A Niche Product

In the past few decades, spelt has undergone a renaissance as a niche product. This may be due to the perception that it is a "healthier," more "natural," or less "overbred" grain than modern wheat. Consequently, there are an increasing number of international publications on spelt food quality, spelt proteins, rheology of spelt dough or gluten, or comparisons of spelt and modern wheat. Unfortunately, very few differences between spelt and modern wheat have been confirmed experimentally. In respect to food quality, most of the studies found higher protein contents for spelt than for modern wheat, but in some other studies, the opposite was reported and in some cases differences were not significant. Overall, the values found for proximate compositions and minor components in spelt are within the range found among modern wheats.

Spelt may have a role for speciality breads and other food products with characteristics different from regular wheat products or for organic food. For example, in southern Germany, traditional spelt breads are produced and breeding spelt cultivars with typical properties, different from modern wheat but specific for such speciality breads, might be desirable. Agronomically, spelt may be more resistant to disease and do better under less advantageous growing conditions, such as wet, cold soils and at high altitudes. Because of the protection provided by the hulls, chemical treatment of hulled seeds used for sowing may not be required. Additionally, excess nitrogen fertilization is not possible due to the incidence of lodging of the long, less stable straw. This low-nitrogen tolerance may thus be seen as an advantage in providing a more environmentally friendly crop. For the same reason, it is not easy to compare spelt and modern wheat grown under identical conditions, because optimum growth conditions for modern wheat would include more nitrogen fertilization than for spelt.

Spelt, Uncooked

Table of nutritional values per 100 g of spelt

Energy	1415 kJ	(338 kcal)
Protein	14.57 g	
Total fat	2.43 g	
Saturated	0.406 g	
Monounsaturated	0.445 g	
Polyunsaturated	1.258 g	
Carbohydrates	70.19 g	
Starch	53.92 g	
Dietary fiber	10.7 g	

Thiamine (B_1)	0.364 mg	(32% DV)
Riboflavin (B_2)	0.113 mg	(9% DV)
Niacin (B_3)	6.843 mg	(46% DV)
Pantothenic acid (B_5)	1.068 mg	(11% DV)
Vitamin B_6	0.230 mg	(18% DV)
Folate (B_9)	45 μg	(11% DV)
Vitamin B_{12}	0 μg	(0% DV)
Vitamin E	0.79 mg	(5% DV)
Vitamin K	3.6 μg	(4% DV)
Calcium	27 mg	(3% DV)
Iron	4.44 mg	(34% DV)
Magnesium	136 mg	(38% DV)
Manganese	3.0 mg	(143% DV)
Phosphorus	401 mg	(57% DV)
Potassium	388 mg	(8% DV)
Selenium	11.7 μg	(17% DV)
Sodium	8 mg	(0% DV)
Zinc	3.28 mg	(35% DV)

Source: USDA National Nutrient Database

8.4 Oats

The oat (*Avena sativa*), sometimes called the *common oat*, is a species of cereal grain known by the same name (usually in the plural, unlike other cereals and pseudocereals). While oats are suitable for human consumption as oatmeal and rolled oats, one of the most common uses is as livestock feed. Oats have numerous uses in foods; most commonly, they are rolled or crushed into oatmeal or ground into fine oat flour. Oatmeal is chiefly eaten as porridge but may also be used in a variety of baked goods, such as oatcakes, oatmeal cookies, and oat bread. Oats are also an ingredient in many cold cereals, in particular muesli and granola. Oats are also occasionally used in several different drinks. In Britain, they are sometimes used for brewing beer. Oatmeal stout is one variety brewed using a percentage of oats for the wort. A cold, sweet drink called *avena* made of ground oats and milk is a popular refreshment throughout Latin America. Oatmeal caudle, made of ale and oatmeal with spices, was a traditional British drink and a favorite of Oliver Cromwell.

8.4.1 History

The wild ancestor of *Avena sativa* and the closely related minor crop, *A. byzantina*, is the hexaploid wild oat *A. sterilis*. Genetic evidence shows the ancestral forms of *A. sterilis* grew in the Fertile Crescent of the Near East. Domesticated oats appear relatively late, and far from the Near East, in Bronze Age Europe. Oats, like rye, are usually considered a secondary crop, i.e., derived from a weed of the primary cereal domesticates wheat and barley. As these cereals spread westward into cooler, wetter areas, this may have favored the oat weed component and have led to its domestication.

8.4.2 Nutrients

Oats are generally considered healthy due to their rich content of several essential nutrients. In a 100 g serving, oats provide 389 calories and are an excellent source of protein (34% DV), dietary fiber (44% DV), several B vitamins, and numerous dietary minerals, especially manganese (233% DV) (see table "**Oats**"). Oats are 66% carbohydrates, including 11% dietary fiber and 4% beta-glucans, 7% fat, and 17% protein (see table "**Oats**").

Oats, after corn (maize), have the highest lipid content of any cereal, e.g., greater than 10% for oats and as high as 17% for some maize cultivars compared to about 2–3% for wheat and most other cereals.

Oats are the only cereal containing a globulin or legume-like protein, avenalin, as the major (80%) storage protein. Globulins are characterized by solubility in dilute saline as opposed to the more typical cereal proteins, such as gluten and zein, the prolamines (prolamins). The minor protein of oat is a prolamine, avenin. Oat protein is nearly equivalent in quality to soy protein, which World Health Organization research has shown to be equal to meat, milk, and egg protein. The protein content of the hull-less oat kernel (groat) ranges from 12 to 24%, the highest among cereals. Some cultivars of pure oat (*pure oat refers to oats uncontaminated with other gluten-containing cereals*) could be a safe part of a gluten-free diet, requiring knowledge of the oat variety used in food products for a gluten-free diet.

8.4.3 Soluble Fiber

Oat contains almost 11% fiber and the majority of this fiber is the soluble fiber beta-glucans, a class of indigestible polysaccharides widely found in nature and also in other sources such as grains, barley, yeast, bacteria, algae, and mushrooms. Oats contain more soluble fiber than other grains, leading to slower digestion, increased satiety, and suppression of appetite. The oat beta-glucan is a viscous polysaccharide made up of units of the monosaccharide D-glucose. Oat beta-glucan is composed of mixed-linkage polysaccharides. This means the bonds between the D-glucose or D-glucopyranosyl units are either beta-1, 3 linkages or beta-1, 4 linkages. This type of beta-glucan is also referred to as a mixed-linkage (1 → 3), (1 → 4)-beta-D-glucan. The (1 → 3)-linkages break up the uniform structure of the beta-D-glucan molecule and make it soluble and flexible. In comparison, the indigestible polysaccharide cellulose is also a beta-glucan but is not soluble because of its (1 → 4)-beta-D-linkages. The percentages of beta-glucan in the various whole oat products are oat bran, from 5.5 to 23.0%; rolled oats, about 4%; and whole oat flour, about 4%. Oats contain also insoluble fibers, including lignin, cellulose, and hemicellulose.

Beta-glucans are known to lower cholesterol levels and increase excretion of bile acids. They are also believed to cause a reduction in blood sugar and insulin levels after a carbohydrate-rich meal [15, 16]. The cholesterol-lowering effects of oat beta-glucans [17] have led to acceptance of oats as a health food [18]. After reports of research finding that dietary oats can help lower cholesterol, the US Food and Drug Administration (FDA) issued a final rule that allows food companies to make health claims on food labels of foods that contain soluble fiber from whole oats (oat bran, oat flour, and rolled oats), noting that 3.0 g of soluble fiber daily from these foods may reduce the risk of heart disease. To qualify for the health claim, the whole oat-containing food must provide at least 0.75 g of soluble fiber per serving.

Oats

Table of nutritional values per 100 g of oats

Energy	1628 kJ	(389 kcal)
Protein	16.9 g	
Total fat	6.9 g	
Saturated	1.22 g	
Monounsaturated	2.18 g	
Polyunsaturated	2.54 g	
Carbohydrates	66.3 g	
Starch	53.92 g	
Dietary fiber	10.6 g	

Thiamine (B_1)	0.763 mg	(66% DV)
Riboflavin (B_2)	0.139 mg	(12% DV)
Niacin (B_3)	0.961 mg	(6% DV)
Pantothenic acid (B_5)	1.349 mg	(27% DV)
Vitamin B_6	0.120 mg	(9% DV)
Folate (B_9)	56 μg	(5% DV)
Vitamin B_{12}	0 μg	(0% DV)
Vitamin E	0.0 mg	(0% DV)
Vitamin K	0.0 μg	(0% DV)

Calcium	54 mg	(3% DV)
Iron	5.0 mg	(38% DV)
Magnesium	177 mg	(50% DV)
Manganese	4.9 mg	(233% DV)
Phosphorus	523 mg	(75% DV)
Potassium	429 mg	(9% DV)
Sodium	2 mg	(0% DV)
Zinc	4 mg	(42% DV)

Source: USDA National Nutrient Database

8.5 Rye

Rye (*Secale cereale*) is a grass grown extensively as a grain. It is a member of the wheat tribe (Triticeae) and is closely related to barley (genus *Hordeum*) and wheat (*Triticum*). Rye grain is used for flour, rye bread, rye beer, crisp bread, some whiskeys, some vodkas, and animal fodder.

8.5.1 History

Rye is one of a number of species that grow wild in central and eastern Turkey and in adjacent areas. Domesticated rye occurs in small quantities at a number of Neolithic sites in (Asia Minor) Turkey but is otherwise absent from the archaeological record until the Bronze Age of Central Europe, c. 1800–1500 BC. It is possible that rye traveled west from (Asia Minor) Turkey as a minor admixture in wheat and was only later cultivated in its own right. Although archaeological evidence of this grain has been found in Roman contexts along the Rhine, Danube, and in Ireland and Britain, Pliny the Elder was dismissive of rye, writing that it "is a very poor food and only serves to avert starvation" and spelt is mixed "to mitigate its bitter taste, and even then is most unpleasant to the stomach."

Since the Middle Ages, people have cultivated rye widely in Central and Eastern Europe. It serves as the main bread cereal in most areas east of the French-German border and north of Hungary. In Southern Europe, it was cultivated on marginal lands.

8.5.2 Uses and Nutrition

Rye bread is a widely eaten food in Northern and Eastern Europe. Rye is also used to make crisp bread. Rye flour is high in gliadin but low in glutenin. It therefore has a lower gluten content than wheat flour. Anyway, rye contains gluten, which makes it an unsuitable grain for consumption by people with gluten-related disorders, such as celiac disease, non-celiac gluten sensitivity, and wheat allergy, among others. Nevertheless, some wheat allergy patients can tolerate rye. It also contains a higher proportion of soluble fiber. Alkylresorcinols are phenolic lipids present in high amounts in the bran layer (e.g., pericarp, testa, and aleurone layers) of wheat and rye (0.1–0.3% of dry weight).

Ergotism is an illness that can result from eating rye and other grains infected by ergot fungi (which produce LSD-25-like toxins in infected products). Although it is no longer a common illness because of modern food safety efforts, it was common before the twentieth century, and it can still happen today if food safety vigilance breaks down (see table "**Rye**").

Rye

Nutritional value per 1 cup (169 g)

Energy	2370 kJ	(566 kcal)
Protein	24.9 g	
Total fat	4.2 g	
Saturated	0.5 g	
Monounsaturated	0.5 g	
Polyunsaturated	1.9 g	
Total omega-3	265 mg	
Total omega-6	1619 mg	
Carbohydrates	118 g	
Sugars	1.8 g	
Dietary fiber	24.7 g	

Vitamin A	18.6 IU	(0% DV)
Thiamine (B_1)	0.5 mg	(36% DV)
Riboflavin (B_2)	0.4 mg	(25% DV)
Niacin (B_3)	7.2 mg	(36% DV)
Pantothenic acid (B_5)	2.5 mg	(25% DV)
Vitamin B_6	0.5 mg	(25% DV)
Folate (B_9)	101 μg	(25% DV)
Vitamin B_{12}	0 μg	(0% DV)
Vitamin E	2.2 mg	(11% DV)
Vitamin K	10.0 μg	(12% DV)

Calcium	55.8 mg	(6% DV)
Iron	4.5 mg	(25% DV)
Magnesium	204 mg	(51% DV)
Manganese	4.5 mg	(226% DV)
Phosphorus	632 mg	(63% DV)
Potassium	446 mg	(13% DV)
Selenium	59.7 mcg	(85% DV)
Sodium	10.1 mg	(0% DV)
Zinc	6.3 mg	(42% DV)

Source: USDA SR-21

8.5.3 The Health Effects of Rye

Rye is accounted for numerous beneficial actions on health. Rye is a good source of fiber richly endowed with noncellulose polysaccharides, which have exceptionally high water-binding capacity and quickly give a feeling of fullness and satiety, making, for example, the rye bread a real help for anyone trying to lose weight.

Another important property of fiber from rye and from other food sources is its ability to bind to toxins in the colon and then remove them from the body. When it binds to cancer-causing chemicals, fiber helps protect the cells of the colon from damage. This is one possible reason why a high-fiber diet has been shown to prevent colon cancer. Moreover, fiber binds to bile salts in the intestines and removes them from the body, so forcing the body to make more bile salts. This is good for serum cholesterol levels, because the body must break down cholesterol to make bile. This explains why a good intake of fiber can help to lower high cholesterol levels.

However, the most important effect of rye and other whole grains is its impact on type 2 diabetes mellitus risk.

8.5.4 Rye Bread, Glucose Metabolism, and Diabetes

Rye products, particularly rye bread, have demonstrated to reduce the risk of diabetes. A study published in the *American Journal of Clinical Nutrition* [19] found that bread made from wheat triggers a greater insulin response than rye bread does. In this study the effects of eating refined wheat bread was compared with the effects of eating endosperm rye bread, traditional rye bread, and high-fiber rye bread on several markers of blood sugar control including plasma glucose, insulin, glucose-dependent insulinotropic polypeptide (GIP), glucagon-like peptide 1 (GLP1), and serum C-peptide in 19 healthy postmenopausal women (*GIP and GLP1 are hormones secreted within the gastrointestinal tract during meals that boost the effects of insulin; C-peptide is a marker of insulin secretion*). All of these markers were evaluated in blood samples taken both before and after the women ate each of the breads. Results showed that after the women had eaten any of the rye breads, their insulin, GIP, and C-peptide responses were significantly lower than after they ate wheat bread. Among the different rye breads, no significant differences were seen in insulin and C-peptide response despite their varying levels of fiber. Researchers felt this lower after-meal insulin response could, therefore, not be attributed only to the fiber content of the rye breads but also to the fact that the starch granules in rye bread form a less porous and mechanically firmer matrix than in wheat bread. This would translate into a much greater particle size being swallowed when rye bread is eaten compared to wheat, which would slow the rate at which the starch could be digested into sugar.

These data have been confirmed by another recent study [20] on disintegration of rye and wheat breads during in vitro gastric digestion and its relation to the postprandial glucose and insulin responses. Breads with distinct composition and texture characteristics were prepared with refined or whole grain wheat and rye flour by using either straight dough or sourdough process. After chewing and gastric digestion in vitro, 100% wholemeal and refined rye breads prepared by sourdough method were disintegrated to a much lower extent than the wheat breads, having more bread digesta larger particles, with size over 2 or 3 mm. Microstructure of the digesta particles of rye sourdough bread revealed more aggregated and less degraded starch granules when compared to refined wheat bread. The postprandial insulin responses, but not those of glucose, to the 100% rye breads made with sourdough method were lower than the responses to the refined wheat bread. PCA (principal component analysis) confirmed that the insulin response had a negative correlation with the number of larger particles after in vitro digestion as well as amount of soluble fiber and sourdough process.

Definitely, the larger-sized starch particles of wholemeal rye bread after gastric digestion have been demonstrated to be associated with low postprandial insulin responses. This mechanism most likely synergizes with the effects of fiber and wholemeal cereal in reducing the diet-induced diabetes risk. It is known from the literature that diets containing rapidly absorbing carbohydrates and low in dietary fiber (DF) are associated with increased risk of type 2 diabetes [21, 22], whereas consumption of whole grain cereal foods reduces the risk of type 2 diabetes and heart disease, partly via the effects on insulin metabolism [23, 24]. Starchy foods like breakfast cereals, standard wheat breads, and potato products result in high glycemic responses, whereas intact cereal grains, pasta, and dense breads produce lower responses [25, 26]. Thus the fiber content and the form of cereal-based starch-rich food products appear to be important factors for postprandial response of a carbohydrate-rich diet. To this purpose, also the bread structure has been shown to be important in the postprandial glycemic and insulinemic response.

8.5.5 The Structure of Bread and Its Impact on Glucose Metabolism

The bread structure has been shown to have a role in glucose metabolism. The regular refined wheat flour bread have very porous structure and thus low density, while acidic or fiber-enriched solid foam structures (typical for rye products) have high density [27]. Wheat bread is based on continuous gluten network, which provides viscoelastic network trapping gas inside the product. Presence of nondigestible carbohydrates, especially soluble arabinoxylan and beta-glucan, results in higher viscosity, macro density, and hardness. In 100% rye bread, protein cannot form a continuous network and elastic dough similar to wheat protein [28], and arabinoxylan is the main water-binding substance having larger effect than protein on dough rheology and gas-holding properties. Besides compositional differences of wheat and rye flour, lactic acid bacteria fermentation process generally used in rye bread making results in dense structure and altered starch properties and a high number of starch-protein interactions [29]. The distinct structures of rye and wheat breads have been related to starch digestibility and postprandial glucose metabolism [19]. In refined wheat bread, highly gelatinized starch and porous structure result in rapid degradation of starch in the small intestine and rapid rise of blood glucose and insulin levels. Rye and wheat-based bread prepared by fermentation with lactic acid bacteria, i.e., sourdough technology, on the contrary, have been reported to induce reduced GI values [30]. The reduced postprandial responses of rye sourdough breads have been attributed to biochemical factors of rye [31–33] and acidity induced by solubilization of dietary fiber, acidity-mediated reduction of starch digestion, and stepwise degradation of protein phase of the bread [19, 29, 30]. However, among these factors, the most important has been shown to be the formation of larger-sized starch particles of rye products during gastric digestion and the consequent slower absorption of starch digesta in the intestine [20].

8.6 Maize (Corn)

Maize, also known as corn, is a large grain plant first domesticated by indigenous people in Mexico about 10,000 years ago. Major types of corn are dent corn, flint corn, pod corn, popcorn, flour corn, and sweet corn.

The word *maize* derives from the Spanish form of the indigenous *Taíno (the indigenous people of the Caribbean and Florida)* word for the plant, *mahiz*. The word "corn" outside North America, Australia, and New Zealand refers to any cereal crop, its meaning understood to vary geographically to refer to the local staple. In the United States, Canada, Australia, and New Zealand, *corn* primarily means maize; this usage started as a shortening of "Indian corn." "Indian corn" primarily means maize (the staple grain of indigenous Americans).

8.6.1 History

Maize (corn) was domesticated in south-central Mexico. A large corpus of data indicates that maize was dispersed into lower Central America by 5600 BC and had moved into the inter-Andean valleys of Colombia between 5000 and 4000 BC. An influential 2002 study by Matsuoka et al. has demonstrated that all maize arose from a single domestication in southern Mexico about 9000 years ago.

After the arrival of Europeans in 1492, Spanish settlers consumed maize and explorers and traders carried it back to Europe and introduced it to other countries. Spanish settlers far preferred wheat bread to maize or potatoes. Maize flour could not be substituted for wheat for communion bread, since in Christian belief only wheat could undergo transubstantiation and be transformed into the body of Christ. At another level, Spaniards worried that by eating indigenous foods, which they did not consider nutritious, not only would they weaken, but they risked turning into Indians. "In the view of Europeans, it was the food they ate, even more than the environment in which they lived, that gave Amerindians and Spaniards both their distinctive physical characteristics and their characteristic personalities" [34]. Despite these worries, Spaniards did consume maize and archaeological evidence from Florida sites indicates they cultivated it as well.

Presently, maize and cornmeal (ground dried maize) constitute a staple food in many regions of the world. Maize is central to Mexican foods (tortillas, tostadas, tamales, pozole, tacos, and so forth). Popcorn are widespread everywhere and consist of kernels of maize that explode when heated, forming fluffy pieces that are eaten as a snack.

8.6.2 Nutrients and Phytochemicals

In a 100 g serving, maize kernels provide 86 calories and are a good source (10–19% of the Daily Value) of B vitamins, thiamin, niacin, pantothenic acid (B5), and folate. In moderate amounts, they also supply dietary fiber and the essential minerals, magnesium and phosphorus, whereas other nutrients are in low amounts (see table "**MAIZE (CORN): Sweetcorn, Yellow Raw**").

MAIZE (CORN): Sweetcorn, Yellow Raw
Nutritional value per 1 cup (166 g)

Energy	2537 kJ	(606 kcal)
Total fat	7.9 g	
Saturated	1.1 g	
Monounsaturated	2.1 g	
Polyunsaturated	3.6 g	
Total omega-3	108 g	
Total omega-6	3481 g	
Carbohydrates	123 g	
Sugars	1.1 g	
Starch	8.5 g	
Dietary fiber	12.1 g	
Protein	15.6 g	

Vitamin A	355 IU	(7% DV)
Lutein zeaxanthin	644 μg	
Thiamine (B_1)	0.6 mg	(43% DV)
Riboflavin (B_2)	0.3 mg	(20% DV)
Niacin (B_3)	6 mg	(30% DV)
Pantothenic acid (B_5)	0.7 mg	(7% DV)
Vitamin B_6	1 mg	(52% DV)
Folate (B_9)	31.5 μg	(8% DV)
Vitamin C	0 mg	(0% DV)
Vitamin E	0.8 mg	(4% DV)
Vitamin K	0.5 μg	(1% DV)

Calcium	11.6 mg	(1% DV)
Copper	0.5 mg	(26% DV)
Iron	4.5 mg	(25% DV)
Magnesium	211 mg	(53% DV)
Manganese	0.8 mg	(40% DV)
Phosphorus	349 mg	(35% DV)
Potassium	476 mg	(14% DV)
Selenium	25.7 μg	(37% DV)
Sodium	58.1 mg	(2% DV)
Zinc	3.7 mg	(24% DV)

Source: USDA SR-21

8.6.3 Risk Factors for Pellagra

When maize was first introduced into farming systems other than those used by traditional Native American peoples, it was generally welcomed with enthusiasm for its productivity. However, a widespread problem of malnutrition soon arose wherever maize was introduced as a staple food. This was a mystery, since these types of malnutrition were not normally seen among the indigenous Americans, for whom maize was the principal staple food.

It was eventually discovered that the indigenous Americans had learned to soak maize in alkaline water—made with ashes and lime (calcium oxide) since at least 1200–1500 BC by Mesoamericans and North Americans—which liberates the B vitamin niacin, the lack of which was the underlying cause of the condition known as pellagra [35]. Maize was introduced into the diet of nonindigenous Americans without the necessary cultural knowledge acquired over thousands of years in the Americas. In the late nineteenth century, pellagra reached epidemic proportions in parts of the southern United States, as medical researchers debated two theories for its origin: the deficiency theory (which was eventually shown to be true) said that pellagra was due to a deficiency of some nutrient and the germ theory said that pellagra was caused by a germ transmitted by stable flies. A third theory, promoted by the eugenicist Charles Davenport, held that people only contracted pellagra if they were susceptible to it due to certain "constitutional, inheritable" traits of the affected individual. Once alkali processing and dietary variety were understood and applied, pellagra disappeared in the developed world. The development of high lysine maize and the promotion of a more balanced diet have also contributed to its demise. Pellagra still exists today in food-poor areas and refugee camps where people survive on donated maize.

8.6.4 Corn Oil

Corn oil (maize oil) is oil extracted from the germ of corn (maize). Its main use is in cooking, where its high smoke point makes refined corn oil a valuable frying oil. It is also a key ingredient in some margarines. Corn oil is generally less expensive than most other types of vegetable oils. Corn oil is also a feedstock used for biodiesel. Other industrial uses for corn oil include soap, salve, paint, inks, textiles, nitroglycerin, and insecticides. It is sometimes used as a carrier for drug molecules in pharmaceutical preparations.

Corn oil contains 12% saturated fatty acids [80% palmitic acid (C 16:0), 14% stearic acid (C 18:0), and 3% arachidic acid (C 20:0)], 28% monounsaturated fatty acids [99% oleic acid (C 18:1)], and 55% polyunsaturated fatty acids [(2% omega-3 linolenic acid C 18:3; 58% omega-6 linoleic acid C18:2; 28% omega-9 oleic acid)] (Table 8.1).

8.6.4.1 Corn Oil and Serum Cholesterol Level

Corn oil is an important source of polyunsaturated fats. The main corn oil's fatty acid is linoleic acid, an omega-6 (n-6) polyunsaturated fatty acid, which represents 55% of corn oil's total fat (Table 8.1). Many studies have shown the significant impact of linoleic acid on serum cholesterol and triglycerides, and this effect is part of a quite complex fascinating story started beginning 1960s.

After the results of the study "Seven Countries Study" by Ancel Keys et al. [36–38] demonstrating a significant correlation between saturated fatty acids (SFA) with elevated serum cholesterol levels and polyunsaturated fatty acids (PUFA) with

Table 8.1 Fat constituents as % of total fat for corn oil compared to other vegetable oils and beef fat

	Palmitic (C-16:0)	Stearic (C-18:0)	Oleic (C-18:1) (omega-9)	Linoleic (C-18:2) (omega-6)	α-Linolenic (18:3) (omega-3)
Corn oil	11	2	25	55	1
Palm oil	45	5	38	10	0
Canola oil	5	2	53	22	10
Linseed oil	3	7	21	16	53
Olive oil	12	3	75	10	0
Sunflower oil	6	4	24	65	1
Safflower oil	7	3	15	75	0
Walnut oil	7	2	15	60	10
Beef fat	26	17 + 3(°)	47 + 3(°°)	3	1

(°) 3% myristic acid, (°°) 3% palmitoleic acid

lower serum cholesterol levels, restriction of intakes of SFA and trans-fatty acids and consumption of PUFA in cholesterol-lowering, heart-healthy diets has been greatly emphasized. The *Seven Countries Study* found that the per capita consumption of dietary cholesterol and saturated fat correlated with mortality from coronary heart disease, and studies in animals also pointed to dietary lipids as a risk factor for atherosclerosis. These studies spawned the widespread recommendations for decreasing dietary cholesterol, decreasing the percentage of dietary calories obtained from fat, and replacing dietary saturated fat with polyunsaturated fat. Therefore, the primary target for reduction of myocardial infarction and coronary heart disease in that time was the reduction of high serum cholesterol level.

Previous studies from Ancel Keys and others [39, 40] performed in the early 1960s had shown that the serum cholesterol level increases when dietary carbohydrates are replaced by certain saturated fatty acids and decreases when carbohydrates are replaced by *n-6* polyunsaturated fatty acids. Quite soon an important problem emerged: these and other studies did not differentiate between the effects of diet and polyunsaturated fats on LDL and HDL lipoprotein cholesterol. This distinction was relevant because LDL and HDL cholesterol had opposite effects on the risk for ischemic heart disease, and other studies had suggested that the cholesterol-decreasing effect of *n-6* polyunsaturated fatty acids was not limited to LDL but extended to HDL cholesterol [41, 42]. In other words, *n-6* polyunsaturated fatty acids decrease not only LDL ("bad") cholesterol but also HDL ("good") cholesterol. Anyway, this controversy was overcome by later studies.

A meta-analysis of 27 trials on the effect of dietary fatty acids on serum lipids and lipoproteins [43] showed that all fatty acids elevate HDL cholesterol when substituted for carbohydrates, but the effect diminishes with increasing unsaturation of the fatty acids. Replacement of saturated by unsaturated fatty acids raises the HDL to LDL cholesterol ratio, whereas replacement by carbohydrates has no effect. Thus, under isocaloric, metabolic ward conditions, the most favorable lipoprotein risk profile for coronary heart disease was achieved if saturated fatty acids were replaced by unsaturated fatty acids, with no decrease in total fat intake.

In the Nurses' Health Study [44, 45], the relation between dietary intake of specific types of fat and the risk of coronary disease was prospectively studied in 80,082 women 34–59 years of age free from coronary disease, stroke, cancer, hypercholesterolemia, or diabetes in 1980. During 14 years of follow-up, 939 cases of nonfatal myocardial infarction or death from coronary heart disease were documented (Fig. 8.1). Each increase of 5% of energy intake from saturated fat, as compared with equivalent energy intake from carbohydrates, was associated with a 17% increase in the risk of coronary disease (relative risk, 1.17; 95% confidence interval, 0.97–1.41; $P = 0.10$), while a 2% increment in energy intake from trans unsaturated fat was associated with a 93% increase of the CHD risk (RR = 1.93; 95% confidence interval, 1.43–2.61; $P = 0.001$). A 5% increment in energy from monounsaturated fat was associated with a 19% decrease of CHD risk (RR = 0.81; 95% confidence interval, 0.65–1.00; $P = 0.05$), and a 5% increment in energy from polyunsaturated fat was associated with a reduction of 38% of the risk (RR = 0.62; 95% confidence

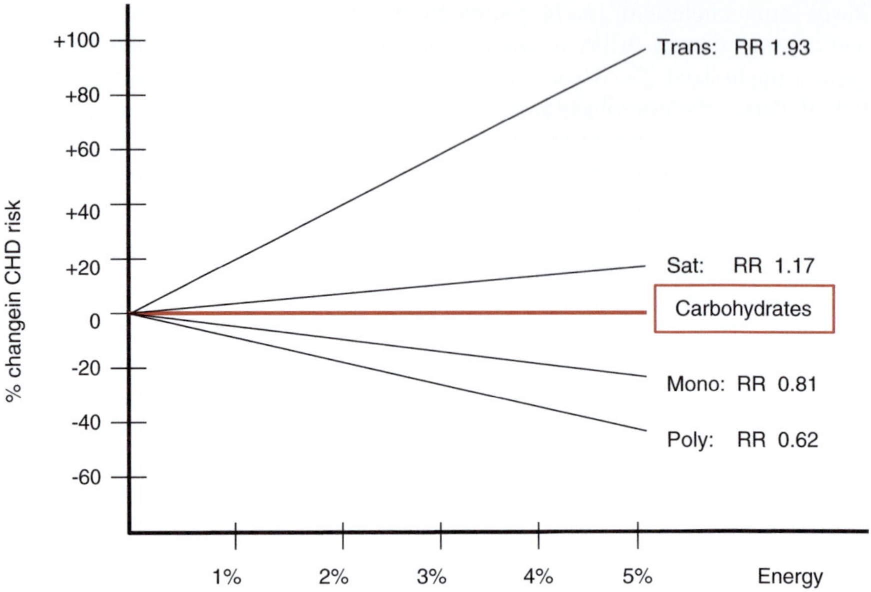

Fig. 8.1 CHD risk modification after replacing carbohydrates with saturated or unsaturated fat in the diet

interval, 0.46–0.85; $P < 0.003$). The replacement of 5% of energy from saturated fat with energy from unsaturated fats reduced risk by 42% (95% confidence interval, 23–56, $P < 0.001$).Total fat intake was not significantly related to the risk of coronary disease (for a 5% increase in energy from fat, the relative risk was 1.02). These data suggested that replacing saturated and trans unsaturated fats with unhydrogenated monounsaturated and polyunsaturated fats is more effective in preventing coronary heart disease in women than reducing overall fat intake.

In a recent pooled analysis of 11 cohort studies [46], the polyunsaturated fatty acids' effects were confirmed: for a 5% lower energy intake from SFAs and a concomitant higher energy intake from PUFAs, a significant inverse association between PUFAs and risk of coronary events was found (hazard ratio, 0.87; 95% CI, 0.77, 0.97); the hazard ratio for coronary deaths was 0.74 (95% CI, 0.61, 0.89). The authors concluded that replacing SFA intake with PUFA intake rather than MUFA or carbohydrate intake prevents CHD over a wide range of intakes and among all middle-aged and older women and men.

8.6.4.2 The Data of the Sydney Diet Heart Study on Linoleic Acid

A recently published evaluation of recovered data from the Sydney Diet Heart Study with an updated meta-analysis, however, has led to intriguing and unexpected conclusions on linoleic acid [47]. The objective of this study was the re-evaluation of recovered data from the Sydney Diet Heart Study, a single-blinded, parallel group, randomized controlled trial conducted in 1966–1973, and an updated meta-analysis including these previously missing data. The aim of the study was to evaluate the effectiveness of replacing dietary saturated fat with omega-6 linoleic acid for the secondary prevention of coronary heart disease and death. The participants were 458 men aged 30–59 years with a recent coronary event. The intervention consisted in replacement of dietary saturated fats (from animal fats, common margarines, and shortenings) with omega-6 linoleic acid (LA) (from safflower oil and safflower oil polyunsaturated margarine). This recent re-evaluation of participants to the study unexpectedly showed that the intervention group ($N = 221$) had higher rates of death than controls ($n = 237$): all cause mortality 17.6 versus 11.8%, hazard ratio 1.62 (95% confidence interval 1.00–2.64, $P = 0.05$); cardiovascular disease 17.2 versus 11.0%, 1.70 (1.03–2.80, $P = 0.04$); coronary heart disease 16.3 versus 10.1%, 1.74 (1.04–2.92, $P = 0.04$). Restriction of the analysis to the intervention group, which was provided safflower oil (a concentrated source of n-6 LA lacking n-3 PUFAs), allowed to estimate the specific effects of increasing n-6 LA only. Among patients in this intervention group, the increase in n-6 LA was associated with higher all-cause and cardiovascular mortality, providing supporting evidence that LA itself was a key component mediating the unfavorable effects.

To explain these unfavorable effects of LA on morbidity and mortality from CHD, the authors have proposed a mechanistic model linking dietary LA to cardiovascular pathogenesis: omega-6 linoleic acid (LA) is the most abundant fatty acid in native low-density lipoprotein particles. Oxidized LA metabolites (OXLAMs) are the most abundant oxidized fatty acids in oxidized low-density lipoprotein [48, 49], which is potentially more atherogenic than unmodified low-density lipoprotein. A potential mechanism contributing to higher cardiovascular mortality in the LA intervention group could be a diet-induced increase in the production of bioactive OXLAMs, including 9- and 13-hydroperoxyoctadecadienoic acid and 9- and 13-hydroxyoctadecadienoic acid. These OXLAMs are enriched in the lipid laden, macrophage foam cells, vascular endothelial cells, and migrating vascular smooth muscle cells of atherosclerotic lesions [50–53]. OXLAMs, particularly the isomers and enantiomers produced by free radical-mediated oxidation [50, 54], have been mechanistically linked to cardiovascular disease pathogenesis. Mechanisms include the formation of macrophage foam cells; endothelial cell activation; migration, proliferation, and foam cell formation of vascular smooth muscle cells; and inhibition of lysosomal hydrolysis of low-density lipoprotein cholesteryl esters.

Major sources of free radical-mediated oxidative stress, such as cigarette smoking and chronic alcohol exposure, increase the oxidation of low-density lipoprotein fatty acids; smokers and drinkers are reported to have increased concentrations of LA oxidation products in atherosclerotic lesions [54]. To conclude, the model proposed by the authors predicts that oxidative stress combined with diets high in n-6 LA facilitates this oxidation, leading to OXLAM-mediated atherosclerotic progression and increased cardiovascular mortality. Consistent with this model, the link between the magnitude of increase in LA and mortality was robust in smokers and drinkers in the Sydney Diet Heart Study, suggesting that diets high in n-6 LA may be particularly detrimental in the context of oxidative stress induced by smoking or alcohol.

After these contrasting results on LA, the advice to substitute polyunsaturated fats for saturated fats remains a key component of worldwide dietary guidelines for coronary heart disease risk reduction. However, there is currently no clinical trial evidence indicating that replacing SFAs with n-6 LA, without a concurrent increase in n-3 PUFAs and antioxidants, lowers the risk of cardiovascular disease or death. Thus, benefits attributed to PUFAs as a general category might be due to n-3 PUFAs specifically, particularly eicosapentaenoic acid and docosahexaenoic acid, particularly if associated to natural antioxidants (e.g., polyphenols from olive oil, fruit, vegetables, and so forth).

8.7 Bread in the Tradition of the Mediterranean Diet

Cereals and complex carbohydrates were the most important source of daily calories in Southern Italian and Greek population in the early 1960s, at the time when these cohorts were enrolled in the Seven Countries Study. In a study of our group on a rural population of South Italy in 1999 [1], the daily caloric intake from complex carbohydrates was 47–50% as yet, 65–70% of which derived from bread.

The bread in the traditional Mediterranean diet of the early 1960s was a staple food of middle-aged population of southern Mediterranean countries. The diet of the middle-aged men sampled enrolled in the Crete, Corfu, and Nicotera cohorts of the Seven Countries Study in the early 1960s had a high percentage of total daily energy intake from bread (Crete in 1960, mean 28.9 ± 7.1%; Corfu in 1961, mean 38.1 ± 7.0% [55]; Nicotera in 1960, median 32.1%) [56]. In the Crete cohort, the bread consumption was 380 g/person/day; in Corfu it was 450 g/person/day and in Nicotera 455 g/person/day.

Ancel Keys commented that the bread these populations consumed was generally brown bread, made from whole wheat often mixed with barley, stone ground in the mills of the town, and consumed at every meal. In that time, in Nicotera (South Italy), bread was leavened with a sourdough starter, probably a type I traditional sourdough. It is likely that bread was leavened with sourdough also in Crete and Corfu in the early 1060s. It has been reported that it was a feature of the traditional Greek diet until the end of 1950s [57]. It should be noted, however, that the westernization of dietetic habits, which started at the beginning of the 1960s, was slower in the poor rural areas than in the richer areas of the country and in the lower social classes than in the upper ones.

8.7.1 Sourdough Leavened Bread

The bread these southern populations consumed in that time had some peculiar characteristics: it was prepared with a homemade, spontaneous sourdough and not with commercial yeast. Spontaneous sourdough is a dough of flour and water that, left for several hours at room temperature, allows the growth of a composite ecosystem of lactic acid bacteria and yeasts. The continuous daily refreshments with the addition of new flour and water keep the microorganisms in an active state. Yeasts are the major producers of CO_2 in sourdough, so they are primarily responsible for leavening [58]. The lactic acid bacteria, both homofermentative and heterofermentative species, are responsible for dough acidification, the former producing lactic acid, the latter lactic acid plus CO_2, acetic acid, and/or ethanol [58]. The final pH is about 4.0, and the fermentation quotient (lactic/acetic acid ratio) is ranging from 3.3 to 5.6.

The sourdough fermentation of wheat flour lowers significantly the *Glycemic Index* (GI) of bread, reducing starch digestibility, mostly through the formation of organic acids, which slowed the absorption of starch [59, 60]. The mechanism responsible for the slow absorption of starch in the presence of lactic acid is the inhibition of amylolytic enzymes [61] or a reduction of starch bioavailability, because of the interaction between starch and gluten [30], whereas acetic acid delays the gastric emptying rate [62]. The whole wheat bread average GI is 71, and the *Glycemic Load* (GL) for a 30-g serving size is nine [63]; the white wheat flour bread GI is 71, and the GL of a 30-g serving size is 10 [63]; the GI of sourdough wheat bread, on the contrary, is 54, and its GL for a 30-g serving size is eight [63]. If we take into consideration the international table of glycemic index and glycemic load values 2002 [25] that ranks food GIs ≤55 as low, between 56 and 69 as moderate, and ≥70 as high GI foods, sourdough wheat bread appears to be a low GI food.

Whole wheat bread and white wheat bread give the same postprandial response of glucose and insulin in type 2 diabetic patients [64]; however, the inclusion of a high percentage of intact or partially milled cereal kernels in the flour reduces the glycemic response of bread [65–67]. These data have a possible biological and technical explanation: wheat germ contains a natural amylase inhibitor that is destroyed by the passage through the roller mill. Standard wholemeal flour (not stone ground meal flour) is a reconstituted flour after passage through the roller mill. Therefore, wholemeal flour is hydrolyzed at a rate identical to white flour.

In a recent study [68], the metabolic effects of four breads prepared from two different wheat flours (whole or white) through two different leavening techniques (sourdough and *Saccharomyces cerevisiae*) were evaluated. Both sourdough fermented breads gave glycemic responses significantly lower than the corresponding breads leavened with *Saccharomyces cerevisiae* in eight healthy volunteers. The presence of fiber did not influence the glycemic potential of breads [68].

In another study [69] conducted on 16 glucose-intolerant subjects, who had randomly received either a meal containing bread (70% durum wheat semolina and 30% corn flour) leavened with sourdough or a meal containing bread leavened with baker's yeast, sourdough bread induced a significantly lower plasma glucose response at 30 min and a significantly smaller incremental area under the curve at 0–30 and 0–60 min in comparison to bread leavened with baker's yeast. Accordingly, the plasma insulin response of sourdough bread showed significantly lower values at 30 min and a significantly smaller incremental area under the curve at 0–30 min [69]. The sourdough wholemeal wheat breads resulted in the lowest postprandial glucose and insulin response among four tested breads (white wheat bread, wholemeal wheat bread, sourdough wholemeal bread, and wholemeal bread made with xylanase) [33].

It has been shown that sourdough fermentation is more efficient than yeast fermentation in reducing phytate content in whole wheat bread (−62% and −38%, respectively) [70], because the reduction of the pH value provides favorable conditions for the endogenous cereal phytase activity [71]. Phytate, which is widely represented in whole grains and legumes but also in oil seeds and nuts [72], strongly bound to metal cations of Ca, Fe, K, Mg, Mn, and Zn, making them insoluble and, thus, unavailable as nutritional factors [73]. It has been commented: "With sourdough processes, the mouthfeel and the palatability of wholemeal bread can be improved without removing any nutritionally important components" [74].

8.7.2 Sourdough Leavened Bread and Body Weight

The traditional Mediterranean diet with sourdough wholemeal bread can be qualified as a low GI diet. Low GI/GL diets offer many health advantages in comparison with high GI/GL diet on body weight, blood lipid levels, and risk of type 2 diabetes mellitus (T2DM), coronary heart disease, and cancer. Regarding the effects of high GI diet on body weight, this diet raises glucose and insulin in the early postprandial period (0–2 h) more than low GI diet, and the excess of insulin lowers blood glucose in the postprandial period (3–5 h), thus leading to excessive hunger. The decrease of plasma glucose and the increased hunger have been associated with increased activity in specific brain regions related to food intake, reward, and craving in overweight or obese men. The assessment has been done by using arterial spin-labeling functional magnetic resonance imaging [75]. In 14 healthy subjects, an activation of limbic-striatal brain regions with a concomitant increasing desire for high-calorie foods was evident when a mild hypoglycemia occurred during hyperinsulinemic euglycemic-hypoglycemic clamp [76]. A recent meta-analysis of clinical trials evaluated the relationship between glycemic response and markers of health. When food intake was limited controlled or ad libitum, low GL diets were significantly associated with lower body weight under free-living conditions if a GL reduction by ≥17 g glucose equivalent/day occurred and most consistently when the GL reduction was by >42 g glucose equivalent/day [77]. Other observational studies, however, have shown conflicting results about the relationship between GI/GL and body mass index [78–81].

8.7.3 GI, GL, and Serum Lipid Profile

High GI/GL diets have an unfavorable effect on serum lipid, influencing cardiovascular disease. In cross-sectional analyses of two large cohort studies [82, 83], a large trial [84] and a sample of the Nurses' Health Study [85], GL was inversely associated with HDL cholesterol and directly associated with triglycerides. In 5830 nondiabetic subjects aged 20–70 of the Health Worker Cohort Study, the adjusted odds ratios in the highest versus the lowest quartile of dietary GL were 1.78 for low HDL cholesterol (<40 mg/dL for men; <50 mg/dL for women) (p for a trend of 0.002) and 1.85 for high triglycerides (≥150 mg/dL) (p for a trend of 0.01) [83]. In two studies [83, 84], high dietary GI was positively associated with both lower HDL cholesterol and higher triglyceride concentrations. In a small cross-sectional study in which dietary GI/GL were calculated accurately from 3-day dietary records, the highest concentration of HDL cholesterol and the lowest of triglycerides and insulin were observed in the lowest GI tertile ($p < 0.01$) [86]. An increase in insulin resistance, which, in turn, causes an increase in triglycerides and a decrease in HDL cholesterol, can explain the effects of high GI/GL diets on blood lipids. In the early postprandial period (0–2 h after the meal), the rapid absorption of carbohydrates after a high GI meal leads to a relatively high blood glucose level and a high insulin/glucagon ratio. In the late postprandial period (4–6 h after the meal), the counter-regulatory hormones restore normal glycemia and cause a marked increase in free fatty acid concentration [86]. Elevated glucose, insulin, and free fatty acids induce insulin resistance [87].

8.7.4 Glycemic Index (GI), Glycemic Load (GL), and the Risk of Type 2 Diabetes Mellitus (T2DM)

High GL diet has been associated with an increased risk of developing T2DM in several large prospective studies. In a systematic review and meta-analyses of 24 prospective cohort studies, the GL ranged from ~60 to ~280 g per daily intake of 2000 kcal (8.4 MJ); in a fully adjusted meta-analysis model, the GL was positively associated with RR of T2DM of 1.45 (95% CI: 1.31, 1.61) for a 100 g increment in GL ($P < 0.001$; $n = 24$ studies; 7.5 million person-years of follow-up) [88]. These findings from prospective cohort studies relating the GL to T2D appear robust and consistently indicate strong and significantly lower T2D risk in persons who consume lower GL diets [88].

The potential mechanisms whereby high GL diets, over a period of years, could increase the risk of T2DM include an increase in insulin demand following hyperglycemia that, in turn, leads to a loss of pancreatic function (due to β-cell exhaustion or toxicity of hyperglycemia) and an increased insulin resistance induced by free fatty acids, produced in the late postprandial period by counter-regulatory hormones. The progressively higher glucose levels induced by a high GL depend on the degree of underlying insulin resistance being more evident in obese, inactive, or genetically susceptible people [89].

Actually, the mechanism by which GL, hyperinsulinemia, and insulin resistance lead to T2DM appears to be more complex and strongly related to the increase of abdominal-perivisceral fat [90].

In presence of a positive caloric balance, adipocytes undergo excessive hypertrophy, which causes adipocyte dysfunction, as well as adipose tissue endocrine and immune responses (see Chap. 4, Fig. 4.1). A preferential site of fat accumulation is the abdominal-perivisceral region, due to peculiar factors of the adipose tissue in

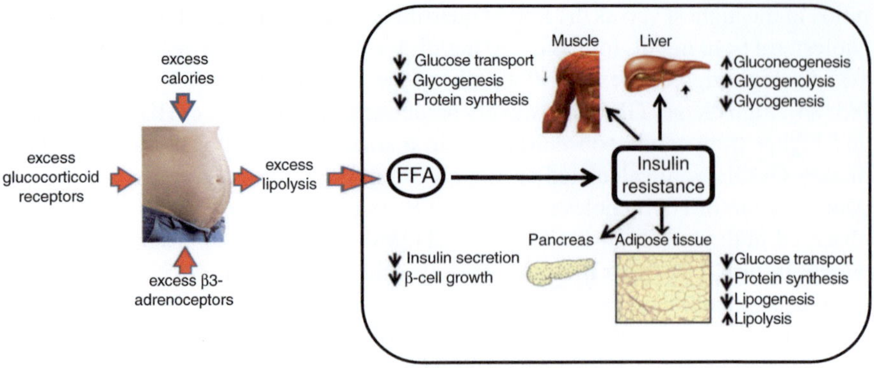

Fig. 8.2 Peripheral insulin resistance induced by abdominal obesity

such sites, namely, an excess of glucocorticoid activity, which promotes the accumulation of fat, and the greater metabolic activity and sensitivity to lipolysis, due to increased number and activity of β_3-adrenoceptors and, partly, to reduced activity of α_2-adrenoceptors. As a consequence, an increased lipolysis takes place and more free fatty acids (FFA) are released into the portal system, causing insulin resistance in several organs and tissues, i.e., the liver, muscle, adipose tissue, and pancreas (Fig. 8.2). Hypertrophic adipocytes begin to secrete low levels of TNF-α, which stimulate preadipocytes and endothelial cells to produce MCP-1, in turn responsible for attracting macrophages to the adipose tissue, thus developing a state of chronic low-grade inflammation which is causally linked to insulin resistance (see Chap. 4, Fig. 4.1). Excess of circulating FFA, TNF-α, and other factors induces insulin resistance (Fig. 8.2). FFA cause insulin resistance by inhibiting insulin signaling through the activation of serine kinases, i.e., protein kinase C-Θ, and the kinases JNK and IKK, which promote a mechanism of serine phosphorylation of insulin receptor substrates (IRS), leading to interruption of the downstream insulin receptor (IR) signaling. TNF-α, secreted by hypertrophic adipocytes and adipose tissue macrophages, also inhibits IR signaling by a double mechanism of serine phosphorylation and tyrosine dephosphorylation of IRS-1, causing inactivation and degradation of IRS-1 and a consequent stop of IR signaling (Fig. 8.3). Such mechanisms explain the transition from excess adiposity to insulin resistance, key to the further development of T2DM [90].

8.7.5 GI, GL, and the Risk of Coronary Heart Disease (CHD)

Several prospective studies have evaluated the relationship between dietary GI/GL and the risk of CHD. Four systematic reviews and meta-analyses [91–94], including an Italian prospective study [95], showed that high dietary GL significantly increases the risk of coronary heart disease in women, but not in men. A greater decrease in HDL cholesterol and a greater increase in triglycerides in women than in men in response to a high GI/GL diet [96], due to sex-related differences in lipid

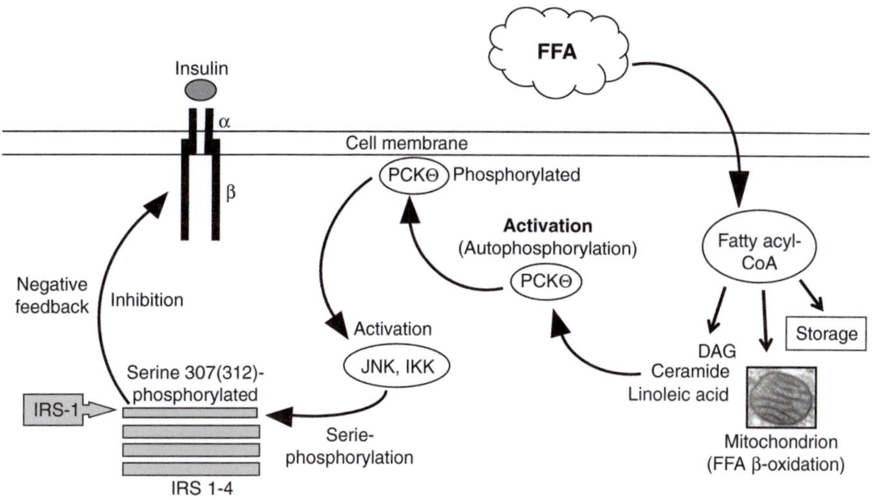

Fig. 8.3 Derangement of intracellular insulin signalling induced by excess of circulating FFA

metabolism, can explain these results. Furthermore, the hazards ratio for coronary heart disease is higher in diabetic women than in men [97]. Interestingly, in the EPICOR (long-term follow-up of antithrombotic management patterns in acute coronary syndrome patients) study, increasing carbohydrate intake from high GI foods was significantly associated with greater risk of coronary heart disease in women, whereas increasing carbohydrate intake from low GI foods was not [95]. The dietary GI can influence the risk of coronary heart disease through inflammation and oxidative stress. Low GI diets are associated with lower C-reactive protein [84] and lipid peroxidation markers [98] in comparison to high GI diets in cross-sectional studies.

8.7.6 GI, GL, and Cancer Development

Several case–control and prospective epidemiological studies have investigated the relationship between GI/GL, diets, and cancer development. Chronic hyperinsulinemia may promote cancer through abnormal stimulation of multiple cellular signaling cascades and increasing the bioactivity of insulin-like growth factor 1. Concerning breast cancer, insulin, by reducing sex hormone-binding globulin levels, increases the estrogens bioavailability that, in turn, promotes cellular proliferation and inhibits apoptosis in breast epithelium and endometrium [99]. Moreover, hyperinsulinemia increases pro-inflammatory cytokines and oxidative stress that, in turn, can promote malignancy and neoplastic progression [99]. Systematic reviews and meta-analysis however have shown conflicting results regarding the cancer sites [100–104]. However, a large nationwide population-based case–control study showed that GI is positively associated with the risk of prostate cancer, and a high GL significantly increases the risk of colorectal and pancreatic cancers [105].

8.7.7 The Fiber in Sourdough Bread

The richness in fiber of wholemeal sourdough bread is an important peculiarity to consider (see also Chap. 9, Sect. 9.5.3.9). It has been shown that high intake of cereal fiber reduces the risk of coronary heart disease [106], T2DM [107], obesity [108], and colorectal cancer [109]. Cereal fiber reduces inflammatory markers [110, 111] and improves insulin sensitivity [112]. Whole grain cereals, but not refined grains, reduce the risk of coronary heart disease, gastrointestinal cancer [113], and T2DM [113, 114]. The protective mechanisms of whole grain cereals against the risk of developing chronic diseases depend on bioactive compounds and dietary fiber, mainly contained in the bran and germ fractions that are lost in the milling process [115]. Interestingly, fiber and oligosaccharides of whole grain wheat have also a prebiotic effect on gut microbiota [8, 116] involved in systemic low-grade inflammation and progression of chronic metabolic diseases [117].

References

1. Solfrizzi V, Panza F, Torres F, Mastroianni F, Del Parigi A, Venezia A, Capurso A. High monounsaturated fatty acids intake protects against age-related cognitive decline. Neurology. 1999;52:1563–9.
2. Aune D, Keum N, Giovannucci E, Fadnes LT, Boffetta P, Greenwood DC, Tonstad S, Vatten LJ, Riboli E, Norat T. Whole grain consumption and risk of cardiovascular disease, cancer, and all cause and cause specific mortality: systematic review and dose-response meta-analysis of prospective studies. Br Med J. 2016;353:i2716.
3. Whole grains and fiber. American Heart Association; 2016.
4. Health claim notification for whole grain foods. Bethesda, MD: Food and Drug Administration, US Department of Health and Human Services; 1999. Accessed 4 Dec 2016.
5. Stevenson L, Phillips F, O'Sullivan K, Walton J. Wheat bran: its composition and benefits to health, a European perspective. Int J Food Sci Nutr. 2012;63:1001–13.
6. Topping D. Cereal complex carbohydrates and their contribution to human health. J Cereal Sci. 2007;46:220–9.
7. Chen HL, Haack VS, Janecky CW, Vollendorf NW, Marlett JA. Mechanisms by which wheat bran and oat bran increase stool weight in humans. Am J Clin Nutr. 1998;68:711–9.
8. Costabile A, Klinder A, Fava F, Napolitano A, Fogliano V, Leonard C, Gibson GR, Tuohy KM. Whole-grain wheat breakfast cereal has a prebiotic effect on the human gut microbiota: a double-blind, placebo-controlled, crossover study. Br J Nutr. 2008;99:110–20.
9. Laddomada B, Caretto S, Mita G. Wheat bran phenolic acids: bioavailability and stability in whole wheat-based foods. Molecules. 2015;20:15666–85.
10. Mateo Anson N, van den Berg R, Havenaar R, Bast A, Haenen GR. Ferulic acid from aleurone determines the antioxidant potency of wheat grain (Triticum aestivum L.). J Agric Food Chem. 2008;56:5589–94.
11. Adom KK, Sorrells ME, Liu RH. Phytochemicals and antioxidant activity of milled fractions of different wheat varieties. J Agric Food Chem. 2005;53:22972306.
12. Qu H, Madl RL, Takemoto DJ, Baybutt RC, Wang W. Lignans are involved in the antitumor activity of wheat bran in colon cancer SW480 cells. J Nutr. 2005;135:598–602.
13. Shan BE, Wang MX, Li RQ. Quercetin inhibit human SW480 colon cancer growth in association with inhibition of cyclin D1 and survivin expression through Wnt/beta-catenin signaling pathway. Cancer Investig. 2009;27:604–12.

14. Schober TJ, Bean SR, Kuhn M. Gluten proteins from spelt (Triticum aestivum ssp. spelta) cultivars: a rheological and size-exclusion high-performance liquid chromatography study. J Cereal Sci. 2006;44:161–73.
15. CS1 maint: Uses authors parameter (link), Behall KM, Scholfiels DJ, Hallfrisch JG. Barley B. Glucan reduces plasma glucose and insulin responses compared with resistant starch in men. Nutr Res. 2006;26:644–650.
16. Lia A, Hallmans G, Sandberg AS, Sundberg B, Aman P, Andersson H. Oat beta-glucan increases bile acid excretion and a fiber-rich barley fraction increases cholesterol excretion in ileostomy subjects. Am J Clin Nutr. 1995;62:1245–51.
17. Whitehead A, Beck EJ, Tosh S, Wolever TM. Cholesterol-lowering effects of oat β-glucan: a meta-analysis of randomized controlled trials. Am J Clin Nutr. 2014;100:1413–21.
18. Nutrition for everyone. Centers for Disease Control and Prevention, US Department of Health and Human Services; 2014.
19. Juntunen KS, Laaksonen DE, Niskanen LK, Holst JJ, Savolainen KE, Liukkonen K-H, Poutanen KS, Mykkanen HM. Structural differences between rye and wheat bread but not total fiber content may explain the lower postprandial insulin response to rye bread. Am J Clin Nutr. 2003;78:957–64.
20. Nodlund E, Katina K, Mykkänen H, Poutanen K. Distinct characteristics of rye and wheat breads impact on their in vitro gastric disintegration and in vivo glucose and insulin responses. Foods. 2016;5:24.
21. Bhupathiraju SN, Tobias DK, Malik VS, Pan A, Hruby A, Manson JE, Willett WC, Hu FB. Glycemic index, glycemic load, and risk of type 2 diabetes: results from 3 large US cohorts and an updated meta-analysis. Am J Clin Nutr. 2014;100:218–32.
22. Raben A. Glycemic index and metabolic risks: how strong is the evidence? Am J Clin Nutr. 2014;100:1–3.
23. Mellen PB, Walsh TF, Herrington DM. Whole grain intake and cardiovascular disease: a meta-analysis. Nutr Metab Cardiovasc Dis. 2008;18:283–90.
24. Chanson-Rolle A, Meynier A, Aubin F, Lappi J, Poutanen K, Vinoy S, Braesco V. Systematic review and meta-analysis of human studies to support a quantitative recommendation for whole grain intake in relation to type 2 diabetes. PLoS One. 2015;10:e0131377.
25. Foster-Powell K, Holt SH, Brand-Miller JC. International table of glycemic index and glycemic load values: 2002. Am J Clin Nutr. 2002;76:5–56.
26. Eelderink C, Noort MW, Sozer N, Koehorst M, Holst JJ, Deacon CF, Rehfeld JF, Poutanen K, Vonk RJ, Oudhuis L, Priebe MG. The structure of wheat bread influences the postprandial metabolic response in healthy men. Food Funct. 2015;6:3236–328.
27. Autio K, Parkkonen T, Fabritius M. Observing structural differences in wheat and rye breads. Cereal Foods World. 1997;42:702–5.
28. Lorenz K. Rye bread: fermentation processes ABD products in the United States. In: Kulp K, Lorenz K, editors. Handbook of dough fermentations. New York, NY: Marcel Dekker Inc; 2003. p. 159–91.
29. De Angelis M, Rizzello CG, Alfonsi G, Arnault P, Cappelle S, Di Cagno R, Gobbetti M. Use of sourdough lactobacilli and oat fibre to decrease the glycaemic index of white wheat bread. Br J Nutr. 2007;98:1196–205.
30. Östman EM, Nilsson M, Liljeberg Elmståhl HGM, Molin G, Björck IME. On the effect of lactic acid on blood glucose and insulin responses to cereal products: mechanistic studies in healthy subjects and *in Vitro*. J Cereal Sci. 2002;36:339–46.
31. Rosén LA, Östman EM, Shewry PR, Ward JL, Andersson AA, Piironen V, Lampi AM, Rakszegi M, Bedö Z, Björck IM. Postprandial glycemia, insulinemia, and satiety responses in healthy subjects after whole grain rye bread made from different rye varieties. 1. J Agric Food Chem. 2011;59:12139–48.
32. Rosén LA, Blanco Silva LO, Andersson UK, Holm C, Östman EM, Björck IME. Endosperm and whole grain rye breads are characterized by low post-prandial insulin response and a beneficial blood glucose profile. Nutr J. 2009;8:42.

33. Lappi J, Selinheimo E, Schwab U, Katina K, Lehtinen P, Mykkänen H, Kolehmainen M, Poutanen K. Sourdough fermentation of wholemeal wheat bread increases solubility of arabinoxylan and protein and decreases postprandial glucose and insulin responses. J Cereal Sci. 2010;51:152–8.
34. Earle R. The body of the conquistador: food, race, and the colonial experience in Spanish America, 1492–1700. New York: Cambridge University Press; 2012.
35. Staller JE, Carrasco M. Pre-Columbian Foodways: interdisciplinary approaches to food, culture, and markets in Ancient Mesoamerica, vol. 317. Berlin: Springer-Verlag; 2009.
36. Menotti A, Keys A, Anderson JT, Grande F. Prediction of serum-cholesterol responses of man to changes in fats in the diet. Lancet. 1957;273:959–66.
37. Keys A. Seven countries. A multivariate analysis of death and coronary heart disease. Cambridge: Harvard University Press; 1980.
38. Keys A, Blackburn H, Kromhout D, Karvonen M, Nissinen A, Pekkanen J, Punsar S, Fidanza F, Giampaoli S, Seccareccia F, Buzina R, Mohacek I, Nedeljkovic S, Aravanis C, Dontas A, Toshima H, Lanti M. Comparison of multivariate predictive power of major risk factors for coronary heart diseases in different countries: results from eight nations of the seven countries study, 25-year follow-up. J Cardiovasc Risk. 1996;3:69–75.
39. Keys A, Anderson JT, Grande F. Serum cholesterol response to changes in the diet: IV. Particular saturated fatty acids in the diet. Metabolism. 1965;14:776–86.
40. Hegsted DM, McGandy RB, Myers ML, Stare FJ. Quantitative effects of dietary fat on serum cholesterol in man. Am J Clin Nutr. 1965;17:281–95.
41. Vega GL, Groszek E, Wolf R, Grundy SM. Influence of polyunsaturated fats on composition of plasma lipoproteins and apolipoproteins. J Lipid Res. 1982;23:811–22.
42. Shepherd J, Packard CJ, Grundy SM, Yeshurun D, Gotto AM Jr, Taunton OD. Effects of saturated and polyunsaturated fat diets on the chemical composition and metabolism of low density lipoproteins in man. J Lipid Res. 1980;21:91–9.
43. Mensink RP, Katan MB. Effect of dietary fatty acids on serum lipids and lipoproteins. Arterioscler Thromb. 1992;12:911–9.
44. Hu FB, Stampfer MJ, Manson JE, Rimm E, Colditz GA, Rosner BA, Hennekens CH, Willett WC. Dietary fat intake and the risk of coronary heart disease in women. New Engl J Med. 1997;337:1491–9.
45. Willet WC. Dietary fats and coronary heart disease. J Intern Med. 2012;272:13–24.
46. Jakobsen MU, O'Reilly EJ, Heitmann BL, Pereira MA, Bälter K, Fraser GE, Goldbourt U, Hallmans G, Knekt P, Liu S, Pietinen P, Spiegelman D, Stevens J, Virtamo J, Willett WC, Ascherio A. Major types of dietary fat and risk of coronary heart disease: a pooled analysis of 11 cohort studies. Am J Clin Nutr. 2009;89:1425–32.
47. Ramsden CE, Zamora D, Leelarthaepin B, Majchrzak-Hong SF, Faurot KR, Suchindran CM, Ringel A, Davis JM, Hibbeln JR. Use of dietary linoleic acid for secondary prevention of coronary heart disease and death: evaluation of recovered data from the Sydney diet heart study and updated meta-analysis. Br Med J. 2013;346:e8707.
48. Folcik VA, Cathcart MK. Predominance of esterified hydroperoxy-linoleic acid in human monocyte-oxidized LDL. J Lipid Res. 1994;35:1570–82.
49. Lenz ML, Hughes H, Mitchell JR, Via DP, Guyton JR, Taylor AA, et al. Lipid hydroperoxy and hydroxy derivatives in copper-catalyzed oxidation of low density lipoprotein. J Lipid Res. 1990;31:1043–50.
50. Shibata N, Toi S, Shibata T, Uchida K, Itabe H, Sawada T, et al. Immunohistochemical detection of 13(R)-hydroxyoctadecadienoic acid in atherosclerotic plaques of human carotid arteries using a novel specific antibody. Acta Histochem Cytochem. 2009;42:197–203.
51. Harland WA, Gilbert JD, Steel G, Brooks CJW. Lipids of human atheroma. 5. Occurrence of a new group of polar sterol esters in various stages of human atherosclerosis. Atherosclerosis. 1971;13:239.
52. Carpenter KL, Taylor SE, van der Veen C, Williamson BK, Ballantine JA, Mitchinson MJ. Lipids and oxidised lipids in human atherosclerotic lesions at different stages of development. Biochim Biophys Acta. 1995;1256:141–50.

53. Kuhn H, Belkner J, Wiesner R, Schewe T, Lankin VZ, Tikhaze AK. Structure elucidation of oxygenated lipids in human atherosclerotic lesions. Eicosanoids. 1992;5:17–22.
54. Waddington EI, Croft KD, Sienuarine K, Latham B, Puddey IB. Fatty acid oxidation products in human atherosclerotic plaque: an analysis of clinical and histopathological correlates. Atherosclerosis. 2003;167:111–20.
55. Keys A, Aravanis C, Sdrin H. The diets of middle-aged men in two rural areas of Greece. In: Den Hartog C, Buzina K, Fidanza F, Keys A, Roine P, editors. Dietary studies and epidemiology of heart diseases. The Hague: Stichting tot Wetenschappelijke Voorlichting op Voedingsgebied; 1968. p. 57–68.
56. Alberti-Fidanza A, Fidanza F, Chiuchiù MP, Verducci G, Fruttini D. Dietary studies on two rural Italian population groups of the seven countries study. 3. Trend of food and nutrient intake from 1960 to 1991. Eur J Clin Nutr. 1999;53:854–60.
57. Simopoulos AP. The Mediterranean diets: what is so special about the diet of Greece? The scientific evidence. J Nutr. 2001;131:3065–73.
58. Corsetti A, Settanni L. Lactobacilli in sourdough fermentation. Food Res Int. 2007;40:539–58.
59. Björck I, Elmståhl HL. The glycaemic index: importance of dietary fibre and other food properties. Proc Nutr Soc. 2003;62:201–6.
60. Poutanen K, Flander L, Katina K. Sourdough and cereal fermentation in a nutritional perspective. Food Microbiol. 2009;26:693–9.
61. Liljeberg HG, Lönner CH, Björck I. Sourdough fermentation or addition of organic acids or corresponding salts to bread improves nutritional properties of starch in healthy humans. J Nutr. 1995;125:1503–11.
62. Liljeberg H, Björck I. Delayed gastric emptying rate may explain improved glycaemia in healthy subjects to a starchy meal with added vinegar. Eur J Clin Nutr. 1998;52:368–71.
63. Atkinson FS, Foster-Powell K, Brand-Miller JC. International tables of glycemic index and glycemic load values: 2008. Diabetes Care. 2008;31:2281–3.
64. Breen C, Ryan M, Gibney MJ, Corrigan M, O'Shea D. Glycemic, insulinemic, and appetite responses of patients with type 2 diabetes to commonly consumed breads. Diabetes Educ. 2013;39:376–86.
65. Jenkins DJ, Wesson V, Wolever TM, Jenkins AL, Kalmusky J, Guidici S, Csima A, Josse RG, Wong GS. Wholemeal *versus* wholegrain breads: proportion of whole or cracked grain and the glycaemic response. BMJ. 1988;297:958–60.
66. Holt SH, Miller JB. Particle size, satiety and the glycaemic response. Eur J Clin Nutr. 1994;48:496–502.
67. Liljeberg H, Granfeldt Y, Björck I. Metabolic responses to starch in bread containing intact kernels *versus* milled flour. Eur J Clin Nutr. 1992;46:561–75.
68. Scazzina F, Del Rio D, Pellegrini N, Brighenti F. Sourdough bread: starch digestibility and postprandial glycemic response. J Cereal Sci. 2009;49:419–21.
69. Maioli M, Pes GM, Sanna M, Cherchi S, Dettori M, Manca E, Farris GA. Sourdough leavened bread improves postprandial glucose and insulin plasma levels in subjects with impaired glucose tolerance. Acta Diabetol. 2008;45:91–6.
70. Lopez HW, Krespine V, Guy C, Messager A, Demigne C, Remesy C. Prolonged fermentation of whole wheat sourdough reduces phytate level and increases soluble magnesium. J Agric Food Chem. 2001;49:2657–62.
71. Reale A, Konietzny U, Coppola R, Sorrentino E, Greiner R. The importance of lactic acid bacteria for phytate degradation during cereal dough fermentation. *J Agric Food Chem.* 2007;55:2993–7.
72. Schlemmer U, Frølich W, Prieto RM, Grases F. Phytate in foods and significance for humans: food sources, intake, processing, bioavailability, protective role and analysis. Mol Nutr Food Res. 2009;53:330–75.
73. Bohn L, Meyer AS, Rasmussen SK. Phytate: impact on environment and human nutrition. A challenge for molecular breeding. J Zhejiang Univ Sci B. 2008;9:165–91.

74. Katina K, Arendt E, Liukkonen K-H, Autio K, Flander L, Poutanen K. Potential of sourdough for healthier cereal products. Trends Food Sci Tech. 2005;16:104–12.
75. Lennerz BS, Alsop DC, Holsen LM, Stern E, Rojas R, Ebbeling CB, Goldstein JM, Ludwig DS. Effects of dietary glycemic index on brain regions related to reward and craving in men. Am J Clin Nutr. 2013;98:641–7.
76. Page KA, Seo D, Belfort-DeAguiar R, Lacadie C, Dzuira J, Naik S, Amarnath S, Constable RT, Sherwin RS, Sinha R. Circulating glucose levels modulate neural control of desire for high-calorie foods in humans. J Clin Investig. 2011;121:4161–9.
77. Livesey G, Taylor R, Hulshof T, Howlett J. Glycemic response and health. A systematic review and meta-analysis: relations between dietary glycemic properties and health outcomes. Am J Clin Nutr. 2008;87:258–68.
78. Lau C, Toft U, Tetens I, Richelsen B, Jørgensen T, Borch-Johnsen K, Glümer C. Association between dietary glycemic index, glycemic load, and body mass index in the Inter99 study: is underreporting a problem? Am J Clin Nutr. 2006;84:641–5.
79. Murakami K, McCaffrey TA, Livingstone MB. Associations of dietary glycaemic index and glycaemic load with food and nutrient intake and general and central obesity in British adults. Br J Nutr. 2013;9:1–11.
80. Rossi M, Bosetti C, Talamini R, Lagiou P, Negri E, Franceschi S, La Vecchia C. Glycemic index and glycemic load in relation to body mass index and waist to hip ratio. Eur J Nutr. 2010;49:459–64.
81. Mendez MA, Covas MI, Marrugat J, Vila J, Schröder H. Glycemic load, glycemic index, and body mass index in Spanish adults. Am J Clin Nutr. 2009;89:316–22.
82. Ford ES, Liu S. Glycemic index and serum high-density lipoprotein cholesterol concentration among US adults. Arch Intern Med. 2001;161:572–6.
83. Denova-Gutiérrez E, Huitrón-Bravo G, Talavera JO, Castañón S, Gallegos-Carrillo K, Flores Y, Salmerón J. Dietary glycemic index, dietary glycemic load, blood lipids, and coronary heart disease. J Nutr Metab. 2010;2010:170680.
84. Levitan EB, Cook NR, Stampfer MJ, Ridker PM, Rexrode KM, Buring JE, Manson JE, Liu S. Dietary glycemic index, dietary glycemic load, blood lipids, and C-reactive protein. Metabolism. 2008;57:437–43.
85. Liu S, Manson JE, Stampfer MJ, Holmes MD, Hu FB, Hankinson SE, Willett WC. Dietary glycemic load assessed by food-frequency questionnaire in relation to plasma high-density lipoprotein cholesterol and fasting plasma triacylglycerols in postmenopausal women. Am J Clin Nutr. 2001;73:560–6.
86. Amano Y, Kawakubo K, Lee JS, Tang AC, Sugiyama M, Mori K. Correlation between dietary glycemic index and cardiovascular disease risk factors among Japanese women. Eur J Clin Nutr. 2004;58:1472–8.
87. Ludwig DS. The glycemic index: physiological mechanisms relating to obesity, diabetes, and cardiovascular disease. JAMA. 2002;287:2414–23.
88. Livesey G, Taylor R, Livesey H, Liu S. Is there a dose-response relation of dietary glycemic load to risk of type 2 diabetes? Meta-analysis of prospective cohort studies. Am J Clin Nutr. 2013;97:584–96.
89. Willett W, Manson J, Liu S. Glycemic index, glycemic load, and risk of type 2 diabetes. Am J Clin Nutr. 2002;76:274–80.
90. Capurso C, Capurso A. From excess adiposity to insulin resistance: the role of free fatty acids. Vasc Pharmacol. 2012;57:91–7.
91. Dong JY, Zhang YH, Wang P, Qin LQ. Meta-analysis of dietary glycemic load and glycemic index in relation to risk of coronary heart disease. Am J Cardiol. 2012;109:1608–13.
92. Fan J, Song Y, Wang Y, Hui R, Zhang W. Dietary glycemic index, glycemic load, and risk of coronary heart disease, stroke, and stroke mortality: a systematic review with meta-analysis. PLoS One. 2012;7:e52182.
93. Mirrahimi A, de Souza RJ, Chiavaroli L, Sievenpiper JL, Beyene J, Hanley AJ, Augustin LS, Kendall CW, Jenkins DJ. Associations of glycemic index and load with coronary heart

disease events: a systematic review and meta-analysis of prospective cohorts. J Am Heart Assoc. 2012;1:e000752.
94. Mirrahimi A, Chiavaroli L, Srichaikul K, Augustin LS, Sievenpiper JL, Kendall CW, Jenkins DJ. The role of glycemic index and glycemic load in cardiovascular disease and its risk factors: a review of the recent literature. Curr Atheroscler Rep. 2014;16:1–10.
95. Sieri S, Krogh V, Berrino F, Evangelista A, Agnoli C, Brighenti F, Pellegrini N, Palli D, Masala G, Sacerdote C, et al. Dietary glycemic load and index and risk of coronary heart disease in a large Italian cohort: the EPICOR study. Arch Intern Med. 2010;170:640–7.
96. Knopp RH, Paramsothy P, Retzlaff BM, Fish B, Walden C, Dowdy A, Tsunehara C, Aikawa K, Cheung MC. Gender differences in lipoprotein metabolism and dietary response: basis in hormonal differences and implications for cardiovascular disease. Curr Atheroscler Rep. 2005;7:472–9.
97. The Emerging Risk Factors Collaboration, Sarwar N, Gao P, Seshasai SR, Gobin R, Kaptoge S, di Angelantonio E, Ingelsson E, Lawlor DA, Selvin E, Stampfer M, et al. Diabetes mellitus, fasting blood glucose concentration, and risk of vascular disease: a collaborative meta-analysis of 102 prospective studies. Lancet. 2010;375:2215–22.
98. Hu Y, Block G, Norkus EP, Morrow JD, Dietrich M, Hudes M. Relations of glycemic index and glycemic load with plasma oxidative stress markers. Am J Clin Nutr. 2006;84:70–6.
99. Arcidiacono B, Iiritano S, Nocera A, Possidente K, Nevolo MT, Ventura V, Foti D, Chiefari E, Brunetti A. Insulin resistance and cancer risk: an overview of the pathogenetic mechanisms. Exp Diabetes Res. 2012;2012:789174.
100. Gnagnarella P, Gandini S, la Vecchia C, Maisonneuve P. Glycemic index, glycemic load, and cancer risk: a meta-analysis. Am J Clin Nutr. 2008;87:1793–801.
101. Mulholland HG, Murray LJ, Cardwell CR, Cantwell MM. Dietary glycaemic index, glycaemic load and endometrial and ovarian cancer risk: a systematic review and meta-analysis. Br J Cancer. 2008;99:434–41.
102. Mulholland HG, Murray LJ, Cardwell CR, Cantwell MM. Glycemic index, glycemic load, and risk of digestive tract neoplasms: a systematic review and meta-analysis. Am J Clin Nutr. 2009;89:568–76.
103. Aune D, Chan DS, Greenwood DC, Vieira AR, Rosenblatt DA, Vieira R, Norat T. Dietary fiber and breast cancer risk: a systematic review and meta-analysis of prospective studies. Ann Oncol. 2012;23:1394–402.
104. Dong JY, Qin LQ. Dietary glycemic index, glycemic load, and risk of breast cancer: meta-analysis of prospective cohort studies. Breast Cancer Res Treat. 2011;126:287–94.
105. Hu J, la Vecchia C, Augustin LS, Negri E, de Groh M, Morrison H, Mery L, Canadian Cancer Registries Epidemiology Research Group. Glycemic index, glycemic load and cancer risk. Ann Oncol. 2013;24:245–51.
106. Pereira MA, O'Reilly E, Augustsson K, Fraser GE, Goldbourt U, Heitmann BL, Hallmans G, Knekt P, Liu S, Pietinen P, Spiegelman D, Stevens J, Virtamo J, Willett WC, Ascherio A. Dietary fiber and risk of coronary heart disease: a pooled analysis of cohort studies. Arch Intern Med. 2004;164:370–6.
107. Schulze MB, Schulz M, Heidemann C, Schienkiewitz A, Hoffmann K, Boeing H. Fiber and magnesium intake and incidence of type 2 diabetes: a prospective study and meta-analysis. Arch Intern Med. 2007;167:956–65.
108. Koh-Banerjee P, Franz M, Sampson L, Liu S, Jacobs DR Jr, Spiegelman D, Willett W, Rimm E. Changes in whole-grain, bran, and cereal fiber consumption in relation to 8-y weight gain among men. Am J Clin Nutr. 2004;80:1237–45.
109. Aune D, Chan DS, Lau R, Vieira R, Greenwood DC, Kampman E, Norat T. Dietary fibre, whole grains, and risk of colorectal cancer: systematic review and dose-response meta-analysis of prospective studies. Br Med J. 2011;343:d6617.
110. Esposito K, Nappo F, Giugliano F, di Palo C, Ciotola M, Barbieri M, Paolisso G, Giugliano D. Meal modulation of circulating interleukin 18 and adiponectin concentrations in healthy subjects and in patients with type 2 diabetes mellitus. Am J Clin Nutr. 2003;78:1135–40.

111. Chuang SC, Vermeulen R, Sharabiani MT, Sacerdote C, Fatemeh SH, Berrino F, Krogh V, Palli D, Panico S, Tumino R, et al. The intake of grain fibers modulates cytokine levels in blood. Biomarkers. 2011;16:504–10.
112. Weickert MO, Möhlig M, Schöfl C, Arafat AM, Otto B, Viehoff H, Koebnick C, Kohl A, Spranger J, Pfeiffer AF. Cereal fiber improves whole-body insulin sensitivity in overweight and obese women. Diabetes Care. 2006;29:775–80.
113. Gil A, Ortega RM, Maldonado J. Wholegrain cereals and bread: a duet of the Mediterranean diet for the prevention of chronic diseases. Public Health Nutr. 2011;14:2316–22.
114. Aune D, Norat T, Romundstad P, Vatten LJ. Whole grain and refined grain consumption and the risk of type 2 diabetes: a systematic review and dose-response meta-analysis of cohort studies. Eur J Epidemiol. 2013;28:845–58.
115. Fardet A. New hypotheses for the health-protective mechanisms of whole-grain cereals: what is beyond fibre? Nutr Res Rev. 2010;23:65–134.
116. Slavin J. Fiber and prebiotics: mechanisms and health benefits. Forum Nutr. 2013;5:1417–35.
117. Nakamura YK, Omaye ST. Metabolic diseases and pro- and prebiotics: mechanistic insights. Nutr Metab. 2012;9:60.

Vegetables

9

9.1 Premises

Vegetables are crucial part of the Mediterranean diet, which is principally founded on plant-based foods with occasional inclusion of land or sea animals. In addition to whole grains, legumes and pulses, fresh fruit, cheese, and olive oil, the Mediterranean diet places a major emphasis on vegetables, which are included abundantly in the daily eating plan.

Today, nearly everyone is aware of the importance of eating vegetables, especially dark green leafy ones, which are packed with vitamins and are nutrient-dense and incredibly healthy.

As noted above, most of the benefits of the Mediterranean diet derive from vegetables, which are particularly rich in vitamins and antioxidants that have an important impact on human health.

This chapter is dedicated to some of the many benefits of the vegetables currently used in the Mediterranean diet of south Europe and south Italy, i.e., *Cruciferae,* leafy vegetables, and *Solanaceae*.

9.2 Cruciferae: Brassicaceae

Cruciferae is a family of *Brassicaceae* containing 372 genera and 4060 accepted species. The family of *Brassicaceae, or Cruciferae*, includes species, such as *Brassica oleracea* (e.g., cauliflower, cabbage, kale, broccoli, collards), *Brassica rapa* (turnip, Chinese cabbage), *Brassica napus* (rapeseed), *Raphanus sativus* (common radish), *Armoracia rusticana* (horseradish), and others.

Brassica oleracea is a widely cultivated vegetable species including many different foods, such as cauliflower, cabbage, kale, turnip greens, broccoli, collard greens, brussels sprouts, and similar green leafy vegetables. At present, cruciferous vegetables are the one of the most dominant food crops worldwide. Ten of the most

A. Capurso et al., *Benefits of the Mediterranean Diet in the Elderly Patient*, Practical Issues in Geriatrics, https://doi.org/10.1007/978-3-319-78084-9_9

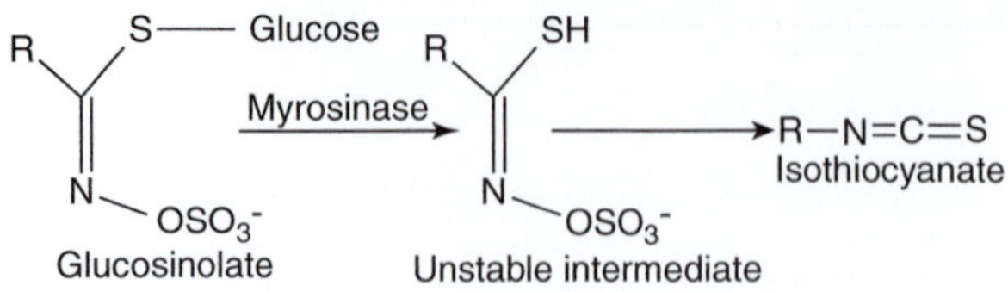

Fig. 9.1 Hydrolysis of glucosinolate to isothiocyanate

common cruciferous vegetables, known colloquially in North America as *cole crops,* belong to the single species of *Brassica oleracea.*

Cruciferae vegetables all have high levels of vitamin C and K, often exceeding the minimum daily value and recommended intake. It should be noted that up to two-thirds of Americans don't meet the daily recommended goal for vitamin K (90 μg for women and 120 μg for men).

The high content of glucosinolate in *Cruciferous* vegetables is another important fact that merits attention. Glucosinolates are sulfur-containing compounds that impart a pungent aroma and spicy (some say bitter) taste. The hydrolysis (breakdown) of glucosinolates by a class of plant enzymes called myrosinase leads to the formation of biologically active compounds, such as indoles and isothiocyanates (Fig. 9.1). Myrosinase is physically separated from glucosinolates in intact plant cells. But, when cruciferous vegetables are chopped or chewed, myrosinase comes in contact with glucosinolates and catalyzes their hydrolysis to isothiocyanate. Scientists are currently studying the potential effects of high intakes of cruciferous vegetables as well as of several sources of glucosinolate and their hydrolysis products for their cancer prevention properties.

The complete list of cruciferous vegetables includes 27 different species. Some of them, the most commonly used in the Mediterranean diet, will be described below.

9.2.1 Collard Greens and Kales

Collard greens (collards) and kale are some loose-leafed cultivars of *Brassica oleracea.* The cultivar group called *Acephala* ("without head" in Greek) refers to the fact that these varieties of *Brassica oleracea* do not have the usual close-knit core of leaves (a "head") like cabbage. Collard greens and kales help to reinforce several systems of human metabolism. There is not a lot of differences between kale and collard greens, because they both belong to the same cultivar group, Acephala of the *Brassica oleracea* species, and the fact that they are also almost identical genetically makes identifying their differences even more difficult.

A 100 g serving of cooked collard greens or kale is composed 90% of water, 3% of protein, 6% of carbohydrates, and less than 1% of fat and provides 33 calories. In terms of % Daily Value (DV), 1 cup (190 g) provides 85% of vitamin K, 80% of vitamin A, 49% of manganese, 46% of vitamin C, and 30% of fiber. It should be noted that as far as vitamin K is concerned, up to two-thirds of Americans do not meet the daily recommended goal (90 μg for women and 120 μg for men). Cooked kale is a vitamin K powerhouse, packing 550 μg in a one-half cup. Raw kale in a salad or a smoothie provides 274 μg for the same half-cup serving.

9.2.1.1 Historical Notes

People have been eating collard greens for at least 2000 years; there is some evidence showing that the ancient Greeks cultivated several forms of both collard greens and kale.

9.2.1.2 Nutrients and Phytochemicals

Collard greens and kale are excellent sources of vitamin A, vitamin C, vitamin K, and manganese, and moderate sources of calcium and vitamin B_6 (see tables). A 100 g serving of cooked collard greens provides about 30 calories, 90% water, 2–3% protein, 6% carbohydrates, and less than 1% fat.

Collard Greens, Cooked, Boiled, Drained
Vitamins and mineral content per 100 g
Source: USDA Database entry

Energy	137 KJ (33 kcal)
Carbohydrates	5.6 g
Sugars	0.4 g
Protein	2.7 g
Fat	0.7 g
Dietary fiber	4.0 g

Vitamin A equiv.	380 μg	(5% DV)
β-Carotene	4513 μg	(4% DV)
Lutein zeaxanthin	6197 μg	
Thiamine (B_1)	0.04 mg	(12% DV)
Riboflavin (B_2)	0.11 mg	(8% DV)
Niacin	0.58 mg	(5% DV)
Pantothenic acid	0.22 mg	(6% DV)
Folate	16 μg	(15% DV)
Vitamin C	18 mg	(102% DV)
Vitamin E	0.9 mg	(6% DV)
Vitamin K	407 μg	(400% DV)

Calcium	141 mg	(14% DV)
Iron	1.13 mg	(9% DV)
Magnesium	21 mg	(6% DV)
Manganese	0.51 mg	(24% DV)
Phosphorus	32 mg	(5% DV)
Potassium	117 mg	(2% DV)
Sodium	0.15 mg	(1% DV)
Zinc	0.23 mg	(2% DV)

DV = Daily Value

Kale, Raw
Nutritional value per 100 g
Source: USDA Database entry

Energy	207 KJ (49 kcal)
Carbohydrates	8.8 g
Sugars	2.3 g
Protein	4.3 g
Fat	0.9 g
Dietary fiber	3.6 g

Vitamin A equiv.	500 μg	(63% DV)
Lutein zeaxanthin	8198 μg	
Thiamine (B_1)	0.11 mg	(10% DV)
Riboflavin (B_2)	0.13 mg	(11% DV)
Niacin	1.0 mg	(7% DV)
Pantothenic acid	0.9 mg	(18% DV)
Vitamin B_6	0.27 mg	(21% DV)
Folate	141 μg	(35% DV)
Vitamin C	120 mg	(145% DV)
Vitamin E	1.54 mg	(10% DV)
Vitamin K	705 μg	(671% DV)

Calcium	150 mg	(15% DV)
Iron	1.5 mg	(12% DV)
Magnesium	47 mg	(13% DV)
Manganese	0.66 mg	(31% DV)
Phosphorus	491 mg	(10% DV)
Sodium	0.38 mg	(3% DV)
Zinc	0.6 mg	(6% DV)

DV = Daily Value

9.2.1.3 Antioxidant Activity

In addition to vitamin A, vitamin C, vitamin E, and manganese, which are four core conventional antioxidants, collard greens and kale also provide caffeic acid, ferulic acid, quercetin, and kaempferol, which are some of the key polyphenolic antioxidant phytonutrients provided by vegetables. This broad spectrum of antioxidant support helps lower the risk of oxidative stress in the cells. To note, chronic oxidative stress is considered an important risk factor for the development of most types of cancer and other diseases.

9.2.1.4 Anti-inflammatory Properties

Collard greens and kale are an excellent source of vitamin K and a good source of omega-3 fatty acids (in the form of alpha-linolenic acid = ALA), two hallmark anti-inflammatory nutrients. In this respect, vitamin K acts as a direct regulator of inflammatory response, and ALA is the building block for several of the body's most widely used families of anti-inflammatory messaging molecules. In addition to these two anti-inflammatory components, there is a third with glucosinolate-derived anti-inflammatory properties. In fact, one of the glucosinolates found in collard greens and kale—glucobrassicin—is readily converted into an isothiocyanate molecule called I3C, or indole-3-carbinol. I3C is an anti-inflammatory compound that can actually operate at the genetic level, thus preventing the initiation of inflammatory responses at a very early stage. Glucoraphanin is another glucosinolate compound of kale promptly converted into sulforaphane, an active isothiocyanate.

The anti-inflammatory nature of glucosinolates/isothiocyanates and other nutrients found in collard greens and kale has been examined by new studies on inflammation-related health problems and the potential use of these *Brassicaceae* in their prevention. Research examining the association of collard greens and kale with the risk of the following inflammation-related conditions is currently underway: Crohn's disease, ulcerative colitis, irritable bowel syndrome, type 2 diabetes, insulin resistance, metabolic syndrome, and obesity.

To note, boiling decreases the level of sulforaphane, whereas steaming, microwaving, or stir-frying does not lead to significant loss.

9.2.1.5 Cardiovascular Benefits

Collard greens and kale both reduce blood cholesterol levels. These commonly eaten cruciferous vegetables appear to be the ones with the greatest cholesterol-lowering properties. They work to reduce cholesterol since their fibers are able to bind bile acids in the intestine. The liver must thus replace the lost bile acids by drawing upon the existing supply of cholesterol, thus causing the cholesterol level to drop. Collard greens and kale have this cholesterol-lowering activity both when they are raw or cooked. But, it has been recently shown that the cholesterol-lowering ability of raw collard greens improves significantly when they are steamed. It has been demonstrated, in fact, that steamed collard greens are more active in binding bile acids in the digestive tract than steamed kale, mustard greens, broccoli, Brussels sprouts, or cabbage.

Interestingly, high blood cholesterol levels promote the formation of atherosclerotic plaques in the vessels, which are characterized, when there are *active plaque* or *inflamed plaques*, by a rich infiltration of inflammatory cells (mostly macrophages and lymphocytes), which secrete in situ several inflammatory cytokines. It is for this reason that atherosclerosis is considered an inflammatory process of the vessel wall.

In this context, isothiocyanate (ITC) sulforaphane derived from glucoraphanin of collard greens has interesting properties. Glucoraphanin is a glucosinolate found in *Brassicaceae*, mostly in broccoli, cauliflower, and kale, particularly in the young sprouts. When these foods are chopped or chewed, the enzyme myrosinase transforms glucoraphanin into raphanin, which is an antibiotic, and then into sulforaphane, which has exhibited anticancer and antimicrobial properties in experimental models. Not only does this ITC trigger anti-inflammatory activity in the cardiovascular system, it may also be able to help prevent and even possibly help reverse blood vessel damage.

9.2.1.6 Cancer Prevention

The most impressive effect of collard greens and kale is probably linked to their cancer-protection properties which are largely related to the four specific glucosinolates found in these cruciferous vegetables: glucobrassicin, glucoraphanin, gluconasturtiin, and glucotropaeolin. Each of these glucosinolates can be converted into an isothiocyanate (ITC) that helps lower cancer risk by supporting detox and anti-inflammatory systems. In fact, collard greens and kale provide special nutrient support for three body systems that are closely connected with cancer development as well as cancer prevention. The three systems are (1) the body's detox system, (2) its antioxidant system, and (3) its inflammatory/anti-inflammatory system. Chronic imbalances in any of these three systems can increase the risk of cancer, and when imbalances in all three systems occur simultaneously, the risk of cancer increases significantly. Prevention of the following types of cancer is closely associated with the intake of collard greens and kale: bladder cancer, breast cancer, colon cancer, lung cancer, prostate cancer, and ovarian cancer.

9.2.2 Turnip Greens and Turnip Tops

Turnips, scientifically known as *Brassica rapa*, belong to the *Cruciferae* family, a cousin to other health-protective giants including kale, collards, cabbage, and broccoli. Turnip greens are the leaves of the turnip plant, which is known for its tasty root. Turnip tops are the inflorescences of turnips which are typically used in the south Italy, where they are called "*cime di rapa*," to prepare delicious dishes in perfect Mediterranean style.

9.2.2.1 Historical Notes

Turnips are a very ancient vegetable. The exact origins of turnip greens are not known, but some evidence shows that they were first domesticated in ancient Greek, Hellenistic and Roman times. Archaeological records show that mustard greens and radishes, two crops related to turnips, were both growing wildly in parts of western Asia and Europe thousands of years ago, suggesting that this is where turnips first started to grow. Other sources date turnip greens to the fifteenth century BC when they were grown in regions throughout India.

Turnips were introduced to North America by the early European settlers and colonists. They grew well in the South and became a popular food in the local cuisine of that region. Turnip greens, which became an integral part of Southern African-American cuisine, are thought to have been adopted into that food culture because of the role they played during the days of slavery. Supposedly, the slave owners would reserve the turnip roots for themselves, leaving the leaves for the slaves. As Western African cuisine traditionally utilizes a wide variety of green leaves in its cooking, the African slaves adopted turnip greens as a substitute and incorporated them into their food culture.

9.2.2.2 Nutrients and Phytochemicals

Turnip leaves (turnip greens) are smaller and more tender than their cousin, collards. Turnip greens are a storehouse of many vital nutrients. The green tops contain several times more minerals and vitamins than in the roots. The greens are a very good source of antioxidants such as vitamin A, vitamin C, carotenoid, xanthin, and lutein. Moreover, the leafy tops are an excellent source of vitamin K. In addition, its top greens are also a good source of the B-complex group of vitamins such as folates, riboflavin, pyridoxine, pantothenic acid, and thiamin and they are also an excellent source of important minerals like calcium, copper, iron, potassium, and manganese.

The slightly bitter flavor of turnip greens and inflorescences is linked to its calcium content. On an ounce-for-ounce basis, turnip greens contain about four times more calcium than a much less bitter-tasting cruciferous vegetable such as cabbage. According to the food rating system, turnip greens rank as the fourth most concentrated source of this mineral. It is not calcium per se that is associated with the bitterness of turnip greens (and many other plant foods), but the varying forms of calcium contained within them (i.e., included in these forms might be calcium chloride, calcium sulfate, calcium lactate, calcium pectate, and others). High calcium content is by no means the only reason for the noticeable bitterness of turnip greens. Numerous other naturally present constituents—including alkaloids, glucosinolates, terpenoids, flavonoids, tannins, sulfimides, and lactones—can contribute to the bitter taste that most people associate with these greens in their raw form.

As far as the total glucosinolate content is concerned, turnip greens outscore cabbage, kale, cauliflower, and broccoli as the most commonly eaten cruciferous vegetables. Such a healthy glucosinolate content brings with it numerous health benefits. As we have already mentioned, glucosinolates are phytonutrients that can be converted into isothiocyanates (ITCs) with cancer-preventing properties. All cruciferous vegetables have long been known to contain glucosinolates, but only recent research has been able to show to what extent turnip greens are beneficial.

Turnip Greens, Cooked, Boiled, Drained
Vitamin and mineral content per 100 g
Source: USDA National Nutrient data base

Energy	84 KJ (20 kcal)
Carbohydrates	4.4 g
Dietary fiber	3.5 g
Protein	1.1 g
Fat	0.2 g

Vitamin A equiv.	381 μg	(48% DV)
β-Carotene	4575 μg	(42% DV)
Lutein zeaxanthin	8440 μg	

Thiamine	0.045 mg	(4% DV)
Riboflavin	0.072 mg	(6% DV)
Niacin	0.411 mg	(3% DV)
Pantothenic acid	0.274 mg	(5% DV)
Vitamin B_6	018 mg	(14% DV)
Folate	118 μg	(30% DV)
Vitamin C	27.4 mg	(33% DV)

Calcium	137 mg	(14% DV)
Iron	0.8 mg	(6% DV)
Magnesium	22 mg	(6% DV)
Manganese	0.337 mg	(16% DV)
Phosphorus	29 mg	(4% DV)
Potassium	203 mg	(4% DV)
Sodium	29 mg	(2% DV)

DV = Daily Value

To note, the root and its top contain small amounts of oxalic acid (0.21 g/100 g), a naturally occurring substance found in some vegetables belonging to the Brassica family, which can crystallize as oxalate stones in the kidneys and urinary tract in some individuals. Those persons with known oxalate urinary tract stones should probably avoid these vegetables. And, in any case, an ample intake of water is advisable to maintain a normal urine output in these individuals to minimize the risk of stone.

The high quantity of vitamin K in turnip greens seems to make these vegetables unsuitable to patients under anticoagulant therapy with vitamin K antagonists (VKA), i.e., warfarin. In fact, it is current opinion that consuming excessive Cruciferae may not be appropriate in patients taking vitamin k antagonists, although recent research has uncovered new data about these assumptions. Patients treated with VKA have on average only about 60% of their international normalized ratio (INR) values within the therapeutic range; INR instability is associated with an increased risk of thrombosis and bleeding events. However, recent findings suggest that a low dietary vitamin K intake may affect anticoagulation control.

A recent review of the literature assessed the role of vitamin K dietary intake in VKA stability and the potential effect of daily vitamin K supplements on VKA therapy. Fifteen studies evaluating a total of 1838 patients were included in the systematic review [1]. The observational studies reviewed suggested that there is an increased risk of unstable anticoagulation control in patients with a lower daily vitamin K intake. The daily use of vitamin K supplementation appears, instead, to be associated with a clinically relevant increase in time in therapeutic range (TTR) in patients with unstable anticoagulation control. Although other large prospective studies are necessary to confirm these findings, it would seem that the intake of vitamin K rich vegetables helps to stabilize anticoagulant control in patients taking warfarin, particularly in those showing an unstable control.

WH Foods Recommendations: Turnip greens should be considered vegetables that should be eaten on a regular basis, in view of the health benefits associated to the cruciferous vegetable family. A minimum of 3/4 cup of cruciferous vegetables should be consumed on a daily basis (one cup = 144 g), meaning the equivalent to approximately 5 cups/week. An intake of 1–1/2 cups/day, or about 10 cups/week, would provide even greater benefits.

9.2.2.3 Health Benefits

Turnip greens and turnip tops share the health benefits of other *Brassicaceae*, particularly collard greens (see Sect. 9.2).

Detox Activity: The detox support provided by turnip greens includes antioxidant nutrients to boost Phase 1 detoxification activities and sulfur-containing nutrients to boost Phase 2 activities. Turnip greens also contain phytonutrients called glucosinolates that can help activate detoxification enzymes and regulate their activity. Two key glucosinolates that have been clearly identified in turnip greens in significant amounts are gluconasturtiin and glucotropaeolin. Glucoraphanin instead, a glucosinolate found in many cruciferous vegetables and a precursor of sulforaphane (an isothiocyanate with important anti-inflammatory properties) does not appear to be present in turnip greens in significant quantities.

Antioxidant Activity: The antioxidant activity of turnip greens depends on the high vitamin content, i.e., vitamin C, vitamin E and β-carotene, and on the high content of polyphenols, i.e., hydroxycinnamic acid, quercetin, myricetin, isorhamnetin, and kaempferol. This broad spectrum of antioxidant support helps lower the risk of oxidative stress in the cells. Chronic oxidative stress is a risk factor for development of many diseases including atherosclerosis and most types of cancer.

Cholesterol-Lowering Activity: As far as cholesterol metabolism is concerned, the fiber-related nutrients in turnip greens bind with bile acids in the intestine and are excreted in the feces rather than being absorbed along with the fat they have emulsified. As a consequence, the liver must replace the lost bile acids by drawing upon the supply of cholesterol, thus leading to lower blood cholesterol levels.

Hyperhomocysteinemia: The high level of folate in turnip greens deserves a special mention. These greens provide 575 μg of folate for every hundred calories, the highest amount for all the commonly eaten cruciferous vegetables. Folate is a crucial B-vitamin that supports cardiovascular health and contributes to preventing hyperhomocysteinemia.

9.2.3 Cauliflower

Cauliflower is one of the several vegetables in the *Brassica oleracea* species, in the Brassicaceae family. Typically, only the head (the *white curd*) is eaten. The cauliflower head is composed of a white inflorescence, the *meristem.*

9.2.3.1 Historical Notes

The oldest record of cauliflower dates back to the sixth century BC. In the first century AD, Pliny included what he called *cyma* in his descriptions of cultivated plants in the *Natural History*: "*Ex omnibus brassicae generibus suavissima est cyma.*"

Cauliflower can be found in many different colors, white, brown, green yellow, and purple. The last color is the result of the presence of anthocyanins, a water-soluble polyphenol that is found in many other plants and plant-based products such as red cabbage and red wine.

9.2.3.2 Nutrients and Phytochemicals

One hundred grams of raw white cauliflower provides 25 calories, and thus is low in fat, carbohydrates, dietary fiber, and protein (see Box). It has a high content (20% or more of the Daily Value, DV) of vitamin C and moderate levels (10–19% DV) of several B vitamins and vitamin K. Boiling reduces the levels of cauliflower compounds, with losses of 20–30% after 5 min, 40–50% after 10 min, and 75% after 30 min. Other preparation methods, however, such as steaming, microwaving, and stir-frying, have no significant effect on the compounds.

Cauliflower also contains several phytochemicals, common in the cabbage family, including glucosinolates and isothiocyanates. As far as isothiocyanates are concerned, the *phenethyl isothiocyanate* is particularly important. It has been shown to inhibit carcinogenesis and tumorigenesis in some conditions [2]. The mechanism of action proposed involves inhibition of cytochrome P450 enzymes, which oxidize compounds such as benzo[*a*]pyrene and other polycyclic aromatic hydrocarbons into more polar epoxy-diols, which can then cause mutation and induce anticarcinogenic activity [3].

Phenethyl isothiocyanate has also been shown to induce apoptosis in certain cancer cell lines, and, in some cases, it is even able to induce apoptosis in cells that are resistant to some currently used chemotherapeutic drugs, for example, in drug-resistant leukemia cells that produce the powerful apoptosis inhibitor protein *Bcl-2* [4]. Other isothiocyanates have been shown to bind to mutated *p53 proteins* found in many types of tumors, causing an increase in the rate of cell death [5].

Cauliflower, Raw

Vitamin and mineral content per 100 g

Source: USDA Database entry

Energy	104 KJ (25 kcal)
Carbohydrates	5 g
Protein	1.9 g
Fat	0.3 g

Thiamine	0.05 mg	(4% DV)
Riboflavin	0.06 mg	(5% DV)
Niacin	0.507 mg	(3% DV)
Pantothenic acid	0.667 mg	(13% DV)
Vitamin B_6	0.184 mg	(14% DV)
Folate	57 μg	(14% DV)
Vitamin C	48.2 mg	(58% DV)

Thiamine	0.05 mg	(4% DV)
Vitamin E	0.08 mg	(1% DV)
Vitamin K	15.5 μg	(15% DV)

Calcium	22 mg	(22% DV)
Iron	0.42 mg	(3% DV)
Magnesium	15 mg	(4% DV)
Manganese	0.155 mg	(7% DV)
Phosphorus	44 mg	(6% DV)
Potassium	299 mg	(6% DV)
Sodium	30 mg	(2% DV)
Zinc	0.27 mg	(3% DV)

DV = Daily Value

9.2.4 Broccoli

The word *broccoli* comes from the Italian plural of *broccolo*, which means "the flowering crest of a cabbage," and is the diminutive form of *brocco*, meaning "small nail" or "sprout." Broccoli is generally boiled or steamed, but it can also be eaten raw.

9.2.4.1 Historical Notes

Broccoli is the offshoot of the careful breeding of cultivated *Brassica* crops in the northern Mediterranean starting in about the sixth century BC. Since the time of the Roman Empire, broccoli has been considered a uniquely valuable food by Italians. Broccoli was first introduced to the United States by Southern Italian immigrants, but it did not become widely popular until the 1920s.

9.2.4.2 Nutrients and Phytochemicals

A 100 g serving of raw broccoli provides 34 kcal and is an excellent source of vitamin C and vitamin K (20% or higher of the Daily Value, DV). Raw broccoli also contains moderate amounts (10–19% DV) of several B vitamins and the dietary mineral manganese, whereas other essential nutrients are in low content. Broccoli has low content of carbohydrates, protein, fat, and dietary fiber (see Box). Broccoli also contains the carotenoid compounds lutein and zeaxanthin, but in amounts that are six times lower than those in kale.

Boiling broccoli reduces the levels of sulforaphane, with losses of 20–30% after 5 min, 40–50% after 10 min, and 77% after 30 min. Other preparation methods, however, such as steaming, microwaving, and stir-frying, do not seem to have significant effects on the compounds.

The perceived bitterness of broccoli, like that of other cruciferous vegetables, is connected to the presence of isothiocyanates and polyphenols of the vegetable. Some research reports that the gene TAS2R38 may in part be responsible for the bitter taste characterizing the vegetable.

Broccoli, Raw
Vitamin and mineral content per 100 g
Source: USDA Database entry

Energy	141 KJ (34 kcal)
Carbohydrates	6.64 g
Sugars	1.7 g
Protein	2.82 g
Fat	0.37 g
Dietary fibers	2.6 g

Vitamin A equiv	31 μg	(4% DV)
β-Carotene	361 μg	(3% DV)
Lutein-zeaxanthin	1403 μg	
Thiamine	0.071 mg	(6% DV)
Riboflavin	0.117 mg	(10% DV)
Niacin	0.639 mg	(4% DV)
Vitamin C	89.2 mg	(107% DV)
Vitamin K	101.6 μg	(97% DV)
Riboflavin	0.117 mg	(10% DV)
Pantothenic acid	0.573 mg	(11% DV)
Vitamin B_6	0.175 mg	(13% DV)
Folate	63 μg	(16% DV)

Calcium	47 mg	(5% DV)
Iron	0.73 mg	(6% DV)
Magnesium	21 mg	(6% DV)
Manganese	0.21 mg	(10% DV)
Phosphorus	66 mg	(9% DV)
Potassium	316 mg	(7% DV)
Sodium	33 mg	(2% DV)
Zinc	0.41 mg	(4% DV)

DV = Daily Value

9.2.5 Cabbage

Cabbage, or headed cabbage, is a leafy green or purple biennial plant, grown as an annual vegetable crop for its dense-leaved heads. Although the exact history of cabbage is not entirely known, it was most likely domesticated somewhere in Europe before 1000 BC. By the Middle Ages, it had become a prominent component of the European cuisine.

9.2.5.1 Historical Notes

Cabbage was considered a table luxury by some Romans, although *Lucullus* considered it unfit for the senatorial table. The more traditionalist *Cato the Elder*, espousing a simple, Republican life, ate his cabbage cooked or raw and dressed with vinegar; he said it surpassed all other vegetables, and distinguished three varieties; he also gave directions for its medicinal use, which extended to the cabbage-eater's urine, in which infants might be rinsed. *Pliny the Elder* listed seven varieties, including Pompeii cabbage, Cumae cabbage, and Sabellian cabbage. *Apicius* gave several recipes for *cauliculi*, tender cabbage shoots. The Greeks and Romans claimed medicinal usages for their cabbage varieties that included relief from gout, headaches, and the symptoms of poisonous mushroom ingestion. Another prescription of cabbage was to be used to treat drunkenness.

9.2.5.2 Nutrients and Phytochemicals

Cabbage is an excellent source of vitamin C and vitamin K, containing more than 20% of the Daily Value (DV) for each of these nutrients per serving. Cabbage is also a good source (10–19% DV) of vitamin B_6 and folate, with no other nutrients having a significant content per 100 g serving (see Box). Cabbage is also a good source for important phytochemicals, such as sulforaphane and other glucosinolate, which stimulate the production of detoxifying enzymes during metabolism. Several studies suggest that cabbage, like other cruciferous vegetables, has protective effects against colon cancer [6]. Purple cabbage contains anthocyanin, an antioxidant polyphenol which protects from oxidative stress and related diseases. It has also been shown that a cabbage leaf treatment can reduce the pain and hardness of engorged breasts, and increase the duration of breast-feeding [7].

Cabbage, Raw

Vitamin and mineral content per 100 g

Source: USDA Database entry

Energy	103 KJ (25 kcal)
Carbohydrates	5.8 g
Dietary fiber	2.5 g
Protein	1.28 g
Fat	0.1 g

Thiamine	0.061 mg	(5% DV)
Riboflavin	0.040 mg	(3% DV)
Niacin	0.234 mg	(2% DV)
Pantothenic acid	0.212 mg	(4% DV)
Vitamin B_6	0.124 mg	(10% DV)
Folate	43 μg	(11% DV)
Vitamin C	36.6 mg	(44% DV)
Vitamin K	76 μg	(72% DV)

Calcium	40 mg	(4% DV)
Iron	0.47 mg	(4% DV)
Magnesium	12 mg	(3% DV)
Manganese	0.16 mg	(8% DV)
Phosphorus	26 mg	(4% DV)
Potassium	170 mg	(4% DV)
Sodium	18 mg	(1% DV)
Zinc	0.18 mg	(2% DV)

DV = Daily Value

9.2.6 Brussels Sprouts

9.2.6.1 Historical Notes

Brussels sprouts are leafy green vegetables typically 2.5–4 cm (0.98–1.6 in.) in diameter that look like miniature cabbages. The forerunners of modern Brussels sprouts were likely cultivated in Ancient Rome. The first written reference dates to 1587. During the sixteenth century, they enjoyed a popularity in the southern Netherlands that eventually spread throughout the cooler areas of Northern Europe. Production of Brussels sprouts in the United States began in the eighteenth century, when the French settlers brought them to Louisiana.

9.2.6.2 Nutrients and Phytochemicals

Raw Brussels sprouts contain high levels of vitamin C and vitamin K, with more moderate amounts of B vitamins, such as folic acid and vitamin B_6; essential minerals and dietary fiber are present in lesser amounts (see Box).

Brussels sprouts, just as broccoli and other Brassicaceae, contain sulforaphane, a phytochemical known for its potential anticancer properties. Eating large quantities of Brussels sprouts may not be suitable for patients taking anticoagulants such as warfarin since they contain vitamin K, a blood-clotting factor. It has nevertheless been shown that the consumption of vitamin-K rich vegetables, such as Brussels sprouts, appears to help stabilize anticoagulant control in patient receiving warfarin particularly in those showing unstable control [1].

Brussels Sprout, Raw

Vitamin and mineral content per 100 g

Source: USDA Database entry

Energy	179 KJ (43 kcal)
Carbohydrates	8.95 g
Sugars	2.2 g
Dietary fiber	3.8 g
Protein	3.48 g
Fat	0.3 g

Vitamin A equiv	38 μg	(5% DV)
β-Carotene	450 μg	(4% DV)
Lutein zeaxanthin	1590 μg	
Thiamine	0.139 mg	(12% DV)
Riboflavin	0.09 mg	(8% DV)
Niacin	0.745 mg	(5% DV)
Pantothenic acid	0.309 mg	(6% DV)
Folate	61 μg	(15% DV)
Choline	19.1 mg	(4% DV)
Vitamin C	85 mg	(102% DV)
Vitamin E	0.88 mg	(6% DV)
Vitamin K	177 μg	(169% DV)

Calcium	42 mg	(4% DV)
Iron	1.4 mg	(11% DV)
Magnesium	23 mg	(6% DV)
Manganese	0.337 mg	(16% DV)
Phosphorus	69 mg	(10% DV)
Potassium	389 mg	(8% DV)
Sodium	25 mg	(2% DV)
Zinc	0.42 mg	(4% DV)

9.3 Non-cruciferae Leafy Vegetables

9.3.1 Lettuce

9.3.1.1 Historical Notes

Lettuce is a leafy vegetable that is used for salads and, less frequently, for soup or grilled. Lettuce was first cultivated by the ancient Egyptians to produce oil from its seeds. From Egypt it spread to the Greeks and Romans, who gave it the name *lactuca*, referring to the white substance, now called latex, exuded by the cut stems. The lettuce was considered a sacred plant as it was thought to help the god "perform the sexual act untiringly".

By 50 AD, multiple types were described, and lettuce together with several other herbals are often mentioned in medieval writings. The sixteenth through eighteenth centuries saw the development of many varieties in Europe and by the mid-eighteenth century cultivars were described that can still be found in gardens. Lettuce was first brought to the Americas from Europe by Christopher Columbus in the late fifteenth century.

At present, the most commonly used lettuce is the Romaine/Cos, but the Iceberg/Crisphead, the Leaf or looseleaf and the Summercrisp are also very popular.

9.3.1.2 Nutrients and Phytochemicals

Depending on the variety, lettuce is an excellent source of vitamin K (97% of the Daily Value, DV) and vitamin A (21% DV) (see table), as it contains higher concentrations of the provitamin A beta-carotene, which is found in darker green lettuces, such as Romaine. With the exception of the iceberg variety, lettuce is also a good source (10–19% DV) of folate and iron (see Box).

Just as other leafy vegetables such as spinach/collard green, or roots like beetroots and carrots, lettuce is also very rich in nitrates. They account for 80–85% of daily dietary nitrate exposure in the average population. Dietary inorganic nitrate has been shown to be an important source of nitric oxide (NO). The beneficial effects of dietary nitrate are thought to be mediated by its reduction to nitrite and then to nitric oxide (NO), a critical regulator of vascular homeostasis. Nitrate and nitrite have been demonstrated to have significant blood-pressure-lowering effects and underpin a cardioprotective effect of vegetables.

The Mediterranean diet appears to provide greater nitrate supplementation than a regular Western diet. It has been reported [8] that a typical Mediterranean meal contains approximately 325 mg of combined nitrate/nitrite per serving, significantly (approximately tenfold) higher in comparison with a typical Western diet (only ~20 mg/serving).

In peripheral resistance vessels, the dietary nitrate-derived nitrite is reduced to NO, the main function of which is to regulate the tone of vascular smooth muscle cells. The endothelium of blood vessels uses NO to signal relaxation in the surrounding smooth muscle cells, thus resulting in vasodilation with increased blood flow and reduced arterial blood pressure (see Fig. 9.4, below).

Lettuce
Vitamin and mineral content per 100 g
Source: USDA Database entry

Energy	55 KJ (13 kcal)
Carbohydrates	2.23 g
Dietary fiber	1.1 g
Protein	1.35 g

Vitamin A	166 μg	(21% DV)
β-Carotene	1987 μg	(18% DV)
Lutein zeaxanthin	1223 μg	
Thiamine	0.057 mg	(5% DV)
Riboflavin	0.062 mg	(5% DV)
Pantothenic acid	0.15 mg	(3% DV)
Vitamin B_6	0.082 mg	(6% DV)
Folate	73 μg	(18% DV)
Vitamin C	3.7 mg	(4% DV)
Vitamin E	0.18 mg	(1% DV)
Vitamin K	102 μg	(97% DV)

Calcium	35 mg	(4% DV)
Iron	1.24 mg	(10% DV)
Magnesium	13 mg	(4% DV)
Manganese	0.179 mg	(9% DV)
Phosphorus	33 mg	(5% DV)
Potassium	238 mg	(5% DV)
Sodium	5 mg	(0% DV)
Zinc	0.2 mg	(2% DV)

DV = Daily Value

9.3.2 Spinach

9.3.2.1 Historical Notes

Spinach is thought to have originated in ancient Persia (modern Iran and neighboring countries). In AD 827 it would appear that the Saracens introduced spinach to Sicily.

Spinach became a popular vegetable in the Arab Mediterranean and arrived in Spain by the latter part of the twelfth century. In the fourteenth century spinach appeared in England and France, probably via Spain, and quickly it gained popularity because it grew in the early spring, when other vegetables were still scarce. Spinach was supposedly the favorite vegetable of *Catherine de' Medici*. Dishes served on a bed of spinach are known as "*Florentine*," reflecting Catherine's birth in Florence.

9.3.2.2 Nutrients and Phytochemicals

Spinach has a high nutritional value, especially when fresh, frozen, steamed, or quickly boiled. It is a rich source (20% or more of the Daily Value, DV) of vitamin A, vitamin C, vitamin K, magnesium, manganese, iron, and folate (see Box). Spinach is also a good source (10–19% of DV) of the B_2 vitamins riboflavin and vitamin B_6, vitamin E, calcium, potassium, and dietary fiber.

Iron: Spinach, along with other green, leafy vegetables, contains an appreciable amount of iron attaining 21% of the Daily Value in a 100-g amount of raw spinach. It also contains iron absorption-inhibiting substances, including high levels of oxalate, which can bind to the iron to form ferrous oxalate rendering much of the iron in spinach unusable by the body. In addition to preventing absorption and use, high levels of oxalates also remove iron from the body [9].

Calcium: Spinach has a moderate calcium content which can be affected by oxalates, decreasing its absorption. The calcium in spinach is among the least bioavailable of food calcium sources [9, 10]. By way of comparison, the human body can absorb about half of the calcium present in broccoli, but only around 5% of the calcium in spinach.

Since 1931 the comics/cartoon character Popeye the Sailor Man has been portrayed as having a strong affinity for spinach, becoming physically stronger after consuming it. It is commonly thought that this portrayal was based on faulty calculations of spinach's iron content. According to this version, the German scientist Emil von Wolff misplaced a decimal point in an 1870 measurement of spinach's iron content, leading to an iron value ten times higher than it is in reality. This faulty measurement was not noticed until the 1930s and led to the popular misconception that spinach is exceedingly high in iron content making the body stronger [11].

Spinach, Raw

Vitamin and mineral content per 100 g

Source: USDA Database entry

Energy	97 KJ (23 kcal)
Carbohydrates	3.6 g
Dietary fiber	2.2 g
Protein	2.9 g
Fat	0.6 g

Vitamin A equiv	469 μg	(59% DV)
β-Carotene	5626 μg	(52% DV)
Lutein zeaxanthin	12,198 μg	
Vitamin A	9377 IU	
Thiamine	0.078 mg	(7% DV)
Riboflavin	0.189 mg	(16% DV)
Niacin	0.724 mg	(5% DV)
Folate	194 μg	(49% DV)
Vitamin C	28 mg	(34% DV)
Vitamin E	2 mg	(13% DV)
Vitamin K	483 μg	(460% DV)

Calcium	99 mg	(10% DV)
Iron	2.71 mg	(21% DV)
Magnesium	79 mg	(22% DV)
Manganese	0.897 mg	(43% DV)
Potassium	558 mg	(12% DV)
Sodium	79 mg	(5% DV)
Zinc	0.53 mg	(6% DV)

DV = Daily Value

9.4 Solanaceae

9.4.1 Bell Peppers

Bell peppers (also known as sweet peppers) belong to the nightshade (*Solanaceae*) family of plants, along with chili peppers, cayenne peppers, eggplant, tomatoes, and potatoes. Their scientific name is *Capsicum annuum*. These delicious vegetables come in a wide variety of colors, including yellow, orange, red, purple, brown, and black. Bell peppers can be eaten at any stage of development. Recent research has nevertheless shown that the vitamin C and carotenoid content of bell peppers tends to increase while the pepper is reaching its optimal ripeness. Bell peppers are also typically more flavorful when optimally ripe.

9.4.1.1 Historical Notes

Native to Mexico, bell peppers have been cultivated for more than 9000 years, with the earliest cultivation appearing in South and Central America. Pepper seeds were imported to Spain in 1493 by the crew of Cristoforo Colombo, and from there spread to other European, African, and Asian countries. The name "pepper" was given to this food by European colonizers of North America who first came across it in the 1500–1600s. For these historical reasons, peppers and the other *Solanaceae* (tomatoes, potatoes) are not ancient historical components of the Mediterranean diet but made their entrance after their arrival from the "*New World,*" becoming a fixed component of the Mediterranean dietary style towards the end of the nineteenth century.

9.4.1.2 Nutrients and Phytochemicals

Bell peppers are a good source of antioxidant and anti-inflammatory phytonutrients, which include flavonoids (luteolin, quercetin, hesperidin) and hydroxycinnamic acids (especially ferulic and cinnamic acids). But the hallmark phytonutrient group found in bell peppers is the carotenoid family, with more than 30 different carotenoids being provided by this vegetable. Alpha-carotene, beta-carotene, cryptoxanthin, lutein, and zeaxanthin are other carotenoids contained in the vegetable. Bell peppers are an excellent source of vitamin A (in the form of carotenoids), vitamin C, and vitamin B_6. They are also a very good source of folate, molybdenum, vitamin E, dietary fiber, vitamin B_2, pantothenic acid, niacin, and potassium. Additionally, they are a good source of vitamin K, manganese, vitamin B_1, phosphorus, and magnesium. Capsicum peppers (spicy) are rich sources of antioxidants and vitamin C. The level of carotene, like lycopene, is nine times higher in red peppers which have twice the vitamin C content of green peppers. Red and green bell peppers are high in para-coumaric acid.

Bell Pepper, Raw

Vitamin and mineral content per 100 g

Source: USDA Database entry

Energy	84 KJ (20 kcal)
Carbohydrates	4.64 g
Dietary fiber	1.8 g
Protein	0.86 g
Fat	0.17 g

Vitamin A equiv.	18 μg	(2% DV)
β-Carotene	208 μg	(2% DV)
Lutein zeaxanthin	341 μg	
Thiamine	0.057 mg	(5% DV)
Riboflavin	0.028 mg	(2% DV)
Niacin	0.48 mg	(3% DV)
Vitamin B_6	0.224 mg	(17% DV)
Folate	10 μg	(3% DV)
Vitamin C	80.4 mg	(97% DV)
Vitamin E	0.37 mg	(2% DV)
Vitamin K	7.4 μg	(7% DV)

Calcium	10 mg	(1% DV)
Iron	0.34 mg	(3% DV)
Magnesium	10 mg	(3% DV)
Manganese	0.122 mg	(6% DV)
Potassium	175 mg	(4% DV)
Sodium	3 mg	(0% DV)
Zinc	0.13 mg	(1% DV)

DV = Daily Value

9.4.2 Tomatoes

The tomato is the edible, red fruit of *Solanum lycopersicum*, commonly known as the tomato plant, which belongs to the nightshade family *Solanaceae,* to which bell peppers and eggplant also belong.

9.4.2.1 Historical Notes

Originating in Mexico, the species can be traced back to the early Aztecs at approximately 700 A.D. It was not until about the sixteenth century that Europeans were introduced to this fruit when the early explorers set sail to discover new lands. Tomatoes spread throughout the world following the Spanish colonization of the Americas. Tomatoes were quickly accepted into the kitchens of south Europe, soon assuming a central role in the Mediterranean alimentary style (see Box).

The word "tomato" originated from the Aztec language, the Nahuatl, which called the fruit "tomati." The word gave rise to the Spanish word "tomate," upon which the English word tomato originates.

Although tomatoes were quickly accepted in the kitchens in southern Europe, they were not so readily welcomed to those in north Europe. In fact, most northern Europeans thought that the tomato was poisonous. In those times, well to do individuals used flatware made of pewter, which has a high-lead content. Foods high in acid, like tomatoes, caused the lead to leech out into the food, resulting to lead poisoning and death. Poor people, who ate from plates made of wood, did not have that problem, and hence did not develop an aversion to tomatoes. This is essentially the reason why tomatoes were only eaten by poor people, particularly in Italy, until the 1800s. At that time, a mass immigration from Europe to America took place leading to a blending of cultures. As many Italian-Americans ate tomatoes they took that custom with them when they immigrated. Moreover, the pizza was invented at that time (in Naples during the late 1880s) and, as anyone knows, there is no pizza without tomato sauce. The story goes that it was created by one restaurateur in Naples to celebrate the visit of Queen Margherita of Savoy, the first Italian monarch since Napoleon conquered Italy. The restaurateur made the pizza using three ingredients that represented the colors of the new Italian flag: tomato sauce is the red ingredient, mozzarella cheese the white one, and the basil topping the green one. The Margherita Pizza was born, and is still today the most popular form of pizza.

9.4.2.2 Nutrients and Phytochemicals

A tomato is 95% water, contains 4% carbohydrates and less than 1% of fat and protein. In a 100 g serving, raw tomatoes supply 18 calories and are a moderate source of vitamin C (17% of the Daily Value). Tomatoes, instead, are rich in lycopene.

Lycopene: A carotenoid, lycopene, is the pigment principally responsible for the characteristic deep-red color of ripe tomato fruits and tomato products. This carotenoid is also found in other red fruits and vegetables, such as red carrots, watermelons, and papayas, although not in strawberries, or cherries. Although lycopene is chemically a carotene, it has no vitamin A activity. The many conjugated double bonds of lycopene make it potentially powerful antioxidant. It has been shown [12] that lycopene has the strongest singlet oxygen-quenching capacity of several carotenoids, with alpha-carotene, beta-carotene, and lutein next in capacity. Investigators have been showing heightened interest in lycopene, as it has a large number of double bonds which make it the most potent scavenger of oxygen free radicals of all the carotenoids.

Studies have demonstrated that lycopene not only scavenge oxygen free radical species, for example, peroxyl radicals, but also interacts with reactive oxygen species such as hydrogen peroxide and nitrogen dioxide and in this manner protects cells from oxidative damage. Interestingly lycopene has been found to be twice as efficient as beta-carotene in scavenging for nitrogen dioxide. Being an acrylic and extremely hydrophobic carotenoid, lycopene is insoluble in water, soluble in fats and better absorbed from the intestine when heated. In fact, studies have shown that lycopene from tomato products appears more readily in the circulation if the tomato has been heated and if a source of fat is included with the meal. It has been shown [13] that while plasma lycopene concentration increases only slightly after unheated tomato juice is ingested, the intake of heated tomato juice mixed with oil increases serum concentration significantly, with a 24–48 h peak after ingestion. This is due to the fact that lycopene, like other carotenoids, is found in tight protein–carotenoid complexes and crystalline aggregates in most foods leading to significant barriers to economic absorption. These tight bonds are dissociated by heating, which greatly improves its intestinal absorption and bioavailability.

Lycopene is known to have 13 conjugated double bonds arranged in a linear fashion (Fig. 9.2). It is the lack of a beta ionone ring that leaves lycopene free of provitamin A activity. The conjugated double bonds give lycopene and indeed all carotenoids the ability to isomerize and thus numerous combinations of cis and trans isomers are possible. The most thermodynamically stable configuration is the all-trans one and it is this isomer of lycopene that is most commonly found in raw foods. However, cooking or other types of food processing cause isomerization of lycopene leading to increased levels of cis-isomers. In biology, the absorption of light, exposure to energy (e.g., heat), or chemical reactions result in isomeric interconversion.

Tomatoes also contain a significant amount of beta-carotene, folate, potassium, and vitamin C, the last being three times higher than lycopene [14]. In the blood, the

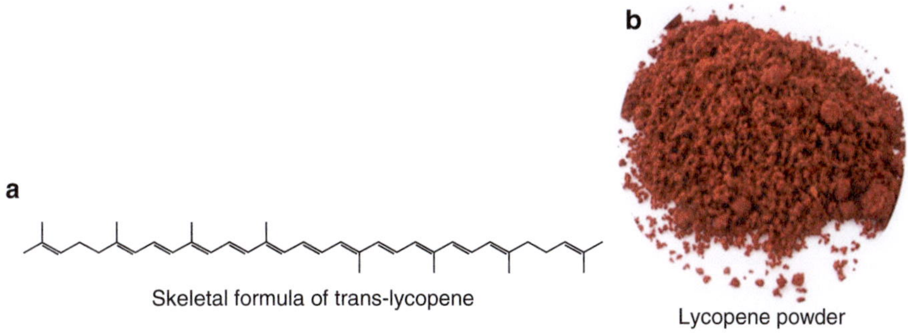

Fig. 9.2 (**a**) Chemical formula of trans-lycopene; (**b**) lycopene powder

carotenoids, including beta-carotene and lycopene, are transported primarily in LDL, which place them in a prime position to protect LDL from oxidation [15]. Studies in smokers and nonsmokers have in fact suggested that lycopene intakes correlated closely with inhibition of LDL oxidation, and in this regard carotenoids may protect against diseases related to oxidative stress [16, 17].

Many studies have suggested that eating lycopene-rich foods or having high blood lycopene levels may be linked to reduced risks of cancer, heart disease, and age-related eye disorders. It must be remembered, however, that lycopene measurements refer to the intake of tomatoes and not on the use of lycopene supplements. Since tomatoes also contain other nutrients, in particular beta-carotene, vitamin C, and potassium, the potential benefits of lycopene alone are still unclear.

Lycopene from tomatoes has been tested in human studies examining cardiovascular diseases and prostate cancer. The studies have, however, produced contrasting results, and its beneficial effects on diseases remain unclear [18]. With regard to the effects of lycopene on prostate cancer, the FDA, in particular, rejected manufacturers' requests in 2005 to allow "*qualified labeling*" for lycopene and the reduction of various cancer risks, and stated: "*A 2011 Cochrane review found insufficient evidence for any effect lycopene might have on prostate symptoms, PSA levels or prostate cancer*" [19].

Red Tomato, Raw

Vitamin and mineral content per 100 g

Source: USDA Database entry

Energy	74 KJ (18 kcal)
Carbohydrates	3.9 g
Dietary fiber	1.2 g
Protein	0.9 g
Fat	0.2 g

Vitamin A equiv	42 µg	(2% DV)
β-Carotene	449 µg	(2% DV)
Lutein zeaxanthin	123 µg	
Thiamine	0.037 mg	(5% DV)
Niacin	0.594 mg	(3% DV)
Vitamin B_6	0.08 mg	(17% DV)
Vitamin C	14 mg	(97% DV)
Vitamin E	0.54 mg	(2% DV)
Vitamin K	7.9 µg	(7% DV)

Magnesium	11 mg	(3% DV)
Manganese	0.114 mg	(5% DV)
Potassium	237 mg	(5% DV)
Phosphorus	24 mg	(3% DV)
Lycopene	2573 µg	
Water	94.5 g	

DV = Daily Value

9.4.3 Eggplant (Aubergine)

Eggplant (aubergine in British English) is a species of nightshade widely used in cooking. The fruit contains numerous small, soft seeds, which, although edible, taste bitter because they contain nicotinoid alkaloids like the close relative, tobacco.

9.4.3.1 Historical Notes

Eggplant has been cultivated in southern and eastern Asia since prehistory. The numerous Arabic and North African names for it, and the fact that there are no ancient Greek and Roman names, indicate that it was introduced throughout the Mediterranean area by the Arabs in the early Middle Ages. There is no mention of aubergine in England until the sixteenth century. Because of the plant's relationship with other nightshades, its fleshy fruit was at one time believed to be extremely poisonous. Given the presence of solanine, its flowers and leaves can in fact be poisonous if they are consumed in large quantities.

9.4.3.2 Nutrients and Phytochemicals

Nutritionally, raw eggplant is low in fat, protein, dietary fiber, and carbohydrates (see Box). It also provides low amounts of essential nutrients; only manganese provides a moderate percentage (11%) of the Daily Value. One of the compounds in eggplant thought to be beneficial to human health is chlorogenic acid. Eggplant flesh turns brown because of the oxidation of *chlorogenic acid,* the most abundant phenolic compound in this fruit. Cooking at higher temperatures however can alter the amount of chlorogenic acid in eggplant to some degree. The purple of the eggplant skin is due to the presence of anthocyanin *nasunin.*

Eggplant, Raw

Vitamin and mineral content per 100 g

Source: USDA Database entry

Energy	104 KJ (25 kcal)
Carbohydrates	5.88 g
Dietary fiber	3 g
Protein	0.98 g
Fat	0.18 g

Thiamine	0.039 mg	(3% DV)
Niacin	0.037 mg	(3% DV)
Vitamin B_6	0.084 mg	(17% DV)
Vitamin C	2.2 mg	(97% DV)
Vitamin E	0.3 mg	(2% DV)
Vitamin K	3.5 μg	(7% DV)

Calcium	9 mg	(1% DV)
Iron	0.23 mg	(2% DV)
Magnesium	14 mg	(4% DV)
Manganese	0.232 mg	(11% DV)
Potassium	229 mg	(5% DV)
Phosphorus	24 mg	(3% DV)
Zinc	0.16 mg	(2% DV)

DV = Daily Value

9.4.4 Potatoes

The potato is a starchy, tuberous crop from the perennial nightshade *Solanum tuberosum*.

9.4.4.1 Historical Notes

The potato is native to southern Peru and to northwestern Bolivia between 8000 and 5000 BC. Following the Spanish conquest of the Inca Empire, the Spanish introduced the potato to Europe in the second half of the sixteenth century. Subsequently, the potato was conveyed by European mariners to territories and ports throughout the world. The potato was slow to be adopted by distrustful European farmers, but soon enough it became an important food staple and field crop that played a major role in the population boom in Europe in the nineteenth century. Due to the limited genetic diversity of the crop, however, the potato was vulnerable to disease, and in 1845, the *late blight*, caused by the water mold *Phytophthora infestans*, spread rapidly through the poorer communities of western Ireland, resulting in crop failures that led to the Great Irish Famine and the mass emigration of the Irish towards North America [20].

9.4.4.2 Nutrients and Phytochemicals

The potato contains vitamins and minerals, as well as numerous phytochemicals, such as carotenoids and natural phenols. Chlorogenic acid constitutes up to 90% of the potato tuber natural phenols. A medium-size 150 g (5.3 oz) potato with the skin provides 27 mg of vitamin C (45% of the Daily Value (DV), 620 mg of potassium (18% of DV), 0.2 mg vitamin B_6 (10% of DV), and trace amounts of thiamin, riboflavin, folate, niacin, magnesium, phosphorus, iron, and zinc.

The potato is best known for its carbohydrate content (approximately 26 g in a medium potato). The predominant form of this carbohydrate is starch. A small but significant amount of this starch is resistant to digestion by enzymes in the stomach and small intestines, and thus reaches the large intestine essentially intact. This resistant starch is considered to have similar physiological effects and health benefits as fiber: in fact, it provides bulk, offers protection against colon cancer and improves glucose tolerance and insulin sensitivity.

The cooking method used can significantly affect the nutrient availability of the potato [21]. In fact, the amount of resistant starch in potatoes depends to a large extent on the preparation methods. Cooking and then cooling potatoes significantly increases resistant starch. For example, cooked potato starch contains about 7%

resistant starch, which increases to about 13% upon cooling [22]. Baking potatoes have more starch (20–22%) than boiling potatoes (16–18%).

Potatoes are often classified as high on the glycemic index (GI) and as a result are often excluded from the diets of diabetics and individuals attempting to follow a low-GI diet. But the GI of potatoes can vary considerably depending on the type of potato, the preparation methods (i.e., cooking method, whether it is eaten hot or cold, whether it is mashed or cubed or consumed whole), and with what it is consumed (i.e., the addition of various high-fat or high-protein condiments).

Potato, Raw, with Skin
Vitamin and mineral content per 100 g
Source: USDA Database entry

Energy	321 KJ (77 kcal)
Carbohydrates	17.47 g
Starch	15.44 g
Dietary fiber	2.2 g
Protein	2 g
Fat	0.1 g

Thiamine	0.08 mg	(7% DV)
Riboflavin	0.03 mg	(3% DV)
Niacin	1.05 mg	(7% DV)
Pantothenic acid	0.296 mg	(6% DV)
Vitamin B_6	0.295 mg	(23% DV)
Folate	16 μg	(4% DV)
Vitamin C	19.7 mg	(24% DV)
Vitamin E	0.01 mg	(0% DV)
Vitamin K	1.9 μg	(2% DV)

Calcium	12 mg	(1% DV)
Iron	0.78 mg	(6% DV)
Magnesium	23 mg	(6% DV)
Manganese	0.153 mg	(7% DV)
Phosphorus	57 mg	(8% DV)
Potassium	421 mg	(9% DV)
Sodium	6 mg	(0% DV)
Zinc	0.29 mg	(3% DV)

DV = Daily Value

9.5 Vegetables and Elderly Persons

9.5.1 Inorganic Nitrates

Data from observational studies and secondary prevention trials have demonstrated that adherence to a Mediterranean-style diet primarily reduces the risk of cardiovascular disease, in addition to cancer, Alzheimer's disease, and Parkinson's disease.

This risk reduction is generally linked to the impact of the components of the Mediterranean diet on the traditional risk factors of atherosclerosis [23–25] and on other risk factors such as markers of oxidation, inflammation, and endothelial dysfunction [23, 25–28].

Although the effect of the Mediterranean diet is generally attributed to the synergistic interaction of its various constituents, numerous in vitro and in vivo studies have shown that single components of the Mediterranean diet may have a direct role in preventing numerous diseases. Among the Mediterranean diet's constituents, the inorganic dietary nitrate contained in some vegetables has been shown to have a significant impact on artery wall-related functions, particularly blood pressure, clotting activity, and endothelial functions.

Here below are some considerations on the role of inorganic dietary nitrate in some vegetables on blood pressure and endothelial functions.

9.5.1.1 Leafy Vegetables and Inorganic Nitrates (Fig. 9.3)

Epidemiological evidence suggests that consuming fruit and vegetables reduces the risk of cardiovascular disease. Although these benefits have been traditionally postulated to derive from antioxidant factors, several studies have proposed other non-antioxidant factors as alternative candidates.

One of the factors that has garnered much scientific and medical interest is inorganic nitrate. Leafy vegetables are the richest source of inorganic nitrates and account for 80–85% of daily dietary nitrate exposure in the average population [29–32].

Dietary nitrate is thought to be a source of the biological messenger nitric oxide (NO), which is used by the endothelium to signal smooth muscle, triggering it to relax. This induces vasodilation, increases blood flow, and lowers blood pressure (BP).

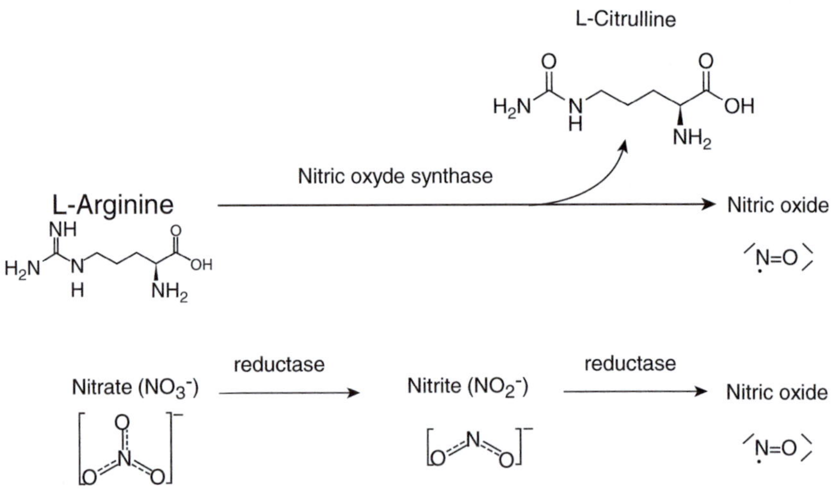

Fig. 9.3 The two-ways synthesis of nitric oxide (NO). NO production by eNOS in the vascular bed in physiologic conditions (*top*) and the alternative NO production by nitrate in tissues (*bottom*). Source: Capurso C, Capurso A. Vasc Pharmacol 2014; 63: 118–126.

Scientific interest in vegetables has been reflected in numerous experimental and clinical studies which have shown that dietary nitrate supplementation at doses that are commonly found in vegetable-rich diets exerts beneficial effects on the cardiovascular system [33–39]. Data in the literature has nevertheless demonstrated that the contribution of fresh fruit to endogenous nitrate levels is almost negligible due to its very low content of inorganic nitrate [29, 30].

Interestingly, although endogenous nitrate and nitrite originate predominantly from the oxidation of endogenously produced NO in biological fluids, a significant portion of body nitrates originates from the diet, and particularly from plant foods, i.e., lettuce, spinach, and beetroot [40].

The beneficial effects of dietary nitrates are mediated at least in part by their reduction to NO, a critical regulator of vascular homeostasis in the body [33–39]. Current available data have shown that nitrate (NO_3^-) undergoes reduction to nitrite (NO_2^-) and then to NO through a nitrate-nitrite pathway which has been postulated to be an alternative pathway to the classical L-arginine-nitric oxide synthase (NOS) pathway for NO production in the body [41–44] (Fig. 9.3).

NO synthesis from the classical L-arginine-nitric oxide pathway involves L-arginine oxidation by three different isoforms of nitric oxide synthase (NOS) enzyme: endothelial (eNOS), neuronal (nNOS), and inducible (iNOS) nitric oxide synthase [45–47]. The three NOS isoforms exhibit different characteristics and produce NO at different rates.

The catalysis of L-arginine oxidation by eNOS requires availability of molecular oxygen and other cofactors, i.e., flavin mononucleotide, flavin adenine dinucleotide, nicotinamide adenine dinucleotide phosphate, and calmodulin [45]. However, unlike NO production from the eNOS whose activity is oxygen-dependent (meaning that endothelial NO-driven processes decline with the depletion of normal oxygen levels), NO production from the nitrate-nitrite-NO pathway increases with diminished oxygen [40, 41, 47–49]. In this context, NO generation from the nitrate-nitrite-NO pathway is viewed as an alternative source for NOS-dependent NO production in the body, a sort of backup system to ensure NO-like bioactivity also in situations when the endogenous L-arginine/NO synthase pathway is dysfunctional [40, 41, 47–49]. Inorganic nitrite, therefore, appears to be a circulating storage pool of NO that selectively donates NO to hypoxic vascular beds [41], and dietary nitrate could be considered a large reservoir for NO production.

9.5.1.2 The Metabolic Fate of Dietary Nitrates (Fig. 9.4)

The dietary nitrate reduction to NO in the body involves its initial reduction to nitrite and then to NO [41–44]. After it is swallowed and absorbed through the stomach wall, about 25% of consumed nitrate (NO_3^-) enters the enterosalivary circulation. The absorbed nitrate (NO_3^-) is then concentrated tenfold in the salivary glands and reduced to nitrite (NO_2^-) by bacterial nitrate reductase contained in facultative anaerobes present on the dorsal surface of the tongue [43, 44]. The bacteria uses nitrate as an alternative electron acceptor to produce energy, thereby effectively reducing it to nitrite. In fact, the use of antibacterial mouthwash after dietary nitrate load has been reported to attenuate the expected rise in systemic nitrite levels [34]. Allopurinol-sensitive tissue

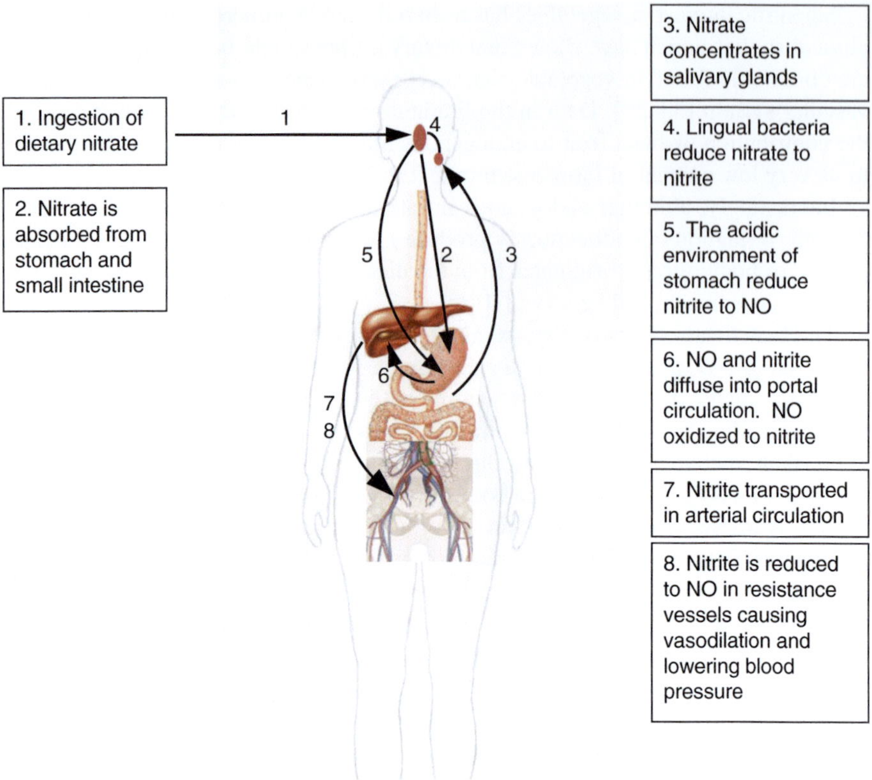

Fig. 9.4 The pathway of dietary nitrate derived consuming leafy vegetables. After it has been absorbed through the stomach wall [1, 2], ~25% of consumed nitrate enters the enterosalivary circulation and is concentrated tenfold in the salivary glands [3] where it is reduced to nitrite by bacterial nitrate reductase from facultative anaerobes present on the dorsal surface of the tongue [4]. Subsequently nitrite is swallowed and in the acidic environment of the stomach is reduced to nitric oxide (NO) [5] or re-enters the circulation as nitrite, then diffuses into portal circulation [6] providing a source of systematically available nitrite/NO. Nitrite is then transported through the arterial circulation to resistance vessels [7, 8], where a lower O_2 tension favors the reduction of nitrite to NO, causing vasodilation and consequent blood pressure lowering. Source: Capurso C, Capurso A – Vasc Pharmacol 2014; 63: 118–126.

nitrate reductase enzymes, which reduce nitrate to nitrite, also seem to contribute to nitrate reduction to nitrite in the body, but the magnitude of this pathway is not clear [36]. Once the nitrite swallowed enters the stomach, it is partly converted to NO by local acidic conditions. Nitrite and NO then diffuse into portal circulation and NO is oxidized to nitrite, which in turn is transported in arterial circulation to resistance vessels, where it lowers O_2 tension and favors the reduction of nitrite to NO which causes vasodilation and thus lowers blood pressure.

Nitrite is reduced to NO by a variety of sources, including deoxyhemoglobin and xanthine oxidoreductase [41–44]. It is noteworthy that the conversion of nitrite to NO requires a reaction with a deoxygenated heme protein, suggesting a novel function of hemoglobin as a deoxygenation-dependent nitrite reductase [41].

Interestingly, unlike NO production from the eNOS whose activity is oxygen-dependent, NO production from the nitrate-nitrite-NO pathway increases with diminished oxygen [41, 42].

NO influences vascular homeostasis in many ways [50–53]. NO enters vascular smooth muscle cells where it increases cyclic guanosine 3′,5′-monophosphate (cGMP) production, leading to smooth muscle relaxation (vasodilation). In addition, NO inhibits platelet aggregation and platelet adhesion to the endothelium. Moreover, NO suppresses the vascular smooth muscle cell proliferation, the adhesion and migration of leukocytes/monocytes into the arterial wall, the activity of inflammatory factors, and the expression of certain adhesion molecules. Increased levels of superoxide anions have been implicated in the reduction of NO bioavailability in the vasculature [54–56].

9.5.1.3 Dietary Nitrates and Blood Pressure

Human studies have shown that dietary nitrate has numerous effects on the cardiovascular system. These are the most important ones.

Larsen et al. [37] showed that a 3-day dietary supplementation with sodium nitrate at a dose corresponding to the amount normally found in 150–250 g of a nitrate-rich vegetable such as spinach, beetroot, or lettuce did not change systolic blood pressure and pulse rate but significantly reduced diastolic blood pressure and mean arterial pressure. The authors agreed with the conclusions of other investigators [57, 58] that a diet rich in vegetables can reduce blood pressure.

Webb et al. [35] demonstrated that the ingestion of a dietary nitrate load (beetroot juice 500 mL; mean nitrate concentration 45 mmol/L) in healthy volunteers significantly reduced systolic blood pressure by 10.4 ± 3 mmHg at 2.5 h after ingestion, an effect that correlated with peak increases in plasma nitrite concentrations. The peak differences in diastolic blood pressure, a drop of 8.1 ± 2.1 mmHg, was seen at 3 h after ingestion. The dietary nitrate load also prevented endothelial dysfunction induced by an acute ischemic insult in the forearm and significantly attenuated the ex vivo platelet aggregation in response to collagen and ADP. The in vivo half-life of nitrite (~1.5 h) in these studies was much longer than the ex vivo half-life of 2 min, suggesting that nitrite is continuously produced from nitrate (which has a long half-life of ~ 8 h) via the enterosalivary circulation [35].

9.5.1.4 Conclusion

Dietary nitrate, contained in particular in green leafy vegetables and beetroot, appears to be a major contributor to vascular effects. Nitrite, the reduced form of nitrate, is an intrinsic signaling molecule, and its ability to form nitric oxide (NO) under hypoxic conditions has transformed this once inert anion into a critical molecule in maintaining NO and nitroso homeostasis throughout the entire physiological oxygen gradient in vivo.

Nitrate and nitrite appear to play a significant role in blood-pressure-lowering effects of vegetable-rich diets, and underlie the cardioprotective effect of vegetables [59]. Interestingly, given that the blood pressure response to a high fruit and vegetable diet appears to be much greater in hypertensives with respect to normotensives [58], it can be hypothesized that the effect of dietary nitrate is heightened particularly in the former.

9.5.2 Cruciferae

9.5.2.1 Cruciferae and Cancer: Biochemical and Experimental Studies

Over the past decades, research on the action of plant bioactive components has been focusing on their benefits on human health. One group of vegetables that has drawn a great deal of attention are those from the *Brassicaceae* family (Cruciferae). The benefits on human health associated to the consumption of cruciferous plants is explained, in part, by their rich composition in secondary metabolites, also called phytochemicals. From this point of view, cruciferous vegetables are unique in that they are a very rich source of sulfur-containing compounds known as glucosinolates that impart a pungent aroma and spicy (some say bitter) taste. The hydrolysis of glucosinolates by a class of plant enzymes called myrosinase results in the formation of bioactive glucosinolate hydrolysis products, such as isothiocyanates and indole-3-carbinol. The enzyme myrosinase is physically separated from glucosinolates in intact plant cells. When cruciferous vegetables are chopped or chewed, myrosinase comes into contact with glucosinolates and catalyzes their hydrolysis.

All glucosinolates have a common core structure that consists of a β-thioglucoside *N*-hydroxysulfate with a side chain R and a sulfur-linked β-D glucopyranoside moiety that derives from different types of amino acid precursors. To date, more than 120 individual glucosinolates have been isolated from the species of the *Brassicaceae* family and allied ones [60]. When cell damage takes place, glucosinolates undergo hydrolysis by myrosinase to yield glucose, sulfate, and aglucones that can undergo fragmentation and/or molecular rearrangement. This process will yield isothiocyanates (ITCs), thiocyanates, and other products, depending on the specific glucosinolate substrate, myrosinase isozyme, reaction pH, and the presence of certain ions. Notably, nearly all of the protective activities of glucosinolates, including those against cancer, can be attributed to their hydrolytic products, of which the ITCs are prominent examples [61–63]. For this reason they have an increased value since they are both therapeutic compounds to be used in medicine and food supplements for the human diet [64].

It had been reported [65] that the risk of cancer is increased in individuals who consume small quantities of Brussels sprouts and broccoli, and decreased in those who eat a lot of these vegetables. These findings are moreover consistent with the lower number of tumors in animals challenged with carcinogens and fed compounds found in the same vegetables. It is now known that this protection is not organ-specific and it has been seen in the lung, esophagus, stomach, colon, breast, bladder, pancreas, and prostate [66]. Likewise, this protective effect is attributed to subtoxic concentrations of glucosinolate degradation products. It has been reported [67] that 3–5 servings of broccoli or cauliflower per week could be cancer-preventive, although the effective therapeutic concentration has not yet been determined by clinical studies.

Recently, ITCs have gained attention as they are responsible for the cancer chemopreventive properties attributed to cruciferous crops [68]. Thus, the anticarcinogenic effects of phenethyl isothiocyanate (PEITC) have become the object of study of several clinical trials. In general, ITCs and glucosinolate hydrolysis products could help prevent cancer by enhancing the elimination of carcinogens before they can damage DNA, or by altering cell-signaling pathways in ways that help prevent normal cells from being transformed into cancerous cell.

Attempts to understand the mechanisms of action of ITCs were initiated in parallel with studies demonstrating their protective effects in animal models of carcinogenesis. It is now recognized that these mechanisms are multiple, meaning that carcinogenesis could be inhibited both at an early and a late state. These mechanisms include at least the following: alterations of carcinogen metabolism due to changes in the activities of drug-metabolizing enzymes; induction of cell cycle arrest and apoptosis; inhibition of angiogenesis and metastasis; changes in histone acetylation status; and oxidant activities [69].

Another growing area of interest regarding the cancer chemopreventive role of glucosinolate breakdown products concerns epigenetics. Different epigenetic changes, such as aberrant DNA methylation, histone modifications, and microRNA profiles, can induce altered gene expression and functional changes, such as tumor suppressor genes silencing and/or activation of oncogenes [70], taking on an important role in carcinogenesis [71–76] (see also the previous Chap. 7). DNA hypomethylation can facilitate genome instability and thus an enhanced expression of oncogenes, whereas DNA hypermethylation can silence tumor suppressor genes, transcription factors, and genes involved in the regulation of the cell cycle and apoptosis [76]. DNA methyltransferases (DNAMTs) are involved in DNA methylation patterns [77] and are overexpressed in many cancers, such as PCa [78], lung cancer [79], leukemia [80], pancreatic cancer [81], or gastric cancer [82]. Histone molecules contribute to genome stability and gene transcription [83], and some transcriptional modifications (acetylation, deacetylation, methylation, phosphorylation, and ubiquitination) can alter them [84] with implications for cancer development [73, 74, 85, 86].

Since epigenetic deregulation that appears at the onset and development of cancer is potentially reversible, many authors have proposed epigenetic intervention strategies for cancer prevention and treatment [71].

Cruciferous vegetables have demonstrated properties against cancer [87] that could be attributed, at least in part, to ITC compounds found in these plants. ITCs may be regulators of DNAMTs, miRNAs, and inhibitors of histone deacetylases (HDACs) [87], affecting the uncontrolled cellular proliferation and the viability of various types of cancer cells such as breast [88, 89], leukemic [90], pancreatic [91], colon [92], or skin [93–95].

Prostate cancer has attracted particular interest since it is a clinically heterogeneous disease (indolent, localized or invasive and metastatic) with multiple mechanisms and signaling pathways involved in its genesis and evolution that could develop resistance to conventional treatment. In vitro studies performed with prostate cancer cells [76, 96] have provided evidence that ITCs may act as epigenetic modulators, thus having consequences on the initiation and progression of carcinogenesis [76, 96, 97]. In fact, ITCs seem to be able to activate cell cycle arrest, apoptosis, and autophagy. ITCs also seem to exhibit activity against metastasis and angiogenesis, acting on epigenetic mechanisms and different signaling pathways.

Sulforaphane (SFN) has been also found to modulate epigenetic mechanisms such as DNAMT expression and DNA methylation in both normal and cancerous (androgen-dependent and androgen-independent) prostate cells [76, 88, 98, 99]. These effects of SFN on DNA methylation can lead to the re-expression of some tumor suppressor genes that had been silenced in cancer cells. Likewise, SFN can also inhibit histone deacetylase (HDAC) activities upregulated in cancer [100, 101]. In particular, SFN can inactivate the HDAC6, influencing the acetylation state of the heat shock protein 90 (HSP90) (a key androgen receptor (AR) chaperone) attenuating AR signaling [101], and finally androgen-dependent prostate cancer cell growth.

These data, and other findings from in vitro and in vivo studies on ITCs encourage investigators to continue to search for innovative approaches to chemoprevention and the treatment of prostate cancer and other types of cancer.

9.5.2.2 Cruciferae and Cancer: Studies in Humans

Beyond the numerous studies in vitro on glucosinolate hydrolysis products, many studies have been carried out on humans to evaluate the real benefits of Cruciferae in preventing human diseases, mostly cancer. An extensive review of case–control studies published prior to 1996 found an inverse association between some type of cruciferous vegetable intake and cancer risk [102]. The inverse association appeared to be most consistent for cancers of the lung and digestive tract. It should be remembered, however, that the results of retrospective case–control studies are prone to be distorted by bias in the selection of participants (cases and controls) and in dietary recall with respect to prospective cohort studies, which collect dietary information from participants before they are diagnosed with cancer [103].

Lung Cancer: A number of case–control studies found that individuals diagnosed with lung cancer had significantly lower intakes of cruciferous vegetables than persons in cancer-free control groups [102]. Prospective studies of Dutch men and women [104], American women [105], and Finnish men [106] found that higher intakes of cruciferous vegetables (more than 3 weekly servings) were associated with significant reductions in lung cancer risk, but prospective studies of American men [105] and European men and women [107] did not find any inverse association. These results suggest that genetic factors affecting the metabolism of glucosinolate hydrolysis products may influence the effects of cruciferous vegetable consumption on lung cancer risk.

Colorectal cancer: Although a number of case–control studies conducted prior to 1990 found that persons diagnosed with colorectal cancer were more likely to have lower intakes of various cruciferous vegetables than individuals without colorectal cancer [65, 108–110], several prospective cohort studies have not found significant inverse associations between cruciferous vegetable intake and the risk of developing colorectal cancer over time [111–116]. One exception was a prospective study examining Dutch adults, which found that the men and women with the highest intakes of cruciferous vegetables (averaging 58 g/day) were significantly less likely to develop colon cancer than those with the lowest intakes (averaging 11 g/day) [117]. The results of several recent epidemiological studies suggest that the protective effects of cruciferous vegetable consumption may be influenced by inherited differences in the capacity of individuals to metabolize and eliminate glucosinolate hydrolysis products.

Breast Cancer: The results of numerous epidemiological studies of cruciferous vegetable intake and breast cancer risk have been found to be inconsistent. A prospective study on 285,526 women found that total vegetable consumption was not related to risk of breast cancer; individual subcategories of vegetable type, including cabbages, root vegetables, and leafy vegetables, were not individually associated with breast cancer in this cohort [118].

Prostate Cancer: A prospective study with the longest follow-up period and the largest number of cases of prostate cancer found a significant inverse association between cruciferous vegetable intake and the risk of prostate cancer when the analysis was limited to men who had a prostate specific antigen (PSA) test [119]. Since men who undergo PSA screening are more likely to be diagnosed with prostate cancer, limiting the analysis in this way is one way to reduce detection bias [120]. Additionally, quite recent prospective study found that the intake of cruciferous vegetables was inversely associated with metastatic prostate cancer that has spread beyond the prostate [67].

The Influence of Genetics: There is evidence that genetic differences in humans may influence the effects of cruciferous vegetable intake on cancer risk. Glutathione *S*-transferases (GSTs) are a family of enzymes that metabolize isothiocyanates in a way that promotes their elimination from the body. Genetic polymorphisms may affect the activity of GST enzymes. Null variants of the *GSTM1* and *GSTT1* genes contain large deletions, and individuals who inherit two copies of the *GSTM1*-null or *GSTT1*-null gene cannot produce the corresponding GST enzyme [121]. Lower GST activity in these individuals results in slower elimination and longer exposure to isothiocyanates after cruciferous vegetable consumption [122]. In support of this idea, several epidemiological studies have found that inverse associations between isothiocyanate intake from cruciferous vegetables and risk of lung cancer [123–125] or colon cancer [126–128] were more pronounced in *GSTM1*-null and/or *GSTT1*-null individuals. These findings suggest that the protective effects of high intakes of cruciferous vegetables may be enhanced in individuals who more slowly eliminate potentially protective compounds such as isothiocyanates.

Carotenoids and Cancer

Carotenoids are the pigments that give fruits and vegetables their vibrant orange, yellow, red, and green colors. They all act as antioxidants with strong cancer-fighting properties. Antioxidants protect cells from free radicals, substances that work to destroy cell membranes and DNA. Carotenoids such as lycopene, alpha-carotene, and beta-carotene, have been shown to lead to a reduction in the risk of cancer, particularly breast and prostate tumors [129].

Breast Cancer: In a meta-analysis [130] of eight cohort studies, examining more than 80% of the world's published data on carotenoids and breast cancer, including 3055 case subjects and 1956 matched control subjects, found a statistically significant inverse association with breast cancer. The relative risk (RR) was: 0.87 for alpha-carotene, 0.83 for beta-carotene, 0.84 for lutein-zeaxanthin, 0.78 for lycopene, and 0.81 for total carotenoids. Beta-cryptoxanthin was not statistically associated with risk. For several carotenoids, associations appeared stronger for estrogen receptor negative (ER^-) than for ER^+ tumors.

According to this comprehensive prospective analysis women with higher circulating levels of alpha-carotene, beta-carotene, lutein+zeaxanthin, lycopene, and total carotenoids seem to be at reduced risk of breast cancer.

Prostate Cancer: The numerous studies that have investigated the association of lycopene intake with prostate cancer have produced contrasting results.

The *Health Professional Follow-up Study* [131] prospective cohort study assessed the dietary intakes over a 1-year period of a cohort of 47,894 eligible subjects initially free of diagnosed cancer. Between 1986 and 1992, 812 new cases of prostate cancer, including 773 non-stage A1 cases, were diagnosed. Intakes of the carotenoids beta-carotene, alpha-carotene, lutein, and beta-cryptoxanthin were not associated with the risk of non-stage A1 prostate cancer; only lycopene intake was related to lower risk (age- and energy-adjusted RR = 0.79; 95% confidence interval [CI] = 0.64–0.99 for high versus low quintile of intake. Of 46 vegetables and fruits or related products, four were significantly associated with lower prostate cancer risk: tomatoes, tomato sauce, tomato juice, and pizza. The combined intake of tomatoes, tomato sauce, tomato juice, and pizza (which accounted for 82% of lycopene intake) was inversely associated with the risk of prostate cancer (multivariate RR = 0.65; 95% CI = 0.44–0.95), for a consumption frequency greater than 10 versus less than 1.5 servings/week, and risk of advanced (stages C and D) prostate cancers (multivariate RR = 0.47; 95% CI = 0.22–1.00; P for trend = 0.03). These results suggest that the intake of lycopene or other compounds in tomatoes may reduce prostate cancer risk. The authors of the study concluded that "*these findings support recommendations to increase vegetable and fruit consumption to reduce cancer incidence but suggest that tomato-based foods may be especially beneficial regarding prostate cancer risk*" [131].

It is important to note that this study is one of some 17 that has examined dietary carotenoid intake and the risk of prostate cancer, and while two have found protective effects for beta-carotene, only one [131] has shown an effect related to lycopene. Moreover, of the seven studies that specifically examined whether dietary tomato products can reduce the risk of prostate cancer, only three found this to be the case [131–133]. Another study was inconclusive from a statistical point of view but with a trend supporting that hypothesis [134] and three found no association at all [135–137].

In conclusion, studies on the beneficial effects of lycopene on prostate cancer have produced contrasting results, although several have shown a clear antiprostate cancer activity, as in the case of the prospective, single blind, placebo controlled, randomized study by the Karmanos Cancer Institute of Detroit [138]. In this study, 15 out of 26 men scheduled for radical prostatectomy for organ confined malignancy were given lycopene supplements (15 mg twice a day for 3 weeks preoperatively). Serial measurements confirmed a 22% increase in plasma and tissue lycopene levels and a statistically significant fall in prostate specific antigen (PSA) over the 3 week periods in those taking lycopene. The patients in the supplement arm were also found to have smaller volume tumors and surgical margins were less likely to be positive. Furthermore, analysis of the excised tissue showed that the biomarkers of cellular proliferation decreased; at the same time, biomarkers of cellular differentiation, including connexin 43, and apoptosis increased in the intervention arm. The trial was clearly too small to permit any real conclusions to be drawn, but it nevertheless increases our propensity to believe in lycopene's antiprostate cancer activity.

On the basis of these results, it seems reasonable to recommend to the general population to consume 1 serving/day or 5 servings/week of tomato products as part of an overall healthy dietary pattern that can reduce the risks of prostate cancer, other malignancies, and probably also chronic diseases. This recommendation is consistent with current dietary guidelines which encourage all individuals to increase their fruit and vegetable consumption to lower the risk of heart disease and many types of cancer. It should be remembered that nutritional prevention of prostate cancer is very different from the use of dietary or nutritional treatments for established prostate cancer. The use of lycopene and other extracts for the treatment of prostate cancer is a separate issue that warrants further investigation.

9.5.3 Vegetables and Chronic Diseases

Although vegetables and fruit are extremely important in human nutrition as sources of nutrients and nonnutritive food constituents as well as to reduce in disease risks, there are still uncertainties regarding their relevance for the prevention of some chronic diseases. In order to evaluate the level of validity of studies regarding the impact of fruit and vegetables on numerous chronic pathological conditions, a working group within the German Nutrition Society (DGE) was established in 2006 to evaluate the evidence on the role of vegetables and fruit in preventing certain chronic diseases. A comprehensive analysis of the studies available in the literature was made, and the strength of the evidence for a risk association was judged by using criteria defined in advance. The evaluation of the evidence was published in 2007 in German as a DGE-statement [139].

9.5.3.1 Obesity

With reference to the impact of vegetables on body weight, most studies have been conducted examining an association with vegetables and fresh fruit. We must thus refer to the impact of both vegetables and fruit on obesity and weight loss.

The prevalence of pre-obesity and obesity has been rising in recent decades in European countries. For example, according to the EPIC–DIOGENES study, the prevalence of obesity in 60- to 65-year-olds increased during an 8.6 years follow-up from 21.5 to 27.8%. This cohort study reported that in the current generation of elderly people, once overweight was developed it persisted into old age [140]. Overweight or obesity occurs disproportionately often in individuals who have unfavorable socioeconomic indicators regarding education, income, and professional position [141]. Data from 196,373 adults living in 52 countries who mainly belonged to the low and middle income families interviewed by the World Health Survey (2002–2003) (24-h recall) showed that about 78% of the men and women consumed <5 portions of vegetables and fruit daily as recommended by the World Health Organization (WHO) (according to the WHO: 400 g/day) [142].

Overweight occurs if energy intake is higher than energy expenditure. Compared with many other foods, the volume of vegetables and fruit in relation to energy content is larger. Due to the favorable volume to energy ratio of vegetables and fruit, satiety signals can emerge without consuming a large amount of energy. The extent to which individual constituents of vegetables and fruit, such as dietary fiber, are involved in regulating hunger and saturation and hence body weight is unknown. Recommendations to eat more vegetables and fruit to stabilize weight can lead to wide differences in weight reduction including substantial weight loss. This weight loss had been generally linked to reduced energy density [143]. The majority of studies have shown that an increase in vegetable and fruit consumption might be a suitable measure to facilitate initial weight loss and subsequent weight stability [144]. In this context, it also seems important to address energy reduction.

Extended analysis of prospective and intervention studies [145] leads to the following conclusions: (1) there is *possible* evidence that an increase in the consumption of vegetables and fruit can contribute to weight stability (i.e., no weight increase occurs); (2) there is also *probable* evidence that an increase in vegetable and fruit consumption alone does not result in weight loss; (3) there is *probable* evidence that an increase in the consumption of vegetables and fruit leads to weight reduction, if this replaces foods rich in fat or energy.

9.5.3.2 Type 2 Diabetes Mellitus

Type 2 diabetes mellitus is one of the most common and most expensive chronic diseases. According to the International Diabetes Federation [146], the diabetes prevalence in 20- to 79-year-olds is 6.4% for women with large regional differences (e.g., 3.8% in Africa, 6.9% in Europe, and 10.2% in North America). Due to aging of populations, this prevalence is expected to increase to 7.7% by the year 2030 with an expected 237 million affected individuals.

Type 2 diabetes mellitus develops due to a complex interaction between genetic predisposition and lifestyle. Particularly important among the lifestyle factors that promote or accelerate the manifestation of type 2 diabetes mellitus are unhealthy nutritional habits and a lack of physical activity [147]. However, the most important risk factor for the development of type 2 diabetes mellitus is visceral/abdominal obesity, which also is the result of unfavorable lifestyle habits including overeating and a lack of physical activity.

Two meta-analysis have recently summarized the results of several prospective cohort studies examining whether consumption of vegetables and fruit is associated with the risk of type 2 diabetes mellitus.

The first meta-analysis [148] including a total of 5 cohort studies did not find any relation between fruit and/or vegetables consumption and the risk of diabetes. Individuals who consumed at least 5 portions of vegetables and fruit per day had a relative risk (RR) of 0.96 (95% CI 0.79–1.17) with respect to persons with low consumption (lowest quintile or non-consumers; 3 cohort studies). There was also no association (RR regarding >3 vs. <3 portions/day: fruit consumption: 1.01; 95% CI 0.88–1.15; vegetable consumption: 0.97; 95% CI 0.86–1.10) when vegetables and fruit were analyzed separately.

A second meta-analysis [149] also showed that there was no risk relation to risk regarding the total intake of vegetables and fruit: the RR for the comparison of the highest with the lowest category of consumption was 1.00 (95% CI 0.92–1.09). Nor was the consumption of either fruit (RR 0.93; 95% CI 0.83–1.01) or vegetables alone (RR 0.91; 95% CI 0.76–1.09) associated with any risk. The risk of diabetes was, however, significantly reduced in persons who consumed relatively large amounts of green leafy vegetables.

Other prospective studies did not find a significant correlation between the overall consumption of vegetables and fruit and risk of diabetes. Only the EPIC Norfolk Study [150] found a significant risk reduction with increased fruit consumption (RR for the comparison of highest and lowest quintile: 0.70; 95% CI 0.54–0.90).

In summary, most studies and meta-analyses report that there is no association between the consumption of vegetables and fruit and the risk of diabetes, meaning that the risk of developing type 2 diabetes mellitus is probably not influenced by the consumption of vegetables and fruit. Vegetables and fruit nevertheless indirectly influence the prevention of type 2 diabetes mellitus, as their consumption may lower the risk of weight gain in adults.

9.5.3.3 Hypertension

Hypertension is one of the most relevant public health issues facing society, with a global prevalence of 26% in the adult population in 2000. Due to the increased risks of stroke and CHD [151], and also of renal cancer [152] associated with hypertension, lifelong medication is usually required. Even a slight reduction in the mean blood pressure of the population seems to reduce the incidence of cardiovascular diseases [153, 154]. The American Heart, Lung and Blood Institute stated in 2003 that measures to prevent hypertension are based on a health-promoting lifestyle which, in addition to weight reduction (whenever overweight is present), include adherence to the DASH diet, reduction of sodium and alcohol intake and an increase of physical activity [155]. The ESH–ESC Task Force on the Management of Arterial Hypertension [156] of the European Society of Hypertension considers an increase in the consumption of vegetables and fruit as one of the lifestyle measures that can lower blood pressure in individuals with only a few risk factors for cardiovascular diseases and slightly increased blood pressure.

Vegetarians often show a lower blood pressure with respect to that in general population, and individuals who change from a normal to a vegetarian one often show a reduction in blood pressure [157]. According to cohort studies, there were either inverse relations between the consumption of vegetables and fruit and new cases of hypertension [158, 159] or inverse relations with one of the two food groups considered here or with a dietary pattern including vegetables and fruit [160, 161]. In the cross-sectional and in the longitudinal analysis carried out by the SU.VI.MAX Study, an inverse relation was observed between vegetable and fruit consumption and blood pressure [162]. The Nurses' Health Study (NHS) I and II and the Health Professionals Follow-up Study (HPFS) which examined flavonoid intake using an updated nutrient database from 2010 uncovered a risk reduction in hypertension with increasing intakes of anthocyanins [163].

The DASH diet, which is based on NIH studies, incorporates more fruits and vegetables. The Dietary Approaches to Stop Hypertension (DASH) study was designed as a randomized 8-week intervention in which 459 hypertensive patients were enrolled and divided into groups. One group was instructed to eat a diet rich in vegetables and fruit, and the other group was given the same instructions with additional information on a diet low in fat and high in dietary fiber. Although lower blood pressure was found in both groups at the end of the trial, the blood-pressure-lowering effect was more pronounced in the group receiving more information with respect to the group that was only instructed to eat a diet rich in vegetables and fruit [58].

A 6-month intervention study examining 690 English subjects between the age of 25 and 64 confirmed the results of the DASH study [164]. It found in fact an increase in the consumption of vegetables and fruit to at least 5 portions/day was accompanied by lower blood pressure. Furthermore, the study showed that an increase in vegetable and fruit consumption neither lowered the blood cholesterol concentration nor led to weight loss, but it did keep weight stable.

The biochemical mechanisms by which fruit and vegetables reduce blood pressure are not completely known. However, nitrates, contained in leafy vegetable, have been demonstrated to significantly reduce blood pressure, particularly in hypertensives [35]. The effects of leafy vegetable nitrates on hypertension have been described previously, in another Sect. 9.5.1.3 of this chapter.

9.5.3.4 Coronary Heart Disease

Coronary heart disease (CHD) is still the single largest cause of premature death in the world. Ischemic heart disease has been estimated to account for 12% of all deaths worldwide in 2004. CHD is also a major cause of disease burden in terms of disability-adjusted life years lost (DALY), accounting for 63 million DALYs worldwide in 2004 [165].

In addition to age and gender, modifiable risk factors are important, especially lifestyle factors like smoking and a lack of physical activity and the medical diagnoses of hypertension, diabetes mellitus, obesity, and dyslipoproteinemia [166]. As far as these factors are concerned, the 4 medical diagnoses listed here are clearly nutrition-related and can be influenced by changes in diet.

Two recent meta-analyses examined the results of several cohort studies that investigated if the consumption of vegetables and fruit was associated with the risk of CHD.

In one meta-analysis [167], which examined 9 cohort studies, the risk of CHD was reduced by 4% (RR 0.96; 95% CI 0.93–0.99) per portion of vegetables and fruit and by 7% (RR 0.93; 95% CI 0.89–0.96) per portion of fruit daily. For vegetables, the inverse relation regarding the risk of CHD was stronger for the overall cardiovascular mortality (RR per portion 0.74; 95% CI 0.75–0.84) than for fatal or nonfatal myocardial infarction (RR 0.95; 95% CI 0.92–0.99). A linear dose-response relation was found between mortality and consumption of fruit as well as the total intake of vegetables and fruit.

Another meta-analysis [168] examining 13 cohorts studies found that persons who consumed 3–5 portions of vegetables and fruit per day (RR 0.93; 95% CI 0.86–1.00) or who consumed >5 portions/day (RR 0.83; 95% CI 0.77–0.89) had a lower risk of CHD than individuals who consumed <3 portions. Further analysis revealed a significant inverse relation with the risk of CHD for both fruit and vegetables.

A higher vegetable and fruit intake was inversely associated with the risk of CHD according to the EPIC-Heart Study [169] and the Morgen Study [170]. The Italian arm of the EPIC Study found no association for vegetables and fruit together, but for leafy vegetables [171].

These data also reflect the opinion of the WHO [172] and the current nutritional recommendations of the European Society of Cardiology [166] and the American Heart Association [173]; both recommend consuming vegetables and fruit to reduce the risk of CHD.

Several intervention studies have investigated intermediary clinical markers of the cardiovascular system, with regard to specific kinds of vegetables and fruit. These studies showed that the consumption of vegetables and fruit can improve the regulation of blood vessel dilation [174], prevent platelet aggregation [175–177], and reduce inflammation markers [178, 179].

On the basis of these studies, we can conclude that many cohort studies have shown a protective association between the consumption of vegetables and fruit and the risk of CHD. In addition, some intervention studies have demonstrated a beneficial influence of vegetables and fruit on metabolic pathways that are associated with the risk of CHD. These data appear quite convincing.

9.5.3.5 Stroke

Stroke, which is one of the major causes of death in the world, also leads to a high number of disability-adjusted life years (DALYs), ranking sixth among the leading causes worldwide [165].

In addition to age and gender, modifiable risk factors are important, especially lifestyle factors such as smoking and lack of physical activity as well as postmenopausal hormone replacement therapy, and the diagnoses of hypertension, diabetes mellitus, obesity, dyslipoproteinemia, CHD, arterial occlusion disease, extracranial stenoses or occlusion of arteries supplying the brain [180]. Most of these vascular and metabolic diseases are clearly nutrition-related and can be influenced by a change in nutrition.

According to a meta-analysis of 7 prospective cohort studies, the risk of stroke was reduced by 11% (RR 0.89; 95% CI 0.85–0.93) per portion of fruit per day, by 5% (0.95; 95% CI 0.92–0.97) for vegetable and fruit, and by 3% (RR 0.97; 95% CI 0.92.1.02) for vegetables [181]. This meta-analysis found a linear dose-response relation.

Another meta-analysis [182] examined 9 prospective cohort studies. Compared to individuals with an intake of vegetables and fruit of <3 portions/day, subjects with 3–5 portions/day (RR 0.89; 95% CI 0.83–0.97) and with >5 portions/day (RR 0.74; 95% CI 0.69–0.79) had a significantly lower risk of stroke.

Overall, the available data indicate a risk-reducing effect of vegetable and fruit consumption. This is also reflected in the opinion of the WHO [172] and current dietary recommendations of the European Society of Cardiology [166] and the American Heart Association [180].

These meta-analyses of cohort studies indicate that there is an inverse association between the consumption of vegetables and fruit and the risk of stroke. It can be concluded that there is convincing evidence that a high intake of vegetables and fruit reduces the risk of stroke.

9.5.3.6 Cancer

In 2008, approximately 2,457,610 new cases of cancer were observed in the European Union. For the same year, cancer was recorded as the cause of 1,231,220 deaths.

The occurrence of cancer as a whole increases with age and the pathogenesis often takes several decades. The disease is characterized by chromosomal changes that can be induced by different causes. In addition to age, the most important risk factors include tobacco smoking, consumption of alcohol, overweight, hormonal factors, physical inactivity, and excess food intake [183].

In a report of the World Cancer Research Fund (WCRF) experts published in 1997, based upon data that was collected until the beginning of the 1990s, vegetables and fruit were rated among the most important cancer preventive factors with a calculated prevention potential of 23% and the strength of evidence was rated as *convincing* for many cancer sites [184].

In 2003, the cancer preventive potential of vegetables and fruits was re-examined by an expert panel of the International Agency for the Research on Cancer, that analyzed the data of prospective cohort studies [185]. The analysis led to the conclusion that there was *probable* evidence for a protective effect of vegetables regarding cancer of the esophagus and colon and rectum, and *possible* evidence regarding cancer of the oral cavity, pharynx, stomach, larynx, lung, ovary, and kidney. There was *probable* evidence for a protective effect of fruit regarding cancer of the esophagus, stomach, and lung and *possible* evidence for a protective effect regarding cancer of the oral cavity, pharynx, colon, rectum, larynx, kidney, and bladder.

Quite recently the *EPIC* study [186] and *NIH-AARP Study* [187], each including more than 500,000 participants, and the *Pooling Study*, a pooled analysis of 17 cohort studies have published crucial new findings in this regard. Key [188] summarized the results of these studies collected until the year 2009, both for cancer in general and regarding the most important cancer sites. The data regarding the different cancer sites are characterized by reduced risks in connection with a high consumption of vegetables and fruit; although the risk relations often proved to be not statistically significant or only just significant, and the risks differed depending on the smoking behavior. In fact, the risk reduction was mainly seen in those types of cancer that are associated with smoking [189].

The risk reductions that have been observed in these large cohort studies with increasing consumption of vegetables and fruit still suggest that the consumption of vegetables and fruit influences the risk of cancer. The influence is however detectable only when there are large differences in the consumption of vegetables and fruit between the groups and seems to appear only in case of high exposure to carcinogens, such as, for example, in smokers. These restrictive statements do not directly influence the evidence regarding the inverse relation between the consumption of vegetables and fruit and the risk of cancer, which is considered *probable*.

9.5.3.7 Eye Diseases

Based on WHO data, more than 28 million subjects in Europe are visually impaired, with a 0.3% prevalence for blindness. The main causes for loss of sight in Europe and the United States are age-related macular degeneration (AMD; 50%), glaucoma (18%), diabetic retinopathy (17%), and cataract (5%) [190]. Despite worldwide trends showing reduced prevalence of visual impairment and blindness since the 1990s, the prevalence of eye diseases in the aging population is expected to increase in Western countries. The prevalence for cataract is over 40% in subjects older than 75 [191].

Macular Degeneration: Macular degeneration (AMD) is an age-related degenerative retinal disease that leads to the loss of central vision. Risk factors for the development of AMD include age, smoking, and nutrition. Important protective factors are dietary fiber [192], mono-unsaturated fatty acids [193], certain vitamins [194–196], and especially carotenoids like lutein and zeaxanthin. These carotenoids selectively accumulate in the macula lutea (point of high-resolution vision) and protect the pigment epithelial cells from blue light and damage by short-wave rays [197].

The dietary intake of carotenoids, serum levels, and the supplementation of these carotenoids are associated with a risk reduction for AMD in most studies [198–202]. Some studies nevertheless produced contrasting results and the intake of lutein/zeaxanthin and other carotenoids was not associated with the risk of AMD [203].

In women younger than 75, the risk of AMD was reduced by 52% at a higher intake of vegetables (4 vs. 0.9 portions/day) [204]. A high intake (>5 times/week) of foods rich in lutein, like spinach and collard greens, was associated with a reduction in the AMD risk by 86% in a case–control study [205]. According to Goldberg et al. [206], the intake (>7 times/week) of vegetables and fruit rich in provitamin A was associated with a reduction in the AMD risk by 33% according to a cross-sectional study.

Cataract: A cataract is a clouding of the lens in adults, leading to impaired vision or vision acuity. The risk is influenced by age, ethnic origin, gender, smoking, sunlight, consumption of alcohol, diabetes mellitus, corticosteroid medication, and nutritional factors [207].

Studies examining the correlation between the intake of vitamin C and carotenoids and cataract risk have produced contrasting results. The prospective *Blue Mountains Eye Study* [208] suggested that a high intake of vitamin C, especially from fruit juices, is associated with a significantly reduced risk of cataract. The combined intake of vitamin C and other antioxidants (beta-carotene, vitamin E, zinc) from foods and/or supplements was also associated with a reduction in the cataract risk by 38–49%.

A diet following the recommendations of the *Dietary Guidelines for Americans 2000* was found to be associated with a more than 50% reduction in cataract risk. In fact, a prospective study [209] conducted eye exams in 479 *Nurses' Health Study* participants aged 52–73 who were without previously diagnosed cataract or diabetes, living in the Boston, MA, area. Four food-frequency questionnaires (FFQs), collected during a 9- to 11-y period before evaluation of lens status, were used to define the participants' diet. After adjusting for age, smoking, and other risk factors, women in the highest quartile category of HEI scores, i.e., those with the highest fruit consumption (3.9 portions/day), were significantly less likely to have nuclear opacities than those in the lowest category (1.3 portions/day) (odds ratio (OR) = 0.47; 95% CI: 0.26–0.84).

According to the *Health Professionals Follow-up Study* (*HPFS*), high consumption of broccoli and spinach in men was associated with a reduction in the cataract risk by 23 and 27% [210]. A high intake of vegetables and fruit was likewise associated with a significant reduction (10–15%) in cataract risk in the participants of the *Women's Health Study* [211]. The risk of cataract was 18% and 14% lower in the highest quintile of both lutein/zeaxanthin and vitamin E intake than that in the lowest quintile when an updated analysis of the same study was carried out [212].

According to the *Carotenoids in the Age-Related Eye Disease Study* (CAREDS), the risk was reduced by 26% when individuals were consuming high vegetable intakes [213]. Comparing highest with lowest quintiles, the risk of cataract was reduced by 32% both in connection to the calculated daily intake of lutein and zeaxanthin and the measured plasma concentrations of lutein and zeaxanthin. These findings were confirmed by the results of the prospective POLA Study (*Pathologies Oculaires Liées à l'Age*) [214]. The risk of nuclear cataract was significantly reduced (OR = 0.23; 95% CI: 0.01–0.58; $P = 0.005$) in the group with the highest plasma concentration of zeaxanthin (the highest quintile of plasma zeaxanthin).

Glaucoma: Glaucoma is caused by changes in the intraocular pressure that can damage the optic nerve and may progress to complete blindness. There are very few data on the influence of lifestyle factors on the risk of glaucoma. As far as nutritional factors are concerned, only one study has examined the association between vegetable and fruit intake and the risk of glaucoma [215]. According to this cross-sectional investigation, there was a lower risk when individuals had high intakes of certain kinds of vegetables and fruit, for example, fresh carrots (−64%). However, the evidence regarding the risk of glaucoma has been deemed insufficient due to the lack of data.

9.5.3.8 Dementia

Dementia is a mental disease characterized by a loss of mental ability that is severe enough to interfere with normal activities of daily living. Logical and critical thinking, judgment, retentive memory, and short-term memory are impaired, while remote memory (long-term memory) can remain for a long time. There is 5.4% prevalence in Europe in persons over 60. Due to an increasing life expectancy in industrialized countries and the exponential increase in dementia in old age, the prevalence of dementia in these countries continue to rise steadily.

Worldwide, Alzheimer's disease and vascular dementia are the two most common subtypes of dementia, which respectively account for 50–70 and 15–25% of all dementia cases [216]. Old age and genetic susceptibility are well-established risk factors for dementia and Alzheimer's disease. Vascular risk factors (e.g., diabetes mellitus, hypertension, and smoking) as well as cardio- and cerebrovascular diseases may contribute to the development and progression of dementia, whereas social, physical, and mental activities may delay their onset [216].

There are only a few studies on the association between fruit and vegetables consumption and dementia.

A cohort study examining 3718 participants of the *Chicago Health and Aging Project* (mean age at baseline 74 years) investigated the relation between the consumption of vegetables and fruit and the decrease in cognitive performance (6 years follow-up) [217]. Vegetable and fruit intake analyzed together did not show any association with cognitive functions; an inverse association was found for the consumption of vegetables alone, but not for the consumption of fruit. Other cohort studies showed similar results.

The decline in cognitive performance was investigated in 13,388 women (age at baseline: 30–55 years, follow-up: 19–25 years) by a prospective cohort study [218]. Fruit was not associated with cognition or cognitive decline, while total vegetable intake was significantly associated with less decline. Women in the highest quintile of cruciferous vegetables showed a slower decline with respect to the lowest quintile. Women consuming the most green leafy vegetables also experienced slower decline than those consuming the least amount.

An inverse association was also found by a Dutch cohort ($n = 2613$, age at baseline: 43–70 years, follow-up: 10 years), only between vegetable consumption and cognitive performance, and not with regard to fruit and juices [219]. The study also found an inverse association between the consumption of root vegetables (carrots, beetroot) and the decrease in cognitive performance.

It should be noted that while the results of cross-sectional studies show a protective effect of both fruit and vegetables in maintaining cognitive performance [220, 221], the results of cohort studies suggest a protective effect only in connection to vegetables.

Three cohort studies focusing on dementia or Alzheimer's dementia as a target parameter have also been conducted [222–224]. In the first of these studies [222], the intake of vegetable and fruit juices was analyzed in 1836 Japanese immigrants (mean age, 71 years) between 1992 and 1994 in relation to the incidence of Alzheimer's dementia in 2001. The risk of disease decreased with increasing consumption, independently of the intake of vitamins C, E, and β-carotene.

The frequency of vegetables and fruit consumption was investigated in 8085 subjects (aged >65 years) in Bordeaux, Dijon, and Montpellier (France) by the second cohort study [223]. After a 3.6 year follow-up, it was found that greater frequency of vegetable and fruit consumption reduced the risk of dementia, including the risk of Alzheimer's dementia. Daily consumption compared with rare consumption was associated with a risk reduction of about 30%.

The third study [224], the Swedish Twins (HARMONY) Study which monitored 3779 individuals (mean age at baseline: 48 years) with a follow-up of 30 produced similar results. The study found that a medium or high intake of fruit and vegetables was associated with a decreased risk of dementia and Alzheimer's dementia with respect to a low or no consumption of fruit and vegetables. The difference was nevertheless significant only in fully adjusted models. Compared with the consumption of more than 2 portions of vegetables and fruit per day, the consumption of <2 portions was associated with a significantly higher risk of dementia, adjusting for age and gender.

In summary, the studies on cognitive performance and risk of dementia suggest that there is an inverse relation with the consumption of vegetables and fruit, and that consuming vegetables seems to be more important than eating fruit.

9.5.3.9 Dietary Fiber and Intestine

The chapter on vegetables would not be complete without a section on fiber, a very important component of all vegetables.

Dietary fibers are the nondigestible carbohydrates and lignin that are intrinsic and intact in plants. Functional fibers consist of isolated, nondigestible carbohydrates that have beneficial physiologic effects in humans. Total fiber is the sum of dietary fibers and functional fibers.

Dietary fibers are divided into two types: water-soluble and water-insoluble (see table below)

1. Water-soluble fibers, that generally absorb water to become a gelatinous, viscous substance which is fermented by bacteria in the colon into gases and physiologically active by-products. Some, but not all, soluble plant fibers block intestinal mucosal adherence and translocation of potentially pathogenic bacteria and may therefore modulate intestinal inflammation, an effect that has been termed contrabiotic.
2. Water-insoluble fibers, that generally do not dissolve in water, are metabolically inert and provide bulking. Bulking fibers absorb water as they move through the digestive system, easing defecation. Some insoluble fibers, notably resistant starch, are fully fermented in the large intestine.

Consuming fiber leads to the production of healthful compounds during the fermentation of soluble fiber. Moreover, insoluble fiber is able to increase bulk (via its passive hygroscopic properties), soften stools, and shorten the transit time through the intestinal tract. A disadvantage of a diet high in fiber is the potential for significant intestinal gas production and bloating.

Dietary fibers (Types and source)	
Water-insoluble dietary fibers	
Beta-glucans	
Cellulose	Cereal, fruit, vegetables
Chitin	Fungi, exoskeleton of insects and crustaceans
Hemicellulose	Cereals, pulses and legumes, bran, timber
Hexose	Wheat, barley
Pentose	Rye, oat
Lignin	Vegetable filaments, cereals
Resistant starch	Legumes, bananas, barley, high amylase wheat
Water-soluble dietary fibers	
Arabinoxylan (hemicellulose)	Psyllium
Fructans	(Replace starch as storage carbohydrate in some plants)
Inulin	Banana, chicory, artichoke, onion, garlic, wheat, barley
Pectin	In the fruit skin (apples, quinces), vegetables
Alginic acids	In algae
Raffinose	In legumes

Fiber content in foods		
Food groups	*Serving mean*	*Fiber g/per serving*
Fruit	0.5 cup	1.1
Dark-green vegetables	0.5 cup	6.4
Orange vegetables	0.5 cup	2.1
Cooked dry beans (legumes)	0.5 cup	8.0
Starchy vegetables	0.5 cup	1.7
Other vegetables	0.5 cup	1.1
Whole grains	28 g (1 oz)	2.4
Meat	28 g (1 oz)	0.1

Source: USDA National Nutrient Database for Standard Reference

Sources of soluble and insoluble fibers
Sources of soluble fibers
– Legumes (peas, chickpeas, beans, soya bean, lupins, and other beans)
– Oats, rye, barley
– Some fruits, including plums, berries, ripe bananas, skin of apples and pears
– Certain vegetables, such as broccoli, carrots, turnip tops, artichokes
– Root tubers and root vegetables (e.g., sweet potatoes, onions)
– Flax seeds
– Nuts and almonds are the highest in dietary fibers
Source of insoluble fibers
– Whole grain foods
– Wheat and corn bran
– Legumes such as beans and peas
– Nuts and seeds
– Potato skins
– Vegetables such as green beans, cauliflower, zucchini, celery
– Skins of some fruits including grapes, tomatoes, apples

The biological, chemical, and physical properties of dietary fibers are associated with physiologic actions in the small and large intestines that have important metabolic implications for health. Fiber's properties include water dispersibility, bulk, viscosity, adsorption and binding of compounds and fermentability.

Within the small intestine, properties such as water dispersibility, bulking, and viscosity are associated with slowing the digestion and absorption of carbohydrate and lipid and promoting nutrient absorption along a greater length of the small intestine. Both of these actions are related to cholesterol reduction and blunting of alimentary glycemia. Certain sources of fiber, and in particular digested cereal products (barley, oat, rye and wheat flour; oat bran), interact with bile acids and increase their fecal excretion [225, 226]. A greater excretion of bile acids contributes to the plasma-cholesterol-lowering ability of dietary fiber [227].

Water and electrolytes are absorbed in the large intestine, and microbial action breaks down the macronutrients in the residual material that passes from the small bowel.

Dietary fiber and undigested starch are the primary substrates for microflora growth in the large bowel. Thus the bulk associated with undigested residue contributes directly to stool bulk as undigested material, or indirectly through the growth of microflora, which are a part of the stool weight. The dispersibility of polysaccharides in water and water-holding capacity determine the ability with which microorganisms can penetrate the undigested food residue and gain access to the polysaccharides for metabolism.

Because inulin and oligofructose are dispersible in water, they are likely to be readily degraded by microorganisms present in the large bowel. The fermentability of inulin and oligofructose provides a route by which they can increase stool weight because they increase microbial mass in the colon. In addition, fermentation can lower the pH of colon contents, and the production of short chain fatty acids is likely to affect the health of the intestinal mucosa.

A recent paper described a new interesting healthy aspect of dietary fibers in the large bowel [228]. The article outlines how fiber deprivation impacts the gut microbiota and alters disease risks. Using a gnotobiotic mouse model, in which animals were colonized with a synthetic human gut microbiota composed of fully sequenced commensal bacteria, investigators studied the functional interactions between dietary fiber, the gut microbiota, and the colonic mucus barrier, which serves as a primary defense against enteric pathogens. The trial showed that during chronic or intermittent dietary fiber deficiency, the gut microbiota resorts to host-secreted mucus glycoproteins as a nutrient source, leading to erosion of the colonic mucus barrier. Dietary fiber deprivation, together with a fiber-deprived and a mucus-eroding microbiota, promotes greater epithelial access and lethal colitis by the mucosal pathogen *Citrobacter rodentium.* This study has shed light on some intricate pathways linking diet, the gut microbiome, and intestinal barrier dysfunction. Given the numerous benefits of dietary fiber, it is generally recommended that most men and women should respectively consume about 38 and 25 g of dietary fiber a day. Older men and women typically need respectively about 30 and 21 g, according to the USDA. These general guidelines stem from the basic dietary recommendation that all individuals, regardless of age or gender, should eat 14 g of fiber for every 1000 calories consumed. An individual who averages 2200 calories a day, for example, should get about 31 g of fiber. One small apple, for example supplies about 12% of the recommended amount of fiber.

9.5.4 Conclusive Remarks

The data that is presently available shows that higher intakes of vegetables and fruit can potentially prevent a number of diseases. While the evidence regarding its risk-reducing effect on hypertension, CHD, and stroke appears quite convincing, studies regarding the cancer connection seem less conclusive with respect to what was originally thought.

The scientific basis of the "*5 a day*" campaign, that has been widely promoted in recent years in Europe and nationwide, is strongly supported by the data available on its prevention potential. There seems to be a broader basis for disease prevention than what was thought at the beginning of the campaign when the focus was primarily on cancer. The recommendation to increase the consumption of vegetables and fruit are principally based upon convincing data regarding hypertension, CHD, and stroke and, potentially, many other diseases. Scientific societies have been carefully monitoring the progress of these studies, and, for example, the European Society of Cardiology has included recommendations on the intake of vegetables and fruit in its guidelines about prevention.

As vegetables and fruit and the phytochemicals therein particularly influence inflammatory, cellular redox as well as endothelial and metabolic processes, which are involved in the pathogenesis of various diseases, it is probable that these mechanisms are primarily responsible for the risk-reducing effect of vegetables and fruit consumption on single diseases.

References

1. Dentali F, Crowther M, Galli M, Pomero F, Garcia D, Clark N, Spadafora L, Witt DM, Ageno W, WARPEDI Investigators. Effect of vitamin K intake on the stability of treatment with vitamin K antagonists: a systematic review of the literature. Semin Thromb Hemost. 2016;42:671–81.
2. Hayes JD, Kelleher MO, Eggleston IM. The cancer chemopreventive actions of phytochemicals derived from glucosinolates. Eur J Nutr. 2008;47:73–88.
3. Zhang Y, Kensler TW, Cho CG, Posner GH, Talalay P. Anticarcinogenic activities of sulforaphane and structurally related synthetic norbornyl isothiocyanates. Proc Natl Acad Sci U S A. 1994;91:3147–50.
4. Tsimberidou AM, Keating MJ. Treatment of fludarabine-refractory chronic lymphocytic leukemia. Cancer. 2009;115:2824–36.
5. Wang X, Di Pasqua AJ, Govind S, McCracken E, Hong C, Mi L, Mao Y, Wu JY, Tomita Y, Woodrick JC, Fine RL, Chung FL. Selective depletion of mutant p53 by cancer chemopreventive isothiocyanates and their structure-activity relationships. J Med Chem. 2011;54:809–16.
6. Tse G, Eslick GD. Cruciferous vegetables and risk of colorectal neoplasms: a systematic review and meta-analysis. Nutr Cancer. 2014;66:128–39.
7. Wong BB, Koh S, Hegney DG, He HG. The effectiveness of cabbage leaf application (treatment) on pain and hardness in breast engorgement and its effect on the duration of breastfeeding. The. JBI Database System Rev Implement Rep. 2012;10:1185–213.
8. Bryan NS. Food, nutrition, and the nitric oxide pathway: biochemistry and bioactivity. Lancaster, PA: DEStech Publications, Inc.; 2010.
9. Noonan SC, Savage GP. Oxalate content of foods and its effect on humans (PDF). Asia Pac J Clin Nutr. 1999;8:64–74.

10. Weaver CM, Heaney RP. Calcium in human health. New York: Human Press Inc.; 2006. p. 135. ISBN 1-59259-452.8.
11. Sutton M. Spinach Iron and Popeye. Ironic lessons from biochemistry and history on the importance of healthy eating, healthy scepticism and adequate citation. Int J Criminol. 2010. http://www.internetjournalofcriminology.com/Sutton_Spinach_Iron_and_Popeye_March_2010.pdf.
12. Di Mascio P, Kaiser S, Sies H. Lycopene as the most efficient biological carotenoid singlet oxygen quencher. Arch Biochem Biophys. 1989;274:532_538.
13. Stahl W, Sies H. Uptake of lycopene and its geometrical isomers is greater from heat-processed than from utomato juice in humans. J Nutr. 1992;122:2161–6.
14. Arab L, Steck S. Lycopene and cardiovascular disease. Am J Clin Nutr. 2000;71(suppl): 1691S–5S.
15. Goulinet S, Chapman MJ. Plasma LDL and HDL subspecies are heterogenous in particle content of tocopherols and oxygenated and hydrocarbon carotenoids. Relevance to oxidative resistance and atherogenesis. Arterioscler Thromb Vasc Biol. 1997;17:786–96.
16. Hininger I, Chopra M, Thurnham DI, et al. Effect of increased fruit and vegetable intake on the susceptibility of lipoprotein to oxidation in smokers. Eur J Clin Nutr. 1997;51:601–6.
17. Steinberg FM, Chait A. Antioxidant vitamin supplementation and lipid peroxidation in smokers. Am J Clin Nutr. 1998;68:319–27.
18. Romanchik JE, Harrison EH, Morel DW. Addition of lutein, lycopene or beta-carotene to LDL or serum in vitro: effects on carotenoid distribution, LDL composition, and LDL oxidation. J Nutr Biochem. 1997;8:681–8.
19. Dugas TR, Morel DW, Harrison EH. Impact of LDL carotenoids and alpha-tocopherol content on LDL oxidation by endothelial cells in culture. J Lipid Res. 1998;39:999–1007.
20. Francis JM. Iberia and the Americas. Santa Barbara, CA: ABC-CLIO; 2005. ISBN 1-85109-426-1.
21. Tudela JA, Cantos E, Espín JC, Tomás-Barberán FA, Gil MI. Induction of antioxidant flavonol biosynthesis in fresh-cut potatoes. Effect of domestic cooking. J Agric Food Chem. 2002;50:5925–31.
22. Englyst HN, Kingman SM, Cummings JH. Classification and measurement of nutritionally important starch fractions. Eur J Clin Nutr. 1992;46:S33–50.
23. Esposito K, Marfella R, Ciotola M, Di Palo C, Giugliano F, Giugliano G, et al. Effect of a Mediterranean-style diet on endothelial dysfunction and markers of vascular inflammation in the metabolic syndrome: a randomized trial. JAMA. 2004;292:1440–6.
24. Vincent-Baudry S, Defoort C, Gerber M, Bernard MC, Verger P, Helal O, et al. The Medi-RIVAGE study: reduction of cardiovascular disease risk factors after a 3-mo intervention with a Mediterranean-type diet or a low-fat diet. Am J Clin Nutr. 2005;82:964–71.
25. Estruch R, Martínez-González MA, Corella D, Salas-Salvadò J, Ruiz-Gutiérrez V, Covas MI, et al. Effects of a Mediterranean-style diet on cardiovascular risk factors:a randomized trial. Ann Intern Med. 2006;145:1–11.
26. Fitó M, Guxens M, Corella D, Sàez G, Estruch R, de la Torre R, et al. Effect of a traditional Mediterranean diet on lipoprotein oxidation: a randomized controlled trial. Arch Intern Med. 2007;167:1195–203.
27. Mena MP, Sacanella E, Vázquez-Agell M, Morales M, Fitò M, Escoda R, et al. Inhibition of circulating immune cell activation: a molecular anti-inflammatory effect of the Mediterranean diet. Am J Clin Nutr. 2009;89:248–56.
28. Fuentes F, López-Miranda J, Sánchez E, Sàncez F, Paez J, Paz-Rojas E, et al. Mediterranean and low-fat diets improve endothelial function in hypercholesterolemic men. Ann Intern Med. 2001;134:1115–9.
29. Hord NG, Tang Y, Bryan NS. Food sources of nitrates and nitrites: the physiologic context for potential health benefits. Am J Clin Nutr. 2009;90:1–10.
30. Susin J, Kmecl V, Gregorcic A. A survey of nitrate and nitrite content of fruit and vegetables grown in Slovenia during 1996–2002. Food Addit Contam. 2006;23:385–90.
31. Santamaria P. Nitrate in vegetables: toxicity, content, intake and EC regulation. J Sci Food Agric. 2006;86:10–7.

32. Pennington JAT. Dietary exposure models for nitrates and nitrites. Food Control. 1998;9:385–95.
33. Bryan NS, Calvert JW, Elrod JW, Gundewar S, Ji SY, Lefer DJ. Dietary nitrite supplementation protects against myocardial ischemia-reperfusion injury. Proc Natl Acad Sci U S A. 2007;104:19144–9.
34. Govoni M, Jansson EA, Weitzberg E, Lundberg JO. The increase in plasma nitrite after a dietary nitrate load is markedly attenuated by an antibacterial mouthwash. Nitric Oxide. 2008;19:333–7.
35. Webb AJ, Patel N, Loukogeorgakis S, et al. Acute blood pressure lowering, vasoprotective, and anti-platelet properties of dietary nitrate via bioconversion to nitrite. Hypertension. 2008;51:784–90.
36. Jansson EA, Huang L, Malkey R, et al. A mammalian functional nitrate reductase that regulates nitrite and nitric oxide homeostasis. Nat Chem Biol. 2008;4:411–7.
37. Larsen FJ, Ekblom B, Sahlin K, Lundberg JO, Weitzberg E. Effects of dietary nitrate on blood pressure in healthy volunteers. N Engl J Med. 2006;355:2792–3.
38. Kapil V, Milsom AB, Okorie M, et al. Inorganic nitrate supplementation lowers blood pressure in humans: role for nitrite-derived NO. Hypertension. 2010;56:274–81.
39. Carlstrom M, Larsen FJ, Nystrom T, et al. Dietary inorganic nitrate reverses features of metabolic syndrome in endothelial nitric oxide synthase-deficient mice. Proc Natl Acad Sci U S A. 2010;107:17716–20.
40. Lundberg JO, Weitzberg E, Gladwin MT. The nitrate-nitrite-nitric oxide pathway in physiology and therapeutics. Nat Rev Drug Discov. 2008;7:156–67.
41. Dejam A, Hunter CJ, Schechter AN, Gladwin MT. Emerging role of nitrite in human biology. Blood Cells Mol Dis. 2004;32:423–9.
42. Lundberg JO, Weitzberg E. NO generation from nitrite and its role in vascular control. Arterioscler Thromb Vasc Biol. 2005;25:915–22.
43. Benjamin N, O'Driscoll F, Dougall H, Duncan C, Smith L, Golden M, McKenzie H. Stomach NO synthesis. Nature. 1994;368:502.
44. Lundberg JO, Govoni M. Inorganic nitrate is a possible source forsystemic generation of nitric oxide. Free Radic Biol Med. 2004;37:395–400.
45. Moncada S. Nitric oxide: discovery and impact on clinical medicine. J R Soc Med. 1999;92:164–9.
46. Villanueva C, Giulivi C. Subcellular and cellular locations of nitric oxide synthase isoforms as determinants of health and disease. Free Radic Biol Med. 2010;49:307–16.
47. Chatterjee A, Black SM, Catravas JD. Endothelial nitric oxide (NO) and its pathophysiologic regulation. Vasc Pharmacol. 2008;49:134–40.
48. Kapil V, Webb AJ, Ahluwalia A. Inorganic nitrate and the cardiovascular system. Heart. 2010;96:1703–9.
49. Bryan NS. Cardioprotective actions of nitrite therapy and dietary considerations. Front Biosci. 2009;14:4793–808.
50. Moncada S, Palmer RMJ, Higgs EA. Nitric oxide: physiology, pathophysiology, and pharmacology. Pharmacol Rev. 1991;43:109–42.
51. Radomski MW, Moncada S. Regulation of vascular homeostasis by nitric oxide. Thromb Haemost. 1993;70:36–41.
52. Naseem KM. The role of nitric oxide in cardiovascular diseases. Mol Asp Med. 2005;26:33–65.
53. Llorens S, Jordán J, Nava E. The nitric oxide pathway in the cardiovascular system. J Physiol Biochem. 2002;58:179–88.
54. Cai H, Harrison DG. Endothelial dysfunction in cardiovascular diseases: the role of oxidant stress. Circ Res. 2000;87:840–4.
55. Hadi HAR, Carr CS, Endothelial Dysfunction SJA. Cardiovascular risk factors, therapy, and outcome. Vasc Health Risk Manag. 2005;1:183–98.
56. Hirata Y, Nagata D, Suzuki E, Nishimatsu H, Suzuki J, Nagai R. Diagnosis and treatment of endothelial dysfunction in cardiovascular disease. Int Heart J. 2010;51:1–6.
57. Rouse IL, Beilin LJ, Armstrong BK, Vandoingen R. Blood pressure-lowering effects of a vegetarian diet: controlled trial in normotensive subjects. Lancet. 1983;1:5–10.

58. Appel LJ, Moore TJ, Obarzanek E, Vollmer WM, Svetkey LP, Sacks FM, Bray GA, Vogt TM, Cutler JA, Windhauser MM, Lin PH, Karanja N. A clinical trial of the effects of dietary patterns on blood pressure. DASH Collaborative Research Group. N Engl J Med. 1997;336:1117–24.
59. Appel LJ, Brands MW, Daniels SR, Karanja N, Elmer PJ, Sacks FM. Dietary approaches to prevent and treat hypertension: a scientific statement from the American Heart Association. Hypertension. 2006;47:296–308.
60. Fahey JW, Zalcmann AT, Talalay P. The chemical diversity and distribution of glucosinolates and isothiocyanates among plants. Phytochemistry. 2001;56:5–51.
61. Mithen RF, Dekker M, Verkerk R, Rabot S, Johnson IT. The nutritional significance, biosynthesis and bioavailability of glucosinolates in human foods. J Sci Food Agric. 2000;80:967–84.
62. Talalay P, Fahey JW. Phytochemicals from cruciferous plants protect against cancer by modulating carcinogen metabolism. J Nutr. 2001;131(Suppl. 11):3027S–33S.
63. Traka M, Mithen RF. Glucosinolates, isothiocyanates and human health. Phytochem Rev. 2009;8:269–82.
64. Manchali S, Murthy KNC, Patil BS. Crucial facts about health benefits of popular cruciferous vegetables. J Funct Foods. 2012;4:94–106.
65. Graham S, Dayal H, Swanson M, Mittelman A, Wilkinson G. Diet in the epidemiology of cancer of the colon and rectum. J Natl Cancer Inst. 1978;61:709–14.
66. Gupta P, Kim B, Kim SH, Srivastava SK. Molecular targets of isothiocyanates in cancer: recent advances. Mol Nutr Food Res. 2014;58:1685–707.
67. Kirsh VA, Peters U, Mayne ST, Subar AF, Chatterjee N, Johnson CC, Hayes RB. Prostate, lung, colorectal and ovarian cancer screening trial. Prospective study of fruit and vegetable intake and risk of prostate cancer. J Natl Cancer Inst. 2007;99:1200–9.
68. Juge N, Mithen RF, Traka M. Molecular basis for chemoprevention by sulforaphane: a comprehensive review. Cell Mol Life Sci. 2007;64:1105–27.
69. Fuentes F, Paredes-Gonzalez X, Kong AT. Dietary glucosinolates sulforaphane, phenethyl isothiocyanate, indole-3-carbinol/3,31-diindolylmethane: anti-oxidative stress/inflammation, Nrf2, epigenetics/epigenomics and *in vivo* cancer chemopreventive efficacy. Curr Pharmacol Rep. 2015;1:179–96.
70. Dworkin AM, Huang TH, Toland AE. Epigenetic alterations in the breast: implications for breast cancer detection, prognosis and treatment. Semin Cancer Biol. 2009;19:165–71.
71. Basse C, Arock M. The increasing roles of epigenetics in breast cancer: implications for pathogenicity, biomarkers, prevention and treatment. Int J Cancer. 2015;137:2785–94.
72. Berger SL, Kouzarides T, Shiekhattar R, Shilatifard A. An operational definition of epigenetics. Genes Dev. 2009;23:781–3.
73. Sharma S, Kelly TK, Jones PA. Epigenetics in cancer. Carcinogenesis. 2010;31:27–36.
74. Nowsheen S, Aziz K, Tran PT, Gorgoulis VG, Yang ES, Georgakilas AG. Epigenetic inactivation of DNA repair in breast cancer. Cancer Lett. 2014;342:213–22.
75. Ferguson LR, Chen H, Collins AR, Connell M, Damia G, Dasgupta S, Malhotra M, Meeker AK, Amedei A, Amin A, et al. Genomic instability in human cancer: molecular insights and opportunities for therapeutic attack and prevention through diet and nutrition. Semin Cancer Biol. 2015;35:S5–S24.
76. Wong CP, Hsu A, Buchanan A, Palomera-Sanchez Z, Beaver LM, Houseman EA, Williams DE, Dashwood RH, Ho E. Effects of sulforaphane and 3,31-diindolylmethane on genome-wide promoter methylation in normal prostate epithelial cells and prostate cancer cells. PLoS One. 2014;9:e86787.
77. Denis H, Ndlovu MN, Fuks F. Regulation of mammalian DNA methyltransferases: a route to new mechanisms. EMBO Rep. 2011;12:647–56.
78. Morey Kinney SR, Smiraglia DJ, James SR, Moser MT, Foster BA, Karpf AR. Stage-specific alterations of DNA methyltransferase expression, DNA hypermethylation, and DNA hypomethylation during prostate cancer progression in the transgenic adenocarcinoma of mouse prostate model. Mol Cancer Res. 2008;6:1365–74.

79. Lin RK, Wu CY, Chang JW, Juan LJ, Hsu HS, Chen CY, Lu YY, Tang YA, Yang YC, Yang PC, et al. Dysregulation of p53/Sp1 control leads to DNA methyltransferase-1 overexpression in lung cancer. Cancer Res. 2010;70:5807–17.
80. Mizuno S, Chijiwa T, Okamura T, Akashi K, Fukumaki Y, Niho Y, Sasaki H. Expression of DNA methyltransferases DNMT1, 3A, and 3B in normal hematopoiesis and in acute and chronic myelogenous leukemia. Blood. 2001;97:1172–9.
81. He S, Wang F, Yang L, Guo C, Wan R, Ke A, Xu L, Hu G, Xu X, Shen J, et al. Expression of DNMT1 and DNMT3a are regulated by GLI1 in human pancreatic cancer. PLoS One. 2011;6:e27684.
82. Etoh T, Kanai Y, Ushijima S, Nakagawa T, Nakanishi Y, Sasako M, Kitano S, Hirohashi S. Increased DNA methyltransferase 1 (DNMT1) protein expression correlates significantly with poorer tumor differentiation and frequent DNA hypermethylation of multiple CpG islands in gastric cancers. Am J Pathol. 2004;164:689–99.
83. Sproul D, Gilbert N, Bickmore WA. The role of chromatin structure in regulating the expression of clustered genes. Nat Rev Genet. 2005;6:775–81.
84. Kouzarides T. Chromatin modifications and their function. Cell. 2007;128:693–705.
85. Cedar H, Bergman Y. Linking DNA methylation and histone modification: patterns and paradigms. Nat Rev Genet. 2009;10:295–304.
86. Turner BM. Histone acetylation and an epigenetic code. BioEssays. 2000;22:836–45.
87. Royston KJ, Tollefsbol TO. The epigenetic impact of cruciferous vegetables on cancer prevention. Curr Pharmacol Rep. 2015;1:46–51.
88. Meeran SM, Patel SN, Li Y, Shukla S, Tollefsbol TO. Bioactive dietary supplements reactivate ER expression in ER-negative breast cancer cells by active chromatin modifications. PLoS One. 2012;7:e37748.
89. Gerhauser C. Epigenetic impact of dietary isothiocyanates in cancer chemoprevention. Curr Opin Clin Nutr Metab Care. 2013;16:405–10.
90. Singh SV, Singh K. Cancer chemoprevention with dietary isothiocyanates mature for clinical translational research. Carcinogenesis. 2012;33:1833–42.
91. Forster T, Rausch V, Zhang Y, Isayev O, Heilmann K, Schoensiegel F, Liu L, Nessling M, Richter K, Labsch S, et al. Sulforaphane counteracts aggressiveness of pancreatic cancer driven by dysregulated Cx43-mediated gap junctional intercellular communication. Oncotarget. 2014;5:1621–34.
92. Rajendran P, Kidane AI, Yu TW, Dashwood WM, Bisson WH, Löhr CV, Ho E, Williams DE, Dashwood RH. HDAC turnover, CtIP acetylation and dysregulated DNA damage signaling in colon cancer cells treated with sulforaphane and related dietary isothiocyanates. Epigenetics. 2013;8:612–23.
93. Balasubramanian S, Chew YC, Eckert RL. Sulforaphane suppresses polycomb group protein level via a proteasome-dependent mechanism in skin cancer cells. Mol Pharmacol. 2011;80:870–8.
94. Chew YC, Adhikary G, Wilson GM, Xu W, Eckert RL. Sulforaphane induction of p21(Cip1) cyclin-dependent kinase inhibitor expression requires p53 and Sp1 transcription factors and is p53-dependent. J Biol Chem. 2012;287:16168–78.
95. Su ZY, Zhang C, Lee JH, Shu L, Wu TY, Khor TO, Conney AH, Lu YP, Kong AN. Requirement and epigenetics reprogramming of Nrf2 in suppression of tumor promoter TPA-induced mouse skin cell transformation by sulforaphane. Cancer Prev Res. 2014;7:319–29.
96. Wang LG, Chiao JW. Prostate cancer chemopreventive activity of phenethyl isothiocyanate through epigenetic regulation (review). Int J Oncol. 2010;37:533–9.
97. Traka MH, Melchini A, Mithen RF. Sulforaphane and prostate cancer interception. Drug Discov Today. 2014;19:1488–92.
98. Hsu A, Wong CP, Yu Z, Williams DE, Dashwood RH, Ho E. Promoter de-methylation of cyclin D2 by sulforaphane in prostate cancer cells. Clin Epigenetics. 2011;3:3.
99. Meeran SM, Patel SN, Tollefsbol TO. Sulforaphane causes epigenetic repression of hTERT expression in human breast cancer cell lines. PLoS One. 2010;5:e11457.

100. Myzak MC, Hardin K, Wang R, Dashwood RH, Ho E. Sulforaphane inhibits histone deacetylase activity in BPH-1, LnCaP and PC-3 prostate epithelial cells. Carcinogenesis. 2006;27:811–9.
101. Gibbs A, Schwartzman J, Deng V, Alumkal J. Sulforaphane destabilizes the androgen receptor in prostate cancer cells by inactivating histone deacetylase 6. Proc Natl Acad Sci U S A. 2009;106:16663–8.
102. Verhoeven DT, Goldbohm RA, van Poppel G, Verhagen H, van den Brandt PA. Epidemiological studies on brassica vegetables and cancer risk. Cancer Epidemiol Biomark Prev. 1996;5:733–48.
103. Willett W. Nutritional epidemiology. 2nd ed. New York: Oxford University Press; 1998.
104. Voorrips LE, Goldbohm RA, Verhoeven DT, et al. Vegetable and fruit consumption and lung cancer risk in the Netherlands cohort study on diet and cancer. Cancer Causes Control. 2000;11:101–15.
105. Feskanich D, Ziegler RG, Michaud DS, et al. Prospective study of fruit and vegetable consumption and risk of lung cancer among men and women. J Natl Cancer Inst. 2000;92:1812–23.
106. Neuhouser ML, Patterson RE, Thornquist MD, Omenn GS, King IB, Goodman GE. Fruits and vegetables are associated with lower lung cancer risk only in the placebo arm of the beta-carotene and retinol efficacy trial (CARET). Cancer Epidemiol Biomark Prev. 2003;12:350–8.
107. Miller AB, Altenburg HP, Bueno-de-Mesquita B, et al. Fruits and vegetables and lung cancer: findings from the European prospective investigation into cancer and nutrition. Int J Cancer. 2004;108:269–76.
108. Benito E, Obrador A, Stiggelbout A, et al. A population-based case-control study of colorectal cancer in Majorca. I. Dietary factors. Int J Cancer. 1990;45:69–76.
109. West DW, Slattery ML, Robison LM, et al. Dietary intake and colon cancer: sex- and anatomic site-specific associations. Am J Epidemiol. 1989;130:883–94.
110. Young TB, Wolf DA. Case-control study of proximal and distal colon cancer and diet in Wisconsin. Int J Cancer. 1988;42:167–75.
111. Kojima M, Wakai K, Tamakoshi K, et al. Diet and colorectal cancer mortality: results from the Japan Collaborative Cohort Study. Nutr Cancer. 2004;50(1):23–32.
112. McCullough ML, Robertson AS, Chao A, et al. A prospective study of whole grains, fruits, vegetables and colon cancer risk. Cancer Causes Control. 2003;14:959–70.
113. Michels KB, Edward G, Joshipura KJ, et al. Prospective study of fruit and vegetable consumption and incidence of colon and rectal cancers. J Natl Cancer Inst. 2000;92:1740–52.
114. Steinmetz KA, Kushi LH, Bostick RM, Folsom AR, Potter JD. Vegetables, fruit, and colon cancer in the Iowa Women's Health Study. Am J Epidemiol. 1994;139:1–15.
115. Hsing AW, McLaughlin JK, Chow WH, et al. Risk factors for colorectal cancer in a prospective study among US white men. Int J Cancer. 1998;77:549–53.
116. Pietinen P, Malila N, Virtanen M, et al. Diet and risk of colorectal cancer in a cohort of Finnish men. Cancer Causes Control. 1999;10:387–96.
117. Voorrips LE, Goldbohm RA, van Poppel G, Sturmans F, Hermus RJ, van den Brandt PA. Vegetable and fruit consumption and risks of colon and rectal cancer in a prospective cohort study: The Netherlands cohort study on diet and cancer. Am J Epidemiol. 2000;152:1081–92.
118. van Gils CH, Peeters PH, Bueno-de-Mesquita HB, et al. Consumption of vegetables and fruits and risk of breast cancer. JAMA. 2005;293:183–93.
119. Giovannucci E, Rimm EB, Liu Y, Stampfer MJ, Willett WC. A prospective study of cruciferous vegetables and prostate cancer. Cancer Epidemiol Biomark Prev. 2003;12(12):1403–9.
120. Kristal AR, Stanford JL. Cruciferous vegetables and prostate cancer risk: confounding by PSA screening. Cancer Epidemiol Biomark Prev. 2004;13:1265.
121. Coles BF, Kadlubar FF. Detoxification of electrophilic compounds by glutathione S-transferase catalysis: determinants of individual response to chemical carcinogens and chemotherapeutic drugs? Biofactors. 2003;17:115–30.
122. Seow A, Shi CY, Chung FL, et al. Urinary total isothiocyanate (ITC) in a population-based sample of middle-aged and older Chinese in Singapore: relationship with dietary total ITC and glutathione S-transferase M1/T1/P1 genotypes. Cancer Epidemiol Biomark Prev. 1998;7:775–81.

123. Lewis S, Brennan P, Nyberg F, et al. Re: Spitz, M. R., Duphorne, C. M., Detry, M. A., Pillow, P. C., Amos, C. I., Lei, L., de Andrade, M., Gu, X., Hong, W. K., and Wu, X. Dietary intake of isothiocyanates: evidence of a joint effect with glutathione S-transferase polymorphisms in lung cancer risk. Cancer Epidemiol Biomark Prev. 2000;9:1017–20.
124. London SJ, Yuan JM, Chung FL, et al. Isothiocyanates, glutathione S-transferase M1 and T1 polymorphisms, and lung-cancer risk: a prospective study of men in Shanghai, China. Lancet. 2000;356:724–9.
125. Zhao B, Seow A, Lee EJ, et al. Dietary isothiocyanates, glutathione S-transferase -M1, -T1 polymorphisms and lung cancer risk among Chinese women in Singapore. Cancer Epidemiol Biomark Prev. 2001;10:1063–7.
126. Turner F, Smith G, Sachse C, et al. Vegetable, fruit and meat consumption and potential risk modifying genes in relation to colorectal cancer. Int J Cancer. 2004;112:259–64.
127. Seow A, Yuan JM, Sun CL, Van Den Berg D, Lee HP, Yu MC. Dietary isothiocyanates, glutathione S-transferase polymorphisms and colorectal cancer risk in the Singapore Chinese Health Study. Carcinogenesis. 2002;23:2055–61.
128. Slattery ML, Kampman E, Samowitz W, Caan BJ, Potter JD. Interplay between dietary inducers of GST and the GSTM-1 genotype in colon cancer. Int J Cancer. 2000;87:728–33.
129. Baena Ruiz R, Salinas Hernández P. Cancer chemoprevention by dietary phytochemicals: Epidemiological evidence. Maturitas. 2016;94:13–9.
130. Eliassen AH, Hendrickson SJ, Brinton LA, Buring BJ, Campos H, et al. Circulating carotenoids and rosk of breast cancer: pooled analysis of eight prospective studies. J Natl Cancer Inst. 2012;104:1905–16.
131. Giovannucci E, Ascherio A, Rimm EB, Stampfer MJ, Colditz GA, Willett WC. Intake of carotenoids and retinol in relation to risk of prostate cancer. J Natl Cancer Inst. 1995;87:1767–76.
132. Tzonou A, Signorello LB, Lagiou P, Wuu J, Trichopoulos D, Trichopoulou A. Diet and cancer of the prostate: a case-control study in Greece. Int J Cancer. 1999;80:149–55.
133. Mills PK, Beeson WL, Phillips RL, Fraser GE. Cohort study of diet, lifestyle and prostate cancer in Adventist men. Cancer. 1989;64:598–604.
134. Norrish AE, Jackson RT, Sharpe SJ, Murray Skeaff C. Prostate cancer and dietary carotenoids. Am J Epidemiol. 2000;151:119–23.
135. Key T, et al. A case – control study of diet and prostate cancer. Br J Cancer. 1997;76:678–87.
136. Schuman L, Mandel J, Radke A. Some selected features of the epidemiology of prostate cancer: Minneapolis-St Paul, Minnesota case–control study, 1976–1979. In: Magnus K, editor. Trends in cancer incidence: causes and implications. Washington, DC: Hemisphere Publishing Corporation; 1982. p. 345–54.
137. Schuurman AG, Goldbohm RA, Dorant E, van den Brandt PA. Vegetable and fruit consumption and prostate cancer risk: a cohort study in the Netherlands. Cancer Epidemiol Biomark Prev. 1998;7:673–80.
138. Kucuk O, Sarkar FH, Sakr W, Djuric Z, Pollak MN, Khachik F, Li YW, Banerjee M, Grignon D, Bertram JS, Crissman JD, Pontes EJ, Wood DP Jr. Phase II randomized clinical trial of lycopene supplementation before radical prostatectomy. Cancer Epidemiol Biomark Prev. 2001;10:861–8.
139. DGE (Deutsche Gesellschaft für Ernahrung e. V.; ed.). Obst und Gemüse in der Pravention chronischer Krankheiten. Bonn: Angela Bechthold; 2007.
140. von Ruesten A, Steffen A, Floegel A, et al. Trend in obesity in European adult cohort populations during follow-up since 1996 and their predictions to 2015. PLoS One. 2011;6:e27455.
141. Helmert U, Strube H. Trends in the development and prevalence of obesity in Germany between 1985 and 2002. Gesundheitswesen. 2004;66:409–15.
142. Hall JN, Moore S, Harper SB, Lynch JW. Global variability in fruit and vegetable consumption. Am J Prev Med. 2009;36:402–9.
143. Ledikwe JH, Blanck HM, Kettel Khan L, et al. Dietary energy density is associated with energy intake and weight status in US adults. Am J Clin Nutr. 2006;84:1362–8.
144. Rolls BJ, Ello-Martin JA, Tohill BC. What can intervention studies tell us about the relationship between fruit and vegetable consumption and weight management? Nutr Rev. 2004;62:1–17.

145. Boeing H, Bechthold A, Bub A, Ellinger S, Haller D, Kroke A, Leschik-Bonnet E, Müller MJ, Oberritter H, Schulze M, Stehle P, Watzl B. Critical review: vegetables and fruit in the prevention of chronic diseases. Eur J Nutr. 2012;51:637–63.
146. Thefeld W, Prävalenz d. diabetes mellitus in der erwachsenen Bevölkerung Deutschlands. Gesundheitswesen. 1999;61:S85–9.
147. Schulze MB, Hu FB. Primary prevention of diabetes: what can be done and how much can be prevented? Annu Rev Public Health. 2005;26:445–67.
148. Hamer M, Chida Y. Intake of fruit, vegetables, and antioxidants and risk of type 2 diabetes: systematic review and meta-analysis. J Hypertens. 2007;25:2361–9.
149. Carter P, Gray LJ, Troughton J, et al. Fruit and vegetable intake and incidence of type 2 diabetes mellitus: systematic review and meta-analysis. Br Med J. 2010;341:c4229.
150. Harding AH, Wareham NJ, Bingham SA, et al. Plasma vitamin C level, fruit and vegetable consumption, and the risk of new-onset type 2 diabetes mellitus: the European prospective investigation of cancer—Norfolk prospective study. Arch Intern Med. 2008;168:1493–9.
151. Lewington S, Clarke R, Qizilbash N, et al. Age-specific relevance of usual blood pressure to vascular mortality: a metaanalysis of individual data for one million adults in 61 prospective studies. Lancet. 2002;360:1903–13.
152. Weikert S, Boeing H, Pischon T, et al. Blood pressure and risk of renal cell carcinoma in the European prospective investigation into cancer and nutrition. Am J Epidemiol. 2008;167:438–46.
153. Cook NR, Cohen J, Heber PR, et al. Implications of small reductions in diastolic blood pressure for primary prevention. Arch Intern Med. 1995;155:701–9.
154. Staessen JA, Li Y, Thijs L, Wang JG. Blood pressure reduction and cardiovascular prevention: an update including the 2003–2004 secondary prevention trials. Hypertens Res. 2005;28:385–407.
155. Chobanian AV, Bakris GL, Black HR, et al. The seventh report of the joint national committee on prevention, detection, evaluation, and treatment of high blood pressure: the JNC 7 report. JAMA. 2003;289:2560–72.
156. Mancia G, De Backer G, Dominiczak A, et al. 2007 ESH–ESC practice guidelines for the management of arterial hypertension: ESH–ESC task force on the management of arterial hypertension. J Hypertens. 2007;25:1751–62.
157. Berkow SE, Barnard ND. Blood pressure regulation and vegetarian diets. Nutr Rev. 2005;63:1–8.
158. Ascherio A, Hennekens C, Willett WC, et al. Prospective study of nutritional factors, blood pressure, and hypertension among US women. Hypertension. 1996;27:1065–72.
159. Miura K, Greenland P, Stamler J, et al. Relation of vegetable, fruit, and meat intake to 7-year blood pressure change in middle-aged men: the Chicago Western Electric Study. Am J Epidemiol. 2004;159:572–80.
160. Steffen LM, Kroenke CH, Yu X, et al. Associations of plant food, dairy product, and meat intakes with 15-y incidence of elevated blood pressure in young black and white adults: the Coronary Artery Risk Development in Young Adults (CARDIA) Study. Am J Clin Nutr. 2005;82:1169–77.
161. Schulze MB, Hoffmann K, Kroke A, Boeing H. Risk of hypertension among women in the EPIC-Potsdam Study: comparison of relative risk estimates for exploratory and hypothesis-oriented dietary patterns. Am J Epidemiol. 2003;158:365–73.
162. Dauchet L, Kesse-Guyot E, Czernichow S, et al. Dietary patterns and blood pressure change over 5-y follow-up in the SU.VI.MAX cohort. Am J Clin Nutr. 2007;85:1650–6.
163. Cassidy A, O'Reilly EJ, Kay C, et al. Habitual intake of flavonoid subclasses and incident hypertension in adults. Am J Clin Nutr. 2011;93:338–47.
164. John JH, Ziebland S, Yudkin P, et al. Effects of fruit and vegetable consumption on plasma antioxidant concentrations and blood pressure: a randomised controlled trial. Lancet. 2002;359:1969–74.
165. WHO (World Health Organization). The global burden of disease: 2004 update. Geneva: WHO; 2008.

166. Graham I, Atar D, Borch-Johnsen K, et al. European guidelines on cardiovascular disease prevention in clinical practice: executive summary. Fourth joint task force of the European society of cardiology and other societies on cardiovascular disease prevention in clinical practice (constituted by representatives of nine societies and by invited experts). Eur J Cardiovasc Prev Rehabil. 2007;14(Suppl 2):E1–E40.
167. Dauchet L, Amouyel P, Hercberg S, Dallongeville J. Fruit and vegetable consumption and risk of coronary heart disease: a meta-analysis of cohort studies. J Nutr. 2006;136:2588–93.
168. He FJ, Nowson CA, Lucas M, Macgregor GA. Increased consumption of fruit and vegetables is related to a reduced risk of coronary heart disease: meta-analysis of cohort studies. J Hum Hypertens. 2007;21:717–28.
169. Crowe FL, Roddam AW, Key TJ, et al. European prospective investigation into cancer and nutrition (EPIC)-heart study collaborators. Fruit and vegetable intake and mortality from ischaemic heart disease: results from the European Prospective Investigation into Cancer and Nutrition (EPIC)-Heart Study. Eur Heart J. 2011;32:1235–43.
170. Oude Griep LM, Geleijnse JM, Kromhout D, et al. Raw and processed fruit and vegetable consumption and 10-year coronary heart disease incidence in a population-based cohort study in The Netherlands. PLoS One. 2010;5:e13609.
171. Bendinelli B, Masala G, Saieva C, et al. Fruit, vegetables, and olive oil and risk of coronary heart disease in Italian women: the EPICOR Study. Am J Clin Nutr. 2011;93:275–83.
172. Bazzano LA. Dietary intake of fruits and vegetables and risk of diabetes mellitus and cardiovascular disease. Geneva: World Health Organization; 2005.
173. American Heart Association Primary prevention of cardiovascular disease in adults, 2011. www.americanheart.org/presenter.jhtml?identifier=4704. Accessed 9 Mar 2011.
174. McCall DO, McGartland CP, McKinley MC, et al. Dietary intake of fruits and vegetables improves microvascular function in hypertensive subjects in a dose-dependent manner. Circulation. 2009;119:2153–60.
175. Hubbard GP, Wolffram S, de Vos R, et al. Ingestion of onion soup high in quercetin inhibits platelet aggregation and essential components of the collagen-stimulated platelet activation pathway in man: a pilot study. Br J Nutr. 2006;96:482–8.
176. O'Kennedy N, Crosbie L, Whelan S, et al. Effects of tomato extract on platelet function: a double-blinded crossover study in healthy humans. Am J Clin Nutr. 2006;84:561–9.
177. Erlund I, Koli R, Alfthan G, et al. Favourable effects of berry consumption on platelet function, blood pressure, and HDL cholesterol. Am J Clin Nutr. 2007;87:323–31.
178. Watzl B, Kulling SE, Möseneder J, et al. A 4-week intervention with high intake of carotenoid-rich vegetables and fruit reduces plasma C-reactive protein in healthy, non-smoking men. Am J Clin Nutr. 2005;82:1052–8.
179. Kelley DS, Rasooly R, Jacob RA, et al. Consumption of Bing sweet cherries lowers circulating concentrations of inflammation markers in healthy men and women. J Nutr. 2006;136:981–6.
180. Goldstein LB, Bushnell CD, Adams RJ, et al. Guidelines for the primary prevention of stroke: a guideline for healthcare professionals from the American Heart Association/American Stroke Association. Stroke. 2011;42:517–84.
181. Dauchet L, Amouyel P, Dallongeville J. Fruit and vegetable consumption and risk of stroke: a metaanalysis of cohort studies. Neurology. 2005;65:1193–7.
182. He FJ, Nowson CA, MacGregor GA. Fruit and vegetable consumption and stroke: meta-analysis of cohort studies. Lancet. 2006;367:320–6.
183. WHO (World Health Organization). Diet, nutrition and the prevention of chronic diseases. WHO Tech Rep Ser. 2003;916:55.
184. WCRF (World Cancer Research Fund). Food, nutrition, and the prevention of cancer: a global perspective. Washington, DC: World Cancer Research Fund/American Institute for Cancer Research; 1997.
185. IARC. Fruit and vegetables. IARC handbook of cancer prevention, vol. 8. Lyon: IARC Press; 2003.
186. Riboli E, Hunt KJ, Slimani N, et al. European Prospective Investigation into Cancer and Nutrition (EPIC): study populations and data collection. Public Health Nutr. 2002;5:1113–24.

187. Schatzkin A, Subar AF, Thompson FE, et al. Design and serendipity in establishing a large cohort with wide dietary intake distributions: the National Institutes of Health-American association of retired persons diet and health study. Am J Epidemiol. 2001;154:1119–25.
188. Key TJ. Fruit and vegetables and cancer risk. Br J Cancer. 2011;104:6–11.
189. Boffetta P, Couto E, Wichmann J, et al. Fruit and vegetable intake and overall cancer risk in the European Prospective Investigation into Cancer and Nutrition (EPIC). J Natl Cancer Inst. 2010;102:529–37.
190. Resnikoff S, Pascolini D, Etya'ale D, et al. Global data on visual impairment in the year 2002. Bull World Health Organ. 2004;82:844–51.
191. Sasaki K, Sasaki H, Jonasson F, et al. Racial differences of lens transparency properties with aging and prevalence of age-related cataract applying a WHO classification system. Ophthlamic Res. 2004;36:332–40.
192. Kaushik S, Wang JJ, Flood V, et al. Dietary glycemic index and the risk of age-related macular degeneration. Am J Clin Nutr. 2008;88:1104–10.
193. Parekh N, Voland RP, Moeller SM, et al. Association between dietary fat intake and age-related macular degeneration in the Carotenoids in Age-Related Eye Disease Study (CAREDS): an ancillary study of the women's health initiative. Arch Ophthalmol. 2009;127:1483–93.
194. Evans JR. Antioxidant vitamin and mineral supplements for slowing the progression of age-related macular degeneration. Cochrane Database Syst Rev. 2006;2:CD000254.
195. Evans JR, Heanshaw KS. Antioxidant vitamin and mineral supplements to prevent the development of age-related macular degeneration. Cochrane Database Syst Rev. 2008;1:CD000253.
196. Johnson EJ. Age-related macular degeneration and antioxidant vitamins: recent findings. Cur Opin Clin Nutr Metabol Care. 2010;13:28–33.
197. Krinsky NI, Landrum JT, Bone RA. Biologic mechanisms of the protective role of lutein and zeaxanthin in the eye. Annu Rev Nutr. 2003;23:171–201.
198. Beatty S, Boulton M, Henson D, et al. Macular pigment and age related macular degeneration. Brit J Ophthalmol. 1999;83:867–77.
199. Landrum JT, Bone RA. Lutein, zeaxanthin, and the macular pigment. Arch Biochem Biophys. 2001;385:28–40.
200. Mares-Perlman JA, Fisher AI, Klein R, et al. Lutein and zeaxanthin in the diet and serum and their relation to age-related maculopathy in the third national health and nutrition examination survey. Am J Epidemiol. 2001;153:424–32.
201. Gale CR, Hall NF, Phillips DIW, Martyn CH. Lutein and zeaxanthin status and risk of age-related macular degeneration. Invest Ophthalmol Vis Sci. 2003;44:2461–5.
202. Beatty S, Nolan J, Kavanagh H, O'Donovan O. Macular pigment optical density and its relationship with serum and dietary levels of lutein and zeaxanthin. Arch Biochem Biophys. 2004;430:70–6.
203. Van Leeuwen R, Boekhoorn S, Vingerling JR, et al. Dietary intake of antioxidants and risk of age-related macular degeneration. JAMA. 2005;294:3101–7.
204. Moeller SM, Parekh N, Tinker L, et al. Associations between intermediate age-related macular degeneration and lutein and zeaxanthin in the Carotenoids in Age-Related Eye Disease Study (CAREDS). Arch Ophthalmol. 2006;124:1151–62.
205. Seddon JM, Ajani UA, Sperduto RD, et al. Dietary carotenoids, vitamins A, C, and E, and advanced age-related macular degeneration. Eye disease case-control study group. JAMA. 1994;272:1413–20.
206. Goldberg J, Flowerdew G, Smith E, et al. Factors associated with age-related macular-degeneration. Am J Epidemiol. 1988;128:700–10.
207. Asbell PA, Dualan L, Mindel J, et al. Age-related cataract. Lancet. 2005;365:599–609.
208. Tan JSL, Mitchell P, Flood V, et al. Antioxidant nutrient intake and the long-term incidence of age-related cataract—the Blue Mountains Eye Study. Am J Clin Nutr. 2008;87:1899–905.
209. Moeller SM, Taylor A, Tucker KL, ML MC, Chylack LT Jr, Hankinson SE, Willett WC, Jacques PF. Overall adherence to the dietary guidelines for Americans is associated with reduced prevalence of early age-related nuclear lens opacities in women. J Nutr. 2004;134:1812–9.

210. Brown L, Rimm EB, Seddon JM, et al. A prospective study of carotenoid intake and risk of cataract extraction in US men. Am J Clin Nutr. 1999;70:517–24.
211. Christen WG, Liu SM, Schaumberg DA, Buring JE. Fruit and vegetable intake and the risk of cataract in women. Am J Clin Nutr. 2005;81:1417–22.
212. Christen WG, Liu S, Glynn RJ, et al. Dietary carotenoids, vitamins C and E, and risk of cataract in women. Arch Ophthalmol. 2008;126:102–9.
213. Moeller SM, Voland R, Tinker L, et al. Associations between age-related nuclear cataract and lutein and zeaxanthin in the diet and serum in the Carotenoids in the Age-Related Eye Disease Study (CAREDS), an ancillary study of the women's health initiative. Arch Ophthalmol. 2008;126:354–64.
214. Delcourt C, Carrière I, Delage M, et al. Plasma lutein and zeaxanthin and other carotenoids as modifiable risk factors for age-related maculopathy and cataract: the POLA Study. Invest Ophthalmol Vis Sci. 2006;47:2329–35.
215. Coleman AL, Stone KL, Kodjebacheva G, et al. Glaucoma risk and the consumption of fruits and vegetables among older women in the study of osteoporotic fractures. Am J Ophthalmol. 2008;145:1081–9.
216. Qiu C, De Ronchi D, Fratiglioni L. The epidemiology of the dementias: an update. Curr Opin Psychiatry. 2007;20:380–5.
217. Morris MC, Evans DA, Tangney CC, et al. Associations of vegetable and fruit consumption with age-related cognitive change. Neurology. 2006;67:1370–6.
218. Kang JH, Ascherio A, Grodstein F. Fruit and vegetable consumption and cognitive decline in aging women. Ann Neurol. 2005;57:713–20.
219. Nooyens AC, Bueno-de-Mesquita HB, van Boxtel MP, et al. Fruit and vegetable intake and cognitive decline in middle-aged men and women: the Doetinchem cohort study. Br J Nutr. 2011;106:752–61.
220. Ortega RM, Requejo AM, Andres P, et al. Dietary intake and cognitive function in a group of elderly people. Am J Clin Nutr. 1997;66:803–9.
221. Lee L, Kang SA, Lee HO, et al. Relationships between dietary intake and cognitive function level in Korean elderly people. Public Health. 2001;115:133–8.
222. Dai Q, Borenstein AR, Wu Y, et al. Fruit and vegetable juices and Alzheimer's disease: the Kame project. Am J Med. 2006;119:751–9.
223. Barberger-Gateau P, Raffaitin C, Letenneur L, et al. Dietary patterns and risk of dementia: the three-city cohort study. Neurology. 2007;89:1921–39.
224. Hughes TF, Andel R, Small BJ, et al. Midlife fruit and vegetable consumption and risk of dementia in late life in Swedish twins. Am J Geriatr Psychiatry. 2010;18:413–20.
225. Dongowski G. Interactions between dietary fibre-rich preparations and glycoconjugated bile acids in vitro. Food Chem. 2007;104:390–7.
226. Story JA, Watterson JJ, Matheson HB, Furumoto EJ. Dietary fiber and bile acid metabolism. Adv Exp Med Biol. 1990;270:43–8.
227. Marlett JA. Sites and mechanisms for the hypocholesterolemic actions of soluble dietary fiber sources. Adv Exp Med Biol. 1997;427:109–21.
228. Mahesh S, Desai MS, Seekatz AM, Koroptkin NM, Kamada N, Hickey CA, Wolter M, et al. A dietary fiber-deprived gut microbiota degrades the colonic mucus barrier and enhances pathogen susceptibility. Cell. 2016;167:1339–53.

10 Fresh Fruit

10.1 Premises

Fresh fruit is a fixed component of Mediterranean diet, in that it is an integral part of lunch and dinner and substitutes the dessert.

Fruits are naturally low in fat, sodium, calories, and important sources of many essential nutrients, including potassium, dietary fiber, and folate (folic acid). None have cholesterol. The fruit fiber content is important for proper bowel function: it helps reduce constipation and diverticulosis. Moreover, fiber-containing foods, such as fruits, help provide a feeling of fullness with fewer calories. Whole or cut-up fruits are important sources of dietary fiber; fruit juices contain little or no fiber. Fruits contain also many antioxidants such as polyphenolic flavonoids and vitamin C. These compounds protect from oxidant stress, diseases, and cancers, and help the body develop capacity to fight against these ailments by boosting the immunity level. The high antioxidant values of fruit can be measured as "Oxygen Radical Absorbent Capacity" (ORAC).

According to US Department of Agriculture [1], it is highly advisable to eat a diet rich in fruit, for the following reasons:

- May reduce risk for stroke, other cardiovascular diseases, and type-2 diabetes.
- A fruit containing eating pattern is part of an overall healthy diet and may protect against certain cancers.
- Fruit helps maintain optimum health due to the health promoting phytochemicals it contains—many of which are still being identified.
- One to 2–1/2 cups of fruit are recommended each day, depending on how many calories you need.

In the Healthiest Way of Eating Plan, the consumption of 5–10 servings of fruits-plus-vegetables (combined) each day is encouraged. In particular, they recommend for a more generous amount of fruits and vegetables than the amount recommended by the Centers for Disease Control (CDC) at the U.S. Department of Health and

A. Capurso et al., *Benefits of the Mediterranean Diet in the Elderly Patient*, Practical Issues in Geriatrics, https://doi.org/10.1007/978-3-319-78084-9_10

Human Services (DHHS). The CDC recommends between 1.5–2.5 cups of fruit and 2.5–4.0 cups of vegetables per day, as well as a target goal of at least 5 fruit-plus-vegetable servings (combined) per day. The WHFoods recommend to take closer to 3 fruit servings per day (consisting of one cup's worth of fruit per serving, or 3 cups total per day) to provide with optimum health benefits.

With respect to berries (grapes are included among the berry fruits), it is recommended to include berries at least 3–4 times per week within fruit servings. In several sample meal plans, berries are included on a daily basis. It would definitely not be a mistake to include a serving of either grapes, raspberries, blueberries, strawberries, cranberries, or other berries in a daily meal plan! When including grapes among daily fruit servings, one should treat one cup as the equivalent of approximately 15–20 grapes.

Here, the most common fruit of the daily Mediterranean diet are briefly described.

10.2 Apples

10.2.1 History and Mythology

The original wild ancestor of *Malus pumila* was *Malus sieversii*, found growing wild in the mountains of Central Asia in southern Kazakhstan, Kyrgyzstan, Tajikistan, and Xinjiang, China. Cultivation of the species progressed over a long period of time and permitted secondary acquisition of genes from other species into the open-pollinated seeds. Significant exchange with *Malus sylvestris*, the crabapple resulted in current populations of apples being more related to crabapples than to the more morphologically similar progenitor *Malus sieversii*.

In 2010, an Italian-led consortium announced they had sequenced the complete genome of the apple in collaboration with horticultural geneticists at Washington State University, using the Golden delicious variety [2]. It had about 57,000 genes, the highest number of any plant genome studied to date and more genes than the human genome (about 30,000).

In the Greek mythology, the Greek goddess of discord, Eris, became disgruntled after she was excluded from the wedding of Peleus and Thetis. In retaliation, she tossed a golden apple inscribed Καλλίστη (*Kalliste*), ("For the most beautiful one") into the wedding party. Three goddesses claimed the apple: Hera, Athena, and Aphrodite. Paris of Troy was appointed to select the recipient. After being bribed by both Hera and Athena, Aphrodite tempted him with the most beautiful woman in the world, Helen of Sparta. He awarded the apple to Aphrodite, thus indirectly causing the Trojan War. The apple was thus considered, in ancient Greece, to be sacred to Aphrodite, and to throw an apple at someone is to symbolically declare one's love, and similarly, to catch it was to symbolically show one's acceptance of that love.

10.2.2 Nutrients and Phytochemicals

Apples are a rich source of various phytochemicals including flavonoids (e.g., catechins, flavanols, and quercetin) and other phenolic compounds (e.g., epicatechin and procyanidins) found in the skin, core, and pulp of the apple. *Ideain* (cyanidin 3-*O*-galactoside) is an anthocyanin, a type of pigment, which is found in some red apple varieties. Apple fruit contains also good quantities of *vitamin C* and *beta-carotene.* Vitamin C is a powerful natural antioxidant. Consumption of foods rich in vitamin C helps the body develop resistance against infectious agents and scavenge harmful, pro-inflammatory free radicals from the body. Further, apple fruit is a good source of B-complex vitamins such as riboflavin, thiamin, and pyridoxine (vitamin B-6). Together, these vitamins help as cofactors for enzymes in metabolism as well as in various synthetic functions inside the human body.

Apples carry also a small amount of minerals like potassium, phosphorus, and calcium. Potassium is an important component of cell and body fluids, which helps in controlling heart rate and blood pressure, thus counters the bad influences of sodium. Finally, apples are also a rich source of dietary soluble fibers; a medium-sized apple contains about 4.4 g of fiber, particularly in the skin.

Apple Fruit (*Malus domestica*), Raw, with Skin
Vitamins and mineral content per 100 g
ORAC value: 5900
Source: USDA National Nutrient Data base

Energy	218 KJ (52 kcal)
Carbohydrates	13.81 g
Sugars	10.39 g
Protein	0.26 g
Fat	0.17 g
Dietary fiber	2.4 g

Vitamin A equiv.	3 μg	(0% DV)
β-Carotene	27 μg	(0% DV)
Lutein zeaxanthin	29 μg	
Thiamine (B1)	0.017 mg	(1% DV)
Riboflavin (B2)	0.026 mg	(2% DV)
Niacin	0.091 mg	(1% DV)
Pantothenic acid	0.061 mg	(1% DV)
Folate	3 μg	(1% DV)
Vitamin C	4.6 mg	(6% DV)
Vitamin E	0.18 mg	(1% DV)
Vitamin K	2.2 μg	(2% DV)

Calcium	6 mg	(1% DV)
Iron	0.12 mg	(1% DV)
Magnesium	5 mg	(1% DV)
Manganese	0.035 mg	(2% DV)
Phosphorus	11 mg	(2% DV)
Potassium	107 mg	(2% DV)
Sodium	1 mg	(0% DV)
Zinc	0.04 mg	(0% DV)
Fluoride	3.3 μg	
Water	85.56 g	

DV = Daily Value
ORAC: Oxygen Radical Absorbance Capacity = antioxidant strength

10.2.3 The Health Benefits of Apples

Everyone has heard the old adage "*An apple a day keeps the doctor away.*" There are more than 7500 varieties of this delicious fruit, and it comes in a variety of colors, including red, yellow, and green. The nutrients are in the flesh and the skin, which is a rich source of anthocyanins and various tannins that give its color. Apple fruit contains good quantities of vitamin C and beta-carotene. It is hardly necessary to recall that the vitamin C is a powerful natural antioxidant. Apple fruit is also a good source of B-complex vitamins such as riboflavin, thiamin, and pyridoxine (vitamin B6). Together, these vitamins help as cofactors for enzymes in metabolism as well as in various synthetic functions inside the human body.

Apple fruit is also rich in dietary fiber. A small, raw, unpeeled apple weighing just over 5 ounces (about 140 g) provides 77 calories and 3.6 g of fiber, an amount equivalent to about 14% of the daily value for fiber. Without skin, a small apple has 63 calories and just 1.7 g of fiber, according to USDA data. Whole, unpeeled apples are a good source of both soluble and insoluble fiber.

Apple skins are richest in the insoluble fiber, while approximately 80% of the fiber found in the fruit's flesh is soluble. Because the skin is a more concentrated source of fiber than the flesh, however, the fiber ratio of a raw, unpeeled apple is about 30% soluble and 70% insoluble. Because it's high in insoluble fiber, the skin of an apple is particularly beneficial for bowel health and regularity. Insoluble fiber binds to water rather than dissolving in it, a quality that allows it to make stools larger, softer, and easier to pass. It also promotes more frequent bowel movements by keeping material moving through the intestinal tract.

Most of the soluble fiber in an apple's flesh is a type known as pectin. Like other soluble fibers, pectin dissolves in water to form a viscous substance capable of adhering to fatty acids and cholesterol. Pectin in fact is particularly efficient in binding cholesterol. Eating one large apple every day has been shown to reduce blood cholesterol levels by as much as 11%.

A recent research [3] has evaluated the long-term cardioprotective effects of daily consumption of apple in postmenopausal women. This study randomly assigned 160 women aged 45–65 to one of two dietary intervention groups: one received dried apples daily (75 g/day for 1 year) and the other group ate dried prunes every day for a year. Blood samples were taken at 3, 6, and 12 months. Women who consumed dried apple had significantly lower serum levels of total cholesterol and low-density lipoprotein cholesterol by 9% and 16%, respectively, at 3 months compared with baseline. These values were further decreased to 13% and 24%, respectively, after 6 months but stayed constant thereafter. The within-group analysis reported that daily apple consumption profoundly improved atherogenic risk ratios. On the contrary, in the group consuming dried plums there were no significant changes in lipid profile or atherogenic risk ratios. Both dried fruits were able to lower serum levels of lipid hydroperoxide and C-reactive protein. Serum C-reactive protein levels, however, were significantly lower in the dried plum group compared with the dried apple group at 3 months.

Apples are also rich in antioxidant flavonoids and polyphenols. The total measured antioxidant strength (ORAC value) of 100 g apple fruit is 5900 TE. Important flavonoids of apples are quercetin, epicatechin, and procyanidin B2. Apples are good in tartaric acid that gives tart flavor to them. Altogether, these compounds help the body protect from deleterious effects of free radicals.

It is recommended that most men and women should get about 38 g and 25 g of dietary fiber a day, respectively. Older men and women typically need about 30 g and 21 g, respectively, according to the USDA. These general guidelines stem from the principle dietary recommendation that all individuals, regardless of age or gender, should eat 14 g of fiber for every 1000 calories consumed. An individual who averages 2200 calories a day, for example, should get about 31 g of fiber. One small apple supplies about 12% of the recommended amount of fiber.

For a more detailed description of fibers, see the Sect. 10.11 of this chapter: "Dietary Fibers and Fresh Fruit."

10.3 Oranges

The sweet orange (*Citrus sinensis*) is an hybrid between pomelo (*Citrus maxima*) and mandarin (*Citrus reticulata*). The sweet orange has gene that are 25% pomelo and 75% mandarin.

Citrus fruits are notable for their fragrance, partly due to flavonoids and limonoids (which in turn are terpenes) contained in the rind, and most are juice-laden. The juice contains a high quantity of citric acid giving them their characteristic sharp flavor. The genus is commercially important as many species are cultivated for their fruit, which is eaten fresh, pressed for juice, or preserved in marmalades and pickles. They are also good sources of vitamin C and flavonoids. The flavonoids include various flavanones and flavones.

Blood oranges are a natural mutation of *Citrus sinensis.* High concentration of anthocyanin gives the rind, flesh, and juice of the fruit their characteristics dark red color. Blood orange were first discovered and cultivated in the fifteenth century in Sicily.

10.3.1 History

The orange was first cultivated in China. Sweet oranges were mentioned in Chinese literature in 314 BC. The European oranges (such as the bitter orange) were originally brought from India at around the time of Alexander the Great. In the ninth century, during the Emirate of Sicily, the bitter orange was introduced in Sicily. Subsequently the Muslims domination, the *Moors*, introduced to Spain in Andalucía the sour orange with large scale cultivation starting in the tenth century. The sweet orange was unknown until late fifteenth century, when Italian and Portuguese merchants brought orange trees into the Mediterranean area. Shortly afterwards, the sweet orange quickly was adopted as an edible fruit. On his second voyage in 1493, Christofer Columbus may have planted the fruit in Hispaniola. Subsequent expeditions in the mid-1500 brought sweet oranges to south America and Mexico, and to Florida in 1565. Spanish missionaries brought orange trees to Arizona between 1707 and 1710, while the Franciscans did the same in San Diego, California, in 1769. As oranges are rich in vitamin C and do not spoil easily, during the *Age of Discovery* Portuguese, Spanish and Dutch sailors planted orange trees along trade routes to prevent scurvy.

10.3.2 Nutrients and Phytochemicals

Orange pulp is an excellent source of vitamin C, providing 64% of the Daily Value in a 100 g serving. Numerous other essential nutrients are present in low amounts. Oranges contain numerous phytochemicals including carotenoids (beta-carotene, lutein, and beta-cryptoxanthin), flavonoids (nanigenin), and numerous volatile organic compounds producing orange aroma, including aldehydes, esters terpenes, alcohols, and ketones. (For a more detailed description of Flavonoids in fresh fruit, see Sect. 10.10 of this chapter: "Active Phytochemicals in Fresh Fruits").

Orange, Raw
Nutritional values per 100 g
Source: USDA National Nutrient Data base

Energy	197 KJ (47 kcal)
Carbohydrates	11.75 g
Sugars	9.35 g
Protein	0.94 g
Fat	0.12 g
Dietary fiber	2.4 g

Vitamin A equiv.	11 µg	(1% DV)
Thiamine (B1)	0.087 mg	(8% DV)
Riboflavin (B2)	0.04 mg	(3% DV)
Niacin	0.282 mg	(2% DV)
Pantothenic acid	0.25 mg	(5% DV)
Vitamin B6	0.06 mg	(5% DV)
Folate	30 µg	(8% DV)
Vitamin C	53.2 mg	(64% DV)
Vitamin E	0.18 mg	(1% DV)

Calcium	40 mg	(4% DV)
Iron	0.1 mg	(1% DV)
Magnesium	10 mg	(3% DV)
Manganese	0.025 mg	(1% DV)
Phosphorus	14 mg	(2% DV)
Potassium	181 mg	(4% DV)
Zinc	0.07 mg	(1% DV)
Water	86.75 g	

DV = Daily Value

10.4 Pears

The word "pear" probably derives from vulgar Latin "*pira*," the plural form of "*pirum*" meaning fruit.

10.4.1 History

Pear cultivation extends to the remotest antiquity, with evidences of its use as a food since prehistoric times. The word "*pear*" occurs in all the Celtic languages and in Slavic dialects. The pear cultivation is thought to have originated in present-day Western China, and to have spread to the north and the south evolving into diverse group of over 20 widely recognized primary species.

The pear was largely cultivated by the Romans, who ate the fruit raw or cooked, just like apples. In his "*Natural history,*" Pliny the Elder, mentioning at least three dozen of varieties, recommended to stew the pears with honey. The Roman "*De re cocquinaria*" contained a recipe for a spiced, stewed-pear.

10.4.2 Nutrients and Phytochemicals

A small pear of 100 g (small pear) is a god source of dietary fibers but otherwise provides very low amounts of essential nutrients (see table below). Concerning the fiber content, one pear (178 g) contains 3.1 g in 100 g, and 5.5 g of fibres, corresponding to 22% of Daily Value.

Pear, Raw
Vitamins and mineral content per 100 g
Source: USDA Database entry

Energy	239 KJ (39 kcal)
Carbohydrates	15.23 g
Sugars	9.75 g
Dietary fiber	3.1 g
Protein	0.36 g
Fat	0.14 g

Thiamine	0.012 mg	(1% DV)
Riboflavin	0.026 mg	(2% DV)
Niacin	0.161 mg	(1% DV)
Pantothenic acid	0.049 mg	(1% DV)
Vitamin B_6	0.029 mg	(2% DV)
Folate	7 μg	(2% DV)
Choline	5.1 mg	(1% DV)
Vitamin C	4.3 mg	(5% DV)
Vitamin E	0.12 mg	(1% DV)
Vitamin K	4.4 μg	(4% DV)

Calcium	9 mg	(1% DV)
Magnesium	7 mg	(2% DV)
Manganese	0.048 mg	(2% DV)
Potassium	116 mg	(2% DV)
Phosphorus	12 mg	(2% DV)
Iron	0.18 mg	(1% DV)
Zinc	0.1 mg	(1% DV)

DV = Daily Value

10.5 Peaches

The scientific name *persica*, along with the word peach itself and its cognates in many European languages, derives from an early European belief that peaches were native to Persia (present Iran). The fruit has yellow or whitish flesh, a delicate aroma, and a skin that is either velvety (peaches) or smooth (nectarines).

10.5.1 History

Genetic studies suggest peaches originated in China, where they have been cultivated since the early days of Chinese culture. Recent evidences indicate that domestication of peaches occurred as early as 6000 BC. From China, peaches cultivation went to Europe through Persia and reached Greece by 300 BC. Peaches were well known to the Romans in first century AD, and peaches trees were portrayed in wall paintings of *Pompei*, the Roman town destroyed by the Vesuvius eruption of 79 AD.

10.5.2 Nutrients and Phytochemicals

A medium peach weighing 100 g contains small amounts of essential nutrients, but none is a significant proportion of the Daily Value.

Peaches, Raw
Vitamins and mineral content per 100 g
Source: USDA Database entry

Energy	165 KJ (39 kcal)
Carbohydrates	9.54 g
Sugars	8.39 g
Dietary fiber	1.5 g
Protein	0.91 g
Fat	0.25 g

Vitamin A equiv	16 μg	(2% DV)
β-Carotene	162 μg	(2% DV)
Thiamine	0.024 mg	(2% DV)

Vitamin A equiv	16 μg	(2% DV)
Riboflavin	0.031 mg	(3% DV)
Niacin	0.806 mg	(5% DV)
Pantothenic acid	0.153 mg	(3% DV)
Vitamin B_6	0.025 mg	(2% DV)
Folate	4 μg	(1% DV)
Choline	6.1 mg	(1% DV)
Vitamin C	6.6 mg	(8% DV)
Vitamin E	0.73 mg	(5% DV)
Vitamin K	2.6 μg	(2% DV)

Calcium	6 mg	(1% DV)
Magnesium	9 mg	(3% DV)
Manganese	0.061 mg	(3% DV)
Potassium	190 mg	(4% DV)
Phosphorus	20 mg	(3% DV)
Iron	0.25 mg	(2% DV)
Zinc	0.17 mg	(2% DV)
Fluoride	4 μg	

DV = Daily Value

Total polyphenols in mg per 100 g of fresh weight are 14–102 in white-flesh nectarines, 18–54 in yellow-flesh nectarines, 20–111 in white-flesh peaches, and 21–61 in yellow-flesh peaches [4].The major phenolic compounds identified in peach are chlorogenic acid, catechins, epicatechins, gallic acid, ellagic acid, rutin and isoquercetin. Red-fleshed peaches are rich in anthocyanin, particularly cyaniding glucosides.

Peach is a good source of fibers. A small peach provides 2 g of fibers, while larger peaches can contain between 2.6 and 3.4 g.

Peaches can cause allergy. Peach allergy or intolerance is a relatively common form of hypersensitivity to proteins contained in peaches and related fruits, such as almonds. These adverse reactions are related to the "freshness" of the fruit: peeled or canned fruit may be tolerated.

10.6 Plums and Prunes

Plum belongs to the plant genus which is a relative of the peach, apricot, cherry, and almond. It is a drupe, which is a fruit that has a hard stone pit around its seeds which does not easily separate from the flesh. Plums are eaten either fresh or dried. When dried, plums are called prunes, although the prune fruit comes from a different type of plant than plums. Although of the same genus (prunus) as plums, prunes have pits that are easier to remove from the flesh unlike plums. Moreover, prunes are oval-shaped and are blue or purple when ripe.

There are over 2000 varieties of plums which come in different shapes and colors, some are oval-shaped and others are heart-shaped.

10.6.1 History

The European plum is thought to have been discovered around two thousand years ago, originating in the area near the Caspian Sea. Even in ancient Roman times there were already over 300 varieties of European plums. European plums made their way across the Atlantic Ocean with the pilgrims, who introduced them into the United States in the seventeenth century.

The process of drying plums to make prunes is thought to have originated thousands of years ago in an area near the Caspian Sea, the same region where the prune-producing European plums originated. They spread throughout Europe with the migration of different cultures and civilizations.

The process of drying plums to produce prunes took hold in California, now the leading producer of prunes worldwide, in the mid-nineteenth century when Louis Pellier planted grafted plum tree cuttings brought back with him from his native France. Among these trees were those belonging to the Agen variety, the type of plum that is extremely well suited to be dried to make prunes.

10.6.2 Nutrients and Phytochemicals

Dried prunes and prune juice are well known for their ability to prevent constipation. Due to their high content in soluble and insoluble fibers, prunes provide bulk and decrease the transit time of fecal matter, thus decreasing the risk of colon cancer and hemorrhoids. Prunes contain also other mild laxatives including sorbitol, dihydrophenylsatin, neochlorogenic acid, and chlorogenic acid, which all work together to get intestine moving.

Sorbitol, a sugar alcohol with a sweet taste which the human body metabolizes slowly, exerts its laxative effect by drawing water into the large intestine, thereby stimulating bowel movements.

For all these reasons, prunes are usually eaten by the elderly as medication for constipation and so they are associated with them.

Beyond the laxative action, chlorogenic and neo-chlorogenic acids of prunes, esters of caffeic acid, are primarily phenols functioning as potent antioxidants. These damage-preventing phenols are particularly effective in neutralizing a particularly dangerous oxygen radical called superoxide anion radical. Chlorogenic acid has also the property of slowing the release of glucose into the bloodstream after a meal [5].

Insoluble fibers of prunes, in addition to their laxative properties, provide food for the "friendly" bacteria in the large intestine. When these helpful bacteria ferment prunes' insoluble fibers, they produce a short-chain fatty acid, the butyric acid, which serves as the primary fuel for the cells of the large intestine and helps maintain a healthy colon. These helpful bacteria also create two other short-chain fatty acids, propionic and acetic acid, which are used as fuel by the cells of the liver and muscles. In addition to producing the helpful short-chain fatty acids described above, friendly bacteria play an important protective role by crowding out pathogenic bacteria and preventing them from surviving in the intestinal tract.

Soluble fibers of prunes, on other hands, help to lower cholesterol by binding to bile acids and removing them from the body via the feces. Bile acids are compounds that are manufactured by the liver from cholesterol. When they are excreted along with prunes' fiber and lost with feces, the liver must manufacture new bile acids and uses up more cholesterol, thus lowering the amount of circulating cholesterol.

Plums are also a god source of vitamin C, vitamin A, vitamin B_2, and potassium. They are full of carbohydrates, sodium, minerals, and amino acids.

Plums and prunes have been demonstrated to increase absorption of iron into the body. This ability of plums and prunes to make iron more available may be related to the vitamin C content of this fruit. These fruits, in fact, are qualified as a very good source of vitamin C. Vitamin C is also needed for a strong immune system, so getting a little extra vitamin C around cold and flu season is highly recommended. Being a potent antioxidant, vitamin C prevents the oxidation of numerous substrates, including cell membranes, brain cells, and cholesterol.

Dried Plums (Prunes) Uncooked

Nutritional value per 100 g

Source: USDA Database entry

Energy	1.006 KJ (240 kcal)
Carbohydrates	63.88 g
Sugars	38.13 g
Dietary fiber	7.1 g
Protein	2.18 g
Fat	0.38 g

Vitamin A equiv	39 μg	(5% DV)
β-Carotene	394 μg	(4% DV)
Lutein zeaxanthin	148 μg	
Thiamine	0.051 mg	(4% DV)
Riboflavin	0.186 mg	(16% DV)
Niacin	1.182 mg	(13% DV)
Pantothenic acid	0.422 mg	(8% DV)
Vitamin B_6	0.205 mg	(16% DV)
Folate	4 μg	(1% DV)
Choline	10.1 mg	(2% DV)
Vitamin C	0.6 mg	(1% DV)
Vitamin E	0.43 mg	(3% DV)
Vitamin K	59.5 μg	(57% DV)

Calcium	43 mg	(4% DV)
Magnesium	41 mg	(12% DV)
Manganese	0.299 mg	(14% DV)
Potassium	732 mg	(16% DV)
Phosphorus	69 mg	(10% DV)
Iron	0.93 mg	(7% DV)
Zinc	0.44 mg	(5% DV)
Fluoride	4 μg	

DV = Daily Value

10.7 Grapes

Grapes are one of the most important fruits, from nutritional and commercial point of view. Internationally, more grapes are being traded than apples, pears, and oranges combined. However, the majority of the grapes are used for wine production. Only about 10% are sold as table grapes for fresh consumption and about 5% are dried to make raisins.

Grapes are usually classified as either table or wine grapes, based on their intended method of consumption: eaten raw (table grapes) or used to make wine (wine grapes).

While almost all of them belong to the same species, *Vitis vinifera*, table and wine grapes have significant differences, brought about through selective breeding. Table grape cultivars tend to have large, seedless fruit with relatively thin skin. Wine grapes are smaller, usually seeded, and have relatively thick skins, a desirable characteristic in winemaking, since much of the aroma in wine comes from the skin. Wine grapes also tend to be very sweet: they are harvested at the time when their juice is approximately 24% sugar by weight.

Raisins are a product of grapes. A raisin is a dried grape. Raisins are produced in many regions of the world and may be eaten raw or used in cooking, baking, and brewing. Raisin varieties depend on the type of grape used, and are made in a variety of sizes and colors including green, black, brown, blue, purple, and yellow. Raisins can contain up to 72% sugars by weight, most of which is fructose and glucose. They also contain about 3% protein and 3.7–6.8% dietary fiber. Raisins, like prunes and apricots, are also high in antioxidants, but have a lower vitamin C content than fresh grapes.

10.7.1 History

Grapes belong to the oldest plants on earth, much older than the human being. Archeological finds indicate that several varieties of wild vines existed already 130 million years ago.

The exact origin of grape is unknown. The most likely origin is from the regions around the Caspian Sea, where grapes have been cultivated when the Mesopotamian town Ur was at the peak of its development. The earliest "wine-culture" in the world has been found in the mountainous regions of Transcaucasia, modern Georgia, Armenia, and Azerbaijan, and refers to the Neolithic period (c. 8000–4000 BC). Permanent Neolithic communities had been established there by at least 6000 BC, a place in which other essential preconditions for this momentous innovation (e.g., pottery-making) came together for the first time in human history [6].

Via the countries around the Black Sea grapes were eventually introduced into Greece. From here they reached France, when Greek colonists settled around Marseille in the sixth century BC. From there the Romans spread them further throughout Europe and the Spaniards took them along their explorations to the New World.

Grapes, Red Or Green
Nutritional value per 100 g
Source: USDA Database entry

Energy	288 KJ (69 kcal)
Carbohydrates	18.1 g
Sugars	15.48 g
Dietary fiber	0.9 g
Protein	0.72 g
Fat	0.16 g

Thiamine	0.069 mg	(6% DV)
Riboflavin	0.07 mg	(6% DV)
Niacin	1.188 mg	(1% DV)
Pantothenic acid	0.05 mg	(1% DV)
Vitamin B_6	0.086 mg	(7% DV)
Folate	2 µg	(1% DV)
Choline	5.6 mg	(1% DV)
Vitamin C	3.2 mg	(4% DV)
Vitamin E	0.19 mg	(1% DV)
Vitamin K	14.6 µg	(14% DV)

Calcium	10 mg	(1% DV)
Magnesium	7 mg	(2% DV)
Manganese	0.071 mg	(3% DV)
Potassium	191 mg	(4% DV)
Phosphorus	20 mg	(3% DV)
Iron	0.36 mg	(3% DV)
Zinc	0.07 mg	(1% DV)

DV = Daily Value

10.7.2 Nutrients and Phytochemicals

The three main species of grapes grown around the world are: European (*Vitis vinifera*), North American (*Vitis labrusca* and *Vitis rotundifolia*), and French hybrids.

The color of the berry is because of the presence of polyphenolic pigments in them. Red or purple berries are rich in anthocyanins while white-green berries contain more of tannins, especially, catechin. Interestingly, these antioxidant compounds are densely concentrated in the skin and seeds. To be emphasized is the high content of the antioxidant resveratrol in red/blue grapes, mostly concentrated in the skin. Table 10.1. gives a general view of the phytonutrient richness of grapes. While a single grape variety is unlikely to contain all of the phytonutrients listed in the table, grapes as a group have been shown to provide the health-supportive nutrients listed in the table.

In a recent study [7] the presence of flavonols, the product of the flavonoid biosynthetic pathway, was investigated in the berry skins of 91 grape varieties. In red grapes, the main flavonol was quercetin (mean = 43.99%), followed by myricetin

Table 10.1 Phytonutrients of grapes

• Stilbenes
– Resveratrol
– Piceatannol
– Pterostilbene
• Flavanols
– Catechins
– Epicatechins
– Procyanidins
– Proanthocyanidins
– Viniferones
• Flavonols
– Quercetin
– Kaempferol
– Myricetin
– Isorhamnetin
• Phenolic acids
– Caffeic acid
– Coumaric acid
– Ferulic acid
– Gallic acid
• Carotenoids
– Beta-carotene
– Lutein
– Zeaxanthin

All phytonutrients listed are potent antioxidants

(36.81%), kaempferol (6.43%), laricitrin (5.65%), isorhamnetin (3.89%), and syringetin (3.22%). In white grapes, the main flavonol was quercetin (mean = 81.35%), followed by kaempferol (16.91%) and isorhamnetin (1.74%) (for a complete list of flavonoids, see Fig. 10.2, below).

Grapes are rich source of micronutrient minerals like copper, iron, and manganese. Copper and manganese are an essential cofactor of antioxidant enzyme superoxide dismutase. Iron is especially concentrated in raisins. In addition, 100 g of fresh grapes contain about 191 mg of health benefiting electrolyte, potassium. They are also good source of vitamin C, vitamin A, vitamin K, carotenes, and B-complex vitamins such as pyridoxine, riboflavin, and thiamin (see table of nutritional values) (see Table 10.1.)

The most important phytochemical of grapes are the polyphenols flavonoids, including resveratrol, anthocyanins, and catechins. Some of these potent antioxidants are produced by grapes in response to mechanical injuries, ultraviolet radiation, and as a defense for viral and fungal infections. Resveratrol in particular is produced by grapes when they are stressed particularly by fungal pathogens, i.e., *Botrytis cinerea.* It seems that grapes use the resveratrol to increase their resistance to fungal growth and survive this stress.

The effects of these polyphenols on human health are described in Chap. 14—"Red and white wine": *resveratrol* (cancer, glucose metabolism and diabetes mellitus, cognitive functions, cardiovascular, longevity); *anthocyanins* (blood pressure, total and LDL cholesterol, myocardial infarction, ischemic stroke, and anti-inflammatory effect); *proanthocyanidins* (blood lipids, collagen, and on free radicals); *thyrosol* (oxidative stress, myocardial ischemic stress, and myocardial infarction); *caffeic acid* (oxidative stress and inflammation).

It should be emphasized that in addition to polyphenols, the presence in grapes of a new phytochemical first believed to be present only in vertebrates has been found: the melatonin.

10.7.3 Melatonin

Melatonin is an indoleamine, a hormone secreted in human by the pineal gland especially in response to darkness, and has been linked to the regulation of circadian rhythms. In human, melatonin is synthesized from tryptophan and serotonin, and modulates circadian and circannual physiological functions, such as the sleep/wake cycle, reproductive function, bone metabolism and turnover, via cell receptor-mediated mechanisms.

In addition to receptor-mediate functions, a receptor-independent activity of melatonin has been also reported, mainly because of melatonin's powerful antioxidant activity. Melatonin can directly scavenge free radical species (both reactive oxygen and nitrogen species) and stimulate the activity of antioxidant enzymes; thus, it is involved in immune response and the pathogenesis of chronic-degenerative disorders. Endogenously produced melatonin declines with age and its loss contributes to degenerative conditions of aging. Recently, it was reported [8] that melatonin also activates *Sirtuins*, similarly to *Resveratrol* (see Chap. 14: "Red and White Wine").

Melatonin biosynthesis has been first described in the pineal gland (epiphysis), but it also occurs in other tissues outside the central nervous system, such as the gastrointestinal tract, bone marrow, and lymphocytes. The aromatic amino acid tryptophan is the precursor of melatonin and other indoleamines, including serotonin (Fig. 10.1).

Outside the animal kingdom, the presence of melatonin in food plants has been recently reported. Melatonin in fact has been detected and quantified in roots, shoots, leaves, flowers, fruits, and seeds of a considerable variety of spermatophyte species, and its presence in plants has been unequivocally confirmed [9]. Among the Mediterranean diet components, melatonin has been first reported in grapes and then in olives and olive oil. In the berry exocarp (skin) of different wine grape cultivars, high melatonin concentrations have been detected in Italian and French wine grape cultivars, with levels ranging from 0.005 to 0.96 ng g^{-1} [10]. Higher levels of melatonin have been recently found in the whole berry of Sangiovese red and Albana white grapes (1.5 and 1.2 ng g^{-1}, respectively), from central Italy [11]. In a recent study, melatonin has been also found in the wines produced with these grape varieties.

In a recent screening of Italian mono- and polyvarietal red, white, and dessert wines from different geographical areas, melatonin was found at concentrations around or less than 0.5 ng mL^{-1} [12]. In this study the linear correlation coefficient

Fig. 10.1 Biosynthetic pathway of melatonin in living organisms

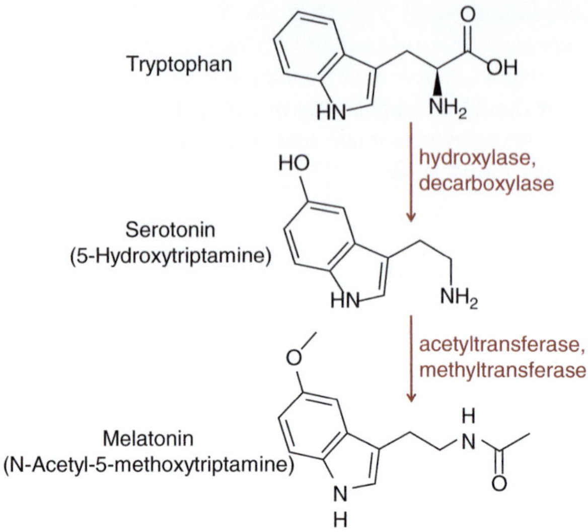

between the melatonin content in wines and their antiradical capacity was higher compared with the weak correlation found between *trans*-resveratrol-3-*O*-glucoside (*trans*-piceid) and the same activity, even though the levels of resveratrol and other stilbenes (around or less than 1 mg mL^{-1}) were three orders of magnitude higher than the levels of indoleamine (melatonin) [12]. In these terms, it was hypothesized that melatonin possesses a higher antioxidant activity than resveratrol.

The possibility of modulating the circulating levels of melatonin in mammals, which are basically very low (~200 pg mL^{-1} at the maximum night-time peak and lower than 10 pg mL^{-1} during the day) [13], with melatonin in grape products (near 1 ng g^{-1} and 0.5 ng mL^{-1} in berry skin and wine respectively) through the intake of plant foods, represents an exciting promise. Actually, a very efficient uptake and bioavailability of dietary melatonin have been demonstrated in both animals and humans [14–18].

Although data from studies on melatonin of berry tissues are still fragmentary and somewhat contrasting, it is likely that neither polyphenols nor melatonin possess "per se" thaumaturgic properties, but their synergy with other bioactive phytochemicals (e.g., carotenoids and polyphenols) contributes greatly to maximizing the benefits of healthy dietary styles rich in fresh fruit, including Mediterranean diet.

10.8 Cherries

The English word cherry, French *cerise*, Spanish *cereza*, Italian *ciliegia*, and Turkish *kiraz* all derive from the Latin *cerasum*, which referred to an ancient Greek region which today is the city of Giresun, Turkey, from which cherries were first thought to be exported to Europe.

10.8.1 History

The indigenous range of the sweet cherry extends through most of Europe, western Asia, and parts of northern Africa, and the fruit has been consumed throughout its range since prehistoric times. A cultivated cherry is recorded as having been brought to Rome by *Lucius Licinius Lucullus* from northeastern Anatolia, also known as the Pontus region, in 72 BC.

Cherries were introduced into England at Teynham, near Sittingbourne in Kent by order of Henry VIII who had tasted them in Flanders.

10.8.2 Nutrients and Phytochemicals

As raw fruit, sweet cherries provide little nutrient content per 100 g serving. Dietary fiber and vitamin C are present in moderate content while other vitamins and dietary minerals each supply less than 10% of the Daily Value (DV) per serving, respectively.

Compared to sweet cherries, raw sour cherries contain slightly higher content per 100 g of vitamin C (12% DV) and vitamin A (8% DV).

Cherry, Sweet, Red, Raw
Nutritional value per 100 g
Source: USDA Database entry

Energy	263 KJ (63 kcal)
Carbohydrates	16 g
Sugars	12.8 g
Dietary fiber	2.1 g
Protein	1.1 g
Fat	0.2 g

Vitamin A equiv.	3 μg	(0% DV)
Beta-carotene	38 μg	(0% DV)
Lutein zeaxanthin	85 μg	
Thiamine	0.027 mg	(2% DV)
Riboflavin	0.033 mg	(3% DV)
Niacin	1.154 mg	(1% DV)
Pantothenic acid	0.199 mg	(4% DV)
Vitamin B_6	0.049 mg	(4% DV)
Folate	4 μg	(1% DV)
Choline	6.1 mg	(1% DV)
Vitamin C	7 mg	(8% DV)
Vitamin K	2.1 μg	(2% DV)

Calcium	13 mg	(1% DV)
Magnesium	11 mg	(3% DV)
Manganese	0.07 mg	(3% DV)
Potassium	222 mg	(5% DV)
Phosphorus	21 mg	(3% DV)

Calcium	13 mg	(1% DV)
Iron	0.36 mg	(3% DV)
Zinc	0.07 mg	(1% DV)

DV = Daily Value

10.8.3 Polyphenols in Cherries

In cherry, as in other red fruits, the ripening process is related to a change from the initial green color to red, with accumulation of polyphenolic compounds, anthocyanins, and degradation of chlorophyll. Phenolic compounds are concentrated in the skin and contribute to sensory and organoleptic qualities of fruits, such as taste and astringency.

The phenols contained in sour and sweet cherries have been characterized [7]. Cyanidin 3- glucoside, cyanidin 3-rutinoside, cyanidin 3-sophoroside, pelargonidin 3-glucoside, pelargonidin 3- rutinoside, 3-glucoside, and peonidin 3-rutinoside are the polyphenols that have been identified in sweet and sour cherries.

Among phenolic acids, hydroxycinnamates (neochlorogenic acid and p-coumaroylquinic acid) have been quantified either in sweet and sour cherries. Flavonols and flavan-3-ols such as catechin, epicatechin, quercetin 3-glucoside, quercetin 3-rutinoside, and kaempferol 3-rutinoside were also found in sweet and sour cherries. The higher levels of total phenolics in sour cherries have been attributed to higher concentrations of anthocyanins and hydroxycinnamic acids.

10.9 Wild and Cultivated Berries

A berry fruit generally refers to any small fruit that lacks seeds and can be eaten whole. Berries are usually juicy, rounded, brightly colored, sweet or sour, and do not have a stone or pit, although many pips or seeds may be present. Common examples are strawberries, raspberries, blueberries, and red- and blackcurrants. Some berries such as raspberries and strawberries have been bred for hundreds of years and are distinct from their wild counterparts, while other berries, such as blackcurrant, lingonberries, and cloudberries, grow almost exclusively in the wild.

10.9.1 History

Wild berries have been valuable as a food source for humans since before the start of agriculture and remain among the primary food sources of other primates. They were a seasonal staple for early hunter-gatherers for thousands of years, and wild berry gathering remains a popular activity in Europe and North America today. In time, humans learned to store berries so that they could be used in the winter, and they may be made into fruit preserves, and among Native Americans, mixed with meat and fats as pemmican.

Berries also began to be cultivated in Europe and other countries. Some species of blackberries and raspberries have been cultivated since the seventeenth century, while smooth-skinned blueberries and cranberries have been cultivated in the United States for over a century.

Strawberry is mentioned by ancient Romans, who thought it had medicinal properties, but it was then not a staple of agriculture. Woodland strawberries began to be grown in French gardens in the fourteenth century. The musky-flavored strawberry began to be grown in European gardens in the late sixteenth century. In the early 1800s, English breeders of strawberry made varieties of *F. ananassa* which were important in strawberry breeding in Europe, and hundreds of cultivars have since been produced through the breeding of strawberries.

10.9.2 Nutrients and Phytochemicals

Once ripened, berries are typically of a contrasting color to their background (often of green leaves), making them visible and attractive to frugivorous animals and birds. This assists the wide dispersal of the plants' seeds.

Berry colors are due to natural plant pigments, such as anthocyanins, together with other flavonoids localized mainly in berry skins, seeds, and leaves. Among fruits, wild berries are the richest in antioxidants, as measured according to ORAC values (Table 10.2). Although berry pigments have antioxidant properties *in vitro* [19], it is current opinion that there is insufficient physiological evidence established to date that berry pigments have actual antioxidant or any other functions within the human body.

Table 10.2 ORAC (antioxidant) values of some berries and fruits

FRUITS	ORAC
Prunes	5770
Goji berries	3290
Blueberries	2400
Blackberries	2036
Cranberries	1750
Strawberries	1540
Pomegranates	1245
Raspberries	1220
Plums	949
Oranges	750
Grapes (red)	739
Cherries	670
Kiwifruit	602
Grapes (white)	446
Banana	221
Apple	218
Apricots	164
Peach	158
Pear	134

ORAC values refer to the Oxygen Radical Absorbance Capacity of a food, as determined by the U.S. Department of Agriculture (DOA). By testing the ability of foods and other compounds to subdue oxygen free radicals, the DOA was able to determine each compound's antioxidant capability.

Although the contrasting opinions on the beneficial effects of berry pigments and their antioxidant properties on human diseases, the berries phenolic compounds have been shown to exert other effects beyond the antioxidant activity. Numerous studies have demonstrated that besides their in vitro antioxidant capacity, certain phenolic compounds, such as anthocyanins, catechins, proanthocyanidins, and other noncolored flavonoids, may regulate different signaling pathways involved in cell survival, growth, and differentiation [20].

Blueberries are rich in flavonoids, particularly in anthocyanin, the natural pigments responsible for the blue, purple, red, and orange colors of many fruits and vegetables. More than 500 different anthocyanins have been described in the literature. Depending on the number and position of hydroxyl and methoxyl groups as substituents, different anthocyanins have been described and six of them are commonly found in fruits and vegetables: pelargonidin, cyanidin, delphinidin, petunidin, peonidin, and malvid. Anthocyanins are some of the few polyphenols that can be detected in plasma in the native form found in plant foods (glycosides).

Anthocyanins have clearly demonstrated, in animal and humans, in vitro and in vivo, to provide significant protection against many chronic diseases, some of which will be considered below.

A mention deserves the bright red color of goji berries. The red flesh and pulp contain carotenoids, such as zeaxanthin. In fact, nearly 75% of the carotenoids in goji are zeaxanthin, the rest are beta-carotene (vitamin A). Zeaxanthin has been most studied for its benefits to the eyes, which is why goji are often recommended as part of a healthy diet for those suffering from age-related macular degeneration and a whole host of other vision-related diseases.

10.10 Active Phytochemicals in Fresh Fruits: Polyphenols

Fresh fruit is an important component of Mediterranean diet. Fresh fruits have many positive effects on human health. These effects are generally attributed to two components of fresh fruit: polyphenols and fibers (soluble and insoluble).

10.10.1 Polyphenols

Polyphenols, or poly-hydroxy-phenol, are a group of plant metabolites thought to provide health benefits in humans through cell signaling pathways and antioxidant effects. Most often, they are considered as antioxidant phytochemicals that tend to prevent or neutralize the damaging effects of free radicals, the oxidative stress. Oxidative stress is considered to be substantial, if not crucial, in the initiation and development of many current conditions and diseases, including: inflammation, autoimmune diseases, cataract, cancer, Parkinson's disease, arteriosclerosis, and aging. Oxidative stress plays a role also in heart diseases, neurodegenerative diseases, cancer, and in the aging process. This theory is supported by increasing evidence suggesting that oxidative damage plays a role in the development of chronic, age-related degenerative diseases, and that dietary antioxidants oppose this and lower the risk of disease.

Polyphenols are present in fruits and vegetables, but the highest concentrations are found in the outer part of ripe fruits, concentrations that decrease during ripening, while the total amount increases as the size of the fruits increases.

All polyphenols have similar ring-shaped chemical structures, but they differ in the number of rings and molecules that are attached to those rings. Thus, polyphenols are grouped into four different categories based on those differences: *phenolic acids, stilbenes, lignans, and flavonoids*. The first three (phenolic acids, stilbenes, and lignans) are also called "*non-flavonoids*," to distinguish from "*flavonoids*" (Fig. 10.2).

Phenolic acids include hydroxybenzoic acids, such as gallic acid found in tea, and hydroxycinnamic acids found in coffee, mangos, blueberries, kiwis, plums, apples, citrus fruits, and cherries. Phenolic acids are also present in good quantity in numerous vegetables: chicory, artichokes carrots, lettuce, eggplant, wheat, and coffee are among the richest sources. Phenolic acids are contained also in flour

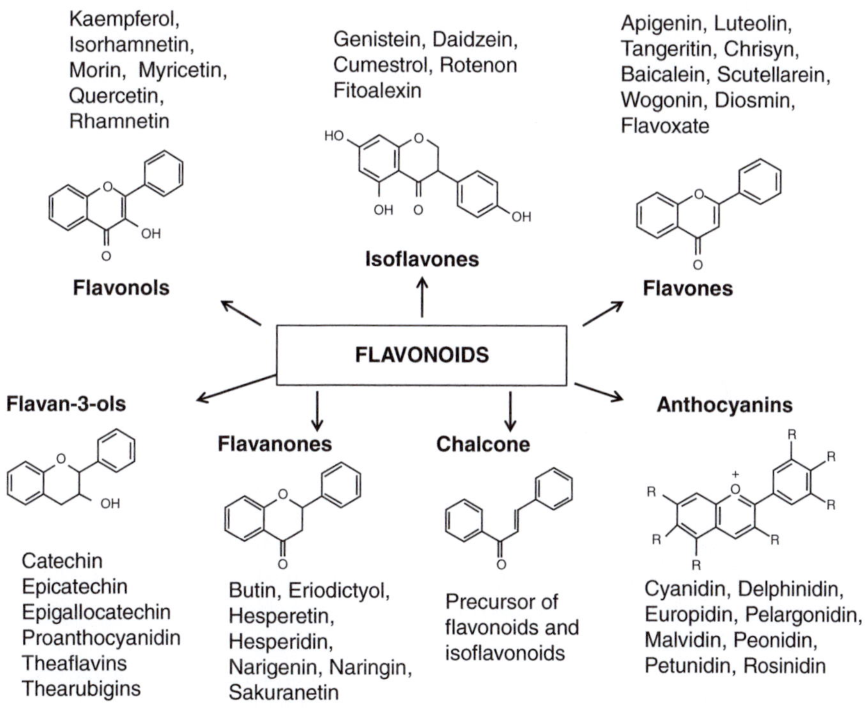

Fig. 10.2 Flavonoids

made from whole wheat, rice, corn, or oats. Phenolic compounds confer unique taste, flavor, and health-promoting properties found in vegetables and fruits. Therefore, increasing the phenolic content in these plants enhances their quality. Phenolic compounds are crucial for plants growth and reproduction, and are produced as a response to environmental factors (light, chilling, pollution, etc.) and to defend injured plants.

Stilbenes are a small group of phenolic compounds, essentially resveratrol and pterostilbene. Resveratrol is the most important stilbene. Red wine, red-grape skin, peanuts, blueberries, and cranberries are the richest source of resveratrol. Pterostilbene is found in blueberries and grapes. It's an antioxidant that has shown promise in the treatment and prevention of cancer and cardiovascular disease, but (like resveratrol) it's only been tested in lab animals. Currently, there aren't any studies in humans.

Lignans: Plant lignans are co-passengers of dietary fiber, and therefore fiber-rich food items are often good sources of lignans. Flax seed and sesame seed contain higher levels of lignans than most other foods. Other sources of lignans include cereals (rye, wheat, oat, and barley), soybeans, cruciferous vegetables such as broccoli and cabbage, and some fruit, particularly apricots and strawberries.

Flavonoids: There are several types of flavonoids: flavones, flavonols, flavanones, isoflavones, anthocyanidins, catechins, and chalcones (Fig. 10.2). They're found in a wide variety of plant-based foods, including fruits, vegetables, legumes, red wine, and green tea. Flavonoids work primarily as antioxidants. Nowadays, it is widely accepted that if flavonoids have any preventive or curative activity through their ingestion, this effect must involve not only their antioxidant potential, but also the modulation of multiple cellular pathways that are crucial in the pathogenesis of those diseases [21]. Their dietary intake has been associated with the prevention of the development of chronic diseases such as type-2 diabetes, cardiovascular disease, and cancer (Fig. 10.3).

10.10.2 Flavonoids and Diabetes

In diabetic male rats, blueberry anthocyanins (BA) given orally prevented diabetes-induced weight loss and increased blood glucose. BA also upregulated the antioxidant capacity of the retina, increased the content of glutathione (GSH) and glutathione peroxidase (GPx) activity, and decreased malondialdehyde (MDA) and reactive oxygen species (ROS) levels. Vascular endothelial growth factor (VEGF) and interleukin-1β (IL-1β), two pro-inflammatory cytokines upregulated in the serum of diabetes model rats, were significantly reversed by BA [22].

In a double-blinded, randomized, and placebo-controlled clinical study design [22], insulin sensitivity was measured on 32 obese, nondiabetic, and insulin-resistant subjects. Participants were randomized to consume either a smoothie containing 22.5 g blueberry bioactives (blueberry group, $n = 15$) or a smoothie of equal nutritional value without added blueberry bioactives (placebo group, $n = 17$) twice daily for 6 week. The mean change in insulin sensitivity improved more in the blueberry

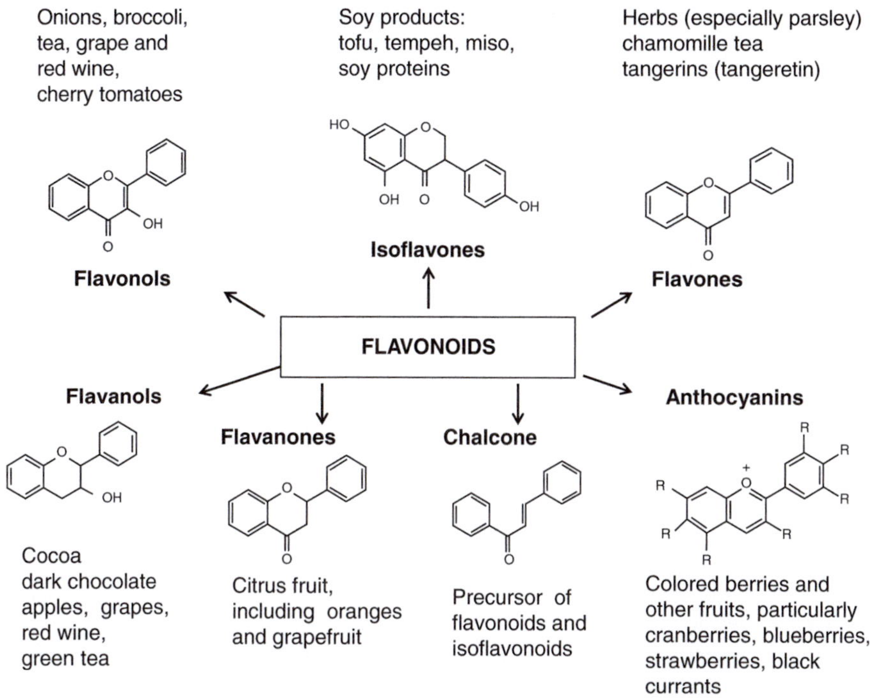

Fig. 10.3 Fruit, vegetables, and beverages containing flavonoids

group (1.7 ± 0.5 mg kg FFM^{-1} min^{-1}) than in the placebo group (0.4 ± 0.4 mg kg FFM^{-1} min^{-1}) ($P = 0.04$). Insulin sensitivity was enhanced in the blueberry group at the end of the study without significant changes in adiposity, energy intake, and inflammatory biomarkers. The conclusions were that daily dietary supplementation with bioactives from whole blueberries improved insulin sensitivity in obese, non-diabetic, and insulin-resistant participants [23].

The effects of dietary intakes of major flavonoid subclasses (i.e., flavonols, flavones, flavanones, flavan-3-ols, and anthocyanins) were assessed in a study that included three important epidemiological studies, to see whether flavonoids intakes were associated with the risk of type 2 diabetes in US adults [24]. The authors studied a total of 70,359 women in the Nurses' Health Study (NHS; 1984–2008), 89,201 women in the NHS II (1991–2007), and 41,334 men in the Health Professionals Follow-Up Study (1986–2006) who were free of diabetes, cardiovascular disease, and cancer at baseline. During 3,645,585 person-years of follow-up, 12,611 incident cases of type 2 diabetes were documented. Higher intakes of anthocyanins were significantly associated with a lower risk of type 2 diabetes (pooled HR for the 3 cohorts from a comparison of extreme quintiles: 0.85; 95% CI: 0.80, 0.91; *P*-trend <0.001) after multivariate adjustment for age, BMI, and lifestyle and dietary factors. Consumption of anthocyanin-rich foods, particularly blueberries (pooled HR: 0.77 from a comparison of ≥2 servings/week with

<1 serving/mo; 95% CI: 0.68, 0.87; *P*-trend <0.001) was also associated with a lower risk of type 2 diabetes. No significant associations were found for total flavonoid intake or other flavonoid subclasses [24].

10.10.3 Flavonoids and Cardiovascular Disease

Polyphenols have been shown to reduce cardiovascular (CVD) risk in atherosclerotic subjects.

Several epidemiological studies have suggested that the regular consumption of foods and beverages rich in flavonoids is associated with a reduction in the risk of several cardiovascular pathological conditions ranging from hypertension to coronary heart disease, stroke, and dementia. The major polyphenols shown to have these protective effects in humans are primarily from cocoa, wine, grape seed, berries, tea, tomatoes (polyphenolics and nonpolyphenolics), soy, and pomegranate. Also flavonoids from apples and onions appear to impact positively on some CVD risk factors, e.g., blood pressure, vascular function, and serum lipid levels. A recent prospective study reported that anthocyanidins, flavanones, and foods rich in flavonoids (including apples, pears, strawberries, red wine, chocolate, and bran) were associated with lower CVD mortality in women [25].

Atherosclerosis is a chronic inflammatory disease that develops in lesion-prone regions of medium-sized arteries. Atherosclerotic lesions may be present and clinically silent for decades before becoming active and producing clinical events such as acute myocardial infarction, unstable angina, or sudden cardiac death. Such events are often caused by acute rupture or erosion of a vulnerable plaque, which exposes the highly thrombogenic sub-endothelium to flowing blood. The development of a vulnerable plaque and the subsequent ischemic events represent a profound loss of endothelial homeostasis. Dyslipidemia, hypertension, diabetes mellitus, smoking, aging, physical inactivity, systemic inflammation and infectious processes, hyperhomocysteinemia, and the postmenopausal state are all associated with endothelial dysfunction. Lipid-lowering therapy, angiotensin converting enzyme inhibitors, angiotensin receptor blockers, smoking cessation, and exercise have all been shown to reverse endothelial dysfunction among patients with atherosclerosis or cardiovascular risk factors.

Flavonoids have been shown to reverse the CVD acting primarily on endothelial dysfunction and platelet aggregation.

10.10.3.1 Flavonoids and Endothelial Dysfunction

There is increasing evidence that flavonoids have beneficial effects on endothelial control of thrombosis, inflammation, and vascular tone.

Tea contains an assortment of water-soluble antioxidant flavonoids, including catechins, quercetin, kaempferol, and other polyphenols, including thearubigins. The short-term and long-term effects of tea consumption on flow-mediated dilation were studied in the brachial artery among 50 subjects with angiographically proven coronary artery disease, in a placebo-controlled, crossover study [26]. Short-term effects of tea were examined by measuring flow-mediated dilation before and 2 h after the subjects consumed 450 mL of freshly brewed black tea. Long-term effects were examined by measuring flow-mediated dilation again after the subjects had consumed 900 mL of black tea per day for 30 day. Both short-term and long-term tea consumption improved significantly endothelial function.

In another study [27], the effect of tea consumption on brachial artery flow-mediated dilation was studied in a group of otherwise healthy subjects with modest hypercholesterolemia. It was observed that consumption of 5 cups of black tea per day for 5 week led to improved flow-mediated dilation. Interestingly, tea consumption was also associated with an improvement in nitroglycerin-mediated dilation, which suggested that tea improved the bioactivity of endothelium-derived nitric oxide and/or had a beneficial effect on the function of vascular smooth muscle.

Other flavonoid-containing beverages, particularly grape products, have been shown to improve endothelial function. It was observed [28] that consumption of grape juice for 14 day was associated with improved brachial artery flow-mediated dilation among 15 adults with angiographically proven coronary artery disease. In that study, the susceptibility of LDL to ex vivo oxidation was reduced, which suggested an antioxidant effect. A second study from the same group also indicated beneficial effects of purple grape juice on endothelial function [29].

In another study [30] the effects of cocoa on flow-mediated dilation were examined. Among patients with at least one cardiovascular disease risk factor, impaired endothelial function was observed. Two hours after the patients consumed cocoa containing 176 mg/dL flavan-3-ols, the investigators observed a significant increase in flow-mediated dilation. They also observed increases in nitrosylated and nitrosated species in plasma, which suggested an increase in nitric oxide production.

10.10.3.2 Flavonoids and Plateled Aggregation

In a study on dogs [31] the effects of grape juice on platelet function in vivo were examined. The investigators used the Folts model of unstable coronary stenosis, which involves the creation of endothelial injury and sub-occlusive stenosis in a dog coronary artery. In this model, transient platelet aggregation and release are reflected in cyclic variations in coronary blood flow; therefore, the model closely mimics a ruptured atherosclerotic plaque causing unstable angina. In this model, acute intragastric administration of red wine or grape juice was associated with marked reductions in cyclic flow variations, which indicates an important antiplatelet effect that is relevant to cardiovascular disease events [31].

There are mixed data regarding the effects of tea consumption on platelet function. Animal studies of the effects of tea consumption on platelet aggregation in the Folts model suggested that tea may have benefits comparable to those of grape juice, although rather high doses of tea were required. It was also observed that tea consumption reduces plasma concentration of *P*-selectin, a marker of in vivo platelet aggregation [32].

Other polyphenolic compounds have been reported to reduce cardiovascular disease risk and to have beneficial effects on endothelial and platelet function. For example, soy products, which are rich sources of isoflavones such as genistein and daidzein, have been reported to improve endothelial function, possibly through an effect on the estrogen receptor [33].

There is growing evidence that polyphenolic compounds may have anti-inflammatory effects. For example, the grape and wine component resveratrol inhibits adhesion molecule expression and monocyte adhesion in vitro [34].

10.10.3.3 Other Effects of Flavonoids

Because of their antioxidant and chelating properties, flavonoids inactivate reactive oxygen species (ROS) and this way counteract plasma LDL oxidation and ameliorate inflammation of the blood vessel endothelium. Furthermore, flavonoids decrease activity of xanthine oxidase, NADPH oxidase, and lipoxygenase, i.e., the enzymes that increase ROS production. Anti-arteriosclerotic action of flavonoids is related also to the reduction of inflammation in the blood vessel wall through inhibition of the influx of leucocytes. Flavonoids also decrease activity of such enzymes as 15-lipoxygenase (15-LOX) and cyclooxygenase (COX, particularly COX-2). These enzymes participate in formation of prostaglandins and leukotrienes, substances that mediate inflammation, from arachidonic acid. Decline in their secretion results in reduction of synthesis of prostaglandin PGE2, leukotriene B4, and thromboxane A2, what in turn leads to decrease in inflammation and platelet aggregation [35].

Beyond the protection of blood vessels against ox-LDL, anti-atheromatous action of flavonoids results also from suppression of 3-hydroxy-3-methylglutaryl-coenzyme A reductase (HMG-CoA) activity. This enzyme plays a key role in the synthesis of cholesterol in the human body, and thereby influences its plasma levels. Inhibition of its activity lowers intracellular cholesterol concentrations and results in the following increase in expression of LDL receptors. This in turn raises the cellular lipoprotein uptake and removal of cholesterol from the circulation. Hesperetin is a good example of a flavonoid, found in lemons and oranges, which reduces blood cholesterol level in the aforementioned way [36].

Improved endothelial function, antiplatelet effects, and anti-inflammatory effects are among the important mechanisms to be considered for the observed benefits of flavonoids on cardiovascular atheromatous disease. Overall, the findings of available studies fit well with the recommendations of the American Heart Association that Americans should increase their consumption of fresh fruit and vegetables and other foods with high polyphenol contents [37].

10.10.4 Flavonoids and Cancer

Numerous studies in animals have demonstrated the efficacy of some polyphenols in preventing cancer. Much attention, in this respect, has been focused on flavonoids. It seems that biologically active substances found in foodstuffs may affect such stages of carcinogenesis as initiation, promotion, and progression [38]. Numerous mechanisms of flavonoid action have been discovered. In the initiation and promotion stages, they include: inactivation of the carcinogen, inhibition of cell proliferation, enhancement of DNA repair processes, and reduction of oxidative stress. In the progression phase flavonoids may induce apoptosis, inhibit angiogenesis, and exhibit antioxidant activity and cytotoxic or cytostatic action against cancer cells [38–41].

Prevention of metabolic activation of pro-carcinogens appears to be related to flavonoid interaction with phase I enzymes that are responsible for metabolism of various endogenous or exogenous substrates. This results from the inhibition of the cytochrome P450 enzymes, such as CYP1A1 and CYP1A2. To note, P450 enzymes are involved in metabolizing numerous substances, including aromatic hydrocarbons and estradiol to potentially carcinogenic intermediates; moreover, it is overexpressed in human cancer cells. Flavonoids selectively inhibit CYP1 enzymes, and are thus useful as chemoprotective agents in cancer prevention. Flavonoids thus protect against cellular damage arising from the activation of carcinogenic factors. Another mechanism of their action is related to reinforcement of mutagen detoxification through induction of the phase II enzymes, such as glutathione S-transferase (GST) and UDP-glucuronyl transferase (UDP-GT), which detoxify and eliminate carcinogens from the body [39, 42].

The studies quoted above were performed in animals, and so the conclusions should be extrapolated to humans with caution. Observational studies conducted on various human populations have shown contrasting results [43–45].

The Iowa Women's Health Study [46] investigated the effect of dietary flavonoid consumption on the incidence of cancer of the lung, colon, breast, and pancreas in 34,708 postmenopausal women who were observed from 1986 to 2004. Their dietary habits were determined by means of a food frequency questionnaire. Results showed that regular flavonoid consumption significantly reduced the risk of the lung cancer, particularly in the women who had stopped smoking. However, there was no evident effect of flavonoid consumption on the risk of other cancers.

Another study, performed in 34,408 women (aged above 45 years), demonstrated no significant links between intake of foods rich in flavonoids and the risk of cancer [45].

Despite of these findings, a meta-analysis of 12 studies showed a reduced risk of breast cancer in women, especially postmenopausal, who consumed large amounts of flavonoids, such as flavonols and flavones [44]. Further studies are therefore required to assess the promising influence of flavonoids on the human body.

10.10.5 The Synergy of Phytochemicals

It should be emphasized that numerous epidemiological studies have consistently demonstrated that regular consumption of fruits and vegetables is associated with reduced risk of developing chronic diseases, such as cancer and cardiovascular disease. So, dietary modification by increasing the consumption of a wide variety of fruits, vegetables, and whole grains daily should be considered a practical strategy for consumers to optimize their health and to reduce the risk of chronic diseases.

The Cancer Formation and Progression [47]

Cancer proceeds through three stages: initiation, promotion, and progression.

The initiation stage takes place in a very short period of time, even minutes. It is the time required for the chemical carcinogen to be consumed, absorbed into the blood, transported into cells, changed into its active product, bonded to DNA, and passed on to the daughter cells. These daughter cells and all their progeny will forever be genetically damaged, giving rise to the potential for cancer. The completion of initiation phase is in most cases irreversible.

The second growth stage is called promotion stage. It takes place when newly formed cancer-prone cells are ready to grow and multiply until they become a visibly detectable cancer. This stage occurs over a far longer period of time than initiation, often many years. It is when the newly initiated cluster multiply and grows into larger masses. A clinically visible mass is formed. The promotion phase is reversible, depending on whether the early cancer growth is given the right conditions in which to grow. This is where certain dietary factors become so important. There are dietary factors called "promoters" that feed cancer growth. Other dietary factors called "anti-promoters" slow cancer growth. Cancer growth flourishes when there are more promoters than anti-promoters. When anti-promoters prevail, cancer growth slows or stops.

The third phase is the progression stage and begins when a bunch of advanced cancer cells progress in their growth until they have done their final damage. The developing cancer tumor wanders away from its initial site in the body and invades neighboring or distant tissues. When cancer breaks away from its initial home and wanders, it is metastasizing. This final stage of cancer results in death.

Phytochemical extracts from fruits and vegetables have demonstrated to have a strong antioxidant and antiproliferative activities in vitro. However, it is believed that the actions of the antioxidant nutrients alone do not explain the observed health benefits of diets rich in fruits and vegetables, because taken alone, the individual antioxidants studied in clinical trials have not demonstrated to have consistent preventive effects. Other studies however have shown that most antioxidant and antiproliferative activity is due to the combination of phytochemicals [48]. It has been suggested that the additive and synergistic effects of phytochemicals in fruits and vegetables are responsible for the antioxidant and anticancer activities and that these benefits should be actually attributed to the complex mixture of phytochemicals present in whole foods [48]. This explains why no single antioxidant can replace the combination of natural phytochemicals in fruits and vegetables to achieve the observed health benefits. The evidence suggests that antioxidants or bioactive compounds are best acquired through whole-food consumption, not from expensive dietary supplements. Eating 5 to 10 servings of a wide variety of fruits and vegetables daily is an appropriate strategy for significantly reducing the risk of chronic diseases and to meet the nutrient requirements for optimum health.

10.11 Dietary Fibers and Fresh Fruit

Dietary fibers are the second most important component of fresh fruit, besides phytochemical antioxidants. The role of dietary fibers has been described extensively in Chap. 9: Vegetables—Sect. 9.5.3.9: "Dietary fibers and intestine," this book.

Briefly, dietary fibers are the nondigestible carbohydrates and lignin that are intrinsic and intact in plants. Functional fibers consist of isolated, nondigestible carbohydrates that have beneficial physiologic effects in humans. Total fiber is the sum of dietary fibers and functional fibers. Dietary fibers are divided into water-soluble and water-insoluble (see table "Dietary Fiber (Types and Source)" in Chap. 9)

(1) Water-soluble fibers, which generally absorb water to become a gelatinous, viscous substance which is fermented by bacteria in the colon into gases and physiologically active by-products. Some, but not all, soluble plant fibers block intestinal mucosal adherence and translocation of potentially pathogenic bacteria and may therefore modulate intestinal inflammation, an effect that has been termed contrabiotic. (2) Water-insoluble fibers, which in general do not dissolve in water, are metabolically inert and provide bulking. Bulking fibers absorb water as they move through the digestive system, easing defecation. Some insoluble fibers, notably resistant starch (e.g., in potatoes), are fully fermented in the large intestine.

Advantages of consuming fiber are the production of healthful compounds during the fermentation of soluble fiber, and insoluble fiber's ability (via its passive hygroscopic properties) to increase bulk, soften stool, and shorten transit time through the intestinal tract. A disadvantage of a diet high in fiber is the potential for significant intestinal gas production and bloating.

Dietary fiber and undigested starch are the primary substrates for growth of the microflora in the large bowel. Thus the bulk associated with undigested residue contributes directly to stool bulk as undigested material or indirectly through the growth of microflora, which are a part of the stool weight.

Given the numerous benefit of dietary fiber, it is generally recommended that most men and women should get about 38 g and 25 g of dietary fiber a day, respectively. Older men and women typically need about 30 g and 21 g, respectively, according to the USDA. These general guidelines stem from the principle dietary recommendation that all individuals, regardless of age or gender, should eat 14 g of fiber for every 1000 calories consumed. An individual who averages 2200 calories a day, for example, should get about 31 g of fiber. One small apple supplies about 12% of the recommended amount of fiber.

References

1. U.S. Department of Agriculture. ChooseMyPlate.gov Website. Washington DC. Why is it Important to Eat Fruit?
2. Velasco R, Zharkikh A, Affourtit J, Dhingra A, Cestaro A, Kalyanaraman A, et al. The genome of the domesticated apple (Malus × domestica Borkh.). Nat Genet. 2010;42:833–9.
3. Chai SC, Hooshmand S, Saadat RL, Payton ME, Brummel-Smith K, Arjmandi BH. Daily apple versus dried plum: impact on cardiovascular disease risk factors in postmenopausal women. J Acad Nutr Diet. 2012;112:1158–68.
4. Gil MI, Tomàs-Barberàn FA, Hess-Pierce B, Kader AA. Antioxidant capacities, phenolic compounds, carotenoids, and vitamin C contents of nectarine, peach, and plum cultivars from California. J Agricol Food Chem. 2002;50:4976–82.
5. Johnston KL, Clifford MN, Morgan LM. Coffee acutely modifies gastrointestinal hormone secretion and glucose tolerance in humans: glycemic effects of chlorogenic acid and caffeine. Am J Clin Nutr. 2003;78:728–33.

6. McGovern PE. Ancient wine. The search for the origins of viniculture. Princeton, NJ: Princeton University Press; 2003.
7. Serrano M, Guillen F, Martınez-Romero D, Castillo S, Valero D. Chemical constituents and antioxidant activity of sweet cherry at different ripening stages. J Agric Food Chem. 2005;53:2741–5.
8. Ramis MR, Esteban S, Miralles A, Tan DX, Reiter RJ. Caloric restriction, resveratrol and melatonin: role of SIRT1 and implications for aging and related-diseases. Mech Ageing Dev. 2015;146–148:28–41.
9. Paredes SD, Korkmaz A, Manchester LC, Tan D-X, Reiter RJ. Phytomelatonin: a review. J Exp Bot. 2009;60:57–69.
10. Iriti M, Rossoni M, Faoro F. Melatonin content in grape: myth or panacea? *J Sci Food Agric.* 2006;86:1432–8.
11. Mercolini L, Addolorata Saracino M, Bugamelli F, Ferranti A, Malaguti M, Hrelia S, et al. HPLC-F analysis of melatonin and resveratrol isomers in wine using an SPE procedure. J Separ Sci. 2008;31:1007–114.
12. Vitalini S, Gardana C, Simonetti P, Fico G, Iriti M. Melatonin, melatonin isomers and stilbenes in Italian traditional grape products and their antiradical capacity. J Pineal Res. 2013;54:322–33.
13. Bonnefont-Rousselot D, Collin F. Melatonin: action as antioxidant and potential applications in human disease and aging. Toxicology. 2010;278:55–67.
14. Reiter RJ, Manchester LC, Tan D-X. Melatonin in walnuts: influence on levels of melatonin and total antioxidant capacity of blood. Nutrition. 2005;21:920–4.
15. Maldonado MD, Moreno H, Calvo JR. Melatonin present in beer contributes to increase the levels of melatonin and antioxidant capacity of the human serum. Clin Nutr. 2009;28:188–91.
16. Sae-Teaw M, Johns J, Johns NP, Subongkot S. Serum melatonin levels and antioxidant capacities after consumption of pineapple, orange, or banana by healthy male volunteers. J Pineal Res. 2013;55:58–64.
17. Nagata C, Nagao Y, Shibuya C, Kashiki Y, Shimizu H. Association of vegetable intake with urinary 6-sulfatoxymelatonin level. Cancer Epidemiol Biomark Prev. 2005;14:1333–5.
18. Oba S, Nakamura K, Sahashi Y, Hattori A, Nagata C. Consumption of vegetables alters morning urinary 6-sulfatoxymelatonin concentration. J Pineal Res. 2008;45:17–23.
19. Wu X, Beecher GR, Holden JM, Haytowitz DB, Gebhardt SE, Prior RL. Lipophilic and hydrophilic antioxidant capacities of common foods in the United States. J Agric Food Chem. 2004;52:4026–37.
20. de Pascual-Teresa S, Moreno DA, García-Viguera C. Flavanols and anthocyanins in cardiovascular health: a review of current evidence. Int J Mol Sci. 2010;11:1679–703.
21. Williams RJ, Spencer JP, Rice-Evans C. Flavonoids: antioxidants or signalling molecules? Free Radic Biol Med. 2004;36:838–49.
22. Song Y, Huang L, Yu J. Effects of blueberry anthocyanins on retinal oxidative stress and inflammation in diabetes through Nrf2/HO-1 signaling. J Neuroimmunol. 2016;301:1–6.
23. Stull AJ, Cash KC, Johnson WD, Champagne CM, Cefalu WT. Bioactives in blueberries improve insulin sensitivity in obese, insulin-resistant men and women. J Nutr. 2010; 140:1764–8.
24. Wedick NM, Pan A, Cassidy A, Rimm EB, Sampson L, Rosner B, Willett W, Hu FB, Sun Q, van Dam RM. Dietary flavonoid intakes and risk of type 2 diabetes in US men and women. Am J Clin Nutr. 2012;95:925–33.
25. Mink PJ, Scrafford CG, Barraj LM, et al. Flavonoid intake and cardiovascular disease mortality: a prospective study in postmenopausal women. Am J Clin Nutr. 2007;85:895–909.
26. Duffy SJ, Keaney JF Jr, Holbrook M, et al. Short- and long-term blacktea consumption reverses endothelial dysfunction in patients with coronary artery disease. Circulation. 2001;104:151–6.
27. Hodgson JM, Puddey IB, Burke V, Watts GF, Beilin LJ. Regular ingestion of black tea improves brachial artery vasodilator function. Clin Sci (Lond). 2002;102:195–201.

28. Stein JH, Keevil JG, Wiebe DA, Aeschlimann S, Folts JD. Purple grape juice improves endothelial function and reduces the susceptibility of LDL cholesterol to oxidation in patients with coronary artery disease. Circulation. 1999;100:1050–5.
29. Chou EJ, Keevil JG, Aeschlimann S, Wiebe DA, Folts JD, Stein JH. Effect of ingestion of purple grape juice on endothelial function in patients with coronary heart disease. Am J Cardiol. 2001;88(5):553.
30. Heiss C, Dejam A, Kleinbongard P, Schewe T, Sies H, Kelm M. Vascular effects of cocoa rich in flavan-3-ols. JAMA. 2003;290:1030–1.
31. Demrow HS, Slane PR, Folts JD. Administration of wine and grape juice inhibits in vivo platelet activity and thrombosis in stenosed canine coronary arteries. Circulation. 1995;91:1182–8.
32. Hodgson JM, Puddey IB, Mori TA, Burke V, Baker RI, Beilin LJ. Effects of regular ingestion of black tea on haemostasis and cell adhesion molecules in humans. Eur J Clin Nutr. 2001;55:881–6.
33. Squadrito F, Altavilla D, Morabito N, et al. The effect of the phytoestrogen genistein on plasma nitric oxide concentrations, endothelin-1 levels and endothelium dependent vasodilation in postmenopausal women. Atherosclerosis. 2002;163:339–47.
34. Carluccio MA, Siculella L, Ancora MA, et al. Olive oil and red wine antioxidant polyphenols inhibit endothelial activation: antiatherogenic properties of Mediterranean diet phytochemicals. Arterioscler Thromb Vasc Biol. 2003;23:622–9.
35. Kozłowska A, Szostak-Wegierek D. Flavonoids-food sources and health benefits. Rocz Panstw Zakl Hig. 2014;65:79–85.
36. Majewska-Wierzbicka M, Czeczot H. Flavonoids in the prevention and treatment of cardiovascular diseases. Pol Merk Lek. 2012;32:50–4.
37. Krauss RM, Eckel RH, Howard B, et al. AHA dietary guidelines, revision 2000: a statement for healthcare professionals from the Nutrition Committee of the American Heart Association. Circulation. 2000;102:2284–99.
38. Olejnik A, Tomczyk J, Kowalska K, Grajek W. The role of natural dietary compounds in colorectal cancer chemoprevention. Postępy Hig Med Dosw. 2010;64:175–87.
39. Chahar MK, Sharma N, Dobhal MP, Joshi YC. Flavonoids: a versatile source of anticancer drugs. Pharmacogn Rev. 2011;5:1–12.
40. Majewski G, Lubecka-Pietruszewska K, Kaufman-Szymczak A, Fabianowska-Majewska K. Anticarcinogenic capabilities of plant polyphenols: flavonoids and stilbene. Pol J Public Health. 2012;122:434–9.
41. Zalega J, Szostak-Węgierek D. Nutrition in cancer prevention. Part I. Plant polyphenols, carotenoids, dietary fiber. Probl Hig Epidemiol. 2013;94:41–9.
42. Krajka-Kuźniak V. Induction of phase II enzymes as a strategy in the chemoprevention of cancer and other degenerative diseases. Postępy Hig Med Dosw. 2007;61:627–38.
43. Dong H, Lin W, Jing W, Taosheng C. Flavonoids activate pregnane x receptor-mediated CYP3A4 gene expression by inhibiting cyclin-dependent kinases in HepG2 liver carcinoma cells. BMC Biochem. 2010;11:23.
44. Hui C, Qi X, Xiaoli P, Jundong Z, Mantian M. Flavonoids, flavonoid subclasses and brest cancer risk: a meta-analysis of epidemiologic studies. PLoS One. 2013;8:e54318.
45. Wang L, Lee I, Zhang SM, Blumberg JB, Buringj E, Sesso HD. Dietary intake of selected flavonols, flavones, and flavonoid-rich foods and risk of cancer in middle-aged and older women. Am J Clin Nutr. 2009;89:905–12.
46. Cutler GJ, Nettleton JA, Ross JA, Harnack LJ, Jacobs DR, Scrafford CG, Barraj LM, Mink PJ, Robien K. Dietary flavonoid intake and risk of cancer in postmenopausal women: The Iowa Women's Health Study. Int J Cancer. 2008;123:664–71.
47. Colin Campbell T, Capbell TM II. The China Study. Dallas, TX: BenBella Books; 2006.
48. Liu RH. Potential synergy of phytochemicals in cancer prevention: mechanism of action. J Nutr. 2004;134(12 Suppl):3479S–85S.

Nuts

11

11.1 Premises

The nuts are fruits composed of a hard shell and a seed, which is generally edible. In a general context, however, a wide variety of dried seeds are called nuts, but in a botanical context, there is an additional requirement that the shell does not open to release the seed.

Most seeds come from fruits that naturally free themselves from the shell, unlike nuts such as hazelnuts and chestnuts, which have hard shell walls and originate from a compound ovary. The general and original usage of the term is less restrictive, and many nuts (in the culinary sense), such as almonds, pecans, pistachios, walnuts, and Brazil nuts, are not nuts in a botanical sense. Common usage of the term often refers to any hard-walled, edible kernel as a nut.

Nuts are the source of energy and nutrients for the new plant (see Table 11.1). They contain a relatively large quantity of calories, essential unsaturated and monounsaturated fats including linoleic acid and linolenic acid, vitamins, and essential amino acids. Many nuts are good sources of vitamin E, vitamin B_2, folate, fiber, and the essential minerals magnesium, phosphorus, potassium, copper, and selenium. Nuts are most healthy in their raw unroasted form, because roasting can significantly damage and destroy fats during the process. Unroasted walnuts have twice as many antioxidants as other nuts or seeds.

Walnuts are the best source of polyunsaturated fats (linoleic and linolenic acid), while pistachios and peanuts are the best source of proteins (23–25 g%). Almonds

Table 11.1 Percentage of various nutrients in five unroasted nuts

Name	Protein	Total fat	PUFA	MUFA	Carbohydrate
Walnuts	15.23	65.21	47.17	8.933	19.56
Almonds	21.26	50.64	3.881	32.15	28.10
Peanuts	23.68	49.66	6.893	24.64	26.66
Pistachio	25.30	54.70	16.45	28.31	34.95
Hazelnut	14.95	60.75	7.80	45.00	16.70

PUFA = polyunsaturated fat, MUFA = monounsaturated fat

A. Capurso et al., *Benefits of the Mediterranean Diet in the Elderly Patient*, Practical Issues in Geriatrics, https://doi.org/10.1007/978-3-319-78084-9_11

are a good source of monounsaturated fats (32 g%) and proteins (21 g%). Hazelnut are a good source of MUFA (45 g%).

Nuts have been shown to have beneficial effects on health. They have been first linked to protection against myocardial infarction. In fact, people who consume nuts regularly are less likely to develop coronary heart disease. Moreover, regular nuts consumptions is associated with lower mortality from ischemic heart disease, cardiovascular disease and all causes [1]. Consumption of various nuts such as walnuts and almonds lowers serum cholesterol and LDL-cholesterol concentrations. The hypolipidemic response is essentially due to the high content of mono- and polyunsaturated fatty acids, i.e., n-9, n-6, and n-3 fatty acids [2].

11.2 Walnuts

11.2.1 History

Walnuts (*Juglans regia*) have a rich history dating back thousands of years. Walnuts are the oldest tree food known to man, dating back to 7000 B.C. The Romans called walnuts "Jupiter's royal acorn." Early history indicates that English walnuts came from ancient Persia, where they were reserved for royalty. Thus, the walnut is often known as the "Persian Walnut." Walnuts were traded along the Silk Road route between Asia and the Middle East. Caravans carried walnuts far off lands and eventually through sea trade, spreading the popularity of the walnut around the world. English merchant marines transported the product for trade to ports around the world and they became known as "English Walnuts." England, in fact, never grew walnuts commercially. The outer shell provided a natural protective layer helping to maintain the quality of the nut.

In California, the walnut was first cultivated by the Franciscan Fathers in the late 1700s. The earliest walnuts to enter California were known as "mission" walnuts. Unlike today's walnuts, these first entries were small with hard shells. The trees flourished in the Mediterranean-like climate zones of California, and by the 1870s modern walnut production had begun with orchard plantings in southern California, near Santa Barbara. In the next 70 years the center of California's walnut production shifted with successful plantings in the central and northern parts of the state.

11.2.2 Nutrients and Phytochemicals

Walnuts without shells are 4% water, 15% protein, 65% fat, and 14% carbohydrates, including 7% dietary fiber (see table "**Walnut**"). In a 100 g serving, walnuts provide 2740 kilojoules (654 kcal) and a rich content (more than 19% of the Daily Value or DV) of several dietary minerals, particularly manganese at 163% DV, and B vitamins (see table "**Walnut**"). Among the fruits and nuts, walnuts are the richest in manganese.

Unlike most nuts that are high in monounsaturated fatty acids, walnut oil is composed largely of polyunsaturated fatty acids (72% of total fats), particularly 14% alpha-linolenic acid (a n-3 fatty acid) and 58% linoleic acid (a n-6 fatty acid), but it does contain also oleic acid (a n-9 fatty acid) as 13% of total fats.

Walnut fresh hull contains polyphenols. Seven phenolic compounds, including ferulic acid, vanillic acid, coumaric acid, syringic acid, myricetin, and juglone, have been identified in walnut husks. Juglone, the predominant phenolic, was found in concentrations of 2–4% fresh weight. Walnuts also contain ellagitannin pedunculagin. Juglone, regiolone, betulinic acid, and sitosterol have been isolated from the stem bark of *J. regia* [3, 4].

11.2.3 Bioactive Compounds of Walnuts

Walnuts have been extensively studied mostly for their cardiovascular disease prevention effects, due to their elevated content in polyunsaturated fatty acids (see also Chap. 8, Sect. 8.6.4.2, this book). Walnuts contain also polyphenols, whose numerous effects have been discussed in other chapters of this book. However, Juglone and ellagic acid, two polyphenols contained in high quantity in walnuts deserve a mention.

Juglone is generally extracted from the husk of walnut fruit of which it contains 2–4% by fresh weight. Juglone is an allelopathic compound, a substance that is produced by a plant to stunt the growth of another. Landscapers have long known that gardening underneath or near black walnut trees can be difficult. This polyphenol exerts its effect by inhibiting certain enzymes needed for metabolic function. Juglone is currently being studied for its anticancer properties. One of the potential pathways through which juglone achieves its anticancer properties is through the formation of the semiquinone radical; the semiquinone radical causes superoxide anion radicals to form which can lead to apoptosis when present in large concentrations [5]. This conversion from juglone to semiquinone radical that causes the superoxide anion radical to form takes place in the mitochondria as well as the cytosol [6].

Ellagic acid (EA) is a polyphenol found in nuts and other fruits including berries, pomegranates, and grapes. EA has been investigated extensively because of its antiproliferative action in some cancers, along with its anti-inflammatory effects. A growing body of evidence suggests that the intake of EA is effective in attenuating obesity and ameliorating obesity-mediated metabolic complications, such as insulin resistance, type 2 diabetes, nonalcoholic fatty liver disease, and atherosclerosis [7].

Walnut

Nutritional value per 100 g

Source: USDA National Nutrient Data base

Energy	2738 KJ (654 kcal)
Carbohydrates	13.71 g
Sugars	2.61 g
Dietary fiber	6.70 g

Fat	65.21 g	
Saturated	6.126 g	
Monounsaturated	8.933 g	
Polyunsaturated	47.17 g	
Omega-3 (linolenic) 9.08 g		
Omega-6 (linoleic)	38.09 g	
Protein	15.23 g	
Essential amino acids		
Histidine	0.391 g	(56%)
Isoleucine	0.625 g	(45%)
Leucine	1.170 g	(43%)
Lysine	0.424 g	(20%)
Methionine	0.236 g	
Phenylalanine	0.711 g	
Threonine	0.596 g	(57%)
Tryptophan	0.170 g	(61%)
Valine	0.753 g	(41%)
Nonessential amino acids		
Arginine	2.278 g	
Alanine	0.696 g	
Aspartate	1.829 g	
Cystine	0.208 g	
Glutamate	2.816 g	
Glycine	0.816 g	
Proline	0.706 g	
Serine	0.934 g	
Tyrosine	0.406 g	
Vitamins		
Vitamin A equiv.	1 μg	(0% DV)
β-Carotene	12 μg	(0% DV)
Lutein zeaxanthin	9 μg	
Vitamin A	20 IU	
Thiamine (B_1)	0.341 mg	(30% DV)
Riboflavin (B_2)	0.15 mg	(13% DV)
Niacin (B_3)	1.125 mg	(8% DV)
Pantothenic acid (B_5)	0.570 mg	(11% DV)
Vitamin B_6	0.537 mg	(41% DV)
Folate (B_9)	98 μg	(25% DV)
Vitamin B_{12}	0 μg	(0% DV)
Vitamin C	1.3 mg	(2% DV)
Vitamin E	0.7 mg	(5% DV)
Vitamin K	2.7 μg	(3% DV)
Minerals		
Calcium	98 mg	(10% DV)
Iron	2.91 mg	(22% DV)
Magnesium	158 mg	(45% DV)
Manganese	3.414 mg	(163% DV)
Phosphorus	346 mg	(49% DV)
Potassium	441 mg	(9% DV)
Sodium	2 mg	(0% DV)
Zinc	3.09 mg	(33% DV)

DV = Daily Value

11.2.4 The Health Benefits of Walnuts

Having evaluated the scientific literature on the potential health value of consuming walnuts, the US Food and Drug Administration (FDA) provided guidance described as a *Qualified Health Claim* to manufacturers for labeling of food and dietary supplement products, stating: "*Supportive but not conclusive research shows that eating 1.5 ounces per day of walnuts, as part of a low saturated fat and low cholesterol diet and not resulting in increased caloric intake, may reduce the risk of coronary heart disease.*" [8].

The husks of the black walnut *Juglans nigra* were once used to make an ink for writing and drawing, having been used by artists including Leonardo da Vinci and Rembrandt.

Walnut husk pigments are used as a brown dye for fabric as once applied in classical Rome and medieval Europe for dyeing hair.

11.2.5 Briefly

Walnuts in an important nutrient due to its high content of unsaturated fats reaching 65% of the whole hull. Due to the high content in unsaturated fatty acids, the regular use of walnuts has been shown to reduce significantly total serum cholesterol and LDL cholesterol, as well as the risk of acute myocardial infarction and mortality for cardiovascular disease and all causes. Its regular use should be recommended to aging people, particularly to undernourished ones. However, due to the high content of the polyunsaturated linoleic acid (45%), walnuts should be associated to an antioxidant-rich Mediterranean diet, to prevent lipid peroxide formation and consequently LDL oxidation.

11.3 Almonds

The almond (*Prunus dulcis*, syn. *Prunus amygdalus*) is a species of tree native to the Middle East, the Indian Subcontinent and North Africa. Almond is also the name of the edible and widely cultivated seed of this tree. Within the genus *Prunus*, it is classified with the peach in the subgenus *Amygdalus*. The fruit of the almond is a drupe, consisting of an outer hull and a hard shell with the seed, which is not a true nut, inside. Shelling almonds refers to removing the shell to reveal the seed. Almonds are sold shelled or unshelled. Blanched almonds are shelled almonds that have been treated with hot water to soften the seed coat, which is then removed to reveal the white embryo.

11.3.1 History

The almond is native to the Mediterranean climate region of the Middle East, eastward as far as the Yamuna River in India. In Iran, India, Pakistan, Afghanistan, Azerbaijan, and other Central Asian countries, it is known as *bādām*. It was spread by humans in ancient times along the shores of the Mediterranean into northern Africa and southern Europe, and more recently transported to other parts of the world, notably California, United States.

Almonds were one of the earliest domesticated fruit trees due to the ability of the grower to raise attractive almonds from seed. Domesticated almonds appear in the Early Bronze Age (3000–2000 BC) such as the archaeological sites of Numeria (Jordan), or possibly a little earlier. Another well-known archaeological example of the almond is the fruit found in Tutankhamun's tomb in Egypt (c.1325 BC), probably imported from the Levant.

11.3.2 Sweet and Bitter Almonds

The seeds of *Prunus dulcis* var. *dulcis* are predominantly sweet but some individual trees produce seeds that are somewhat more bitter. The fruits from *Prunus dulcis* var. *amara* are always bitter, as are the kernels from other *Prunus* species, such as peach and cherry. The bitter almond contains the enzyme emulsin which, in the presence of water, acts on soluble glucosides, amygdalin and prunasin, yielding glucose, cyanide, and the essential oil of bitter almonds, which is nearly pure benzaldehyde, the chemical causing the bitter flavor. Bitter almonds may yield from 4–9 mg of hydrogen cyanide per almond and contain 42 times higher amounts of cyanide than the trace levels found in sweet almonds. The origin of cyanide content in bitter almonds is via the enzymatic hydrolysis of amygdalin.

Extract of bitter almond was once used medicinally but even in small doses, effects are severe or lethal, especially in children; the cyanide must be removed before consumption. The acute oral lethal dose of cyanide for adult humans is reported to be 0.5–3.5 mg/kg of body weight (approximately 50 bitter almonds), whereas for children, consuming 5–10 bitter almonds may be fatal [9].

11.3.3 Nutrients and Phytochemicals

11.3.3.1 Oil

Almonds are a rich source of oil, with 50% of kernel dry mass as fat (see table "**Almonds, Raw**"). Almond oil contains 32% monounsaturated oleic acid (an n-9 fatty acid), 13% linoleic acid (a polyunsaturated n-6 essential fatty acid), and 5% saturated fatty acid. Linolenic acid, a polyunsaturated n-3 fat, is not present. Almond oil is also a rich source of vitamin E providing 261% of the Daily Value per 100 mL (see table "**Almonds, Raw**").

The almond oil is frequently used for application to the skin as emollient, and has been traditionally used by massage therapists to lubricate the skin during a massage session.

11.3.3.2 Proteins

Almonds are also a rich source of proteins and amino acids. With 21.22 g of proteins per 100 g, almonds are second only to peanuts and pistachios, which contain 24 g% and 25 g% proteins, respectively. Almonds contain also relevant amount of several vitamins and minerals (see table "**Almonds, Raw**"), particularly magnesium, manganese, and phosphorus.

11.3.3.3 Fibers

Almonds are high in soluble and insoluble fiber, which makes up to 12.5% of their weight. Advantages of fiber are: (1) the production of healthful compounds during the fermentation of soluble fiber, and (2) insoluble fiber's ability (via its passive hygroscopic properties) to increase bulk, soften stool, and shorten transit time through the intestinal tract. A disadvantage of a diet high in fiber is the potential for significant intestinal gas production and bloating. Fiber also helps moderate blood sugar by slowing absorption of carbohydrates. It has many other benefits as well, such as improved digestive health (see also Chap. 10, Sect. 10.11: "Dietary Fibers and Fresh Fruit").

11.3.3.4 Antioxidants: Impact on Health

Almonds are also rich in antioxidants, i.e., resveratrol (a stilbene contained mostly in grapes and red wine), kaempferol, quercetin, catechin, and epicatechin (see also Chap. 10, Figs. 10.2 and 10.3).

Resveratrol: This antioxidant polyphenol found in a number of plant-based foods such as red wine and grapes has received a great deal of attention for its diverse array of healthful effects. Beneficial effects of resveratrol include improvement of mitochondrial function, protection against obesity and obesity-related diseases such as type-2 diabetes, suppression of inflammation and cancer cell growth, and protection against cardiovascular dysfunction [10]. In insects, resveratrol has been found to be involved in life span duration, through interaction with sirtuins (see also Chap. 14: "Red and White Wine").

Epicatechin: This flavonoid helps in reducing some CVD risk factors. In a study on thirty-seven healthy men and women, daily supplementation with 100 mg epicatechin for 4 weeks improved plasma insulin and insulin resistance, but no effects on plasma glucose [11].

Kaempferol: Epidemiological studies have shown an inverse relationship between kaempferol intake and cancer. Kaempferol, a flavonoid phytoestrogen (plant estrogen) found in grapes, broccoli, and yellow fruits as well as in almonds, has been demonstrated to increase the body's antioxidant defense against free radicals, which promote the development of cancer. At the molecular level, kaempferol has been reported to modulate a number of key elements in cellular signal transduction pathways linked to apoptosis, angiogenesis, inflammation, and metastasis. Significantly, kaempferol inhibits cancer cell growth and angiogenesis and induces cancer cell apoptosis, but on the other hand, kaempferol appears to preserve normal cell viability, in some cases exerting a protective effect [12, 13].

Quercetin: In a study of 12 weeks on mice fed a high-fat diet (HF), the weight gain induced by HF was significantly lowered by several flavonoids (17–29%), but mostly by quercetin. Quercetin significantly lowered HF-induced hepatic lipid accumulation (71%), mesenteric adipose tissue weight, and serum leptin [14].

Many of the antioxidants in almonds are concentrated in the skin. Therefore, almonds should be eaten with the skin to maximize the health benefits. The combination of high content of vitamin E and antioxidants in almonds is particularly active, having synergistic effects against lipids oxidation [15]. The almond skin flavonoid bioactivity in fact was assessed in vitro by their capacity to increase the resistance of human LDL to oxidation induced by 10 micromol/L Cu^{2+}. Combining almond skin flavonoids with vitamin E or ascorbic acid extended the lag time > 200% of the expected additive value [15].

To note, almonds are susceptible to aflatoxin-producing molds. Aflatoxins are potent carcinogenic chemicals produced by moulds such as *Aspergillus flavus* and *Aspergillus parasiticus.* The mold contamination may occur from soil, previously infested almonds, and almond pests such as navel-orange worm. High levels of mold growth typically appear as gray to black filament like growth. It is unsafe to eat mold infected tree nuts.

Almonds, Raw

Nutritional value per 100 g

Source: USDA National Nutrient Data base

Energy	2408 KJ (576 kcal)
Carbohydrates	21.69
Sugars	3.89
Dietary fiber	12.2

Fat	49.42 g
Saturated	3.731 g
Monounsaturated	30.88 g
Polyunsaturated	12.07 g
Omega-3 (linolenic)	0 g
Omega-6 (linoleic)	12.07 g

Protein	21.22 g
Tryptophan	0.214 g
Threonine	0.598 g
Isoleucine	0.702 g
Leucine	1.488 g
Lysine	0.580 g
Methionine	0.151 g
Cystine	0.189 g
Phenylalanine	1.120 g
Tyrosine	0.452 g

Protein	21.22 g
Valine	0.817 g
Arginine	2.446 g
Histidine	0.557 g
Alanine	1.027 g
Aspartic acid	2.911 g
Glutamic acid	6.810 g
Glycine	1.469 g
Proline	1.032 g
Serine	0.948

Vitamins		
Vitamin A equiv.	1 μg	(0% DV)
β-Carotene	1 μg	(0% DV)
Vitamin A	1 IU	
Thiamine (B_1)	0.211 mg	(18% DV)
Riboflavin (B_2)	1.014 mg	(85% DV)
Niacin (B_3)	3.385 mg	(23% DV)
Pantothenic acid (B_5)	0.469 mg	(9% DV)
Vitamin B_6	0.143 mg	(11% DV)
Folate (B_9)	50 μg	(13% DV)
Vitamin B_{12}	0 μg	(0% DV)
Vitamin C	0 mg	(0% DV)
Vitamin D	0 μg	(0% DV)
Vitamin E	26.2 mg	(175% DV)
Vitamin K	0 μg	(0% DV)

Minerals		
Calcium	264 mg	(26% DV)
Iron	3.72 mg	(29% DV)
Magnesium	268 mg	(75% DV)
Manganese	2.285 mg	(109% DV)
Phosphorus	484 mg	(69% DV)
Potassium	705 mg	(15% DV)
Sodium	1 mg	(0% DV)
Zinc	3.08 mg	(32% DV)

DV = Daily Value

11.4 Peanuts

Peanut is a legume grown mainly for its edible seeds. As a legume, the peanut belongs to the botanical family of *Fabaceae*. This family is also known as *Leguminosae*, and commonly known as the *bean*, or *pea*, family. Therefore, the peanut is not a true nut, but rather a legume. However, for culinary purposes and in common English language usage, peanuts are usually referred to as nuts.

11.4.1 History

The use of peanuts dates to the Aztecs and Incas [16]. The oldest known archeological remains of pods have been dated at about 7600 years old. The initial domestication may have taken place in north western Argentina, or in south-eastern Bolivia, where the peanut landraces with the most wild-like features are grown today. From this primary center of origin, cultivation spread and formed secondary and tertiary centers of diversity in Peru, Ecuador, Brazil, Paraguay, and Uruguay.

Many pre-Columbian cultures, such as the Moche, depicted peanuts in their art. Cultivation was well established in Mesoamerica before the Spanish arrived. There, the conquistadors found the "*tlalcacahuatl*" being offered for sale in the marketplace of Tenochtitlan. The peanut was later spread worldwide by European traders, and cultivation is now very widespread in tropical and subtropical regions.

11.4.2 Nutrients and Phytochemicals

Peanuts are used to help fight malnutrition. Plumpy Nut, MANA Nutrition, and Medika Mamba are high-protein, high-energy, and high-nutrient peanut-based pastes developed to be used as a therapeutic food to aid in famine relief. The World Health Organization UNICEF, Project Peanut Butter, and Doctors Without Borders have used these products to help save malnourished children in developing countries.

Due to their high content in proteins (~25 g per cent), peanuts were used to improve childhood malnutrition among the poor in Philippines, in a decennial project funded by the U.S. Agency for International Development and developed by Virginia Tech in the sixties [17]. Peanuts were chosen because of their high content of protein, in substitution of animal proteins that were not available in that very poor country.

Peanuts are also rich in essential nutrients (see table "**Peanut, Raw**"). In a 100 g serving, peanuts provide 570 calories and are an excellent source (defined as more than 20% of the Daily Value, DV) of several B vitamins, vitamin E, several dietary minerals, such as manganese (95% DV), magnesium (52% DV), and phosphorus (48% DV), and dietary fiber. They also contain about 25 g protein per 100 g serving, a higher proportion than in many tree nuts.

Some studies have shown that regular consumption of peanuts is associated with a lower risk of mortality specifically from certain diseases. According to the US Food and Drug Administration, "*Scientific evidence suggests but does not prove that eating 1.5 ounces per day of most nuts (such as peanuts) as part of a diet low in saturated fat and cholesterol may reduce the risk of heart disease*" [18].

Peanuts contain polyphenols, polyunsaturated and monounsaturated fats, phytosterols, and dietary fiber in amounts similar to several tree nuts [19]. Peanut skins contain resveratrol which is under preliminary research for its potential effects in humans.

From peanuts an excellent oil rich in unsaturated fatty acid is obtained. This oil is 46% monounsaturated fats (primarily oleic acid), 32% polyunsaturated fats (primarily linoleic acid), and 17% saturated fats (primarily palmitic acid). The peanut oil is being considered by NASA's Advanced Life Support program for future long-duration human space missions.

A very popular product of peanuts is the peanut butter. Peanut butter is a food paste popular in many countries, a spread made primarily from ground dry roasted peanuts, but often containing additional ingredients that modify the taste or texture. The United States is a leading exporter and itself consumes $800 million of peanut butter annually. Peanut butter is a source of saturated (primarily palmitic acid) and unsaturated fats (primarily oleic and linoleic acids), and an excellent source (>19% of the Daily Value, DV) of protein, dietary fiber, vitamin E, pantothenic cid, niacin, and vitamin B_6.

11.4.3 Contamination with Aflatoxin

If peanut plants are subjected to severe drought during pod formation, or if pods are not properly stored, they may become contaminated with the mold *Aspergillus flavus* which may produce carcinogenic substances called "*aflatoxin*." Lower-quality peanuts, particularly where mold is evident, are more likely to be contaminated. The United States Department of Agriculture tests every truckload of raw peanuts for aflatoxin; any containing aflatoxin levels of more than 15 parts per billion are destroyed. The peanut industry has manufacturing steps in place to ensure all peanuts are inspected for aflatoxin.

Aflatoxin has been demonstrated to cause liver cancer, and this cancer was found to kill numerous Philippine's children in the sixties.

Peanut, Raw
Nutritional value per 100 g
Source: USDA National Nutrient Data base

Energy	2385 KJ (570 kcal)
Carbohydrates	21
Sugars	0.0
Dietary fiber	9 g

Fat	48 g
Saturated	7 g
Monounsaturated	24 g
Polyunsaturated	16 g
Omega-3 (linolenic)	0 g
Omega-6 (linoleic)	15.56 g

Protein	25 g
Tryptophan	0.244 g
Threonine	0.859 g

Protein	25 g
Isoleucine	0.882 g
Leucine	1.627 g
Lysine	0.901 g
Methionine	0.308 g
Cystine	0.322 g
Phenylalanine	1.300 g
Tyrosine	1.020 g
Valine	1.052 g
Arginine	3.001 g
Histidine	0.634 g
Alanine	0.997 g
Aspartic acid	3.060 g
Glutamic acid	5.243 g
Glycine	1.5121 g
Proline	1.107 g
Serine	1.236 g

Vitamins		
Thiamine (B_1)	0.6 mg	(52% DV)
Riboflavin (B_2)	0.3 mg	(25% DV)
Niacin (B_3)	12.9 mg	(83% DV)
Pantothenic acid (B_5)	1.8 mg	(36% DV)
Vitamin B_6	0.3 mg	(23% DV)
Folate (B_9)	246 μg	(62% DV)
Vitamin B_{12}	0 μg	(0% DV)
Vitamin C	0 mg	(0% DV)
Vitamin D	0 μg	(0% DV)
Vitamin E	6.6 mg	(44% DV)
Vitamin K	0 μg	(0% DV)

Minerals		
Calcium	62 mg	(6% DV)
Iron	2 mg	(15% DV)
Magnesium	184 mg	(52% DV)
Manganese	2.0 mg	(95% DV)
Phosphorus	336 mg	(48% DV)
Potassium	332 mg	(7% DV)
Sodium	0 mg	(0% DV)
Zinc	3.08 mg	(32% DV)

DV = Daily Value

11.5 Hazelnuts

Hazelnut, the nut of the hazel, is also known as cobnut of filbert nut. The kernel of the seed is edible and used raw or roasted, or ground into a paste. Hazelnut are used in confectionery to make praline, or used in combination with chocolate for chocolate truffles and products such as *Nutella*.

Hazelnuts are rich in protein, monounsaturated fat, vitamin E, manganese, and numerous other essential nutrients.

11.5.1 History

In 1995, evidence of a large scale Mesolithic nut processing was found in a midden pit on the island of Colonsay in Scotland. In a large shallow pit a great quantity of remains of hundreds of thousands of burned hazelnut shells was found. The nuts were radiocarbon dated to circa 7000 BC.

The Romans cultivated hazelnuts, although no evidence indicates they spread specific cultivars. Cultivated varieties have been grown since at least the sixteenth century, with a great increase in varieties during the 1800s. In particular, the first really widespread cultivar, the "Kentish Cobnut," was introduced in 1830.

11.5.2 Nutrients and Phytochemicals

In a 100-g serving, raw hazelnuts supply 2630 kilojoules (628 kcal) and are a rich source (20% or more of the Daily Value, DV) of numerous essential nutrients (see table "**Hazelnut Or Filberts, Raw**"). Particularly in high amounts are protein, dietary fiber, vitamin E, thiamin, phosphorus, manganese, and magnesium, all exceeding 30% DV (see table "**Hazelnut Or Filberts, Raw**"). Several B vitamins have appreciable content. In lesser but still significant amounts (moderate content, 10–19% DV) are vitamin K, calcium, zinc, and potassium. Hazelnuts are a significant source of total fat, accounting for 93% DV in a 100-g serving. The fat components are monounsaturated fat as oleic acid (75% of total), polyunsaturated fat mainly as linoleic acid (13% of total), and saturated fat, mainly as palmitic acid and stearic acid (together, 7% of total) [20].

Fiber: Hazelnuts are rich in dietary fiber, 9.7 g per cent, corresponding to 25% of RDA.

Folate: These nuts are also exceptionally rich in folate, which is a unique feature for the nuts. 100 g fresh nuts carry 113 mg, corresponding to about 28% of the recommended daily intake of this vitamin. Folate is an important B-complex vitamin that helps prevent *megaloblastic anemia,* and most importantly, neural tube defects in the newborn.

Vitamin E: Hazelnuts are an excellent source of vitamin E, contain about 15 g per 100 g (providing 100% of RDA). Vitamin E is a powerful lipid soluble antioxidant required for maintaining the integrity of cell membrane of mucosa and skin by protecting it from oxygen-free radicals.

Minerals: Hazelnuts are rich source of minerals like manganese, potassium, calcium, copper, iron, magnesium, zinc, and selenium. One serving of hazelnuts supplies over 25% of the Daily Recommended Intake (DRI) for copper and more than 90% of the DRI for manganese. Copper is needed for iron absorption. Copper and manganese are essential cofactors for antioxidant enzyme, *superoxide dismutase*. Iron, a fundamental component of *heme*, helps prevent microcytic sideropenic anemia.

Antioxidants: Hazelnuts have the highest proanthocyanidin content of any tree nut. This polyphenol, in addition to being a potent antioxidant, is known for contributing astringent flavor to foods and reduces the risk of thrombosis and urinary tract infections. Other phenols are present in hazelnuts, mostly in the skin, i.e., caffeic acid and quercetin, which contribute to the antioxidant activity associated to hazelnut intake.

11.5.3 The CVD Risk Reduction

The consumption of hazelnut has been associated with a decreased risk of cardiovascular disease events. In a recent systematic review and meta-analysis [21] including nine studies and 425 participants, hazelnut-enriched diet (28–84 days with a dosage of hazelnuts ranging from 29 to 69 g/day) was associated with a decrease of LDL and total cholesterol, while HDL cholesterol, triglycerides, and BMI remained substantially unchanged.

Similar results have been observed in another study [22] on hamsters fed a high-fat diet who received for 8 weeks a hazelnut skin extract, the hazelnut component containing the antioxidant polyphenols. The consumption of hazelnut skin extract reversed the increase in total and LDL plasma cholesterol induced by the high-fat diet and decreased the circulating levels of free fatty acids and triglycerides. The higher excretion of bile acids found in the feces of hamsters fed the hazelnut skin extract suggested that this mechanism is involved in the cholesterol-lowering effects of the extract. A sharply decrease of the lithocholic/deoxycholic bile acid fecal ratio, a risk factor for colon cancer, was also observed [22].

Hazelnuts has been associated with CVD prevention because of their fatty acid composition, mostly based on monounsaturated fatty acids (MUFA), that when incorporated into LDL makes these lipoproteins resistant to oxidation. Moreover, hazelnuts are rich in various bioactive substances such as tocopherols and phytosterols, L-arginine selenium, caffeic acid, fibers, gallic acid, p-hydroxy benzoic acid, epicatechin, sinapic acid, and quercetin.

The antioxidant activity of non-tocopherol hazelnut phenolics, together with high content of monounsaturated fatty acids, is probably the principal factor that could have antiatherogenic effects by means of biological mechanisms acting on various pathways in CVD development [23].

Hazelnut Or Filberts, Raw
Nutritional value per 100 g
Source: USDA SR-21 and 28

Energy	2629 KJ (628 kcal)
Carbohydrates	19.2 g
Sugars	5.0 g
Dietary fiber	11.2 g

Fat	69.9 g	
Saturated	5.1 g	
Monounsaturated	52.5 g	
Polyunsaturated	9.1 g	
Omega-3 (linolenic)	0.100 g	
Omega-6 (linoleic)	9.007 g	

Protein	14.95 g	
Essential amino acids		
Tryptophan	194 mg	(69% DV)
Histidine	434 mg	(62% DV)
Threonine	499 mg	(48% DV)
Isoleucine	548 mg	(39% DV)
Leucine	1069 mg	(39% DV)
Lysine	422 mg	(20% DV)
Methionine	222 mg	(30% DV)
Cystine	278 mg	(97% DV)
Phenylalanine	667 mg	(76% DV)
Nonessential amino acids		
Arginine	2222 mg	
Alanine	733 mg	
Aspartic acid	1687 mg	
Glutamic acid	3728 mg	
Glycine	727 mg	
Proline	563 mg	
Serine	739 mg	

Vitamins		
Vitamin A equiv.	1 μg	(0% DV)
Beta-carotene	11 μg	(0% DV)
Lutein-zeaxanthin	92 μg	
Thiamine (B_1)	0.643 mg	(56% DV)
Riboflavin (B_2)	0.113 mg	(9% DV)
Niacin (B_3)	1.8 mg	(12% DV)
Pantothenic acid (B_5)	0.918 mg	(18% DV)
Vitamin B_6	0.563 mg	(43% DV)
Folate (B_9)	113 μg	(28% DV)
Vitamin B_{12}	0 μg	(0% DV)
Vitamin C	6.3 mg	(8% DV)
Vitamin D	0 μg	(0% DV)
Vitamin E	17.03 mg	(86% DV)
Vitamin K	14.2 μg	(26% DV)

Minerals		
Calcium	131 mg	(13% DV)
Iron	5.4 mg	(30% DV)
Magnesium	187 mg	(47% DV)
Manganese	7.1 mg	(355% DV)
Phosphorus	333 mg	(33% DV)
Potassium	782 mg	(22% DV)
Sodium	0 mg	(0% DV)
Zinc	2.8 mg	(19% DV)
Copper	2.0 mg	(99% DV)
Selenium	2.8 μg	(4% DV)
Phytosterols	110 mg	

DV = Daily Value

11.6 Pistachios

Pistachios are kernels obtained from fruits belonging to the *Anacardiaceae* family, in the genus *Pistacia*. The tree produces seeds that are widely consumed as food.

11.6.1 History

The history of pistachio is rooted in a very remote past. Remains of the Atlantic pistachio and pistachio seed along with nut-cracking tools were discovered by archaeologists at the *Gesher Benot Ya'aqov* site in Israel's Hula Valley dated to 780,000 years ago [24]. Archaeology shows that pistachio seeds were a common food as early as 6750 BC. *Pliny the Elder* writes in his *Natural History* that *pistacia*, "well known among us," was one of the trees unique to Syria, and that the seed was introduced into Italy by the Roman Proconsul in Syria, *Lucius Vitellius the Elder* (in office in 35 AD) and into Hispania at the same time by *Flaccus Pompeius*. The early sixth-century manuscript *De observatione ciborum* ("On the observance of foods") by *Anthimus* implies that *pistacia* remained well known in Europe in Late Antiquity. The Hanging Gardens of Babylon were said to have contained pistachio trees during the reign of King Merodach-Baladan about 700 BC.

More recently, the pistachio has been cultivated commercially in many parts of the English-speaking world, in Australia, and in New Mexico and California of the United States, where it was introduced in 1854 as a garden tree.

11.6.2 Nutrients and Phytochemicals

Pistachios are a nutritionally dense food. In a 100 g serving, pistachios provide 562 calories and are a rich source (~20% of the Daily Value of DV) of protein, dietary fiber, numerous dietary minerals and the B-vitamin thiamine and especially vitamin B_6 at 131% DV. Pistachios are also a good source of calcium, riboflavin, vitamin B_5, folate, vitamin E, and vitamin K (see table "**Pistachio Nuts, Raw**").

The fat profile of raw pistachios consists of saturated (palmitic acid 10% and stearic acid 2%), monounsaturated (oleic acid 51%), and polyunsaturated (linoleic acid 31%) fatty acids. Among nuts, pistachios have a lower fat and energy content and highest levels of oleic acid, vitamin K, certain minerals (Cu, Fe, and MG), gamma-tocopherol, and certain phytochemicals such as xanthophyll carotenoids and phytosterol [25, 26].

Pistachio Nuts, Raw
Nutritional value per 100 g
Source: USDA SR-21

Energy	2868 (685 Cal)
Carbohydrates	34.4 g
Sugars	7.66 g
Dietary fiber	12.7 g

Fat	50.7 g
Saturated	6.7 (12%) g
Monounsaturated	28.7 (60%) g
Polyunsaturated	16.6 (28%) g

Protein	25.3 g
Tryptophan	336 mg
Threonine	828 mg
Isoleucine	1107 mg
Leucine	1911 mg
Lysine	1416 mg
Methionine	416 mg
Cystine	439 mg
Phenylalanine	1306 mg
Tyrosine	510 mg
Valine	1524 mg
Arginine	2495 mg
Histidine	624 mg
Alanine	1133 mg
Aspartic acid	2235 mg
Glutamic acid	4697 mg
Glycine	1172 mg
Proline	999 mg
Serine	1507 mg

Vitamins		
Vitamin A equiv.	13 (266 IU) μg	(5% DV)
Beta-carotene	159 μg	(5% DV)
Thiamine (B_1)	0.87 mg	(76% DV)
Riboflavin (B_2)	0.160 mg	(13% DV)
Niacin (B_3)	1.8 mg	(11% DV)
Pantothenic acid (B_5)	0.918 mg	(18% DV)
Vitamin B_6	1.7 mg	(131% DV)
Folate (B_9)	113 μg	(28% DV)
Vitamin B_{12}	0 μg	(0% DV)
Vitamin C	5.6 mg	(7% DV)
Vitamin D	0 μg	(0% DV)
Vitamin E	2.3 mg	(15% DV)
Vitamin K	13.2 μg	(13% DV)

Minerals		
Calcium	132 mg	(13% DV)
Copper	1.6 mg	(80% DV)
Iron	5.12 mg	(30% DV)
Magnesium	121 mg	(34% DV)
Manganese	1.5 mg	(74% DV)
Phosphorus	603 mg	(60% DV)
Potassium	1261 mg	(36% DV)
Sodium	0 mg	(0% DV)
Zinc	2.7 mg	(18% DV)

DV = Daily Value

11.6.3 Health Impact

Several published randomized cardiovascular trials have shown that pistachios promote heart-healthy blood lipid profiles. Exploratory clinical studies suggest that pistachios help maintain healthy antioxidant and anti-inflammatory activity, glycemic control, and endothelial functions. When consumed in moderation, pistachios may help control body weight because of their satiety and satiation effects and their reduced net metabolizable energy content. One study with subjects in a weight-loss program demonstrated lower body mass index and triglyceride levels in individuals who consumed pistachios compared with those who consumed an isocaloric pretzel snack. Emerging research suggests that the addition of pistachios to high-glycemic meals may lower the overall postprandial glycemic response. Pistachios have also a high antioxidant and anti-inflammatory potential [26, 27].

Epidemiological and clinical trials have suggested the nut consumption has a beneficial impact on health outcomes such as hypertension, diabetes, CVD, cancer, other inflammatory conditions, and total mortality [27].

11.7 Nuts, Serum Lipid Profile, and Coronary Heart Disease Risk Factors

Numerous epidemiologic studies have consistently demonstrated an association between nut consumption and coronary heart disease (CHD) morbidity and mortality [28]. Compared with people who ate nuts <1 time/week, those who ate them 1–4 times/week experience an ~50% reduction in CVD risk [29]. The benefits of nuts have been acknowledged by the U.S. FDA when they approved a qualified health claim that eating nuts (1.5 oz/day, ~42.8 g/day) may reduce the risk of CHD [30].

Nuts have favorable effects on CHD through a variety of mechanisms. The most extensively studied mechanism involves the lipid-lowering effects. Nuts are a good source of unsaturated fatty acids, i.e., monounsaturated (MUFA) and polyunsaturated fatty acids (PUFA), known for their favorable effects on blood lipids. However, numerous evidences have suggested that components of nuts reduce total cholesterol (TC) and LDL cholesterol (LDL-C) concentrations beyond the effects predicted based solely on the fatty acid profiles. In particular, the magnitude of the cholesterol-lowering effects was shown to be 25% greater than would be predicted based on the fatty acid profile of the test diets studied [28]. Therefore, the possible mechanism whereby nuts may improve lipid profiles doesn't appear to rely exclusively on the beneficial action of unsaturated fatty acids MUFA and PUFA but likely include the effects of fiber, micronutrients such as vitamin E, C, folic acid, copper, magnesium, amino acids (e.g., arginine, aspartic acid, glutamic acid), plant sterols, and phenolic components [28].

In a systematic review [31], 23 studies were pooled to evaluate the impact of nuts on serum lipid profile. The results of three almond (50–100 g/day), two peanut (35–68 g/day), one pecan nut, (72 g/day), and four walnut (40–84 g/day) studies showed decreases in total cholesterol between 2% and 16% and LDL cholesterol between 2% and 19%, compared with subjects consuming control diets. This review concluded that consumption of ~50–100 g (~1.5–3.5 servings) of nuts ≥5 times/week as part of a heart-healthy diet with total fat content (high in MUFA and PUFA) of ~35% of energy may significantly decrease total cholesterol and LDL cholesterol in normo- and hyperlipidemic individuals.

11.8 Nuts and the PREDIMED Study Results

In the PREDIMED study, a recent trial based on Mediterranean diet, nuts have demonstrated to have an important role in the reduction of cardiovascular disease (CVD) events.

The PREDIMED (Prevenciòn con Dieta Mediterranea) study [32] was a multicenter, randomized, primary prevention trial in individuals at high risk of CVD, designed to assess the long-term effects of the Mediterranean diet (MeDiet) without any energy restriction on incident CVD. The primary end point was a composite of myocardial infarction, stroke, and death from cardiovascular causes. Secondary end points were stroke, myocardial infarction, death from cardiovascular causes, and death from any cause.

Participants were randomly assigned to three diet groups: (1) MeDiet supplemented with extra-virgin olive oil (EVOO); (2) MeDiet supplemented with nuts; and (3) control diet (advice on a low-fat diet). Participants in the MeDiet supplemented with nuts received 30 g of mixed nuts per day: 15 g of walnuts, 7.5 g of hazelnuts, and 7.5 g of almonds).

After 4.8 year, 288 major CVD events occurred in 7447 participants; crude hazard ratios were 0.70 (95% CI: 0.53, 0.91) for the MeDiet + EVOO and 0.70 (95% CI: 0.53, 0.94) for the MeDiet + nuts, compared with the control group. The results of multivariate analyses showed a similar protective effect of the two Mediterranean diets (supplemented with EVOO and nuts, respectively) versus the control diet with respect to the primary end point. However, as far as the single components of the primary end point was concerned, only the comparisons of stroke risk reached statistical significance (*P* value: 0.005).

The most evident reduction in cardiovascular disease in the PREDIMED study therefore was that of stroke, an outcome that is exceedingly dependent on blood pressure. This result is concordant with those of observational studies, which have shown that Mediterranean style diets and olive oil are associated with reduced risk of stroke [33–35]. Previously, the PREDIMED investigators reported that, at 3 months after randomization, the group receiving extra-virgin olive oil and the group receiving mixed nuts had substantially lowered blood pressure [36]. Indeed, reductions in blood pressure probably contributed to observed reductions in cardiovascular disease, particularly of stroke. So, in the context of a Mediterranean-style diet, increased consumption of mixed nuts or substitution of regular olive oil with extra-virgin olive oil promotes additional beneficial effects on cardiovascular disease.

The PREDIMED study showed also beneficial effects of the MeDiet supplemented with EVOO or nuts on diabetes and metabolic syndrome. In fact, the respective hazard ratios for incident diabetes (273 cases) among 3541 participants without diabetes were 0.60 (95% CI: 0.43, 0.85) and 0.82 (95% CI: 0.61, 1.10) compared with the control group. After 1-year follow-up, participants in the MeDiet + nuts group showed a significant 13.7% reduction in prevalence of metabolic syndrome compared with reductions of 6.7% and 2.0% in the MeDiet + EVOO and control group, respectively.

Analyses of intermediate markers of CVD risk demonstrated beneficial effects of the MeDiet supplemented with EVOO or nuts on blood pressure, lipid profiles, lipoprotein particles, inflammation, oxidative stress, and carotid atherosclerosis, as well as on the expression of proatherogenic genes involved in vascular events and thrombosis.

In nutrigenomic studies beneficial effects of the intervention with MedDiet supplemented with EVOO or nuts showed interactions with several genetic variants (TCF7L2, APOA2, MLXIPL, LPL, FTO, M4CR, COX-2, GCKR, and SERPINE1) with respect to intermediate and final phenotypes [37].

Thus, the PREDIMED trial provided strong evidence that a vegetable-based MeDiet rich in unsaturated fat and polyphenols derived also from nuts can be a sustainable and ideal model for CVD prevention.

In conclusion, the protective effects of the traditional Mediterranean diet appears to be even greater if the health effects of this dietary pattern is upgraded changing the common olive oil used for extra-virgin olive oil, increasing the consumption of nuts, fatty fish, and whole grain cereals, reducing sodium intake, and maintaining a moderate consumption of wine with meals.

References

1. Luo C, Zhang Y, Ding Y, Shan Z, Chen S, Yu M, Hu FB, Liu L. Nut consumption and risk of type 2 diabetes, cardiovascular disease, and all-cause mortality: a systematic review and meta-analysis. Am J Clin Nutr. 2014;100:256–69.
2. Rajaram S, Hasso Haddad E, Mejia A, Sabaté J. Walnuts and fatty fish influence different serum lipid fractions in normal to mildly hyperlipidemic individuals: a randomized controlled study. Am J Clin Nutr. 2009;89:1657S–63S.
3. Cosmulescu SN, Trandafir I, Achim G, Botu M, Baciu A, Gruia M. Phenolics of green husk in mature walnut fruits. Notulae Botanicae Horti Agrobotanici Cluj-Napoca. 2010;38:53–6.
4. Cerdá B, Tomás-Barberán FA, Espín JC. Metabolism of antioxidant and chemopreventive ellagitannins from strawberries, raspberries, walnuts, and oak-aged wine in humans: identification of biomarkers and individual variability. J Agric Food Chem. 2005;53:227–35.
5. Ji YB, Qu ZY, Zou X. Juglone-induced apoptosis in human gastric cancer SGC-7901 cells via the mitochondrial pathway. Exp Toxicol Pathol. 2011;63:69–78.
6. Inbaraj JJ, Chignell CF. Cytotoxic action of Juglone and Plumbagin: a mechanistic study using HaCaT keratinocytes. Chem Res Toxicol. 2004;17:55–62.
7. Kang I, Buckner T, Shay NF, Gu L, Chung S. Improvements in metabolic health with consumption of Ellagic acid and subsequent conversion into Urolithins: evidence and mechanisms. Adv Nutr. 2016;7:961–72.

8. "Qualified Claims About Cardiovascular Disease Risk: Walnuts & Heart Disease Docket No. 02P-0292". US Food and Drug Administration. 9 March 2004.
9. Chaouali N, Gana I, Dorra A, Khelifi F, Nouioui A, Masri W, Belwaer I, Ghorbel H, Hedhili A. Potential toxic levels of cyanide in almonds (Prunus amygdalus), apricot kernels (Prunus armeniaca), and almond syrup. ISRN Toxicol. 2013;2013:610648.
10. Bitterman JL, Chung JH. Metabolic effects of resveratrol: addressing the controversies. Cell Mol Life Sci. 2015;72:1473–88.
11. Dower JI, Geleijnse JM, Gijsbers L, Zock PL, Kromhout D, Hollman PC. Effects of the pure flavonoids epicatechin and quercetin on vascular function and cardiometabolic health: a randomized, double-blind, placebo-controlled, crossover trial. Am J Clin Nutr. 2015;101:914–21.
12. Chen AY, Chen YC. A review of the dietary flavonoid, kaempferol on human health and cancer chemoprevention. Food Chem. 2013;138:2099–107.
13. Kim SH, Choi KC. Anti-cancer effect and underlying mechanism(s) of Kaempferol, a phytoestrogen, on the regulation of apoptosis in diverse cancer cell models. Toxicol Res. 2013;29:229–34.
14. Hoek-van den Hil EF, van Schothorst EM, van der Stelt I, Swarts HJ, van Vliet M, Amolo T, Vervoort JJ, Venema D, Hollman PC, Rietjens IM, Keijer J. Direct comparison of metabolic health effects of the flavonoids quercetin, hesperetin, epicatechin, apigenin and anthocyanins in high-fat-diet-fed mice. Genes Nutr. 2015;10:23.
15. Chen CY, Milbury PE, Lapsley K, Blumberg JB. Flavonoids from almond skins are bioavailable and act synergistically with vitamins C and E to enhance hamster and human LDL resistance to oxidation. J Nutr. 2005;135:1366–1373.2005.
16. Cumo C. Foods that changed history: how foods shaped civilization from the ancient World to the present. Santa Barbara, CA: ABC-CLIO; 2015. p. 284.
17. Campbell TC, Campbell TM. The China study. Dallas, TX: Benbella Books; 2006.
18. Taylor CL. Qualified Health Claims: Letter of Enforcement Discretion–Nuts and Coronary Heart Disease (Docket No 02P-0505). Center for Food Safety and Applied Nutrition, FDA. (14 July 2003).
19. Nuts (including peanuts). Micronutrient Information Center. Corvallis, OR: Linus Pauling Institute, Oregon State University; 2009.
20. Full Report (All Nutrients): 12120, Nuts, hazelnuts of filberts. USDA National Nutrient Database, version SR-27. 2015.
21. Perna S, Giacosa A, Bonitta G, Bologna C, Isu A, Guido D, Rondanelli M. Effects of hazelnut consumption on blood lipids and body weight: a systematic review and bayesian meta-analysis. Nutrients. 2016;8:E747.
22. Caimari A, Puiggròs F, Suárez M, Crescenti A, Laos S, Ruiz JA, Alonso V, Moragas J, Del Bas JM, Arola L. The intake of a hazelnut skin extract improves the plasma lipid profile and reduces the lithocholic/deoxycholic bile acid faecal ratio, a risk factor for colon cancer, in hamsters fed a high-fat diet. Food Chem. 2015;167:138–44.
23. Yurttas HC, Schafer HW, Warthesen JJ. Antioxidant activity of nontocopherol hazelnut (Corylus spp.) phenolics. J Food Sci. 2000;65:276–80.
24. Remains of seven types of edible nuts and nutcrackers found at 780,000-year-old archaeological site. Scienceblog.com. February 2002.
25. Okay Y. The comparison of some pistachios cultivars regarding their fat, fatty acids and protein content. Die Gartenbauwissenschaff. 2002;67:107–13.
26. Dreher ML. Pistachio nuts: composition and potential health benefit. Nutr Rev. 2012;70:234–40.
27. Bullò M, Juanola-Falgarona M, Hernàndez-Alonso P, Salas-Salvadò J. Nutrition attributes and health effects of pistachios nuts. Br J Nutr. 2015;113(suppl 2):S79–93.
28. Kris-Etherton PM, Zhao G, Binkoski AE, Coval SM, Etherton TD. The effects of nuts on coronary heart disease. Nutr Rev. 2001;59:103–11.
29. Dreher ML, Maher CV, Kearney P. The traditional and emerging role of nuts in healthful diets. Nutr Rev. 1996;54:241–5.
30. Brown D. FDA considers health claim for nuts. J Am Diet Assoc. 2003;103:426.

31. Mukuddem-Petersen J, Oosthuizen W, Jerling JC. Systematic review of the effects of nuts on blood lipid profiles in humans. J Nutr. 2005;135:2082–9.
32. Estruch R, Ros E, Salas-Salvadó J, Covas MI, Corella D, Arós F, Gómez-Gracia E, Ruiz-Gutiérrez V, Fiol M, Lapetra J, Lamuela-Raventos RM, Serra-Majem L, Pintó X, Basora J, Muñoz MA, Sorlí JV, Martínez JA, Martínez-González MA, Study Investigators PREDIMED. Primary prevention of cardiovascular disease with a Mediterranean diet. New Engl J Med. 2013;368:1279–90.
33. Samieri C, Féart C, Proust-Lima C, et al. Olive oil consumption, plasma oleic acid, and stroke incidence: the Three-City study. Neurology. 2011;77:418–25.
34. Misirli G, Benetou V, Lagiou P, Bamia C, Trichopoulos D, Trichopoulou A. Relation of the traditional Mediterranean diet to cerebrovascular disease in a Mediterranean population. Am J Epidemiol. 2012;176:1185–92.
35. Sherzai A, Heim LT, Boothby C, Sherzai AD. Stroke, food groups, and dietary patterns: a systematic review. Nutr Rev. 2012;70:423–35.
36. Estruch R, Martinez-González MA, Corella D, et al. Effects of a Mediterranean-style diet on cardiovascular risk factors: a randomized trial. Ann Intern Med. 2006;145(1):11.
37. Martínez-González MA, Salas-Salvadó J, Estruch R, Corella D, Fitó M, Ros E, Predimed Investigators. Benefits of the Mediterranean diet: insights from the PREDIMED study. Prog Cardiovac Dis. 2015;58:50–60.

Legumes and Pulses 12

12.1 Legumes and Pulses

Grain legumes, also called pulses, are plants belonging to the family Leguminosae (alternatively Fabaceae) which are grown primarily for their edible seeds.

Legume: the term "legume" refers to the plants whose fruit is enclosed in a pod. Commonly, legumes are referred to fresh peas and fresh beans. Legumes represent a vast family of plants including more than 600 genera and more than 13,000 species. When growing, legumes fix nitrogen into the soil, which reduces the need for chemical fertilizers.

Pulse: pulses are part of the legume family, but the term "pulse" refers only to the dried seed. Edible beans (including butter beans, haricot (navy) beans, cannellini beans, red kidney beans, adzuki beans, black-eyed beans, and soybeans), dried peas, lentils, and chickpeas are the most common varieties of pulses.

Pulses are very high in protein and fiber, and are low in fat. Like their cousins in the legume family, pulses are nitrogen-fixing crops that improve the environmental sustainability of annual cropping systems. Pulses contain also numerous active compounds including polyphenols, which actively participate in the health protective effects of Mediterranean diet.

Legumes and pulses contain also some "antinutrients." Plants commonly synthesize a range of secondary metabolites as part of their protection against attack by herbivores, insects, and pathogens or as a means to survive in adverse growing conditions. These compounds may cause adverse physiological effects. The terms "antinutrient" or "natural toxicant" have been widely employed to describe plant defense metabolites in the food and nutrition literature. The observed biological effects vary greatly, depending upon the structures of the individual compounds, which can range from high molecular-weight proteins to simple amino acids and oligosaccharides. Legumes are a rich source of antinutrients in the human diet.

A. Capurso et al., *Benefits of the Mediterranean Diet in the Elderly Patient*, Practical Issues in Geriatrics, https://doi.org/10.1007/978-3-319-78084-9_12

Antinutrients commonly found in legumes/pulses are: phytic acid, aponins, lathyrogens, a-galactosides, protease inhibitors, a-amylase inhibitors, lectins, and, to some extent, also polyphenols [1].

Common beans, broad beans (fava bean), peas, and lentils are the legumes/pulses treated in this chapter.

12.2 Common Beans

Black beans and other beans such as pinto beans, navy beans, kidney beans, and white "cannellini" beans are all known scientifically as *Phaseolus vulgaris*. This scientific name refers to the genus and species of the plant; navy, kidney, pinto, etc. are different varieties of beans, all found within the species *vulgaris*. The word "common" is used to describe all of these different varieties, since the word *vulgaris* in Latin means "common."

12.2.1 History

The common bean (*Phaseolus vulgaris*) was native to the Americas and was domesticated separately in Mesoamerica and in the southern Andes region. Along with squash and maize (corn), beans are one of the "Three Sisters" central to indigenous North American agriculture.

Most of the kinds commonly eaten fresh or dried come originally from the Americas, being first seen by a European when Christopher Columbus, during his exploration of what may have been the Bahamas, found them growing in fields. Subsequently they were spread to Africa and Asia by Spanish and Portuguese traders.

Five kinds of *Phaseolus* beans were domesticated by pre-Columbian peoples: common beans (*Phaseolus vulgaris*) grown from Chile to the northern part of what is now the United States; lima and sieva beans (*Phaseolus lunatus*), as well as the less widely distributed teparies (*Phaseolus acutifolius*), scarlet runner beans (*Phaseolus coccineus*), and polyanthus beans (*Phaseolus polyanthus).*

For a wide variety of reasons—including ease of growth, long-term storage ability, taste and texture, and nutrient content (especially protein)—beans have become popular in many cultures throughout the world. Black beans are an important staple in the cuisines of Mexico, Brazil, Cuba, Guatemala, and the Dominican Republic. The white variety of beans, the navy beans or haricot beans are particularly popular in the United Kingdom and the United States. Other white beans include cannellini, a popular variety in central and southern Italy that is related to the kidney bean. White beans are the most abundant plant-based source of phosphatidylserine known.

12.2.2 Nutrients and Phytochemicals

Throughout history, dry beans have been used as a staple of the diet, and the health benefits derived from them have been well recognized. Dry beans are nutrient-dense in that the amount of nutrients provided per calorie is particularly high. Increased intake provides nutritional benefit to the diet, and help to reduce disease risk and enhance longevity.

Among the different varieties of beans, the black beans is particularly rich in nutrients and phytochemicals.

Black Beans, Cooked

Nutritional profile, per 1 cup (172 g)

Calories	227.04
Protein	15.27 g
Carbohydrates	40.78 g

Fat, total	0.93 g
Monounsaturated	0.08 g
Oleic acid	0.08 g
Polyunsaturated	0.40 g
Linoleic	0.22 g
Linolenic	0.18 g
Saturated	0.24 g
Palmitic	0.22 g
Stearic	0.02 g

Dietary fiber	14.96 g
Soluble fiber	4.13 g
Insoluble fiber	10.84 g
Ash	1.98 g

Vitamins	
Vitamin A	10.32 IU
Retinol (Equivalents)	1.03 μg
β-Carotene (Equivalents)	6.19 μg

Minerals		
Calcium	46.44 mg	5% DRI/DV
Copper	0.36 mg	49% DRI/DV
Iron	3.61 mg	20% DRI/DV
Magnesium	120.40 mg	30% DRI/DV
Manganese	0.76 mg	38% DRI/DV
Molybdenum	129.00 μg	287% DRI/DV
Phosphorus	240.80 mg	34% DRI/DV
Potassium	610.60 mg	17% DRI/DV
Selenium	2.06 μg	4% DRI/DV
Zinc	1.93 mg	18% DRI/DV

Amino acids	
Alanine	0.64 g
Arginine	0.94 g
Aspartic acid	1.84 g
Cysteine	0.17 g
Glutamic acid	2.32 g
Glycine	0.60 g
Histidine	0.42 g
Isoleucine	0.67 g
Leucine	1.22 g
Lysine	1.05 g
Methionine	0.23 g
Phenylalanine	0.82 g
Proline	0.65 g
Serine	0.83 g
Threonine	0.64 g
Tryptophan	0.18 g
Tyrosine	0.43 g
Valine	0.80 g

Source: The Food Processor, Version 10.12.0, ESHA Research, Salem, Oregon, USA

12.2.3 Health Impact

In a recent multicultural study called "Food Habits in Later Life Study" (FHLL) promoted by the Committee on Nutrition and Aging of the International Union of Nutrition Sciences (IUNS), and regarding dietary practices of diverse populations of elderly communities in Australia, China, Greece, Japan, Philippines, Sweden, and other communities of Asia, Europe and Central America, the consumption of beans was shown to be the only dietary component related to longevity [2]. In this study, investigators found that for every 20 g intake of legumes (including dry beans), the risk ratio of death was reduced by 6% in the older people (aged 70 and older) studied. This study has given an important contribution to the great need for descriptive research on the health status, lifestyle, and eating habits of the elderly in developed and developing countries.

Among all groups of food commonly eaten worldwide, no group has a more health-supportive mix of protein-plus-fiber than legumes. In a single, one-cup serving (~200 g) of beans there are nearly 15 g of fiber (well over half of the Daily Value) and 15 g of protein (nearly one-third of the Daily Value and equivalent to the amount in 2 ounces (~ 56 g) of a meat like chicken or a fish like salmon). This outstanding protein–fiber combination is never found in fruit, vegetables, grains, meats, dairy products, nuts and seeds, or seafood. This outstanding protein–fiber combination in legumes, including beans, likely explains several important aspects of their health benefits for the digestive tract.

Another important characteristic of legumes and pulses is the relatively low amount of starch. In beans, the total starch is 45 g/100 g dry matter, compared to the total starch in white bread (77 g/100 g) or in spaghetti (78 g/100 g). Contrary to spaghetti and white bread, the starch of beans pulses in general has a low glycemic index. This phenomenon appears to be largely due, other than to the low amount of total starch, to the presence of two peculiar components: resistant starch and alpha-amylase inhibitors in beans.

12.2.4 Resistant Starch

Resistant starches are those that resist digestion in the small intestine, thereby passing into the large intestine, where they act like dietary soluble fiber.

Resistant starches belong to the category of "*low-digestible carbohydrates*" (LDCs). These are carbohydrates that are incompletely or not absorbed in the small intestine but are fermented, at least in part, by bacteria in the large intestine. Fiber and sugar alcohols belong also to LDCs.

Many of the benefits of resistant starch and LCGs (including a reduced caloric content, reduced or no effect on blood glucose levels, non-cariogenic effect) are related to the inability of human digestive enzymes to break down completely the carbohydrates into absorbable saccharides and the subsequent fermentation of unabsorbed carbohydrates in the colon.

As a result, LDCs may affect laxation and cause gastrointestinal effects, including abdominal discomfort, flatus, and diarrhea, especially at higher or excessive intakes. Such responses, though transient, affect the perception of the well-being of consumers and their acceptance of food products containing LDCs. To note, current recommendations for fiber intake do not consider total LDC consumption nor recommend an upper limit for LDC intake based on potential gastrointestinal effects.

The resistant starch are subdivided into three subgroups: RS1, corresponding to physically inaccessible starches, entrapped in a cellular matrix, as in legume seeds [3]; RS2, corresponding to native granules of starch, whose crystallinity makes them less susceptible to hydrolysis, such as raw potato or banana starches [4, 5]; RS3 which are retrograded starch fractions, which may be formed in cooked foods, that are kept at low or room temperature; the cooling of cooked food, particularly potatoes, makes the gelatinized starch to return partially into its crystalline form, which renders starch inaccessible to digestive enzymes [6].

Resistant starch escaping digestion in the small intestine can yield up to 20% of the starch in cereal and legume products. The rate and extent of starch digestion will affect a number of physiological functions and thus will have different effects on health (e.g., reduction of the glycemic and insulinemic response to a food, hypocholesterolemic effects, protective effects against colorectal cancer) [7–10]. Among the factors affecting the rate and extent of starch digestion, food processing, storage time, and botanic origin of the food are also of importance. Starch in raw foods is barely digestible and corresponds to RS2.

Raw and processed legumes have been shown to contain significant amounts of RS in comparison with other products such as cereals, tubers, and unripe fruits [11, 12].

For this reason, the starch digestion rate and therefore the release of glucose into the blood stream are slower after the ingestion of legumes, resulting in reduced glycemic and insulinemic postprandial responses in comparison with cereal grains or potatoes. In addition to starch, legumes contain high amounts of dietary fiber in a form that gives cell walls high resistance toward disintegration during cooking [13, 14]. This, along with the presence of certain antinutrients, may account for the reduced digestibility of starch in pulses.

Although beans are often considered as a problem-causing food in the digestive tract, perhaps largely because of gas production, recent research has shown that beans actually provide special support in the lower large intestine (colon) where gas is often produced. The higher indigestible fraction (IF) (resistant starch) in beans has recently been shown to be larger than the IF in either lentils or chickpeas. It is the perfect mix of substances for allowing bacteria in the colon to produce butyric acid. Cells lining the inside of the colon can use this butyric acid to fuel their many activities and keep the lower digestive tract functioning properly. By delivering a greater amount of IF to the colon, black beans are able to help support this lower part of our digestive tract. Lowered colon cancer risk that is associated with black bean intake in some research studies may be related to the outstanding IF content of this legume.

The Problem of Flatulence
The common beans contain oligosaccharides (particularly raffinose and stachyose), a type of sugar molecule also found in cabbage. An anti-oligosaccharide enzyme is necessary to properly digest these sugar molecules. As a normal human digestive tract does not contain any anti-oligosaccharide enzymes, consumed oligosaccharides are typically digested by bacteria in the large intestine. This digestion process produces flatulence-causing gases as a by-product. Since sugar dissolves in water, a method of reducing flatulence associated with eating beans is to drain the water in which the beans have been cooked. Another effective strategy to reduce gas formation is to soak beans in alkaline (baking soda) water overnight before rinsing thoroughly.

12.2.5 Alpha-Amylase Inhibitors

Anti-alpha-amylase is a plant defense protein, formed by glycosylated polypeptides of 14–19 kDa, characterized by an anti-enzymatic activity in the sense that it prevents hydrolysis of the alpha −1,4 glycoside bond of starch.

Common beans contain discrete amounts of alpha-amylase inhibitors. Amylase inhibitors are known as starch blockers because they prevent dietary starches from being absorbed by the body. In humans, amylase inhibitors have been shown to decrease intestinal absorption of carbohydrates by reducing intestinal amylase activity. Such action has been exploited for reducing the caloric value of the diet.

AMYLASE: The amylase is an enzyme that catalyzes the hydrolysis of starch into sugars. Amylase is present in the saliva of humans and some other mammals, where it begins the chemical process of digestion. The pancreas and salivary gland make amylase (alpha amylase) to hydrolyze dietary starch into disaccharides and trisaccharides which are converted by other enzymes to glucose to supply the body with energy. By acting at random locations along the starch chain, α-amylase breaks down long-chain carbohydrates, ultimately yielding maltotriose and maltose from amylose, or maltose, glucose and "limit dextrin" from amylopectin. Because it can act anywhere on the substrate, α-amylase tends to be faster-acting than β-amylase. In human physiology, both the salivary and pancreatic amylases are α-amylases.

Another form of amylase is the β-amylase, synthesized also by bacteria, fungi, and plants. Working from the nonreducing end, β-amylase catalyzes the hydrolysis of the second α-1,4 glycosidic bond, cleaving off two glucose units (maltose) at a time. During the ripening of fruit, β-amylase breaks starch into maltose, resulting in the sweet flavor of ripe fruit.

It should be mentioned that other plant constituents with enzymatic inhibitory activity have been described, including polyphenolic compounds and glycoproteins [15]. For example, the polyphenol anthocyanins and ellagitannins present in raspberries and strawberries have been reported to inhibit alpha-glucosidase and alpha-amylase activity, respectively [16]. In addition, theaflavins and catechins present in green and black teas have been reported to inhibit alpha-amylase and alpha-glucosidase activity as well as retard starch digestion in an in vitro model [17]. However, the greatest body of research has gone into alpha-amylase inhibitors (glycoproteins) extracted from beans.

The common white bean (Phaseolus vulgaris) produces an alpha-amylase inhibitor, which has been characterized and tested in numerous clinical studies.

A specific and proprietary product of an alpha-amilase inhibitor extracted from beans and named Phase 2® Carb Controller (Pharmachem Laboratories, Kearny, NJ) has demonstrated the ability to cause significant weight loss [18].

The Phase 2® product is a water extract of the white kidney bean (Phaseolus vulgaris) standardized to alpha-amylase inhibiting units. With doses of 500–3000 mg/day, in either a single dose or in divided doses, Phase 2® has demonstrated to induce a significant weight loss. Clinical studies also show that Phase 2 has the ability to reduce the postprandial spike in blood glucose levels. Experiments conducted incorporating Phase 2 into food and beverage products have found that it can be integrated into various products without losing activity or altering the appearance, texture, or taste of the food. There have been no serious side effects reported following consumption of Phase 2. Gastrointestinal side effects are rare and diminish upon extended use of the product. In summary, Phase 2 has the potential to induce weight loss and reduce spikes in blood sugar caused by carbohydrates through its alpha-amylase inhibiting activity [18].

12.2.6 The Problem of Phytic Acid

Cereals and legumes, particularly beans, are rich in phytic acid and phytates. Phytates belong to the category of *antinutrients,* because it is a strong chelator of

Fig. 12.1 Phytic acid

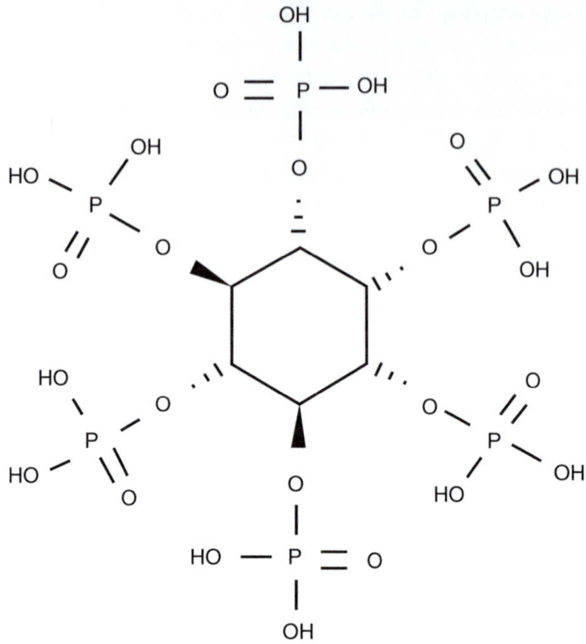

important minerals such as calcium, magnesium, iron, and zinc, and can therefore contribute to mineral deficiencies in people whose diet rely on these foods as basic mineral intake.

When iron and zinc bind to phytic acid they form insoluble precipitate and are far less absorbable in the intestines. This process can therefore contribute to iron and zinc deficiencies in people whose diets rely on these foods for their mineral intake, such as those in developing countries and vegetarians. However, vegetarians and vegans have microbes in their gut that can produce phytase that break down phytic acid [19, 20]. In addition, zinc is well absorbed from meat, even in the presence of phytic acid. Therefore, mineral deficiencies caused by phytic acid are rarely a concern among meat-eaters.

PHYTATES: Phytic acid (known as inositol hexakisphosphate (IP6), inositol polyphosphate, or phytate when in salt form), is a six-phosphate derivative of inositol, which has a glucose-like structure. Inositol and its phosphate derivatives are physiologically inter-convertible and are present in the 0.01–1.0 mM range in almost all living cells. IP6 is found in abundance in high fiber diets. Most cereals, legumes, nuts, oil seeds, and soybean contain 0.5–6.4% (w/w) or even higher levels of IP6. This molecule is *the principal storage form of phosphorus in many plant tissues, especially bran and seeds.*

Although indigestible for many animals, phytic acid and its metabolites as they occur in seeds and grains have several important roles for the seedling plant. Most notably, phytic acid functions as a phosphorus store, as an energy store, as a source of cations, and as a source of myoinositol (a cell wall precursor).

Phytic acid is the principal storage form of phosphorus in plant seeds. The best evidence from numerous studies suggests an intracellular role for phytic acid as a cofactor in DNA repair by nonhomologous end-joining [21]. *Other studies using yeast mutants have also suggested intracellular phytic acid may be involved in mRNA export from the nucleus to the cytosol.*

Phytates require phytase for digestion into absorbable components and humans produce only a small amount of this enzyme (rats, for instance, produce about 30 times more than we do.) However, there's evidence that adaptation occurs over time whereby the more phytate one eats, the more phytase the healthy microbiota in intestines produces.

12.2.7 Phytic Acid (Phytate): Pros and Cons

Phytic acid is contained in numerous foodstuffs (Fig. 12.1). As mentioned above, phytic acid has primarily a strong binding affinity to important minerals, such as iron and zinc. When iron and zinc bind to phytic acid they form insoluble precipitate and are far less absorbable in the intestines. This process can therefore contribute to iron and zinc deficiencies in people whose diets rely on these foods for their mineral intake.

The polyanionic phytate molecule has also a tremendous capacity to chelate cations like Ca forming insoluble Ca–phytate complexes, which are refractory to phytase activity. Therefore, when phytic acid binds these minerals, it makes them unavailable for absorption. The formation of Ca–phytate complex along the gastrointestinal tract, where one phytate (IP_6) molecule binds up to five Ca atoms, assumes importance and approximately one-third of dietary Ca may be bound to phytate in digesta. As a consequence, phytate limits the availability of both P and Ca as a result of insoluble Ca–phytate complex formation. This means that the calcium intake can be lower than expected if one consume notable amounts of food containing phytates. This fact could become a problem for women with osteoporosis. There are data, however, indicating that Ca and phytate interactions occur under acidic conditions with the formation of soluble and insoluble Ca–phytate species. Organic acids, formed during fermentation, promote Ca-phytate complex breakdown. Lactic acid fermentation is the preferred method. Therefore, a good method to overcome the reduced absorption of Ca could be making of sourdough, or to eat yogurt with probacteria lactobacilli, or consider a probiotic supplement with diet.

On the basis of the previous observations, phytate should be considered as a dangerous antinutrients.

However, phytic acid has been shown to be a good example of a nutrient that is both a "friend and foe," depending on the circumstances. In fact, in addition to its strong binding activity to minerals, it has contemporarily antioxidant properties and is protective against kidney stones and several types of cancer. On this basis, phytic acid has been even suggested that might be part of the reason for which whole grains may cut the risk of colon cancer.

Food sources of phytic acid (% of dry weight)		
Food	Minimum	Maximum
Sesame seed flour	5.36	5.36
Brazil nuts	1.97	6.34
Almonds	1.35	3.22
Tofu	1.46	2.90
Linseed	2.15	2.78
Oat meal	0.89	2.40
Beans, pinto	2.38	2.38
Soybeans	1.00	2.22
Corn	0.75	2.22
Peanuts	1.05	1.76
Wheat flour	0.25	1.37
Wheat	0.39	1.35
Oats	0.42	1.16
Whole wheat bread	0.43	1.05
Brown rice	0.84	0.99
Polished rice	0.14	0.60
Chickpeas	0.56	0.56
Lentils	0.44	0.50

Source: Reddy NR and others. Food Phytates, CRC Press, 2001

12.2.7.1 Antioxidant Properties of Phytates

Phytic acid forms an iron chelate which greatly accelerates Fe^{2+}-mediated oxygen reduction, yet blocks iron-driven hydroxyl radical generation and suppresses lipid peroxidation. Furthermore, high concentrations of phytic acid prevent browning and putrefaction of various fruits and vegetables by inhibiting polyphenol oxidase. These observations indicate an important antioxidant function for phytate in seeds during dormancy and suggest that phytate may be a substitute for presently employed preservatives, many of which pose potential health hazards [22].

12.2.7.2 Phytates, Calcifications, and Prevention of Kidney Stone Formation

It is known the extraordinary capacity of phytate (myo-inositol hexaphosphate), a substance present in blood, urine, interstitial and intracellular fluids, to inhibit crystallization of calcium salts (oxalate and phosphate), so preventing calcium renal stone formation. "In vitro" and "in vivo" experiments, as well as clinical studies have clearly demonstrated that phytate plays an important role as a crystallization inhibitor of calcium salts in biological fluids and becomes a clear alternative in the treatment of calcium oxalate renal lithiasis [23].

12.2.7.3 Phytates and Protection against Cancer

In addition to being found in plants, inositol hexaphosphate (IP(6)) is contained in almost all mammalian cells, although in much smaller amounts, where it is important in regulating vital cellular functions such as signal transduction, cell proliferation, and differentiation [24]. Exogenously administered IP(6) is rapidly taken up into cells and dephosphorylated to lower inositol phosphates, which further affect signal transduction pathways resulting in cell cycle arrest. A striking anticancer action of IP(6) has been demonstrated in different experimental models. In addition to reducing cell proliferation, IP(6) also induces differentiation of malignant cells. Enhanced immunity and antioxidant properties also contribute to tumor cell destruction. Preliminary studies in humans show that IP(6) and inositol, the precursor molecule of IP(6), appear to enhance the anticancer effect of conventional chemotherapy, control cancer metastases, and improve quality of life [24].

In rats, a protective effect of wheat bran, rich in phytate, against colon carcinogenesis has been observed [25]. Wheat bran (partly due to its endogenous phytate), and exogenous PA, when added to a low fiber diet, have shown to significantly reduce early biomarkers of colon cancer risk [25].

Consumption of IP6-rich cereals and legumes has been found to be associated with reduction in mammary, colon, and prostate cancers [26–28]. Many laboratories have demonstrated the cancer chemopreventive efficacy of IP6 in different animals, as well as in in vitro cancer models including prostate, skin, mammary, intestine, colon, lung, and liver [28].

As far as the prostate cancer is concerned, it has been suggested [29] that dietary intervention of prostate cancer by IP(6) might be useful in slowing down the growth and progression of the disease in aging males, which would reduce the associated morbidity and mortality, as well as the burden of PCA management on healthcare systems. IP(6) could also be clinically relevant for the human population at high risk of developing prostate cancer as well as those with different stages of this malignancy. Overall, based on its properties, including non-toxicity, high efficacy, low cost and human acceptability, it has been suggested the promise and potential of IP(6) as an ideal preventive and/or therapeutic agent against prostate cancer [29].

12.2.7.4 Broad Spectrum Anticancer Activity of Inositol Hexakisphosphate (IP6)

Deregulated inositol metabolism has been recorded in a number of diseases, including cancer, where inositol modulates different critical pathways. Inositols inhibit pRB phosphorylation, fostering the pRB/E2F complexes formation and blocking progression along the cell cycle. Inositols reduce PI3K levels, thus counteracting the activation of the PKC/RAS/ERK pathway downstream of PI3K activation. Upstream of that pathway, inositols disrupt the ligand interaction between FGF and its receptor as well as with the EGF-transduction processes involving IGF-II receptor and AP-1 complexes. Additionally, Akt activation is severely impaired upon inositol addition. Downregulation of both Akt and ERK leads consequently to NF-kB inhibition and reduced expression of inflammatory markers (COX-2 and PGE2). Remarkably, inositol-induced downregulation of presenilin-1 interferes with the epithelial-mesenchymal transition and reduces Wnt-activation, β-catenin translocation, Notch-1, N-cadherin, and SNAI1 release. Inositols interfere also with the cytoskeleton by upregulating Focal Adhesion Kinase and E-cadherin and decreasing Fascin and Cofilin, two main components of pseudopodia, leading hence to invasiveness impairment. This effect is reinforced by the inositol-induced inhibition on metalloproteinases and ROCK1/2 release [30].

12.3 Broad Beans (Fava Bean)

Vicia faba, also known as the *broad bean, fava bean, faba bean, field bean, bell bean, English bean, horse bean, Windsor bean, pigeon bean,* and *tic(k) bean*, is a species of flowering plant in the family of *Fabaceae*.

The name "broad bean" is used in parts of the English-speaking world for the large-seeded cultivars grown for human food, while "horse bean" and "field bean" refer to cultivars with smaller, harder seeds (more like the wild species) used for animal feed.

The term "fava bean" (from the Italian *fava*, meaning "broad bean") is used in other English-speaking countries such as the United States. "Broad bean" is the most common name in the United Kingdom, Australia, and New Zealand.

12.3.1 History

The origin of this legume is obscure, but it had been cultivated in the Middle East for 8000 years before it spread to Western Europe [31].

Fava beans have been found in the earliest human settlements. They probably originated in the Near East during the Neolithic Age and by the Bronze Age had spread to Northern Italy. They have been found in lakeside settlements in Switzerland and in Britain at Glastonbury. Remains are reported to have been found in Egyptian tombs. In Egypt, the beans were considered commoner food and were shunned by the upper classes [32].

Fava beans were cultivated by the Egyptians, Greeks, and Romans. In ancient Rome, they were used in funeral rites [32]. Like all priests of the Orphic and Eleusinian mysteries who were forbidden from ever touching, mentioning, or looking at Fava beans, Pythagoras forbade his followers from doing the same and some claimed that it was due to his belief that fava beans contained the souls of the dead.

12.3.2 Nutrients and Phytochemicals

Broad beans are very high in protein and a rich source of dietary fiber and plant sterols, particularly isoflavone. They contain also levodopa (L-dopa), a precursor of dopamine, epinephrine, and nor-epinephrine, and good amount of folates, vitamin B_6 (pyridoxine), vitamin B_1 (thiamin), vitamin B_2 (riboflavin), and vitamin B_3 (niacin). Finally, broad beans are a good source of minerals like iron, copper, manganese, calcium, and magnesium. At 1062 mg (corresponding to 23% of daily recommended levels), broad bean is one of the highest plant sources of potassium.

Broad Beans (Fava Beans), Mature Seed, Raw
Nutritional value per 100 g (3.5 oz)

Basic macronutrients	
Calories (kcal)	341
Protein	26.12 g
Total fat	1.53 g
Carbohydrates	58.59 g
Dietary fiber	25 g

Vitamins		
Vitamin A	53 IU	(2% DV)
β-Carotene	32 μg	
Thiamine (B_1)	0.555 mg	(46% DV)
Riboflavin (B_2)	0.333 mg	(25% DV)
Niacin (B_3)	2.832 mg	(18% DV)
Pantothenic acid (B_5)	0.976 mg	(19% DV)
Folate (B_9)	423 μg	(106% DV)
Vitamin B_{12}	0 μg	(0% DV)
Vitamin C	1.4 mg	(2% DV)
Vitamin K	9 μg	(7.5% DV)

Minerals		
Calcium	103 mg	(10% DV)
Copper	0.824 mg	(91% DV)
Iron	6.70 mg	(84% DV)
Magnesium	192 mg	(18% DV)
Manganese	1626 mg	(71% DV)
Phosphorus	421 mg	(60% DV)
Potassium	1062 mg	(23% DV)
Sodium	13 mg	(1% DV)
Selenium	8.2 μg	(4% DV)
Zinc	3.14 mg	(9% DV)

Source: USDA National Nutrient data base

12.3.3 Health Impact

From the safety profile, it should be mentioned that broad (fava) beans should not be eaten from individuals suffering from favism or oxaluria.

Favism is a genetic condition affecting small population with G-6PD (Glucose-6-phosphate dehydrogenase) enzyme deficiency, compromising oxygen-carrying capacity in their blood. The most common clinical manifestations are neonatal jaundice and acute hemolytic anemia. Red cell destruction in these acute hemolytic events is largely intravascular and therefore is associated with hemoglobinuria. The condition is triggered in these individuals on eating fava beans or its products in the diet as well as by some drugs and infections. Prevention mainly includes avoidance of any of these triggering factors, and treatment of acute blood cell lyses.

Oxaluria: Like other class of beans and some Brassica group vegetables, fava too contain oxalic acid, a naturally occurring substance found in some vegetables, which, may crystallize as oxalate stones in the urinary tract in some people. Therefore, people with known oxalate urinary tract stones are advised against eating vegetables belonging to Brassica and Fabaceae family. Adequate intake of water is advised to maintain normal urine output to minimize the stone risk.

In the early twentieth century seedlings of the fava bean were used as an initial source of L-DOPA, a chemical used to increase dopamine concentrations in the treatment of Parkinson's disease and dopamine-responsive dystonia [33]. The amount of levodopa can vary greatly, depending on the species of fava, the area where it's grown, soil conditions, rainfall, and other factors. It appears that the young pod and the immature (green) beans inside the pod contain the greatest amount of levodopa, and the mature, or dried bean, the least. Three ounces (about 84 g or ½ cup) of fresh green fava beans, or three ounces of canned green fava beans, drained, may contain about 50–100 mg of levodopa. If using the young pod as well as the beans, the amount of levodopa may be greater than that in the fresh beans alone.

In a recent paper [34], the phenolic compounds of fava bean sprouts and their antioxidant activity were investigated; structural analysis using NMR and MS revealed that the compounds isolated were kaempferol glycosides. The L-DOPA content was 550.45 mg ± 11.34/100 g of the raw sprouts. L-DOPA showed also high antioxidant activity, while the isolated kaempferol glycosides showed weak activity. Therefore, it was suggested that L-DOPA contributed to the antioxidant activity of fava bean sprouts [34].

Another study [35] evaluated antioxidant and chemopreventative capacities as well as the inhibitory effects on angiotensin-converting enzyme (ACE) and on α-glucosidase and pancreatic lipase, of three Australian-grown faba bean genotypes (Nura, Rossa, and TF). Cell culture-based antioxidant activity assay (cellular antioxidant activity) showed an increase of activity in the colored genotypes after roasting. Faba bean extracts demonstrated cellular protection ability against H_2O_2-induced DNA damage and inhibited the proliferation of all human cancer cell lines (BL13, AGS, Hep G2, and HT-29) evaluated. Flow cytometric analyses showed that faba bean extracts successfully induced apoptosis of HL-60 (acute promyelocytic leukemia) cells. The faba bean extracts also exhibited ACE, α-glucosidase, and pancreatic lipase inhibitory activities. Overall, extracts from Nura (buff-colored) and Rossa (red-colored) were comparable, while TF (white-colored) contained the lowest phenolic content and exhibited the least antioxidant and enzyme inhibition activities.

12.4 Chickpeas

The chickpea or chick pea (*Cicer arietinum*) is a legume of the family Fabaceae. Its different types are variously known as gram, or Bengal gram, garbanzo or garbanzo bean, Egyptian pea, *ceci*, *cece*, *chana*, or *Kabuli chana*. Its seeds are high in protein.

It is one of the earliest cultivated legumes: 7500-year-old remains have been found in the Middle East.

12.4.1 History

Domesticated chickpeas have been found in Pre-Pottery Neolithic Era in Jericho, Middle East, along with Çayönü in Turkey and in Neolithic pottery at Hacilar, Turkey. They were also found in the late Neolithic (about 3500 BCE) at Thessaly, Kastanas, Lerna and Dimini, Greece. In southern France, Mesolithic layers in a cave at L'Abeurador, Aude, have yielded wild chickpeas carbon dated to 6790 ± 90 BCE.

Chickpeas are mentioned in Charlemagne's *Capitulare de villis* (about 800 CE) as *cicer italicum*, as grown in each imperial demesne. Nicholas Culpeper noted "chick-pease or cicers" are less "windy" than peas and more nourishing. Ancient people also associated chickpeas with Venus because they were said to offer medical uses such as increasing sperm and milk, provoking menstruation and urine, and helping to treat kidney stones [36].

In 1793, ground-roast chickpeas were noted by a German writer as a substitute for coffee in Europe [37]. In the First World War, they were grown for this use in some areas of Germany. They are still sometimes brewed instead of coffee.

12.4.2 Nutrients and Phytochemicals

Chickpeas are a nutrient-dense food, providing rich content (20% or higher of the Daily Value, DV) of protein, dietary fiber, folate, and certain dietary minerals such as iron and phosphorus. Thiamin, vitamin B_6, magnesium, and zinc contents are moderate, providing 10–16% of the DV. Chickpeas have a Protein Digestibility Corrected Amino Acid Score of about 0.76, which is higher than many other legumes and cereals. Compared to reference levels established by the United Nations Food and Agricultural Organization and World Health Organization, proteins in cooked and germinated chickpeas are rich in essential amino acids such as lysine, isoleucine, tryptophan, and total aromatic amino acids [38].

A 100-g serving of cooked chickpeas provides 164 kilocalories (690 kJ). Cooked chickpeas are 60% water, 27% carbohydrates, 9% protein, and 3% fat (table). 75% of lipid content is unsaturated fatty acids for which linoleic acid comprises 43% of total fat [39].

Chickpeas, Mature Seed, Cooked, No Salt
Nutritional value per 100 g (3.5 oz)

Energy	686 kJ (164 kcal)	
Protein	8.86 g	
Total fat	2.59 g	
Saturated	0.269 g	
Monounsaturated	0.583 g	
Polyunsaturated	1.156 g	

Energy	686 kJ (164 kcal)	
Carbohydrates	27.42 g	
Sugars	4.8 g	
Dietary fiber	7.6 g	(16% DV)
Vitamin A	1 μg	(0% DV)
Thiamine (B_1)	0.116 mg	(10% DV)
Riboflavin (B_2)	0.063 mg	(5% DV)
Niacin (B_3)	0.526 mg	(4% DV)
Pantothenic acid (B_5)	0.286 mg	(6% DV)
Folate (B_9)	172 μg	(43% DV)
Vitamin B_{12}	0 μg	(0% DV)
Vitamin C	1.3 mg	(2% DV)
Vitamin E	0.35 mg	(2% DV)
Vitamin K	4 μg	(4% DV)

Calcium	49 mg	(5% DV)
Iron	2.89 mg	(22% DV)
Magnesium	48 mg	(14% DV)
Phosphorus	168 mg	(24% DV)
Potassium	291 mg	(6% DV)
Sodium	7 mg	(0% DV)
Zinc	1.53 mg	(16% DV)

Source: USDA National Nutrient data base

12.4.3 Health Benefits

Chickpeas are an excellent source of fiber, containing 16% of daily needs in one half-cup serving. About one-third of the fiber in chickpeas is soluble fiber, making it a heart-healthy food. Chickpeas are also a good source of manganese and folate. They are also a very good source of magnesium, iron, copper, potassium, and thiamin. Chickpeas, like other legumes, contain resistant starch that slows down the digestion of carbohydrates. As mentioned above (see: Common beans – Resistant starch), some resistant starch is not digested in the small intestine at all. It has been shown that replacing more rapidly digested carbohydrates with legumes enhances glycemic control by improving insulin sensitivity in people with diabetes. Consuming foods high in resistant starch improves also colon health, including promoting healthy bowel flora, and prevention of colon cancer [7–10].

Cickpeas, as other legumes of the *Fabaceae* family, contain three important isoflavones that exhibit estrogenic, antiangiogenic, antioxidant, and anticancer activities, and are now popular as dietary supplements:

- Genistein
- Biochanin A
- Formononetin

12.4.3.1 Genistein

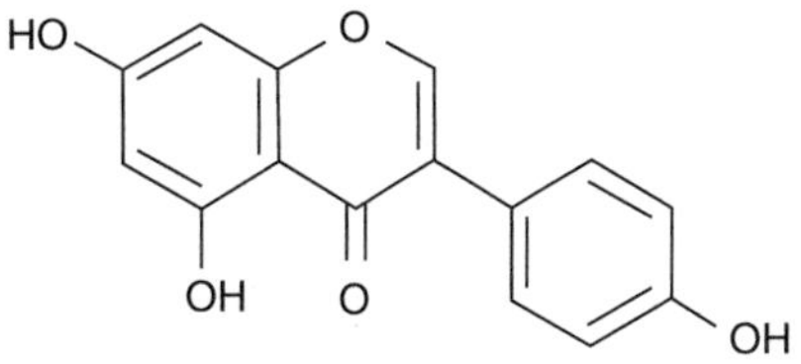

Genistein has been the subject of over 3600 published studies in the last 10 years. Genistein from chickpea has shown to significantly decrease serum insulin levels, total cholesterol, triglycerides, low-density lipoprotein cholesterol, high-density lipoprotein cholesterol, and the ratio of high-density lipoprotein cholesterol to low-density lipoprotein cholesterol, improves glucose tolerance, and reduces serum liver glycogen and muscle glycogen in type 2 diabetic rats [40, 41]. Genistein is beneficial not only to type 2 diabetes but also to type 1 diabetes where it stimulates insulin release [42]. Because of isoflavones structure and the effect of surrounding phenolic hydroxyl, genistein has a low bioavailability.

Genistein has also shown to inhibit cancer cell proliferation, an activity that it shares with biochanin A, as it is described below.

12.4.3.2 Biochanin a

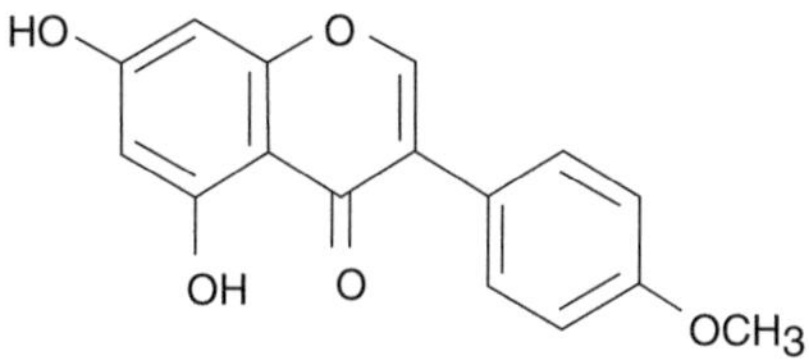

Biochanin A, the 4-methyl ether of genistein, is a natural isoflavone with diverse biological actions, most notably as a phytoestrogen. It can affect hormone levels by inhibiting 5α-reductase and 17β-hydroxysteroid dehydrogenase or altering aromatase (CYP19A1) activity [43, 44]. Also known as 4′-methyl genistein, biochanin A can be metabolized in vivo to genistein, a phytoestrogen with diverse effects [45]. Biochanin A also intersects with signaling through peroxisome proliferator-activated receptors (PPARs), as it activates PPARγ and has also been shown to activate a PPARα promoter [46]. Moreover, it increases the expression of the PPARγ coactivator PGC-1α, promoting mitochondrial biogenesis [47].

In vitro, biochanin A has shown to inhibit the growth of human prostate cancer cell, an activity shared with genistein [48]. The antiproliferative and pro-apoptotic activity of biochanin A has been shown to be due to the inhibition of lipopolysaccharide (LPS)-induced nitric oxide(NO) production, iNOS expression, p38-MAPK and ATF-2 phosphorylation and block of NFκB nuclear translocation [49].

Biochanin A has been shown to have an anti breast cancer activity. Numerous epidemiological studies have shown that the use of exogenous estrogen or an augmented endogenous estrogen concentration is associated with increased breast cancer risk. In both cell and animal models a causal relationship between estrogen exposure and breast cancer has been clearly established. The cancer-inducing mechanisms of estrogen in the breast can be multifaceted, and may participate in either the initiation or promotion stage. Estrogen-induced cell proliferation has been a major focus in breast cancer research. Estrogen is synthesized from cholesterol in several steps, and CYP19 (aromatase) catalyzes the final rate-limiting reaction. Aromatase inhibitors have been shown to be promising agents for breast cancer prevention and therapy. Some flavones have been documented to be aromatase inhibitors. Biochanin A is the only aromatase-inhibitory isoflavone displaying an inhibitory effect with an IC50 value of about 8 mM in the MCF-7aro cells [50]. On the other hands, many studies have documented a biochanin A's chemopreventive effect on breast cancer. Consequently, biochanin A has been proposed as a nutraceutical for preventing breast cancer. It has been suggested that in human subjects an oral dosage of 50 mg/kg could be able to sustain an aromatase-suppressing plasma concentration [50].

12.4.3.3 Formononetin

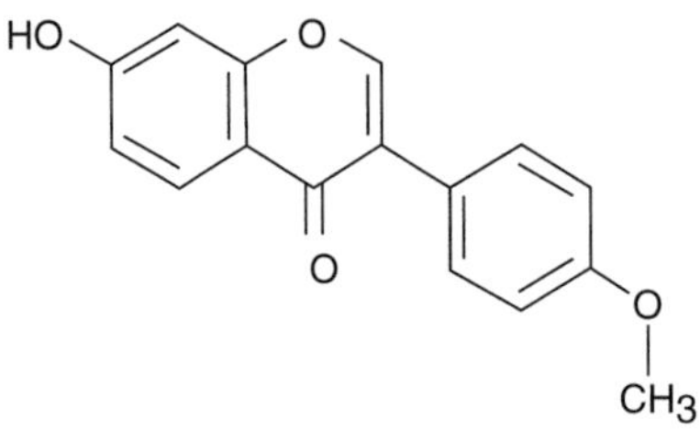

Formononetin is a naturally occurring isoflavone, which can be found in low concentrations in many dietary products, including legumes of the family *Fabaceae* and in Trifolium Pratense (Red Clover). Due to its structural similarity to 17 β -estradiol, it can mimic estradiol's effect and therefore is considered as a "*phytoestrogen*." Phytoestrogens belong to naturally occurring nonsteroidal compounds that have estrogen-like biological activity primarily through binding to estrogen receptors. Administration of formononetin to ovariectomized rats has shown beneficial effect on bone biomechanical features and chemistry, preventing osteoporosis development [51].

In humans, formononetin has been used as an alternative to the hormone replacement therapy. In fact, the potential risks of hormone therapies have prompted an increase in the use of complementary therapies to alleviate postmenopausal osteoporosis [52–54]. Phytoestrogens with estrogen-like biological activity have provided practical hormone therapy alternative [55, 56]. Formononetin has shown to prevent osteoclastogenesis by enhancing bone mechanical properties and bone chemistry improvement during estrogen deficiency [51].

In a recent double-blind, randomized, placebo-controlled trial, 177 women aged 49–65 years received a red clover-derived isoflavone supplement that provided a daily dose of 26 mg biochanin A, 16 mg formononetin, 1 mg genistein and 0.5 mg daidzein, or placebo for one year. There were no significant treatment effects on hip bone mineral content or bone mineral density, markers of bone resorption, or body composition, but bone formation markers were significantly increased ($P = 0.04$ and $P = 0.01$ for bone-specific alkaline phosphatase and N-propeptide of collagen type I, respectively) in the intervention group compared with placebo in postmenopausal women. These data suggest that, through attenuation of bone loss, isoflavones have a potentially protective effect on the lumbar spine in women [57].

12.5 Peas

The pea is the small spherical seed or the seed-pod of the pod fruit *Pisum sativum*. Each pod contains several peas. Pea pods are botanically fruit, since they contain seeds and developed from the ovary of a (pea) flower.

The immature peas (and in snow peas the tender pod as well) are used as a vegetable, fresh, frozen, or canned. Varieties of the species typically called field peas are grown to produce dry peas like the split pea shelled from the matured pod. These are the basis of *pease porridge* and *pea soup*, staples of medieval cuisine. In Europe, consuming fresh immature green peas was an innovation of Early Modern cuisine.

12.5.1 History

The earliest archaeological finds of peas date from the late Neolithic era of current Greece, Syria, Turkey, and Jordan. In Egypt, early finds date from ca. 4800–4400 BC in the Nile delta area, and from ca. 3800–3600 BC in Upper Egypt. The pea was also present in Georgia in the fifth millennium BC. Farther east, the finds are younger. Peas were present in Afghanistan ca. 2000 BC, in Harappa, Pakistan, and in northwest India in 2250–1750 BC. In the second half of the second millennium BC, this pulse crop appears in the Ganges Basin and southern India [58].

In early times, peas were grown mostly for their dry seeds. From plants growing wild in the Mediterranean basin, constant selection since the Neolithic dawn of agriculture improved their yield. In the early third century BC Theophrastus mentions peas among the pulses that are sown late in the winter because of their tenderness. In the first century AD *Columella* (a famous gourmet of ancient Roma) mentions them in *De re rustica*, when Roman legionaries still gathered wild peas from the sandy soils of Numidia and Judea to supplement their rations.

In the Middle Ages, field peas are constantly mentioned, as they were the staple that kept famine at bay, as Charles the Good, count of Flanders, noted explicitly in 1124.

Green "garden" peas, eaten immature and fresh, were an innovative luxury of Early Modern Europe. In England, the distinction between "field peas" and "garden peas" dates from the early seventeenth century.

Green peas were introduced from Genoa to the court of Louis XIV of France in January 1660, with some staged fanfare; a hamper of them were presented before

Table 12.1 Compositional data for peas (*Pisum sativum*) [59–66]

Constituents	Concentration (%)
Protein (% N × 6.25)	21.2–32.9
Starch	36.9–49.0
Resistant starch	2.1–6.3
Amylose	20.7–33.7
Total dietary fiber	14–26
Insoluble fiber	10–15
Soluble fiber	2–9
Soluble sugars	5.3–8.7
Total lipid	1.2–2.4
Ash	2.3–3.4

the King, and then were shelled by the Sovoyan comte de Soissons, who had married a niece of Cardinal Mazarin; little dishes of peas were then presented to the King, the Queen, Cardinal Mazarin and Monsieur, the king's brother. Immediately established and grown for earliness warmed with manure and protected under glass, they were still a luxurious delicacy in 1696, when Mme de Maintenon and Mme de Sevigné each reported that they were "a fashion, a fury."[

12.5.2 Nutrients and Phytochemicals

Peas are starchy, but high in fiber, protein, vitamin A, vitamin B_6, vitamin C, vitamin K, phosphorus, magnesium, copper, iron, zinc, and lutein. Dry weight is about one-quarter protein and one-quarter sugar (see Table 12.1).

Peas have long been recognized as an inexpensive, readily available source of protein, complex carbohydrates, vitamins, and minerals. The high nutrient density of peas makes them a valuable food commodity, capable of meeting the dietary needs of the estimated 800–900 million undernourished individuals worldwide. The US Department of Agriculture My Plate Guidelines recommend consuming at least three cups of dry beans and peas per week.

Peas, Green, Raw

Nutritional value per 1 cup (145 g)

Energy	490 kJ (117 kcal)
Protein	7.9 g
Total fat	0.6 g
Saturated	0.1 g
Monounsaturated	0.1 g
Polyunsaturated	0.3 g
Total omega-3	50.8 mg
Total omega-6	220 mg
Carbohydrates	21.0 g
Sugars	8.2 g
Dietary fiber	7.4 g (30% DV)

Vitamin A	1109 IU	(22% DV)
Thiamine (B_1)	0.4 mg	(26% DV)
Riboflavin (B_2)	0.2 mg	(11% DV)
Niacin (B_3)	3.0 mg	(15% DV)
Pantothenic acid (B_5)	0.2 mg	(2% DV)
Folate (B_9)	94.3 μg	(24% DV)
Vitamin B_{12}	0 μg	(0% DV)
Vitamin C	58.0 mg	(97% DV)
Vitamin E (α-tocopherol)	0.2 mg	(1% DV)
Vitamin K	36.0 μg	(45% DV)
Choline	41.2 mg	
Betaine	0.3 mg	

Calcium	36.2 mg	(4% DV)
Iron	2.1 mg	(12% DV)
Magnesium	47.9 mg	(12% DV)
Phosphorus	157 mg	(16% DV)
Potassium	354 mg	(10% DV)
Sodium	7.3 mg	(0% DV)
Zinc	1.8 mg	(12% DV)
Copper	0.3 mg	(13% DV)
Manganese	0.6 mg	(39% DV)
Selenium	2.6 μg	(4% DV)

Source: USDA SR-21

12.5.2.1 Peas' Proteins

Peas are a valuable source of protein for both man and animals. The majority of pea proteins are storage proteins, or globulins, and the amino acid profile of these proteins determines their nutritional value.

In a study [67] that compared the amino acid composition of proteins isolated from peas with those extracted from lupin and soybeans showed that the amino acid profiles of all products were similar overall, with the greatest contributions from glutamine, followed by aspartic acid, arginine, and lysine, and the lowest contributions from methionine, tryptophan, and cysteine. Products from peas tended to be higher in arginine, valine, and methionine, and lower in glutamic acid and cysteine, than those from lupin and soyabeans.

Relative to human requirements, the protein in peas and other pulses is rich in lysine and marginal or deficient with respect to methionine. The ability of peas to improve CVD and promote weight loss may be attributable to their high protein content [68].

The in vitro digestibility of raw pea protein is reduced by the presence of protease inhibitors. In a recent review [69], the negative physiological and nutritional effects of lectins and protease inhibitors in pulses are described, as are the potential nutraceutical effects of lectins, which include anticancer and immunomodulatory properties. Hydrolysis of pea and other pulse proteins generates peptides with a variety of bioactivities in vitro, including angiotensin I-converting enzyme inhibitor activity, which has an antihypertensive effect, and antioxidant activity [69].

12.5.2.2 Complex Carbohydrates

Starch is composed of amylose, a linear glucan with few branches, and amylopectin, a larger and more highly branched molecule. The ratio of amylose to amylopectin influences the digestibility of starch and thus its impact on the postprandial glucose response [70]. Pea starch, like that of most other starchy pulses, contains an intermediate level of amylose, which is reflected in its higher levels of enzyme-resistant starch and slowly digestible starch (as compared with cereal, root and tuber starches, most of which are lower in amylose).

The relatively low degree of digestibility of starch in pulses has been attributed to the non-availability to amylases of starch granules enclosed in intact cell wall structures, the presence of antinutrients such as amylase inhibitors (phytates and phenolics), and their significant content of dietary fiber [71]. The properties of both their starch and fiber constituents make peas a low-glycemic index food, and hence beneficial in the prevention and management of type 2 diabetes [72]. In addition, fiber may reduce blood cholesterol by decreasing the reabsorption of bile acids [73]. Peas, like other legumes, contain significant concentrations of raffinose-family and other galactose-containing oligosaccharides which may exert prebiotic effects in the large intestine [74].

12.5.2.3 Vitamins and Minerals

Despite the high mineral content of peas, bioavailability may be poor due to high phytate concentrations. Phytate acts as an inhibitor of Zn, Fe, and Ca absorption. In a study [72], however, it was found that phytate content affected Fe but did not influence Zn and Ca availability in pulses; these authors concluded that when Fe availability was low, Ca and Zn availability was high. The study also reported that peas have greater in vitro Ca bioavailability compared with other pulses. If phytate is degraded, peas could be considered a significant source of Ca, Zn, and Fe.

To note, peas contained 101 mg folate per 100 g. Low dietary folate levels have been associated with anemia and neural tube defects in humans.

12.5.2.4 Phytochemicals

Peas, like other pulses, contain a variety of phytochemicals, including phenolic compounds, phytates, saponins, and oxalates. The major phenolic constituents in pulses are tannins, phenolic acids, and flavonoids [75]. Phenolic compounds have been recognized for their ability to act as antioxidants and are the best characterized phytochemicals in peas.

Peas contain a variety of phenolics, with the highest concentrations of most occurring in the seed coat, particularly in dark-seeded varieties. It was found that the antioxidant activity of pea varieties was correlated significantly with seed coat color. Examination of the seed coat and cotyledon in two dark-colored pea varieties has revealed that the seed coat contain glycosides of quercetin, luteolin, and apigenin, along with a variety of simple phenolics and proanthocyanadins. The cotyledon contains mainly hydroxybenzoic and hydroxycinnamic compounds and some of the glycosides found in the seed coat [76].

Peas contain other minor constituents which exhibit bioactivity and which may have positive benefits on human health, including saponins and phytates, which have hypocholesterolaemic and anticarcinogenic activities [75].

Also pea proteins have demonstrated to have antioxidant properties. In a study [77] on pea proteins fractionated by hydrolysis and subsequently separated by HPLC, some peptide fractions of pea proteins showed a very strong radical scavenging and metal chelating activities. In comparison to glutathione, the peptide fractions had significantly higher ability to inhibit linoleic acid oxidation and chelate metals, while glutathione had significantly higher free radical scavenging properties than the peptide fractions.

12.5.3 Health Impact

Epidemiological, in vitro, and interventional studies all have demonstrated the role of peas and pea constituents in maintaining metabolic, cardiovascular, and gastrointestinal health in humans.

12.5.3.1 Glycemic Response and Insulin Resistance

Due to their high fiber content, peas may modulate the glycemic response as compared with low-fiber foods with equal carbohydrate proportions.

A randomized controlled study [78] investigated the use of whole yellow pea flour to create foods with a lower glycemic index than comparable foods made from whole wheat flour. The results demonstrated that foods made with whole yellow pea flour reduced postprandial glucose responses in individuals and, thus, may have a role in the management of type 2 diabetes. Another study from the same group [79] compared the use of whole pea flour (WPF) and fractionated pea flour (FPF; pea hulls) on insulin resistance. WPF and FPF reduced fasting insulin levels by 13.5 and 9.8%, respectively, compared with baseline. Homeostatic model assessment of insulin resistance (HOMA-IR), a method used to quantify insulin resistance and b-cell function, revealed that insulin resistance was reduced by 25% in both the WPF and the FPF groups compared with the control group receiving white wheat flour. HOMA-IR showed no difference in b-cell function among groups.

In a study by Lunde et al. [80], bread containing 17% pea hull fiber significantly reduced glycemic response; however, the fiber breads also contained higher protein.

12.5.3.2 Cardiovascular Health

Fiber-rich diets have been shown to lower blood pressure, improve serum lipid levels, and reduce indicators of inflammation. In a paper illustrating the position of the American Dietetic Association, the health implication of dietary fibers were clearly assessed [81].

The effect of a pea cell wall fiber preparation with a high content of soluble fiber on fasting and postprandial blood lipids was investigated in young healthy subjects [82]. Inclusion of 33 g pea fiber (20 g dietary fiber) in a low fiber diet was tested in five men and six women in randomized crossover intervention study over 2 week separated by a 2-week period of habitual diet consumption. No significant differences in fasting concentrations of total cholesterol, LDL cholesterol, or HDL cholesterol were observed, whereas total and VLDL triglyceride concentrations were lower when subjects consumed the pea fiber diet compared with the low fiber diet ($P < 0.05$). Postprandial response to pea fiber was studied in eight men. Addition of 12 g pea fiber product/10 MJ to a breakfast meal and 15 g/10 MJ to the following lunch meal resulted in significantly lower total triglyceride ($P = 0.01$), chylomicron triglyceride ($P = 0.03$), and insulin ($P = 0.003$) concentrations after the lunch meal compared with results following the same meal without pea fiber. No differences were observed in glycemic response. The conclusions were that pea dietary fiber lowered fasting and postprandial triglyceride concentrations but did not change fasting cholesterol concentrations.

A legume-based hypocaloric diet demonstrated to significantly reduce pro-inflammatory status and improve metabolic features in overweight/obese subjects [83]. In an open study, thirty obese subjects were randomly assigned to a calorie-restricted legume-free diet or to a calorie-restricted legume-based diet, containing 160–235 g of lentils, chickpeas, peas, or beans. The consumption of legumes (4 servings/week) within a hypocaloric diet resulted in a specific reduction in pro-inflammatory markers, such as CRP and C3 and a clinically significant improvement of some metabolic features (total cholesterol and BP).

The effect of a legume-based diet and other types of diets on mitochondrial oxidation, blood pressure, and other biological parameters was assessed on thirty-five obese subjects in a study of 8 weeks [68]. Legumes significantly improved total and LDL cholesterol and specifically activated mitochondrial oxidation.

12.5.3.3 Gastrointestinal Functions and Homeostasis

The effects of peas and pea fractions on gastrointestinal function have been investigated. In a study [84] on residents of a long-term care facility, the addition of 4 g pea hull fiber/day resulted in a significant increase in bowel movement frequency, particularly in those with the lowest frequency. In another study [85] the addition of pea hull fiber to snack foods, in combination with an inulin fiber supplement, provided to children with constipation to significantly increase bowel movement frequency; no adverse symptoms were reported.

Pea proteins often undergo spontaneous glycosylation during storage and processing due to the high concentration of lysine. It was shown [86] that glycosylated pea proteins may escape enzymic breakdown early in the small intestine and may have an impact on the homeostasis of the large intestine by modulating the activity of the microbiota. Using human gastrointestinal tract simulators to predict the effects of glycosylated pea proteins on intestinal bacteria, a significant increase in autochthonic bacteria (Bacteroides, Lactobacillus and Bifidobacterium) and a subsequent increase in their metabolic activity and production of SCFA were observed [87]. Researchers concluded that pea proteins could be used to improve intestinal microbiota homeostasis.

12.5.3.4 Antioxidant Activity

Phenolic compounds are considered natural antioxidants that may help protect against diseases such as cancer and various inflammatory-related diseases. However, current research on the antioxidant activity of peas is limited to in vitro studies.

In an in vitro study [88] the phenolic composition and antioxidant activity of white and colored peas were compared. Phenolic acids were found in both free and esterified form in both white and colored peas, but higher concentrations were seen in the colored varieties.

Condensed tannins, which have been shown to have very high antioxidant activity [89], were detected only in the colored seed coats. The phenolic compounds were extracted with acetone and methanol, and the liposome system was used to measure antioxidant activity via the extent of peroxidation of phosphatidyl choline. The antioxidant activity in the acetone extract from the colored seed coats was significantly higher than in the white coat extract. These properties were slightly altered by cooking the seeds for 30, 60, or 90 min.

Intervention studies are needed to investigate the efficiency of pea antioxidant activity in providing health benefits to humans.

12.6 Lentils

Lentils are a type of pulse, along with beans, field peas, chickpeas, and faba beans. The term "pulse" is used to describe the edible seeds of legumes. It is a bushy annual plant of the legume family, known for its lens-shaped seeds. It is about 40 cm (16 in.) tall, and the seeds grow in pods, usually with two seeds in each.

There are hundreds of varieties of lentils, with as many as fifty or more cultivated for food. Lentil colors range from yellow to red-orange to green, brown and black. Lentils also vary in size, and are sold in many forms, with or without the skins, whole or split. They grow two to a pod and are dried after harvesting.

12.6.1 History

Lentils, botanically known as *Lens culinaris esculenta,* have been a source of sustenance for our ancestors since prehistoric times. They in fact have been part of the human diet since aceramic Neolithic times, being one of the first crops domesticated in the Near East. Archaeological evidence shows they were eaten 9500–13,000 years ago.

The word *lentils* comes from the Latin *lens,* and indeed this bean cousin is shaped like the double convex optic lens which took its name from the lentil.

Lentil artifacts have been found on archeological digs dating back 8000 years, and the Bible's book of Genesis tells the story of Esau, who gave up his birthright for a bowl of crimson lentils and a loaf of bread. As a tasty and plentiful source of protein, lentils graced the tables of peasants and kings alike.

For millennia, lentils have been traditionally been eaten with barley and wheat, three foodstuffs that originated in the same regions and spread throughout Africa and Europe during similar migrations and explorations of cultural tribes. Before the first century AD, they were introduced into India, a country whose traditional cuisine still bestows high regard for the spiced lentil dish known as "*dal*." In many Catholic countries, lentils have long been used as a staple food during Lent. Currently, the leading commercial producers of lentils include India, Turkey, Canada, China, and Syria.

12.6.2 Nutrients and Phytochemicals

Lentils are considered a good source of proteins and are sources of some storage proteins that are described as biologically active proteins for the metabolic needs of the human body.

According to the USDA National Nutrient Database, 100 g of raw lentils (variety unspecified) provide 353 calories; the same weight of cooked lentils provides 116 kcal. Raw lentils are 8% water, 63% carbohydrates including 11% dietary fiber, 25% protein and 1% fat (table).

Total carbohydrates represent the major component of lentils. Among the many pulses, starch yield percent from lentils is the second highest. Furthermore, lentils are a valuable source of total dietary fibers, with insoluble dietary fiber of approximately 93–99%.

Lentils, Whole

Nutritional value g/100 g

Energy	1447 KJ (353 kcal)
Protein	25.8 g
Carbohydrates	63.1 g
Sugars, total	2.0 g
Sucrose	1.5 g

Fat, total	1.4 g
Monounsaturated	23.7%
Polyunsaturated	58.8%
Saturated	16.7%

Dietary fiber	30.5 g
Soluble fiber	1.5 g
Insoluble fiber	29.0 g
Ash	2.7 g

Vitamins		
Vitamin A,IU	39 IU	(1% DV)
Vitamin A, RAE	2 µg	
a-Tocopherol	1.6 mg	(7% DV)
β-γ Tocopherols	4.5 mg	

Thiamine (B_1)	0.9 mg	(76% DV)
Riboflavin (B_2)	0.2 mg	(18% DV)
Niacin (B_3)	2.6 mg	(17% DV)
Pantothenic acid (B_5)	2.1 mg	(10% DV)
Pyridoxine (B_6)	0.5 mg	(2% DV)
Folate (B_9)(Total DFE)	479 μg	(120% DV)
Vitamin B_{12}	0 μg	(0% DV)
Vitamin C	4.4 mg	(5% DV)
Vitamin E (α-tocopherol)	0.5 mg	(1% DV)
ɣ-Tocopherol	4.2 mg	
Vitamin K	5.0 μg	(7% DV)
Choline	96.4 mg	

Minerals		
Calcium	56 mg	6% DRI/DV
Copper	0.5 mg	55% DRI/DV
Iron	7.5 mg	50% DRI/DV
Magnesium	47 mg	13% DRI/DV
Manganese	1.3 mg	55% DRI/DV
Phosphorus	281 mg	40% DRI/DV
Potassium	677 mg	14% DRI/DV
Selenium	8.3 μg	16% DRI/DV
Zinc	3.3 mg	35% DRI/DV

Source: USDA, National Nutrient Database for Standard Reference, Release 23 (2010) [90]

The Oligosaccharides: The total a-galactosides, or raffinose family oligosaccharides, account for 53.0% of the total sugars and oligosaccharides content in lentils [91]. These oligosaccharides are considered soluble dietary fiber, cannot be digested in the human small intestine, and therefore pass through to the large intestine, where they promote the growth of *Bifidobacteria*, which are beneficial to gut health. The functional significance of these carbohydrates, therefore, arises from their ability to work as selective promoters for the growth of beneficial gut microbes. Among these oligosaccharides, stachyose represents the major oligosaccharide, followed by ciceritol and raffinose [91]. Stachyose has several biological functions. Firstly, it is an oligosaccharide that adjusts the intestinal micro-ecological balance and protects the intestinal tract. By proliferation of bifidobacteria, stachyose inhibits cholesterol synthesis and reduces serum cholesterol level. Stachyose improves also immunity and is considered an antiaging. Stachyose in fact significantly increases the activity and content of superoxide dismutase (SOD) in the blood and reduce body aging caused by the free radicals. At the same time, stachyose makes the function of detoxification in vivo significantly enhanced, and slow skin collagen ageing; finally it is quite helpful to repair, moisturize, and nourish the skin. Moreover, stachyose prevent constipation and diarrhea: stachyose in fact is used by Bifidobacterium to produce a large number of short-chain fatty acids, which stimulate intestinal peristalsis, increase fecal humidity, and maintain a certain osmotic pressure, to avoid the dry stool, so as to prevent the occurrence of constipation. Finally, stachyose contains a large number of hydroxyl. It would well absorb water in the intestine, so its effects on diarrhea treatment are also well established.

Lentils have relatively low fat (1.4 g/100) and, therefore, low energy content. Concerning the micronutrients, the mineral content of lentils is composed of relatively high levels of Mg, P, Ca, and S. In addition, lentils have a low Na and relatively high K contents, with a K:Na ratio of about 30:1–90:1 [92]. Iron (Fe) is also present in significant quantity in lentils (mg 7.5/100 g). Because bioavailability of iron from lentils could be adversely affected by natural chelating agents present in pulses, this adverse effect is minimized by cooking of lentils prior to ingestion. In addition, lentils contain Zn, which ranges between 3.2 and 6.3 mg/100 g, and other trace minerals including Cu, Mn, Mo, and B.

Lentils are also a significant dietary source of a plethora of vitamins including folate, thiamin (B_1), and riboflavin (B_2). Other water-soluble vitamins have also been reported in lentils as follows: niacin; pantothenic acid; and pyridoxine. Also vitamin E (α, β, and ɣ tocopherols) have been found in good amounts in lentils (see Table 12.1).

12.6.3 Bioactive Components

Lentils are considered as major source of phytochemicals in the diet [93]. Bioactive components and essential nutrients in lentil seeds could be categorized into different functional compounds according to their chemical structure.

12.6.3.1 Polyphenols

Lentils have the highest total phenolic content in comparison with other common pulses. Among polyphenols, tannins and tannin-related compounds are principal in lentils; lentils in fact are being among the richest leguminous seeds in their condensed tannin content, up to 915 mg/100 g [94]. The total phenolic content and antioxidant activity in lentils exhibit higher or compatible value with those of fruits or vegetables. Lentils have been reported to score the highest values among 14 different types and varieties of pulses for simple polyphenols and the total phenolic contents, with total phenolic content of about 26 mg gallic acid equivalent (GAE)/100 g FM [95]. Green or red whole lentils had a significantly higher phenolic content and antioxidant capacity than that of the pale colored pulses [96]. Catechin glucosides, procyanidin dimers, quercetin diglycoside, and trans-p-coumaric acid have been reported as the dominant phenolics in green lentils, while quercetin diglycoside, catechin, digallate procyanidin, and p-hydroxybenzoic as the dominant phenolics in red lentils. The lentil seed coat contains also trans-resveratrol-3-*O*-glucoside, and large amounts of proanthocyanidins, with the major groups of phenolic.

12.6.3.2 Phytosterols

Pulses are one of the major natural sources of phytosterols, along with cereals. Indeed, phytosterols have been shown to be abundant in lentil seeds. It has been reported that β-sitosterol, representing the predominant phytosterol, ranges 15.0–24.0 mg/100 g in cooked dry pulses [95].

12.6.3.3 Saponins

Saponins are a diverse group of compounds widely distributed in the plant kingdom, which are characterized by their structure containing a triterpene or steroid aglycone and one or more sugar chains. Consumer demand for natural products and the mounting evidence on their biological activity (such as anticancer and anticholesterol activity) has led to the emergence of saponins as commercially significant compounds with expanding applications in food, cosmetics, and pharmaceutical sectors. Lentils, like other pulses, are considered among the best sources of saponins. The lentil content of saponins could be as low as 25 mg/100 g depending on germination conditions [97].

12.6.3.4 Lectins

Lectins or hemagglutinins are a very important group of biologically active proteins bound to carbohydrates (glycoproteins) found in almost all organisms. Lectins specifically binds with glycoproteins and glycolipids on the surface of animal cells, causing agglutination of erythrocytes of certain blood groups or stimulate lymphocyte proliferation. Lectins are found naturally in lentils, with two lectin-binding fractions isolated by affinity chromatography. Lectin has shown different biological activities, such as antimicrobial, antioxidant antihypertensive, and hypocholesterolemic effects. Recently, lectins were tested as cell-proliferation inhibitor showing high activity with an IC_{50} = 0.1 mg/mL. It was suggested that lectins would exert a cytotoxic effect followed by cell apoptosis, in addition to inhibiting cell adhesion [98].

12.6.3.5 Defensins

Defensin has been found and characterized in germinated lentil seeds [99]. Defensins, small cationic cysteine-rich peptides are host defense peptides. Evidence is accumulating that defensins play a central role in defense against pathogens, and they are considered as a part of the innate immune response. They are active against bacteria, fungi, and many enveloped and non-enveloped viruses and consist of 18–45 amino acids including six (in vertebrates) to eight conserved cysteine residues. Cells of the immune system contain these peptides to assist in killing phagocytosed bacteria, for example, in neutrophil granulocytes and almost all epithelial cells. Most defensins function by binding to the microbial cell membrane, and, once embedded, forming pore-like membrane defects that allow efflux of essential ions and nutrients. In human breast milk, defensin play a central role in neonate immunity [100]. An imbalance of defensins in the skin may contribute to acne [101]. A reduction of ileal defensins may predispose to Crohn's disease [102].

12.6.3.6 Protease Inhibitors

Antinutrients are substances that interfere with the absorption of nutrients. Protease inhibitors, present in lentils, belong to this category of substances. Trypsin is one of the digestive system's main protein-digesting enzymes, and seeds probably inhibit it with trypsin inhibitors as a defense against predators. As with all beans and grains, proper soaking of lentils prior of cooking is essential to remove these naturally occurring antinutrients. Trypsin inhibitors have been identified in lentil seeds with a range of 3–8 trypsin inhibitor unit (TIU)/mg in different cultivars. Historically, protease inhibitors were considered as anti-nutritional components of pulse seeds, due to their property of decreasing the digestibility of dietary proteins. Kinetic studies have shown that the trypsin inhibitor isolated from *Lentil culinaria* seeds is characterized by an unusual strong binding affinity to its target and is resistant to thermal denaturation; such stability could explain the potential beneficial effects of lentil's antitrypsin even after the lentils are cooked [103].

12.6.3.7 Resistant Starch

Resistant starches (RS) are those starches that resist the hydrolytic effect of digestive enzymes and could be defined as the sum of starch and starch-degradation products that, on average, reach the human large intestine (see also Sect. 12.2.4 of this chapter). Cooked lentils contain about 25 g of resistant starch/100 g total starch, representing about 48% of total starch content with a value that reaches up to 65.2%. A minimum of 10% of total starch from lentils escapes digestion and absorption in the small intestine (therefore called resistant starch). The low levels of readily digestible starch (5%), and high levels of slowly digested starch, make lentils of potential value to people with diabetes [104]. Among resistant starches, we should include also oligosaccharides (see above, Sect. 12.6.2).

Due to the presence of resistant starch and other sorts of fibers, lentils and other fiber containing food exhibits bifidogenic effect even it is low when compared with that of other pulses such as peas and chickpeas. Further, it has been found that the indigestible fraction of lentils is fermented by colonic bacteria, as shown by in vitro fermentation studies. The starch indigestible fraction from black bean and lentil has been shown to be the best substrate for the fermentative production of short chain fatty acids (SCFA), especially butyric acid, which are important for the intestinal health [105, 106].

12.6.3.8 Dietary Fibers

Lentils are also a valuable source of dietary fibers, most of which are insoluble (93–99%) and less that 7% soluble [90, 107]. The β-glucan component of soluble fibers in lentils is relatively low as compared with its good sources such as oats. However, it is relatively higher than that of peas, winter wheat, and flaxseeds. Further, by virtue of their high fiber content, lentils supplemented to healthy subjects consuming typical western diet had been found to increase their fecal weights significantly, thus aiding in protecting their gut from constipation and its harmful complications [108] (see also Chap. 9—Vegetables, Sect. 9.5.3.9: Dietary Fiber and Intestine).

12.6.3.9 Antioxidant Potential of Lentils

Lentils have shown the highest total antioxidant capacity (TAC) among tested pulses measured by ferric reducing antioxidant power (FRAP) and total radical-trapping antioxidant parameter (TRAP) measures, but came second to broad beans by Trolox equivalent antioxidant capacity (TEAC) measure [109]. In a study [110], lentils showed the highest antioxidant capacity when measured as 2,2-diphenyl-1-picrylhydrazyl (DPPH) free radical scavenging capacity in comparison with green pea, yellow pea, and chickpea. The same study also revealed that the oxygen radical absorbing capacity (ORAC) of lentils was significantly higher than that of green pea, yellow pea, and chickpea. According to the USDA ORAC values 2007 [111], lentils had a higher ORAC value than most of the common fruits and vegetables including apples, plums, blackberries, cherries, figs, peaches, pears, oranges, garlic, cabbage, and almonds.

12.6.4 Health Promoting Effects

12.6.4.1 Impact on Cardiovascular Risk Factors

Among the most compelling effects of pulse including lentils are the hypocholesterolemic and CVD risk-lowering effects. In a meta-analysis [112] of eleven clinical trials that examined the effects of pulses on serum lipoproteins, results revealed that intake of non-soya pulses, including lentils, was associated with reduction in fasting serum total cholesterol (TC), lipoprotein cholesterol (LDL), triglycerides (TG) and an improvement in high density lipoproteins (HDL) cholesterol. The reviewers ascribed the hypocholesterolemic effects of pulses to be related, in estimated order of importance, to soluble dietary fiber, vegetable protein, oligosaccharides, isoflavones, phospholipids and fatty acids, saponins and other factors [112]. In another study [113] the addition of 50 g cooked lentils to diabetic patient's diet led to a significant decrease in TC but not in LDL, HDL and TG. They explained their findings under the light of the low glycemic index (GI) value of lentils. In such low GI foods, the reduction in blood lipids is thought to be due to the greater amounts of amylose in comparison with amylopectin. Digestion and absorption of amylose part of starchy foods are much slower than that of amylopectin. Consequently, GI of amylose is less than that of amylopectin, a matter that could explain the blood lipid-lowering effect of lentils which have higher amylose to amylopectin fraction.

The hypolipidemic effect of lentils had been ascribed also to increased biliary cholesterol and decreased biliary phospholipids in such a way that the biliary cholesterol saturation index rose from 110% to 169% [114]. In a crossover study [115] on nine male subjects housed in a metabolic ward for 6–7 weeks, the consumption of 120 g baked mixed pulses, 60% red, navy and lima beans, 27% peas and 13% lentils, significantly reduced serum LDL-cholesterol by 8% was found at the end of treatment compared to the isoenergetic control diet. It is worth mentioning that because lentils have been quite frequently used as part of a mixed pulse intervention in several studies, the effects of lentils cannot be correctly evaluated and the hypolipidemic effect cannot be ascribed solely to lentils. In this respect, a meta-analysis of randomized controlled trials on the blood cholesterol-lowering effect of non-soy pulse consumption, selected ten randomized, clinical trials [116] including 268 participants who were given diets rich in non-soy pulses: beans, peas, lentils or chickpeas, for a minimum duration of 3 weeks, showed a significant reduction in total and LDL-cholesterol levels. They recommended that dietary modification strategies that target the reduction of risk factors for CVD should include an increase in pulse consumption in addition to other strategies, which have been of proven benefit.

12.6.4.2 The Impact on Diabetes

It has been strongly suggested that eating pulses is beneficial in the prevention and management of diabetes [117]. Therefore, consumption of a wide range of carbohydrate foods from pulses and other rich sources both for the general population and for people with diabetes, especially those with type II diabetes [118], is generally recommended. The ability of lentils to alleviate the glycemic load (GL) has been demonstrated in experimentally induced diabetic rats, healthy volunteers, and insulin-dependent and nondependent diabetic patients [119, 120]. It was demonstrated [113] that addition of 50 g cooked lentils to diabetic patient diet led to a significant decrease in fasting blood glucose. In this study, the administration of lentils significantly decreased serum blood glucose. The glucose lowering effect of lentils was ascribed by the researchers to probable influences of low GI diet on glucose metabolism.

In another relevant study [121], a group of eight healthy volunteers took a series of breakfast test meals containing either lentils, which had been processed in four different ways, or the same amount of carbohydrate as white bread. Of the different types of lentils, boiled lentils resulted in a flattened blood glucose response in comparison with bread. Glycemic index is a measure of the rate at which ingested food causes the level of glucose in the blood to rise. Consumption of foods with high glycemic index and high glycemic load is associated with hyperglycemia and hyperinsulinemia. Lentils showed low glycemic index value in healthy volunteers, with an average value of approximately 29 [122]. This is within the range reported in the International Table of glycemic index and glycemic load [123] in which the values ranged from 18 to 52 depending on the type of lentils as follows: an average value for red lentils of 26 (mean of 4 studies); an average value of 30 for green lentils (mean of 3 studies), 29 for NS type lentils (mean of 2 studies) and 52 (1 study) for green lentils canned in brine. The reported values of glycemic index for lentils have shown noticeable variation between in vitro and in vivo studies. Despite this variation between in vivo and in vitro GI values, lentils have still had the lowest and the slowest rate of hydrolysis of their starches, and the lowest expected glycemic index among tested pulse grains (chickpeas and peas) [124].

12.6.4.3 The Impact on Cancer

Lentils are dietary component traditionally consumed in populations where cancers of the colon, breast, and prostate are low [125]. In a prospective study on 90,630 women, lentils or beans were the only two foods that exhibited an inverse association with the risk of breast cancer [126]. In a case–control study on 186 African-American men and women, the consumption of pulses, including lentils, was negatively associated with risk of developing colorectal cancer [127]. The reasons of the association between lentil consumption and reduced cancer risks and incidence could be ascribed to the constituents of lentils.

Lentils have shown significantly the highest polyphenolic content expressed in terms of TPC (total phenolic content) among different pulses. Polyphenolics have shown chemopreventive ability against cancer with several plausible molecular, genetic, and biochemical mechanisms [128].

The Lectins: Plant lectins are unique group of glycoproteins in lentils with potent biological activity. Several lectins have been found to possess anticancer properties in vitro, in vivo, and in human case studies [129], with different modes of actions including molecular, genetic and epigenetic mechanisms. The mechanisms by which lectins exert their tumor suppressor effects have been summarized [130]. Previous reports have shown in vitro inhibitory effects of lectins from different plant sources, including lentils, on colon cancer. Most studies investigating anticancer effects of lectins used lectins from lentil and various pea varieties, further confirming the uniqueness of lectins from these pulses compared to other natural sources [69]. Hence, lectins from lentils and other pulses have great potential as functional foods for reducing the risk of certain cancers.

The Defensin: A novel peptide called "defensin" has been characterized recently in germinated lentil seeds [99]. Plant defensins are characterized by a broad spectrum of biological activities including antimicrobial activities against bacteria and fungi. They have been suggested to aid in halting tumorigenesis. Indeed, defensin exhibited an antiproliferative activity against more than one tumor cell line [99].

Protease Inhibitors: Protease inhibitors have been widely investigated in pulses. Among the suggested therapeutic applications of protease inhibitors include inhibition of breast cancer cells and hepatoma cells and utilization in acquired immunodeficiency syndrome (AIDS) due to their proteolytic effect against reverse transcriptase enzyme involved in viral replication [131]. Among the protease inhibitors of lentils, the BBI (Bowman-Birk protease Inhibitors) has been proved to have many beneficial biochemical and functional properties, including an anti-tumoral cells activity [130, 132]. Proteases are considered key factors in cancer progression and metastasis; therefore, suppressing their activities by protease inhibitors appears to be contributing to inhibiting carcinogenesis [133]. Mature lentil BBIs were reported to inhibit cell proliferation of colon adenocarcinoma cells in a dose-dependent manner due to their intrinsic abilities to inhibit serine proteases [134].

Phytates: Dietary phytates have been shown to be effective in halting colorectal carcinogenesis [135]. The other anticarcinogenic effects of phytates were critically reviewed elsewhere [24, 136]. Furthermore, preliminary studies in human cancer patients showed that IP6 and inositol, as InoCell, an adjuvant to chemotherapy, appeared to enhance the anticancer effect of the conventional chemotherapy, control cancer metastases, and improve quality of life by reducing the side effects of common chemotherapy [24].

Saponins: Recently saponins have been focused upon, due to increasing evidence of their positive health implications such as hypocholesterolemic and anticancer properties [97]. Anticancer activity of saponins has been reported for many triterpenes and steroid saponins present in pulses, including lentils. Different forms of saponins isolated from different plant sources have been identified as potential anticancer agents by the National Cancer Institute's Anticancer Drug Screen Program

[97]. Soya saponins have been suggested to be potent chemopreventive agents against colorectal cancer, an effect that had been evidenced through several epidemiological, and in vivo and in vitro laboratory studies that were critically reviewed by Gurfinkel and Rao [137]. In a experimental study on colon cancer [138], rats fed with cooked lentils showed a striking 77.8% reduction of the number of small-intestinal adenomas and colonic aberrant crypt foci (ACF), compared to the only 26.8% reduction of ACF observed in rats fed with raw whole lentils. As large ACF have been shown to predict more accurately pre-neoplastic potential, this suggested that the lentils, particularly cooked whole lentils, may act by retarding progression of the early aberrant crypts. It is noteworthy to indicate that the ability to reduce total ACF number reflects the ability lentils to prevent carcinogenesis initiation or working as blocking agents. According to Chen and Kong [139], the blocking agents that inhibit colon carcinogenesis could exert their preventive effect by several mechanisms, including enhancement of detoxification of carcinogens, inhibition of cytochrome P450 (CYP450)-mediated activation of carcinogens, scavenging free radicals and halting antioxidant activity, and finally trapping the carcinogen and preventing their interaction with DNA.

In summary, the vast amount of literature confirms that lentil is one of the most nutritious and health-improving food known to man. According to recent definitions, lentil could be considered a prophylactic and therapeutic functional food due to its considerable content of essential macronutrients, namely functional proteins and carbohydrates, and essential micronutrients, as well as bioactive phytochemicals such as phytates and polyphenols. Indeed, lentils contain an impressive arsenal of secondary metabolites, minerals and bioactive constituents that have shown to be promising in the management and prevention of several human chronic illnesses.

References

1. Khokhar S, Owusu Apenten RK. The role of food, agriculture, forestry and fisheries in human nutrition. In: Squires VR, editor. Antinutritional factors in food legumes and effects of processing, vol. IV. Paris: Encyclopedia of Life Support Systems (EOLSS); 2002–2017.
2. Wahlqvist ML, Hsu-Hage BH-H, Kouris-Blazos A, Lukito W. Food habits in later life. A cross cultural study. Bethesda, MD: Asia Pacific Journal of Clinical Nutrition; 1995.
3. Tovar J, Björck M, Asp NG. Incomplete digestion of legume starches in rats: a study of precookeed flours containing retrograded and physically inaccessible starch fractions. J Nutr. 1992;122:1500–7.
4. Englyst HN, HN CH. Digestion of polysaccharides of potato in the small intestine of man. Am J Clin Nutr. 1987;45:423–31.
5. Faisant N, Gallant DJ, Bouchet B, Champ M. Banana starch breakdown in the human small intestine studied by electron microscopy. Eur J Clin Nutr. 1995;49:98–104.
6. Noah L, Guillon F, Bouchet B, Buleon A, Molis C, Gratas M, Champ M. Digestion of carbohydrate from white beans (Phaseolus vulgaris L.) in healthy humans. J Nutr. 1998;128:977–85.
7. Asp NG, Van Amelsvoort JMM, Hautvast JGA. Nutritional implications of resistant starch. Nutr Res Rev. 1996;9:1–31.
8. Cassidy A, Bingham S, Cummings JH. Starch intake and colorectal cancer risk: and international comparison. Br J Cancer. 1994;69:937–42.

9. De Deckere EAM, Kloots WJ, Van Amelsvoort JMM. Both raw and retrograded starch decrease serum triacylglycerol concentration and fat accretion in the rat. Br J Nutr. 1995;73:287–9.
10. Jenkins DJA, Wolever TMS, Collier GR, Ocana A, Rao AV, Buckley G, Lam Y, Mayer A, Tompson LU. Metabolic effects of a low-glycemic-index diet. Am J Clin Nutr. 1987;46:968–75.
11. Velasco ZI, Rascon A, Tovar J. Enzymic availability of starch in cooked black beans (Phaseolus vulgaris L.) and cowpeas (Vigna spp.). J Agric Food Chem. 1997;45:1548–51.
12. Bravo L, Siddhuraju P, Saura-Calixto F. Composition of underexploited Indian pulses. Comparison with common legumes. Food Chem. 1999;64:185–92.
13. Melito C, Tovar J. Cell walls limit in vitro protein digestibility in processed legumes. Food Chem. 1995;53:305–7.
14. Würsch P, Del Vedovo S, Koellreuter B. Cell structure and starch nature as key determinants of the digestion rate of starch in legumes. Am J Clin Nutr. 1986;43:25–9.
15. Tundis R, Loizzo MR, Menichini F. Natural products as alpha-amylase and alpha-glucosidase inhibitors and their hypoglycaemic potential in the treatment of diabetes: an update. Mini-Rev Med Chem. 2010;10:315–31.
16. McDougall GJ, Stewart D. The inhibitory effects of berry polyphenols on digestive enzymes. Biofactors. 2005;23:189–95.
17. Koh LW, Wong LL, Loo YY, Kasapis S, Huang D. Evaluation of different teas against starch digestibility by mammalian glycosidases. J Agric Food Chem. 2010;58:148–54.
18. Barret ML, Udani JK. A proprietary alpha-amylase inhibitor from white bean (Phaseolus vulgaris): a review of clinical studies on weight loss and glycemic control. Nutr J. 2011;10:24.
19. Markiewicz LH, Honke J, Haros M, Świątecka D, Wróblewska B. Diet shapes the ability of human intestinal microbiota to degrade phytate—in vitro studies. J Appl Microbiol. 2013;115:247–59.
20. Haros M, Carlsson NG, Almgren A, Larsson-Alminger M, Sandberg AS, Andlid T. Phytate degradation by human gut isolated Bifidobacterium pseudocatenulatum ATCC27919 and its probiotic potential. Int J Food Microbiol. 2009;135:7–14.
21. Hanakahi LA, Bartlet-Jones M, Chappell C, Pappin D, West SC. Binding of inositol phosphate to DNA-PK and stimulation of double-strand break repair. Cell. 2000;102:721–9.
22. Graf E, Empson KL, Eaton JW. Phytic acid. A natural antioxidant. J Biol Chem. 1987;262:11647–50.
23. Grases F, Costa-Bauzá A. Phytate (IP6) is a powerful agent for preventing calcifications in biological fluids: usefulness in renal lithiasis treatment. Anticancer Res. 1999;19:3717–22.
24. Vucenik I, Shamsuddin AM. Protection against cancer by dietary IP6 and inositol. Nutr Cancer. 2006;55:109–25.
25. Jenab M, Thompson LU. The influence of phytic acid in wheat bran on early biomarkers of colon carcinogenesis. Carcinogenesis. 1998;19:1087–92.
26. Shamsuddin AM, Wah A. Inositol hexaphosphate inhibits large intestinal cancer in F344 rats 5 months after induction by azoxymethane. Carcinogenesis. 1989;10:625–6.
27. Vucenik I, Yang GY, Shamsuddin AM. Inositol hexaphosphate and inositol inhibits DMBA-induced rat mammary cancer. Carcinogenesis. 1995;16:1055–8.
28. Fox CH, Eberl M. Phytic acid (IP6), novel broad-spectrum anti-neoplastic agent: a systematic review. Complement Ther Med. 2002;10:229–34.
29. Singh RP, Agarwal R. Prostate cancer and inositol hexaphosphate: efficacy and mechanisms. Anticancer Res. 2005;25:2891–904.
30. Bizzarri M, Dinicola S, Bevilacqua A, Cucina A. Broad Spectrum anticancer activity of Myo-inositol and inositol Hexakisphosphate. Int J Endocrinol. 2016;2016:5616807.
31. Vicia faba (Broad bean). Biological Records Centre and Botanical Society of Britain and Ireland.
32. Swenson AA. Foods Jesus ate and how to grow them. New York, NY: Skyhorse Publishing; 2013.
33. Hornykiewicz O. A brief history of levodopa. J Neurol. 2010;257(Suppl 2):S249–52.

34. Okumura K, Hosoya T, Kawarazaki K, Izawa N, Kumazawa S. Antioxidant activity of phenolic compounds from fava bean sprouts. J Food Sci. 2016;8:C1394–8.
35. Siah SD, Konczak I, Agboola S, Wood JA, Blanchard CL. In vitro investigations of the potential health benefits of Australian-grown faba beans (Vicia faba L.): chemopreventative capacity and inhibitory effects on the angiotensin-converting enzyme, α-glucosidase and lipase. Br J Nutr. 2012;108(Suppl1):S123–34.
36. Culpeper, Nicholas. Chick-Pease, or Cicers. The Complete Herbal (1652, originally titled The English Physitian).
37. Internet Archive Way Back Machine. Introduction: Chickpea. International Center for Agricultural Research in the Dry Areas.
38. Milán-Carrillo J, Valdéz-Alarcón C, Gutiérrez-Dorado R, Cárdenas-Valenzuela OG, Mora-Escobedo R, Garzón-Tiznado JA, Reyes-Moreno C. Nutritional properties of quality protein maize and chickpea extruded based weaning food. Plant Foods Hum Nutr. 2007;62:31–7.
39. Nutrition facts for Chickpeas (garbanzo beans, bengal gram), mature seeds, cooked, boiled, without salt, 100 g, USDA Nutrient Database, version SR-21. Conde Nast. 2014.
40. Yang WX, Liang ZS, Wang SW, Zhang L, Xie YH, He ZM. Effect of genistein to FPG and blood lipids on type 2 diabetes rats. J Northwest A & F Univ (Nat Sci Ed). 2009;37:1–6.
41. Li Y. The research about extracting, separating, purifying isoflavone and saponin from *Cicer arietium* L. and their decreasing blood glucose, regulating blood lipid effect. Master's Thesis. Wulumuqi, China: Xin Jiang Agricultural University; 2007.
42. Ayumi H, Katsuhiro T, Kosuke A, Soichiro N, Norio K, Kazuya Y. Genistein stimulates the insulin-dependent signaling pathway. Front Biosci. 2011;3:1534–40.
43. Evans BAJ, Griffiths K, Morton MS. Inhibition of 5α-reductase in genital skin fibroblasts and prostate tissue by dietary lignans and isoflavonoids. J Endocrinol. 1995;147:295–302.
44. Khan SI, Zhao J, Khan IA, et al. Potential utility of natural products as regulators of breast cancer-associated aromatase promoters. Reprod Biol Endocrinol. 2011;9:1–10.
45. Patisaul HB, Jefferson W. The pros and cons of phytoestrogens. Front Neuroendocrinol. 2010;3:400–19.
46. Wang L, Waltenberger B, Pferschy-Wenzig EM, Blunder M, Liu X, Malainer C, Blazevic T, Schwaiger S, Rollinger JM, Heiss EH, Schuster D, Kopp B, Bauer R, Stuppner H, Dirsch VM, Atanasov AG. Natural product agonists of peroxisome proliferator-activated receptor gamma (PPARγ): a review. Biochem Pharmacol. 2014;92:73–89.
47. Rasbach KA, Schnellmann RG. Isoflavones promote mitochondrial biogenesis. J Pharmacol Exp Ther. 2008;325:536–43.
48. Peterson G, Barnes S. Genistein and biochanin a inhibit the growth of human prostate cancer cells but not epidermal growth factor receptor tyrosine autophosphorylation. Prostate. 1993;22:335–45.
49. Kole L, Giri B, Manna SK, Pal B, Ghosh S. Biochanin-a, an isoflavon, showed anti-proliferative and anti-inflammatory activities through the inhibition of iNOS expression, p38-MAPK and ATF-2 phosphorylation and blocking NFκB nuclear translocation. Eur J Pharmcol. 2011;653(1–3):8–15.
50. Wang Y, Man Gho W, Chan FL, Chen S, Leung LK. The red clover (Trifolium pratense) isoflavone biochanin a inhibits aromatase activity and expression. Br J Nutr. 2008;99:303–10.
51. Kaczmarczyk-Sedlak I, Wojnar W, Zych M, Ozimina-Kamińska E, Taranowicz J, Siwek A. Effect of formononetin on mechanical properties and chemical composition of bones in rats with ovariectomy-induced osteoporosis. vEvid Based Complement Alternat Med. 2013;2013:457052.
52. Banu J, Varela E, Fernandes G. Alternative therapies for the prevention and treatment of osteoporosis. Nutr Rev. 2012;70:22–40.
53. Bedell S, Nachtigall M, Naftolin F. The pros and cons of plant estrogens for menopause. J Steroid Biochem Mol Biol. 2014;139:225–36.
54. Zhang DW, Cheng Y, Wang NL, Zhang JC, Yang MS, Yao XS. Effects of total flavonoids and flavonol glycosides from Epimedium Koreanum Nakai on the proliferation and differentiation of primary osteoblasts. Phytomedicine. 2008;15:55–61.

55. Al-Anazi AF, Qureshi VF, Javaid K, Qureshi S. Preventive effects of phytoestrogens against postmenopausal osteoporosis as compared to the available therapeutic choices: an overview. J Nat Sci Bio Med. 2011;2:154–63.
56. Sunita P, Pattanayak SP. Phytoestrogens in postmenopausal indications: a theoretical perspective. Pharmacogn Rev. 2011;5:41–7.
57. Atkinson C, Compston JE, Day NE, Dowsett M, Bingham SA. The effects of phytoestrogen isoflavones on bone density in women: a double-blind, randomized, placebo-controlled trial. Am J Clin Nutr. 2004;79:326.
58. Zohary D, Hopf M. Domestication of plants in the old World. 3rd ed. Oxford: Oxford University Press; 2000.
59. Hood-Niefer SD, Warkentin TD, Chibbar RN, Vandenberg A, Tyler RT. Effect of genotype and environment on the concentrations of starch and protein in, and the hysicochemical properties of starch from, field pea and fababean. J Sci Food Agric. 2012;92:141–50.
60. Tosh SM, Yada S. Dietary fibres in pulse seeds and fractions: characterization, functional attributes, and applications. Food Res Int. 2010;43:450–60.
61. Grosjean F. Combining peas for animal nutrition. In: Hebblethwaite PD, Heath MC, Dawkins TCK, editors. The pea crop: a basis for improvement. London: Butterworths; 1985. p. 453–62.
62. Norton G, Bliss FA, Bressani R. Biochemical and nutritional attributes of grain legumes. In: Summerfield RJ, Roberts EH, editors. Grain legume crops. London: Collins; 1985. p. 73–114.
63. Salunke DK, Kadam SS, Chavan JK. Chemical composition. In: Postharvest biotechnology of food legumes. Boca Raton, FL: CRC Press; 1985. p. 29–52.
64. Savage GP, Deo S. The nutritional value of peas (Pisum sativum). A literature review. Nutr Abstr Rev Ser A: Human Exp Nutr. 1989;59:65–87.
65. Wang N, Daun JK. The chemical composition and nutritive value of Canadian pulses. Winnipeg: Canadian Grain Commission; 2004.
66. Dostalovà R, Horàcek J, Hasalovà I, et al. Study of resistant starch (RS) content in pea during maturation. Czech J Food Sci. 2009;27:S120–4.
67. Tömösközi S, Lásztity R, Haraszi R, Baticz O. Isolation and study of the functional properties of pea proteins. Nahrung/Food. 2001;45:399–401.
68. Abete I, Parra D, Martinez JA. Legume-, fish-, orhigh-protein-based hypocaloric diets: effects on weight loss and mitochondrial oxidation in obese men. J Med Food. 2009;12:100–8.
69. Roy F, Boye JI, Simpson BK. Bioactive proteins and peptides in pulse crops: pea, chickpea and lentil. Food Res Int. 2010;43:432–42.
70. Tahir R, Ellis PR, Bogracheva TY, Meares-Taylor C, Butterworth PJ. Study of the structure and properties of native and dydrothermally processed wild-type, lam and r variant pea starches that affect amylolysis of these starches. Biomacromolecules. 2011;12:123–33.
71. Chung H-J, Liu Q, Hoover R. Effect of single and dual hydrothermal treatments on the crystalline structure, thermal properties, and nutritional fractions of pea, lentil, and navy bean starches. Food Res Int. 2010;43:501–8.
72. Trinidad TP, Mallillin AC, Loyola AS, Sagum RS, Encabo RR. The potential health benefits of legumes as a good source of dietary fibre. Br J Nutr. 2010;103:569–74.
73. Chen WJL, Anderson JW, Jenkins DJA. Propionate may mediate the hypocholesterolemic effects of certain soluble plant fibers in cholesterol-fed rats. Proc Soc Exp Biol Med. 1984;175:215–8.
74. Fernando WMU, Hill JE, Zello GA, et al. Diets supplemented with chickpea or its main oligosaccharide component raffinose modify fecal microbial composition in healthy adults. Benefic Microbes. 2010;1:197–207.
75. Campos-Vega R, Loarca-Pina G, Oomah BD. Minor components of pulses and their potential impact on human health. Food Res Int. 2010;43:461–82.
76. Duenãs M, Estrella I, Hernandez T. Occurrence of phenolic compounds in the seed coat and the cotyledon of peas (Pisum sativum L.). Eur Food Res Technol. 2004;219:116–23.
77. Pownall TL, Udenigwe CC, Aluko RE. Amino acid composition and antioxidant properties of pea seed (Pisum sativum L.) enzymatic protein hydrolysate fractions. J Agric Food Chem. 2010;58:4712–8.

78. Marinangeli CP, Kassis AN, Jones PJ. Glycemic responses and sensory characteristics of whole yellow pea flour added to novel functional foods. J Food Sci. 2009;74:S385–9.
79. Marinangeli CP, Jones PJ. Whole and fractionated yellow pea flours reduce fasting insulin and insulin resistance in hypercholesterolaemic and overweight human subjects. Br J Nutr. 2011;105:110–7.
80. Lunde MS, Hjellset VT, Holmboe-Ottesen G, et al. Variations in postprandial blood glucose responses andsatiety after intake of three types of bread. J Nutr Metab. 2011;2011:437587.
81. Slavin JL. Position of the American dietetic association: health implications of dietary fiber. J Am Diet Assoc. 2008;108:1716–31.
82. Sandström B, Hansen LT, Sørensen A. Pea fiber lowers fasting and postprandial blood triglyceride concentrations in humans. J Nutr. 1994;124:2386–96.
83. Hermsdorff HM, Zulet MA, Abete I, Martinez JR. A legume-based hypocaloric diet reduces proinflammatory status and improves metabolic features in overweight obese subjects. Eur J Nutr. 2011;50:61–9.
84. Dahl WJ, Whiting SJ, Healey AD, Zello GA, Hildebrandt SL. Increased stool frequency and fecal output occurs when finely processed pea hull fiber is added to usual foods consumed by elderly long term care residents. J Am Diet Assoc. 2003;103:1199–202.
85. Flogan C, Dahl WJ. Fiber fortification improves gastrointestinal function and decreases energy intake in children with a history of constipation. Infant Child Adolescent Nutr. 2010;2:312–7.
86. Swiatecka D, Kostyra H, Swiatecki A. Impact of glycosylated pea proteins on the activity of free-swimming and immobilized bacteria. J Sci Food Agric. 2010;90:1837–45.
87. Swiatecka D, Narbad A, Ridgway KP, Kostyra H. The study on the impact of glycosylated pea proteins on human intestinal bacteria. Int J Food Microbiol. 2011;145:267–72.
88. Troszynska A, Ciska E. Phenolic compounds of seed coats of white and coloured varieties of pea (Pisum Sativum L.) and their total antioxidant activity. Czech J Food Sci. 2002;20:15–22.
89. Hagerman AE, Ried KM, Jones GA, Sovik KN, Ritchard NT, Hartzfeld PW, Riechel TL. High molecular weight plant polyphenolics (tannins) as antioxidants. J Agric Food Chem. 1998;46:1887–92.
90. United States Department of Agriculture (USDA). USDA National Nutrient Database for Standard Reference, Release 23; 2011.
91. Vidal-Valverde C, Frias J, Sierra I, Blazquez IF, Lambein F, Kuo YH. New functional legume foods by germination: effect on the nutritive value of beans, lentils and peas. Eur Food Res Technol. 2002;215:472–7.
92. Padovani RM, Lima DM, Colugnati FAB, Rodriguez-Amaya DLB. Comparison of proximate, mineral and vitamin composition of common Brazilian and US food. J Food Compos Anal. 2007;20:733–8.
93. Issa AY, Volate SR, Wargovich MJ. The role of phytochemicals in inhibition of cancer and inflammation: new directions and perspectives. J Food Compos Anal. 2006;19:405–19.
94. Zia-ur-Rehman Salariya AM. The effects of hydrothermal processing on antinutrients, protein and starch digestibility of food legumes. Int J Food Sci Technol. 2005;40:695–700.
95. Kalogeropoulos N, Chiou A, Ioannou M, Karathanos VT, Hassapidou M, Andrikopoulos NK. Nutritional evaluation and bioactive microconstituents (phytosterols, tocopherols, polyphenols, triterpenic acids) in cooked dry legumes usually consumed in the Mediterranean countries. Food Chem. 2010;121:682–90.
96. Xu B, Chang SKC. Phenolic substance characterization and chemical and cell-based antioxidant activities of 11 lentils grown in the Northern United States. J Agric Food Chem. 2011;58:1509–17.
97. Güclü-Üstündag Ö, Mazza G. Saponins: properties, applications and processing. Crit Rev Food Sci Nutr. 2007;47:231–58.
98. Quiroga AV, Barrio DA, Anon MC. Amaranth lectin presents potential antitumor properties. IWT–Food Sci Technol. 2015;60:478–85.
99. Finkina KI, Shramova EI, Tagaev AA, Ovchinnikova TV. A novel defensin from the lentil (lens Culinaris) seeds. Biochem Biophys Res Commun. 2008;371:860–5.

100. Barrera GJ, Sanchez G, Gonzalez JE. Trefoil factor 3 isolated from human breast milk downregulates cytokines (IL8 and IL6) and promotes human beta defensin (hBD2 and hBD4) expression in intestinal epithelial cells HT-29. Bosn J Basic Med Sci. 2012;12:256–64.
101. Philpott MP. Defensins and acne. Mol Immunol. 2003;40:457–62.
102. Wehkamp J, Salzman NH, Porter E, Nuding S, Weichenthal M, Petras RE, Shen B, Schaeffeler E, Schwab M, Linzmeier R, Feathers RW, Chu H, Lima H, Fellermann K, Ganz T, Stange E, Bevins CL. Reduced Paneth cell α-defensins in ileal Crohn's disease. Proc Natl Acad Sci. 2005;102(50):18129–34.
103. Lajolo FM, Genovese M. Nutritional significance of lectins and enzyme inhibitors from legumes. J Agric Food Chem. 2002;50:6592–8.
104. Ramdath D, Renwick S, Duncan AM. The role of pulses in the dietary management of diabetes. Can J Diabetes (Review). 2016;40:355–63.
105. Queiroz-Monici KS, Costa GEA, Silva N, Reis SM, Oliveira AC. Bifidogenic effect of dietary fibre and resistant starch from leguminous on the intestinal microbiota of rats. Nutrition. 2005;21:602–8.
106. Hernandez-Salazar M, Osorio-Diaz P, Loarca-Pina G, ReynosoCamacho R, Tovar J, Bello-Perez LA. In vitro fermentability and antioxidant capacity of the indigestible fraction of cooked black beans (Phaseolus vulgaris L.), lentils (Lens culinaris L.) and chickpeas (Cicer arietinum L.). J Sci Food Agric. 2010;90:1417–22.
107. Bednar GE, Patil AR, Murray SM, Grieshop CM, Merchen NR, GCJ F. Starch and fiber fractions in selected food and feed ingredients affect their small intestinal digestibility and fermentability and their large bowel fermentability in vitro in a canine model. J Nutr. 2001;131:276–86.
108. Stephen AM, Dahl WJ, Sieber GM, Blaricom JA, Morgan DR. Effect of green lentils on colonic function, nitrogen balance, and serum lipids in healthy human subjects. Am J Clin Nutr. 1995;62:1–7.
109. Pellegrini N, Serafini M, Salvatore S, Rio DD, Bianchi M, Brighenti F. Total antioxidant capacity of spices, dried fruits, nuts, pulses, cereals and sweets consumed in Italy assessed by three different in vitro assays. Mol Nutr Food Res. 2006;50:1030–8.
110. Xu BJ, Chang SKC. Effect of soaking, boiling, and steaming on total phenolic content and antioxidant activities of cool season food legumes. Food Chem. 2008;110:1–13.
111. USDA Database for the Oxygen Radical Absorbance Capacity (ORAC) of Selected Foods, Release 2.
112. Anderson JW, Major AW. Pulses and lipemia, short- and long-term effect: potential in the prevention of cardiovascular disease. Br J Nutr. 2002;88:S263–71.
113. Shams H, Tahbaz F, Entezari M, Abadi A. Effects of cooked lentils on glycaemic control and blood lipids of patients with type 2 diabetes. ARYA Athero J. 2008;3:215–8.
114. Kingman SM. The influence of legume seeds on human plasma lipid concentrations. Nutr Res Rev. 1991;4:97–123.
115. Duane WC. Effects of legume consumption on serum cholesterol, biliary lipids, and sterol metabolism in humans. J Lipid Res. 1997;38:1120–8.
116. Bazzano LA, Thompson AM, Tees MT, Nguyen CH, Winham DM. Non-soy legume consumption lowers cholesterol levels: a meta-analysis of randomized controlled trials. Nutr Metab Cardiovasc Dis. 2009;21:94–103.
117. Rizkalla SW, Bellisle F, Slama G. Health benefits of low glycaemic index foods, such as pulses, in diabetic patients and healthy individuals. Br J Nutr. 2002;88:S255–62.
118. Venn BJ, Mann JI. Cereal grains, legumes and diabetes. Eur J Clin Nutr. 2004;58: 1443–146.
119. Al-Tibi AMH, Takruri HR, Ahmad MN. Effect of dehulling and cooking of lentils (Lens culinaris L.) on serum glucose and lipoprotein levels in streptozotocin-induced diabetic rats. Malays J Nutr. 2010;16:83–92.
120. Wolever TMS, Katzman-Relle L, Jenkins AL, Vuksna V, Josse RG, Jenkins DJA. Glycaemic index of 102 complex carbohydrate foods in patients with diabetes. Nutr Res. 1994;14: 651–69.

121. Jenkins DJA, Thorne MJ, Camelon K, Jenkins A, Rao AV, Taylor RH, Thompson LU, Kalmusky J, Reichert R, Francis T. Effect of processing on digestibility and the blood glucose response: a study of lentils. Am J Clin Nutr. 1982;36:1093–101.
122. Jenkins DJA, Wolever TMS, Taylor RH, Barker H, Fielden H, Baldwin JM, Bowling AC, Newman HC, Jenkins AL, Goff DV. Glycaemic index of foods: a physiological basis for carbohydrate exchange. Am J Clin Nutr. 1981;34:362–6.
123. Foster-Powell K, Holt SH, Brand-Miller JC. International table of glycaemic index and glycaemic load values. Am J Clin Nutr. 2002;76:5–56.
124. Chung HJ, Liu Q, Hoover R, Tom D, Warkentin C, Vandenberg A. In vitro starch digestibility, expected glycaemic index, and thermal and pasting properties of flours from pea, lentil and chickpea cultivars. Food Chem. 2008;111:316–21.
125. Correa P. Epidemiological correlations between diet and cancer frequency. Cancer Res. 1981;41:3685–90.
126. Adebamowo CA, Cho E, Sampson L, Katan MB, Spiegelman D, Willett WC, Holmes MD. Dietary flavonols and flavonolrich foods intake and the risk of breast cancer. Int J Cancer. 2005;114:628–33.
127. Agurs-Collins T, Smoot D, Afful J, Makambi K, Adams-Campbell LL. Legume intake and reduced colorectal adenoma risk in African–Americans. J Natl Black Nurses Assoc. 2006;17:6–12. (Abstract).
128. Nichenametla SN, Taruscio TG, Barney DL, Exon JH. A review of the effects and mechanisms of polyphenolics in cancer. Crit Rev Food Sci Nutr. 2006;46:161–83.
129. Mejia EGL, Prisecaru VI. Lectins as bioactive plant proteins: a potential in cancer treatment. Crit Rev Food Sci Nutr. 2005;45:425–45.
130. Scarafoni A, Magni C, Duranti M. Molecular nutraceutics as a mean to investigate the positive effects of legume seed proteins on human health. Trends Food Sci Technol. 2007;18:454–63.
131. Cheung AHK, Ng TB. Isolation and characterization of a trypsin–chymotrypsin inhibitor from the seeds of green lentil (lens Culinaris). Protein Pept Lett. 2007;14:859–64.
132. Losso JN. The biochemical and functional food properties of the Bowman–Birk inhibitor. Crit Rev Food Sci Nutr. 2008;4:94–118.
133. Kennedy AR. The Bowman–Birk inhibitor from soybeans as an anticarcinogenic agent. Am J Clin Nutr. 1998;68:1406S–12S.
134. Caccialupi P, Ceci LR, Siciliano RA, Pignone D, Clemene A, Sonnante G. Bowman-Birk inhibitors in lentil: heterologous expression, functional characterization and anti-proliferative properties in human colon cancer cells. Food Chem. 2010;120:1058–66.
135. Marks G, Aydos RDA, Fagundes DJ, Pontes ERJC, Takita LC, Amaral EGAS, Rossini A, Ynouye AM. Modulation of transforming growth factor beta2 (TGF-beta2) by inositol hexaphosphate in colon carcinogenesis in rats. Acta Cir Bras. 2006;21:51–6.
136. Verghese M, Rao DR, Chawana CB, Walker LT, Shackelford L. Anticarcinogenic effect of phytic acid (IP6): apoptosis as a possible mechanism of action. LWT-Food Sci Technol. 2006;39:1093–8.
137. Gurfinkel DM, Rao AV. Soya saponins: the relationship between chemical structure and colon anticarcinogenic activity. Nutr Cancer. 2003;47:24–33.
138. Faris MAIE, Tacruri HR, Issa AY. Role of lentils (Lens culinaris L.) I human health and nutrition: a review. Mediterr J Nutr Metab. 2013;6:3–16.
139. Chen C, Kong ANT. Dietary cancer-chemopreventive compounds: from signaling and gene expression to pharmacological effects. Trends Pharmacol Sci. 2005;26:318–26.

Fish

13

13.1 Premises

In Mediterranean diet fish has always had a primary role as an important source of animal protein. Fish provides a variety of nutrients, including protein and long-chain omega 3 polyunsaturated fatty acids ($\omega 3$, n-3 PUFAs), as well as micronutrients including selenium, iodine, potassium, vitamin D, and B-vitamins. Intakes of some of these micronutrients, including iodine and vitamin D, are frequently low in some population groups, which makes fish a valuable contributor to intakes of these components. It is recommended that two portions of fish a week should be consumed, one of which should be oily. This is because it is thought that long-chain n-3 PUFAs present in oil-rich fish and fish oil are associated with beneficial health outcomes.

The term "fish" generally includes finfish (vertebrates) and shellfish (invertebrates), whether of marine or freshwater origin, farmed or wild. The terms "fish" and "seafood" are used interchangeably.

13.2 Nutritional Value

The energy content of raw fish varies greatly from 80 kcal (337 kJ)/100 g for cod to 220 kcal (914 kJ)/100 g for mackerel (Table 13.1). This is mainly due to the varying fat content between different species of fish. Based on fat content, fish is classed as either whitefish, oily fish, or shellfish (Table 13.1, Fig. 13.1). Whitefish, such as haddock and seer, contain very little fat (usually less than 1%) whereas oily fish, such as sardines, herrings, mackerel, and salmon, contain 10–25% (Table 13.1, Fig. 13.1). The latter, as a result of its high fat content, contain a range of fat-soluble vitamins (A, D, E, and K) and essential fatty acids, all of which are vital for the healthy functioning of the body. The long-chain n-3 PUFA eicosapentaenoic acid (EPA) and docosahexaenoic acid (DHA), present in oil-rich fish and fish oil are heart-friendly and can make improvements in brain development and reproduction. This has highlighted the role for fish in the functionality of the human body.

A. Capurso et al., *Benefits of the Mediterranean Diet in the Elderly Patient*, Practical Issues in Geriatrics, https://doi.org/10.1007/978-3-319-78084-9_13

Table 13.1 Nutritional content of some fish, cooked (by moist or dry heat with no added ingredients) edible weight portion (serving size: 85 g/3 oz)

	Calories	Total fat	Cholesterol	Protein	Vit. A	Calcium	Iron
		g%	mg%	g%	%DV	%DV	%DV
Clams [1]	110	1.5	80	17	10	8	30
Cod	90	1.0	50	20	1	2	2
Haddock	100	1.0	70	21	2	2	6
Halibut	120	2.0	40	23	4	2	6
Lobster	80	0.5	60	17	2	6	2
Mackerel	140	8.0	54	17	2	2	4
Ocean perch	110	2.0	45	21	0	10	4
Oyster [1]	100	4.0	80	10	0	6	45
Trout	140	6.0	55	20	4	8	2
Salmon (Atlantic)	200	10.0	70	24	4	2	2
Sardines	135	6.1	70	20	4	5	2
Shrimp	100	1.5	170	21	4	6	10
Sole	75	1.0	60	21	0	1	1
Swordfish	120	6.0	40	16	2	0	6
Tuna	130	1.5	50	26	2	2	4

Source: U.S. Food and Drug Administration, January 1, 2008

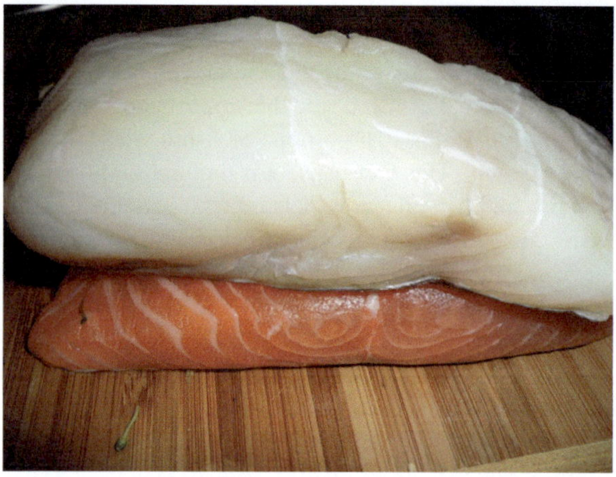

Fig. 13.1 Halibut fillet (a whitefish) on top of a salmon fillet (an oily fish). Source: Wikimedia Foundation

Fish is also a good source of protein containing, on average, 19.5 g of protein per 100 g (Table 13.1). The contribution of fish and fish dishes to total protein intake is 7% in adults aged 19–64 years, 11% in adults aged 65 years and over, and 4% in children aged 4–18 years. Dietary protein is essential for growth, maintenance, and repair of body tissue including muscle and bone, and can also provide energy (Fig. 13.1).

13.3 Omega 3 Fatty Acids

Fish are noteworthy an excellent source of polyunsaturated fatty acids (PUFAs), particularly omega-3 fatty acids ($\omega 3$ FA; n-3 FA) (Table 13.2).

Omega 3 (ω3, n-3) Fatty Acids

The n-3 fatty acids are polyunsaturated fatty acids (PUFAs) with a double bond (C=C) at the third carbon atom from the end of the carbon chain. The fatty acids have two ends, the carboxylic acid (–COOH) end, which is considered the beginning of the chain, thus "alpha," and the methyl (–CH_3) end, which is considered the "tail" of the chain, thus "omega"; the double bond is at omega minus 3 (not dash 3). One way in which a fatty acid is named is determined by the location of the first double bond, counted from the methyl end, that is, the omega (ω-) or the n-end. To note, from the n end the first double bond appears as the third carbon–carbon bond, hence the name "n-3." This is explained by the fact that the n end is almost never changed during physiological transformations in the human body, as it is more energy-stable, and other compounds can be synthesized from the other carbonyl end, for example, in glycerides, or from double bonds in the middle of the chain.

The three types of n-3 fatty acids involved in human physiology are α-linolenic acid (ALA) (found in plant oils), eicosapentaenoic acid (EPA), and docosahexaenoic acid (DHA) (both commonly found in marine oils) (Fig. 13.2). *Marine algae*

Table 13.2 Total fat and fatty acid composition of some types of fish (g/100 g of food, raw)

	Total fat	SFA	MUFA	PUFA	*n*-6 PUFA	*n*-3 PUFA	EPA	DHA
Tuna	0.7	1.5	0.21	0.19	0.04	0.09	0.0127	0.0703
Salmon	11.0	1.9	4.4	3.1	*N*	*N*	0.5	1.3
Cod	0.6	0.16	0.14	0.11	0.03	0.08	0.0240	0.0507
Haddock	0.4	0.09	0.08	0.1	0.01	0.09	0.0192	0.0616
Prawns, king	0.7	0.17	0.08	0.22	0.09	0.12	0.06	0.05
Mackerel	17.9	3.85	6.68	4.46	0.41	4.05	0.9531	1.6466
Sardines	6.1	1.83	1.80	1.56	0.24	1.32	0.4924	0.6228
Scampi	1.3	0.17	0.28	0.43	*N*	*N*	*N*	*N*

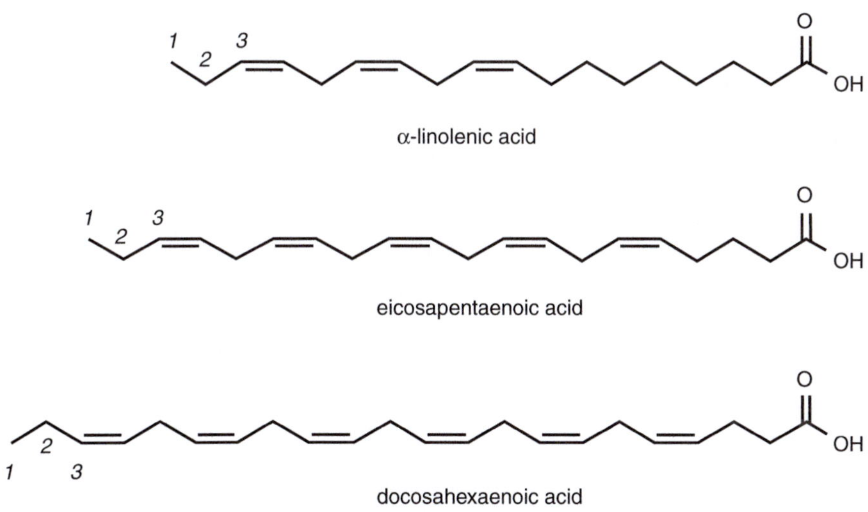

Fig. 13.2 Short-, and long-chain *n*-3 polyunsaturated fatty acids

and phytoplankton are primary sources of n-3 fatty acids. Common sources of plant oils containing the n-3 ALA fatty acid include walnut, edible seeds, clary sage seed oil, algal oil, flaxseed oil, while sources of animal n-3 EPA and DHA fatty acids include fish oils, egg oil, squid oils, and krill oil.

Omega-3 (*n*-3) fatty acids are important for normal metabolism. Mammals are unable to synthesize *n*-6 and *n*-3 fatty acids "de novo," because humans lack the desaturase enzyme that insert double bonds at the *n*-6 and *n*-3 position. For this reason, the *n*-6 and *n*-3 polyunsaturated fatty acids cannot be synthesized by humans and are appropriately called essential fatty acids. The longer-chain *n*-3 fatty acids are assembled from the shorter-chain *n*-3 fatty acid linoleic acid (ALA) (18 carbons and 3 double bonds) derived from diet, which is actually used to form the more important long-chain omega-3 fatty acids, EPA (20 carbons and 5 double bonds) and then from EPA the most crucial DHA (22 carbons and 6 double bonds), through the activity of numerous desaturase and elongase enzymes (Fig. 13.3). Humans can convert short-chain *n*-3 fatty acid ALA to long-chain forms (EPA, DHA) with an efficiency below 5%. However, the conversion of ALA to EPA and further to DHA in humans has been reported to be quite limited, sometimes nearly absent, but it varies with individuals. Women have higher ALA conversion efficiency than men, which is presumed to be due to the lower rate of use of dietary ALA for beta-oxidation. The ability to make the longer-chain *n*-3 fatty acids from ALA is impaired in aging [2].

The closely related *n*-3 and *n*-6 fatty acids act as competing substrates for the same desaturase and elongase enzymes [3], to synthesize inflammatory and regulatory proteins. This outlines the importance of the proportion of *n*-3 to *n*-6 fatty acids in a diet [3].

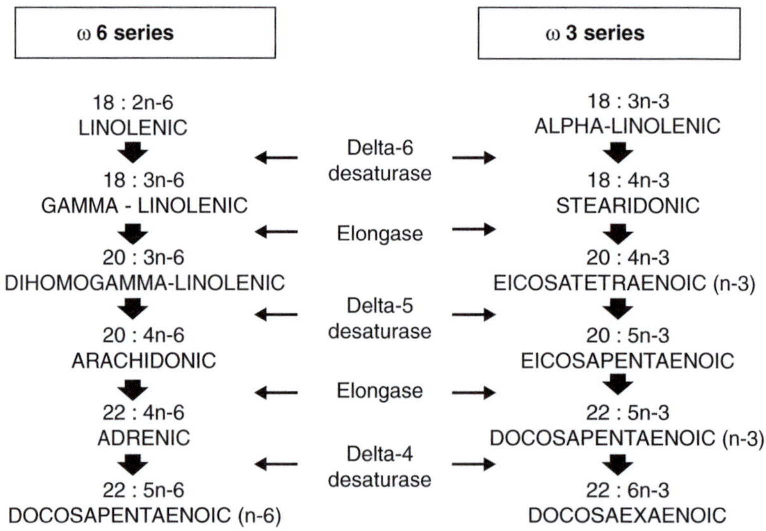

Fig. 13.3 Synthesis of long-chain *n*-6 and *n*-3 from short-chain linoleic and linolenic acids

Human diet has changed rapidly in recent centuries resulting in a reported increased of *n*-6 in comparison to *n*-3. The rapid evolution of human diet away from a 1:1 *n*-3 and *n*-6 ratio, such as during the Neolithic Agricultural Revolution, has presumably been too fast for humans to have adapted to biological profiles adept at balancing omega-3 and omega-6 ratios of 1:1. This is commonly believed to be the reason why modern diets are correlated with many inflammatory disorders. Typical Western diets provide ratios of between 10:1 and 30:1 (i.e., dramatically higher levels of *n*-6 than *n*-3). Metabolites of *n*-6 are more inflammatory (particularly arachidonic acid) than those of *n*-3. This necessitates that *n*-6 and *n*-3 be consumed in a balanced proportion; healthy ratios of *n*-6:*n*-3, according to some authors, range from 1:1 to 1:4. Other authors believe that a ratio of 4:1 (4 times as much *n*-6 as *n*-3) is already healthy. Studies suggest the evolutionary human diet, rich in game animals, seafood, and other sources of *n*-3, may have provided such a ratio.

13.4 The Role of *n*-6 and *n*-3 Fatty Acid Derivatives in Inflammatory Mechanisms

One important aspect of the PUFA functions is that they have to do essentially with inflammation, favoring this important mechanism of defense but also with curtailing inflammation and returning to homeostasis, to preserve tissue integrity.

The *n*-6 PUFA arachidonic acid (AA) can be converted into different families of lipid mediators, the eicosanoids, such as prostaglandins and leukotrienes (Fig. 13.4), which are essentially pro-inflammatory molecules, and Lipoxins (LXs), such as LXA4, which is an anti-inflammatory mediator.

The *n*-3 PUFAs eicosapentaenoic acid (EPA) and docosahexaenoic acid (DHA) act as less-inflammatory and anti-inflammatory molecules. They generate different types of anti-inflammatory molecules, including resolvins, protectins, and maresins, also called *pro-resolution molecules.*

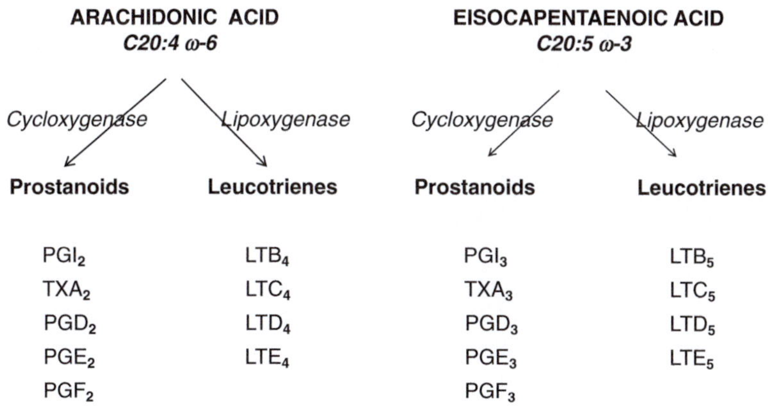

Fig. 13.4 Synthesis of prostanoids and leucotrienes (eicosanoids) from ω-6 and ω-3 fatty acids

Cyclooxygenases and lipoxygenases are key enzymes involved in the conversion of these PUFAs into their respective bioactive mediators. These enzymes, however, have multi-enzymatic activities which regulate different metabolic pathways.

13.4.1 Omega 6 (*n*-6): The Pro-inflammatory Effect of *n*-6 Arachidonic Acid Derivative—The Eicosanoids

Numerous eicosanoids are synthesized from arachidonic acid (AA) (20:2 *n*-6) and eicosapentaenoic acid (20:5 *n*-3) (Fig. 13.4). Eicosanoids are signaling molecules made by the enzymatic or nonenzymatic oxidation of arachidonic acid or other PUFAs (mostly eicosapentaenoic acid). These eicosanoids, i.e., prostaglandins, leukotrienes and thromboxanes, have a different role in inflammation and other diseases, in that eicosanoids of *n*-6 series (arachidonic acid derivatives) have generally pro-inflammatory effects while eicosanoids of *n*-3 series (eicosapentaenoic acid derivatives) have to some extent anti-inflammatory effects (they are just less inflammatory than those made from *n*-6 fats). It has been hypothesized [4] that many diseases are associated with an overproduction of eicosanoids from the *n*-6 arachidonic acid (AA) (20:4 *n*-6). The formation and function of these *n*-6 eicosanoids can be antagonized by dietary *n*-3 fats.

Chronic excessive production of *n*-6 eicosanoids is correlated with arthritis, inflammation, and cancer. Many of the medications used to treat and manage these conditions work by blocking the effects of the cyclooxygenase-2 (COX-2) enzyme [5], the enzyme that convert arachidonic acid into its derivatives prostanoids and leukotrienes (Fig. 13.4). Many steps in formation and action of the pro-inflammatory prostaglandins from *n*-6 arachidonic acid proceed more vigorously than the corresponding competitive steps in formation and action of *n*-3 hormones from *n*-3 eicosapentaenoic acid [6]. The COX-1 and COX-2 inhibitor medications, used to treat inflammation and pain, work by preventing the COX enzymes from turning arachidonic acid into inflammatory compounds [7]. The lipoxygenase (LOX) inhibitor medications, often used to treat asthma, work by preventing the LOX enzyme from converting arachidonic acid into the leukotrienes [8, 9]. Many of the anti-mania medications used to treat bipolar disorder work by targeting the arachidonic acid cascade in the brain [10].

13.4.2 Omega 6 (*n*-6): The Anti-inflammatory Derivatives of *n*-6—Lipoxin A4 (LXA4)

The *n*-6 PUFA arachidonic acid can be converted into different families of lipid mediators: prostaglandins and leukotrienes, which are mostly pro-inflammatory molecules, and lipoxins (LXs) such as LXA4, an anti-inflammation mediator. The 15-lipoxygenase (i.e., ALOX15 and/or possibly ALOX15B)-derived Lipoxin A_4 and B_4 metabolites of the *n*-6 fatty acid, arachidonic acid, are potent anti-inflammatory "*specialized proresolving mediators*" (SPMs).

Lipoxins (LXs), an acronym for "*lipoxygenase interaction products,*" are bioactive autacoid metabolites of arachidonic acid made by various cell types. They are categorized as nonclassic eicosanoids and members of the SPMs family of polyunsaturated fatty acid (PUFA) metabolites. Like other SPMs, LXs form during inflammatory responses and act to resolve them.

Lipoxins are arachidonic acid metabolites containing three hydroxyl residues and four double bonds. This structural definition distinguishes them from other SPMs such as the resolvins, neuroprotectins, and maresins, which are metabolites of the *n*-3 fatty acids eicosapentaenoic acid (EPA) and docosahexaenoic acid (DHA). The lipoxins generally form as a consequence of stimulating the production of pro-inflammatory AA metabolites.

In the initial phases of many acute inflammatory responses, damaged tissues, invading pathogens, and other local events cause nearby cells to make and release arachidonic acid-derived pro-inflammatory metabolites such as leukotrienes hydroxyeicosatetraenoic acid (HETEs), and other pro-inflammatory metabolites. These metabolites proceed to recruit circulating leukocytes and tissue macrophages to the disturbed tissue site. The consequential congregation of the various cell types promotes transcellular pathways in forming *specialized proresolving mediators* (SPMs), including the LXs, which then proceed to stimulate cellular and tissue responses that trend to reverse the actions of the pro-inflammatory mediators, dampen and reverse the inflammatory response, and initiate tissue repair.

LXA4 is a high affinity receptor ligand which activates the FPR2 receptor. This receptor is a G-protein coupled receptor initially identified as a receptor for the leukocyte Chemotactic Factor.

The anti-inflammatory activity of LXA4 includes inhibition of chemotaxis, transmigration, superoxide generation, NF-kB activation, generation of pro-inflammatory cytokines by neutrophils, eosinophils, monocytes, lymphoid cells, and macrophages, as well as suppresses the production of IgM and IgG antibodies by B-lymphocytes. These actions involve stimulation of anti-inflammatory pathways.

13.4.3 Omega-3 (*n*-3): The *n*-3 Anti-inflammatory Mediators—The "*Specialized Proresolving Mediators*" (SPMs)

In addition to the lipoxins, resolvins, protectins, and maresins are three novel families of locally generated lipid mediators derived from *n*-3 fatty acids (EPA and DHA) that display potent anti-inflammatory and proresolving actions in vivo. These lipid mediators belong to the family of the *Specialized Proresolving Mediators* (SPMs).

The SPMs are therefore a large class of cell signaling molecules formed in cells by the metabolism of polyunsaturated fatty acids (PUFA) by one or a combination of lipoxygenase, cyclooxygenase, and cytochrome P450 monooxygenase enzymes. SPMs are locally formed and locally acting cell signaling autacoids which are made by cells and act upon their parent or nearby cells to coordinate functional responses.

SPMs possess potent anti-inflammation, tissue protection, and tissue healing activities and appear to be involved in resolving physiological inflammatory responses.

It has been shown that the *n*-3 bioactive end product produced by the 12/15 lipoxygenases exert pro-resolution functions both at the cellular level involving macrophages and endothelial cells in vitro, and in mouse models engineered to express different levels of lipoxygenase-15 in vivo. The pro-resolution arm of the inflammation homeostatic process is mediated by three SPMs which counteract the potent pro-inflammatory mediators derived from the *n*-6 PUFA arachidonic acid. These SPMs are involved in orchestrating the resolution of inflammation and are very resistant to being metabolically inactivated. These SPMs include resolvins, protectins, and maresins.

Resolvins: Resolvins are dihydroxy or trihydroxy metabolites of *n*-3 fatty acids, primarily EPA and DHA, but also docosapentaenoic acid (DPA). The following oxygenase enzymes are responsible for metabolizing PUFA to resolvins: 15-lipoxygenase-1 (i.e., ALOX15), possibly 15-lipoxygenase-2 (i.e., ALOX15B), 5-lipoxygenase (i.e., ALOX5), cyclooxygenase-2 (i.e., COX-2), and certain Cytochrome P450 mono-oxygenases. The mechanism(s) by which each of the resolvins activate cells has not been fully elucidated. However, many resolvins appear to operate at least in part by acting through the G protein-coupled receptors (GPRs). Regarding the mechanism of action of resolvins, it has been suggested that inflammation provoking insults lead to the production of arachidonic acid metabolites (prostaglandin, leukotrienes) and various inflammatory cytokines (Interleukin 2, interleukin 8, granulocyte macrophage stimulating factor) that orchestrate the ensuing innate immunity-based inflammatory responses. Later in these responses, production of the cited types of arachidonic acid metabolites switches to the production of SPMs, i.e., the resolvin metabolites of EPA, DHA, and DPA and the Maresin and Protectin D1 metabolites of DHA. The SPMs proceed to resolve these responses and initiate healing.

Specific anti-inflammatory actions or resolvins are: (1) to inhibit blood leukocytes from migrating out of the circulation into sites of inflammation; (2) to stimulate macrophages to convert from a M1-like pro-inflammatory phenotype to a tissue repairing and wound healing M2 phenotypes; (3) to stimulate macrophage phagocytosis of apoptotic leukocytes at tissue sites of inflammation; (4) to stimulate Natural Killer T cells to clear leukocytes from inflamed tissues; (5) to stimulate leukocytes to engulf and kill pathogenic microbes at sites of invasion; (6) to inhibit the production of pro-inflammatory cytokines and stimulate the production of anti-inflammatory cytokines; (7) to promote tissue repairing and healing.

Protectins: Protectin D1(PD1), also known as neuroprotectin D1 (NPD1), is another member of the class of SPMs. Protectins are signaling molecules that are produced enzymatically from unsaturated fatty acids. Like other members of this class of polyunsaturated fatty acid metabolites, it possesses strong anti-inflammatory, antiapoptotic, and neuroprotective activity. PD1, like other protectins, is produced by the oxygenation of the *n*-3 polyunsaturated fatty acid docosahexaenoic acid (DHA) and it is found in many tissues, such as the retina, the lungs, and the nervous system. PD1 has a significant role as an anti-inflammatory, antiapoptotic, and neuroprotective molecule.

Studies in Alzheimer's disease animal models, in stroke patients, and in human retina pigment epithelial cells (RPE) have shown that PD1 can potentially reduce inflammation induced by oxidative stress and inhibit the pro-apoptotic signal, thereby preventing cellular degeneration. Recent studies examining the pathogenicity of influenza viruses, including the avian flu (H5N1), have suggested that PD1 can potentially halt the proliferation of the virus, thus protecting respiratory cells from lethal viral infections.

In addition, concerning the antiviral activity of protectins, studies in cultured human lung epithelial cells infected with the influenza virus H1N1 or H5N1 have found that endogenous production of PD1 decreases dramatically during infection due to the inhibition of 15-LO-1. The same studies have subsequently shown that in vivo administration of PD1 to H1N1 infected mice can potentially inhibit both the proliferation of the virus and the inflammation caused by the infection, thus increasing survival. Interestingly, PD1 protects against viral infections by disrupting the virus life cycle. Specifically, PD1 inhibits the binding of viral RNA to specific nuclear export factors in the host cells, thus blocking the export of viral RNA from the nucleus to the cytosol [11].

Maresins: Maresin-1 is a macrophage-derived mediator of inflammation resolution coined from macrophage mediator in resolving inflammation. Maresin-1, more recently defined maresins, are 12-lipoxygenase-derived metabolites of the *n*-3 fatty acid docosahexaenoic acid (DHA), that possess potent anti-inflammatory, proresolving, protective, and pro-healing properties similar to other members of the specialized proresolving mediators (SPM) class of polyunsaturated fatty acid (PUFA) metabolites.

Studies have found that maresins inhibit some pro-inflammatory functions in human neutrophils, reduce the entry of blood neutrophils into the inflamed peritoneum, and promotes the resolution of allergic pulmonary inflammation and wound healing in animal models [1, 12, 13].

13.4.4 Omega 3 (*n*-3): Other Anti-inflammatory Derivatives of *n*-3 DHA—The GPR120 and the β-Arrestin

Another anti-inflammatory effect of *n*-3 derivatives takes place through the G-protein-coupled receptor 120 (GPR120) [14]. The GPR 120 is a *n*-3 fatty acid receptor/sensor that mediates a potent anti-inflammatory and insulin sensitizing effect. GPR120 is known to couple with the Gaq/11 family of G proteins [15]. After ligand binding, GPR120 is phosphorylated and this generates binding sites for β-arrestin 2 [16]. β-Arrestin 2 binds to GPR120 and then interacts with downstream signaling molecules such as extracellular signal-regulated kinase 1/2 (ERK1/2) mitogen-activated protein kinase (MAPK) [17, 18]. This signaling pathway leads to a variety of anti-inflammatory effects attributed to *n*-3 fatty acids.

13.4.5 Omega 3 (*n*-3): The Cytosolic Phospholipase A_2 ($cPLA_2$) Activity

Another anti-inflammatory effect takes place through the cytosolic phospholipases A_2. Cytosolic phospholipase A_2 ($cPLA_2$) is well known to regulate inflammation [19–21], through downstream lipid mediators, as well as having an impact on gene expression [22]. Phospholipases A_2 (PLA_2) are enzymes that hydrolyze the sn-2 ester bond of phospholipids, releasing a free fatty acid such as arachidonic acid and creating a lysophospholipid. $cPLA_2\alpha$ is the only well-characterized PLA_2 that is highly selective for phospholipids containing arachidonic acid at the sn-2 position [19, 20]. $cPLA_2$ is activated by phosphorylation by MAPKs and is translocated to cell membranes by changes in intracellular free calcium levels [23–26]. Arachidonic acid (*n*-6, C20:4), the product of $cPLA_2$ activation, is the precursor for eicosanoid mediators (see Fig. 13.4), including prostaglandins, thromboxanes, leukotrienes, hydroxyeicosatetraenoic acids (HETEs), and epoxyeicosatrienoic acids (EETs), which may have a variety of pro-inflammatory and anti-inflammatory effects [27]. Prostaglandins are generated from arachidonic acid by cyclooxygenases, COX-1 and COX-2 (Fig. 13.5). COX-2 is an inducible enzyme and is involved primarily in the regulation of inflammation.

Prostaglandin E_2 (PGE_2) is one of the major COX-2-derived prostanoids at inflammatory sites [28], which plays an anti-inflammatory role. Docosahexaenoic acid (DHA) regulates $cPLA_2$ activation, so changing arachidonic acid release and modifying its downstream lipid mediator production. In fact, it has been demonstrated [29] that cPLA2 is activated by DHA. This activation leads to activation of COX-2 and production of PGE_2, which plays an anti-inflammatory role by inhibiting nuclear factor-kB (NFkB) signaling through EP4 receptor (Fig. 13.5) [29]. Hence, this new anti-inflammatory mechanism of DHA takes place through the cascade cPLA2–AA–COX-2–PGE2–EP4 (Fig. 13.5).

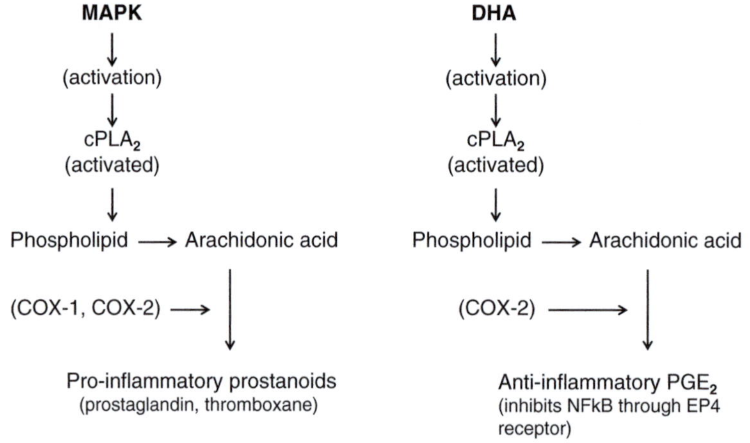

Fig. 13.5 DHA induces the production of antinflammatory PGE_2 from arachidonic acid

13.5 Omega 3 (*n*-3) Fatty Acids and Platelet Functions

Long-chain *n*-3 fatty acids have a significant antiplatelet aggregating activity. The antiplatelet aggregation story started at the end of the 1970s, when Danish workers focused attention on Eskimos from the West Coast of Greenland who had a low incidence of myocardial infarction and stroke as well as a mild tendency to bruise [30]. The dietary fats Eskimos ate were essentially derived from whale, fish, and seal. Compared to Danes, the Eskimos showed lower levels of plasma cholesterol and triglycerides, increased bleeding times, and increased plasma concentrations of *n*-3 very long-chain highly polyunsaturated fatty acids (i.e., eicosapentaenoic and docosahexaenoic acids) characteristic of fish and other marine animals [31].

Actually, arachidonic acid is the *n*-6 fatty acid precursor for prostaglandin synthesis in platelets, endothelial cells, and other tissues, whereas the *n*-3 family is composed of fatty acids such as eicosapentaenoic acid (C20:5 *n*-3) found principally in nature in fish, shellfish, phytoplankton, and in animals that ingest marine life for food. In platelets, arachidonic acid is converted by the enzyme cyclooxygenase to cyclic endoperoxides, which are rapidly transformed by thromboxane synthetase to thromboxane A_2, an extremely potent vasoconstrictor and platelet aggregating substance. In contrast, the vascular endothelial cells convert arachidonic acid via the same endoperoxides to PGI2 (prostacyclin), which is a vasodilator and inhibits platelet aggregation.

To explain the prolonged bleeding times and lack of vascular disease in the Greenland Eskimos, it was suggested that eicosapentaenoic acid (C20:5 *n*-3) competes with arachidonic acid for cyclooxygenase, thereby altering the platelet-vessel interactions [32]. Subsequent numerous papers confirmed the role of *n*-3 EPA and DHA as inhibiting platelet aggregation. In particular, it was observed [33] that diets containing salmon oil led to the incorporation of eicosapentaenoic acid (C20:5 *n*-3) into platelet phospholipids with a reduction in arachidonic acid. The ratio of C20:5/C20:4 (eicosapentaenoic/arachinonic acid) increased from 0.0045 on the control diet to 0.3 on the salmon diet. Bleeding time was prolonged from 6.75 to 10 min, and platelet aggregation in response to dilute concentrations of ADP was inhibited in the subjects ingesting *n*-3 long-chain fatty acids (salmon oil) [33].

This antiplatelet, antithrombotic effect of *n*-3 DHA is a very important anti-atherosclerosis mechanism and is one of the multiple beneficial effects that fish and fish oil have to prevent CHD, stroke, and other cardiovascular diseases.

13.6 Omega 3 (*n*-3) Fatty Acids and Serum Lipids

Numerous studies have documented the efficacy of *n*-3 fatty acids in reducing elevated levels of serum triglycerides. In a randomized, double blind study [34], subjects with serum triglycerides (TG) >500 and <2000 mg/dL were divided into three groups and two of these groups received eicosapentaenoic acid ethyl ester at a dosage of 4 g/day and 2 g/day, the third group receiving placebo as control. For a baseline TG level > 750 mg/dL, eicosapentaenoic acid ethyl ester 4 g/day reduced the placebo-corrected TG levels by 45.4% and 2 g/day by 32.9%. These patients showed also a significant reduction of non-high-density lipoprotein cholesterol, apolipoprotein B, lipoprotein-associated phospholipase A_2, very low-density lipoprotein cholesterol, and total cholesterol.

The US National Lipid Association (NLA) guidelines highlights that for elevated triglycerides (>500 mg/dL), TG lowering becomes the primary management goal, and the immediate use of a TG-lowering drug, including high-dose of *n*-3 [35], is recommended. Also the 2011 AHA scientific statement on triglycerides and CVD recommends the use of pharmacological therapy with a TG-lowering drug, including *n*-3 preparations [36].

The exact TG-lowering mechanisms of action are not completely understood. Results from preclinical and clinical studies suggest that *n*-3 decrease serum TG concentrations by reducing TG synthesis, reducing the incorporation of TG into VLDL, reducing TG secretion, and enhancing TG clearance from VLDL particles [37]. It has been proposed that *n*-3 exert TG-lowering effects via a number of mechanisms:

1. Decrease of hepatic lipogenesis by suppressing the expression of sterol regulatory element-binding protein-1c. This, in turn, leads to decreased expression of cholesterol-, fatty acid-, and TG-synthesizing enzymes [38, 39].
2. Increase of the β-oxidation of fatty acids, resulting in a reduction in available substrate required for TG and VLDL synthesis [37].
3. Inhibition of key enzymes involved in hepatic TG synthesis, such as phosphatidic acid phosphatase and diacylglycerol acyltransferase [40].
4. Finally, *n*-3 have been shown to increase the expression of lipoprotein lipase (LPL), a key lipolytic component of the TRL biosynthetic pathways, leading to increased TG removal from circulating VLDL and chylomicron particles [41, 42].

Recently a potent antioxidant mechanism of eicosapentaenoic acid (EPA) has been also demonstrated [43]. It was shown that EPA, at pharmacologic levels, significantly inhibits glucose-induced lipid peroxidation and cholesterol crystalline domain formation in model membrane lipid vesicles. EPA also potently inhibits lipid oxidation in isolated human LDL. These antioxidant effects have been attributed to the ability of EPA to quench reactive oxygen species (ROS) associated with the phospholipid membrane, thereby preserving normal lipid structure and organization. Following intercalation into the membrane lipid bilayer, the conjugated double bonds associated with EPA facilitate electron stabilization mechanisms that interfere with free radical propagation. These findings indicate a preferred intercalation of the EPA molecule into the membrane where it can trap free radicals. These results also suggested a novel role of EPA in ameliorating the effects of hypertriglyceridemia through its potent antioxidant properties.

13.7 Unsaturated Fatty Acids, Cardiac Arrhythmic Activity, and Sudden Death

Ventricular fibrillation, a cardiac arrhythmia that results in out-of-hospital primary cardiac arrest and a major cause of ischemic heart disease mortality, results in part from an increased myocardial vulnerability to life-threatening arrhythmias.

Numerous studies have found important correlations between fatty acids, cardiac arrhythmia, and sudden cardiac death.

13.7.1 *Trans* Fatty Acids

Trans-fatty acids have been found to be associated with an increased risk of arrhythmia and cardiac arrest. *Trans*-fatty acids are unsaturated fatty acids found in partially hydrogenated oils, beef, and dairy products. They differ from most naturally occurring unsaturated fatty acids by the presence of one or more double bonds in the *trans* configuration instead of the usual *cis* configuration. Like saturated fatty acids, fatty acids with *trans* double bonds pack more tightly than *cis* fatty acids, allowing the processing of oils into margarine.

Population studies have found an increased risk of CHD with higher dietary intake of total *trans*-fatty acids [44, 45]. Because *trans*-fatty acids resemble saturated fatty acids in their biophysical properties, and saturated fatty acids are associated with an increased risk of ventricular fibrillation and sudden cardiac death [46, 47], it has been hypothesized that higher levels of dietary *trans*-fatty acids could be associated with an increased risk of primary cardiac arrest. Based on this hypothesis, a population-based, case control study was done on subjects who had suffered a out-of-hospital primary cardiac arrest [48]. In these subjects the red blood cell levels of *trans* fatty acids were evaluated. Higher total *trans*-fatty acids in red blood cell membranes was associated with a modest increase in the risk of primary cardiac arrest after adjustment for medical and lifestyle risk factors (odds ratio for interquintile range, 1.5; 95% CI, 1.0 to 2.1). However, *trans* isomers of oleic acid were not associated with risk (odds ratio for interquintile range, 0.8; 95% CI, 0.5–1.2), whereas higher levels of *trans* isomers of linoleic acid were associated with threefold increase in risk [48]. The authors concluded that only *trans* isomers of linoleic acid (*trans* linoleic acid, 18:2) which has one *cis* double bond and one *trans* double bond significantly increases the risk of ventricular fibrillation while *trans*-oleic acid with a single *trans* double bond (*trans*-oleic acid, 18:1) is not at risk.

13.7.2 Omega-3 (*n*-3) Fatty Acids

Contrary to saturated fats and *trans*-PUFA, the *n*-3 fatty acids have been shown to protect against fatal arrhythmia and sudden death. In fact, numerous studies in experimental animals have shown that a dietary intake of long-chain *n*-3 PUFAs, compared with an intake of saturated and monounsaturated fatty acids, reduces myocardial vulnerability to ventricular fibrillation, possibly through an effect on myocardial cell membrane composition [46, 47, 49–53]. In vitro experimental studies have confirmed the antiarrhythmic effects of *n*-3 on cardiomyocytes [54]. Infusion of an emulsion of *n*-3 PUFAs just before coronary artery occlusion in an exercising, unanesthetized dog model prevented ischemia-induced sudden cardiac death by preventing ventricular fibrillation. Omega-3 PUFAs prevented induced fibrillation of cultured neonatal rat cardiomyocytes when various cardiotoxins were tested, and after fibrillation was induced, the arrhythmias were terminated by the PUFAs.

Studies in humans have confirmed the antiarrhythmic effects of *n*-3. In a population-based case–control study [55], the dietary intake of long-chain *n*-3 PUFAs from seafood, measured both indirectly with a questionnaire and directly with a biomarker, was found to be associated with a reduced risk of primary cardiac arrest in humans. Compared with no seafood intake, modest intake of *n*-3 PUFAs (5.5 g/month, the equivalent of 1 fatty fish meal/week), was associated with a 50% reduction in the risk of primary cardiac arrest (odds ratio: 0.5; 95% CI: 0.4, 0.8) after adjustment for numerous confounding factors. There was also an inverse correlation between the combined EPA and DHA concentrations of red blood cell membranes and the risk of primary cardiac arrest. Compared with a long-chain *n*-3 PUFA concentration of 3.3% of total fatty acids (the mean value of the lowest quartile), a red blood cell membrane concentration of 5.0% of total fatty acids (the mean of the highest quartile) was associated with a 70% reduction in the risk of primary cardiac arrest (odds ratio: 0.3; 95% CI: 0.2, 0.6), after adjustment for other risk factors. These findings suggested that: (1) compared with no seafood intake, modest dietary intake of long-chain *n*-3 PUFAs from seafood (equivalent to 1 fatty fish meal/week) is associated with a significant reduction in the risk of primary cardiac arrest; (2) compared with modest intake, higher intakes of these fatty acids are not associated with a further reduction in such risk; (3) the reduced risk of primary cardiac arrest could be mediated, at least in part, by the effect of dietary *n*-3 PUFA intake on cell membrane fatty acid composition.

In a Danish study [56], marine *n*-3 PUFA was shown to have a beneficial impact on heart rate variability (HRV) (*The 24-h HRV is considered a surrogate for the risk of developing ventricular arrhythmias and sudden cardiac death. A decreased HRV may predict a poor outcome among healthy subjects due to an increased risk of sudden cardiac death*). The authors found a close positive association between cellular levels of marine *n*-3 PUFA and HRV in healthy men but not in healthy women. Dietary intervention with either 2.0 g or 6.6 g of marine *n*-3 PUFA daily for 12 weeks showed a dose-dependent increase in HRV among men with a low base-line HRV. According to the authors, the results may help explain why dietary marine *n*-3 PUFA may reduce the risk of SCD in healthy men.

Also large prospective cohort studies have shown the protective effects of fish polyunsaturated fats against fatal arrhythmias and sudden death.

In the US Physicians' Health Study [57] a total of 22071 US male physicians 40–84 years of age and free of myocardial infarction, cerebrovascular disease and cancer were enrolled in the study in 1982, to evaluate the incidence of several end points, and the incidence of sudden death. Before randomization, which occurred between August 1982 and December 1984, potential participants were asked to provide base line blood samples, which were processed for long-term storage at 80 °C. Of the randomized study participants, 14,916 (68%) provided base-line blood samples. Over 17 years of follow-up 201 sudden death were documented. Base-line blood levels of long-chain *n*-3 fatty acids were found to be inversely related to the risk of sudden death. As compared with men whose blood levels of long-chain *n*-3 fatty acids were in the lowest quartile, the relative risk of sudden death was significantly lower among men with levels in the third quartile (adjusted relative risk, 0.28; 95% confidence interval, 0.09–0.87), i.e., a 72% lower risk, and the fourth quartile (adjusted relative risk, 0.19; 95% confidence interval, 0.05–0.71), i.e., an 81% lower risk of sudden death. In contrast, the levels of the other fatty acids, including the short-chain *n*-3 polyunsaturated fatty acid (a-linolenic acid), saturated fatty acids, monounsaturated fatty acids, *n*-6 polyunsaturated fatty acids, and trans unsaturated fatty acids, did not differ significantly between men who died suddenly and control subjects. According to the authors, plausible mechanisms for these antiarrhythmic effects included modulation of sodium, potassium, and L-type calcium channels; inhibition of thromboxane production; and beneficial effects on heart-rate variability. Other indirect effects of long-chain *n*-3 fatty acids included lowering of the nonesterified fatty-acid concentration in plasma and cell membranes.

The sense is that the consumption of minimal amount of fish per week is sufficient to substantially reduce the rate of sudden death, due to the potent antiarrhytmic effect of fish omega 3 fatty acids (EPA and DHA) in the Paris Prospective Study [58], nonesterified fatty acids have been shown to have multiple proarrhythmic properties and have been associated with an increased risk of sudden death, but not of fatal myocardial infarction, among men enrolled. Previous data of the same authors [59] had shown that low to moderate intake of fish—at least 1 fish meal per week—was associated with a 52% lower risk of sudden death compared with less than monthly consumption, even after controlling for several confounders. All levels of fish consumption were associated with a decreased risk of sudden death, but the size of the reduction did not appear to differ substantially at levels of consumption greater than 1 fish serving per week, suggesting a threshold effect. This small amount of fish may be sufficient to provide an essential amount of long-chain *n*-3 fatty acids or some unidentified nutrient or both, that decrease sudden death rate.

The GISSI-Prevenzione [59] was a study aimed to assess the time course of the benefit of *n*-3 polyunsaturated fatty acids (PUFAs) on mortality documented by the GISSI-Prevenzione trial in patients surviving a recent (<3 months) myocardial infarction. 11,323 patients were enrolled in this clinical trial aimed at testing the effectiveness of *n*-3 PUFA and vitamin E in preventing sudden death, nonfatal myocardial infarction, total coronary heart disease, and cerebrovascular events. The patients were invited to follow Mediterranean dietary habits, and were treated with up-to-date preventive pharmacological interventions. The events were assessed by right-censoring follow-up data 12 times from the first month after randomization up to 12 months. Survival curves for *n*-3 PUFA treatment (but not for vitamin E) diverged early after randomization, and total mortality was significantly lowered after 3 months of treatment (relative risk 0.59; 95% CI 0.36 to 0.97; $P < 0.037$). The reduction in risk of sudden death was specifically relevant and statistically significant already at 4 months (RR 0.47; 95% CI 0.219–0.995; $P < 0.048$). A similarly significant, although delayed, pattern after 6–8 months of treatment was observed for cardiovascular, cardiac, and coronary deaths. The authors concluded that the early effect of low-dose (1 g/day) *n*-3 PUFAs on total mortality and sudden death supported the hypothesis of an antiarrhythmic effect of *n*-3 PUFAs.

To summarize the effects of *n*-3 EPA and DHA on cardiac arrhythmia, the wealth of data coming from laboratory experiments on isolated myocytes, animal models and epidemiological and clinical studies have conclusively confirmed the potent antiarrhythmic effects of *n*-3 and their particular efficacy in significantly reducing the arrhythmic sudden death. According to the results of electrophysiological studies, *n*-3 PUFAs seem to modulate ion currents (primarily of Na^+ and Ca^{2+}) in the myocyte sarcolemma, shifting the steady-state inactivation potential to more negative values, increasing the depolarizing current necessary to elicit an action potential by ~50% and prolong the refractory period by ~3-fold [54, 60, 61].

13.8 Fish, Omega 3, and CHD Risk Reduction

The observation in the 1980s that native Alaskan and Greenland Inuit, who consume a large amount of fish, had low CHD mortality rates has led to a vast number of studies investigating this association. Several systematic reviews have summarized the evidence around fish consumption and its association with CHD. The results of the numerous studies and meta-analysis have often shown contrasting results, but many studies agreed on a significant reduction of fatal myocardial infarction (MI), while the data on nonfatal MI appeared often inconclusive and contrasting.

A review [62] of evidence from randomized controlled studies (RCTs) and cohort studies suggested that consumption of EPA and DHA (~250–500 mg/day, which equals around one to two 100 g portions of oil-rich fish per week) lowers the RR of fatal CHD by around 25%, but that higher intakes do not substantially further lower CHD mortality, suggesting a threshold of effect [62].

The Monitoring Project on Risk Factors for Chronic Diseases (MORGEN) study [63], was a Dutch population-based cohort study on 22,654 men and women aged 20–65 years. The study contributed to the Dutch part of the EPIC study. The cohort was followed up for 9–14 years (mean 11.3 years). After adjustment for potential confounders, the risk of fatal CHD and fatal MI was inversely associated with EPA and DHA intake, with a 49% lower risk of fatal CHD (RR 0.51; 95% CI, 0.27–0.94) and a 62% reduced risk of fatal MI (RR 0.38; 95% CI, 0.19–0.77) in the top quartile of EPA and DHA intake (median intake 234 mg EPA and DHA per day) compared with the lowest quartile (median intake 40 mg EPA and DHA per day). EPA and DHA intakes were not associated with nonfatal MI [63].

A recent meta-analysis of cohort studies [64] that included 22 cohorts with a total of 256,000 participants, with follow-up periods ranging from 5 to 40 years confirmed this trend. In fact, the meta-analysis of the study outcomes showed that highest compared with lowest fish consumption (or EPA/DHA consumption) was associated with a significantly reduced risk of fatal CHD by 18% (RR 0.82; 95% CI, 0.71–0.94). Fish (or EPA/DHA) consumption was not associated with decreased risk of CHD events (RR 0.87; 95% CI, 0.71–1.06), nonfatal CHD (RR 0.81; 95% CI, 0.59–1.10) or total MI (RR 0.79; 95% CI, 0.53–1.17).

Summarizing, the intake of EPA and DHA EPA reduces significantly the rate of fatal MI but not that of nonfatal MI. These different effects on MI can probably be explained by the different impact of EPA and DHA on MI risk factors. The mild reduction of some atherosclerosis risk factors (i.e., serum triglycerides, platelet aggregation, and inflammation), appears to be insufficient to prevent the nonfatal MI. Different appears the impact of EPA and DHA on fatal MI, which have been shown to be significantly reduced by ~50%. The main cause of fatal MI is a sudden death due to a fatal arrhythmia, i.e., ventricular fibrillation. The wealth of data coming from laboratory experiments on isolated myocytes, animal models and epidemiological and clinical studies have conclusively confirmed the potent antiarrhythmic effect that EPA and DHA exert on myocardial activity. This antiarrhythmic effect clearly explains the substantial reduction of fatal MI rate, whose sudden death is mostly due mostly to a fatal arrhythmia.

To conclude, although many randomized controlled trials have failed to find any positive effects of *n*-3 long-chain fatty acids on primary and secondary MI prevention, data from population studies have shown that a regular consumption of fish (also 1 serving/week) or fish oil significantly reduces the incidence of fatal MI, probably because the main effect of fish and fish oil on the heart is the antiarrhythmic one.

13.9 Fish, Omega 3 (*n*-3), and Stroke

The regular consume of fish has been shown to significantly reduce the cerebrovascular disease and the rate of ischemic stroke.

A meta-analysis [65] that included nine cohorts from eight prospective cohort studies with a total of 200,575 participants and 3491 stroke events, found that fish consumption was associated with a lower risk of stroke. The risk of stroke was 13% lower in those who ate fish once a week (RR 0.87; 95% CI, 0.77–0.98) compared with those who ate no fish or ate fish less than once a month, which was statistically significant. The protective effect on stroke risk appeared to increase with higher fish intakes, with a RR of 0.69 (95% CI, 0.54–0.88) in those who ate fish >5 times/week compared with those who ate no fish or ate fish less than once a month. However, the test for linear trend did not reach statistical significance ($P = 0.06$).

Another systematic review [66] aimed to assess the association between fish and long-chain *n*-3 PUFA intake with cerebrovascular disease, defined as fatal or nonfatal ischemic stroke, hemorrhagic stroke, cerebrovascular accident or transient ischemic attack, included 21 prospective cohort studies totaling 675,048 study participants and 25,320 incident cerebrovascular events. Seven studies were from Europe, seven from North America, and seven from the Asia-Pacific region. Meta-analysis of data from 18 studies (which allowed classifications of comparable fish consumption frequencies) resulted in a modest but significantly reduced risk of cerebrovascular disease when eating 2–4 portions of fish per week compared with ≤1 serving a week (RR 0.94; 95% CI, 0.90–0.98). The risk reduction was larger when comparing >5 servings/week with ≤1 serving a week (RR 0.88; 95% CI, 0.81–0.96; based on data from eight cohort studies). There was no heterogeneity across studies. In a dose-response meta-analysis based on data from 18 cohort studies, an increment of 2 servings/week of any type of fish was associated with a 4% reduced risk of cerebrovascular disease (RR 0.96; 95% CI, 0.93–0.99). When comparing participants in the highest with the lowest category of fish intake in all 21 studies, the RR was 0.88 (95% CI, 0.84–0.93).

The same authors [66] carried out a systematic review and meta-analysis of data from randomized controlled trials (RCTs) investigating the effect of long-chain *n*-3 PUFA supplementation on risk of cerebrovascular disease. Most studies were secondary prevention trials, and two studies were primary prevention trials. The authors found no effect of long-chain *n*-3 supplementation on risk of cerebrovascular disease in any of the trials, regardless of whether they were primary or secondary prevention trials, and found no effect on either stroke subtype. The authors [66] argue from their finding that fish intake is associated with a reduced risk of cerebrovascular disease whereas long-chain *n*-3 PUFA supplementation is not, and that single nutrients may have limited effects on chronic disease risk outside of their original food source. They argue that other nutrients present in fish, such as vitamin D and B-vitamins, may play a role in the protective effect of fish, or that the replacement of other less healthy foods by fish may contribute to the protective effect. They also suggested that fish intake may simply be an indicator of a healthier dietary pattern and lifestyle or higher socioeconomic status.

In summary, evidence suggests that fish consumption is associated with a moderate but statistically significantly decreased risk of cerebrovascular disease, including stroke. The most recent systematic review suggests that this protective effect cannot be explained solely by long-chain *n*-3 PUFAs, but other nutrients or diet and lifestyle factors associated with fish intake may contribute to this effect. Almost all meta-analyses suggest that the association seems stronger for ischemic than hemorrhagic stroke, although one meta-analysis found a protective association for both types of stroke and with a larger effect for hemorrhagic stroke.

13.10 Fish, Omega 3 (*n*-3) PUFA, and Cancer

Several cancers have been associated with diet and other modifiable lifestyle factors. Observational studies have investigated the potential association between fish consumption and/or long-chain *n*-3 PUFA consumption and selected types of cancers.

13.10.1 Colorectal Cancer

Data from prospective cohort studies suggest there may be some protective effect of fish intake on risk of colorectal cancer but the evidence is too inconsistent to draw any firm conclusions. Data from case–control studies have shown a somewhat stronger inverse association, but the studies are generally heterogeneous, and it has been argued that prospective studies are more appropriate to evaluate associations between diet and cancer. Potentially, any protective effects observed may be due to other factors, such as lower meat intakes in fish eaters. Results in some of the meta-analyses were expressed in terms of a 100 g/day increase in fish intake, which is far in excess of typical intakes and may therefore not be relevant for the typical Western diet.

13.10.2 Breast Cancer

The WCRF/AICR expert panel judged the evidence on fish intake and risk of breast cancer to be inconclusive [67]. Altogether, nine studies (six prospective cohort and three nested case–control studies) were included that reported on breast cancer risk in association with fish irrespective of menopausal status (i.e., pre- and postmenopausal combined). One study reported a nonsignificant inverse association, four reported a nonsignificant positive association, three reported no association, and one study reported a significantly increased risk with increasing levels of fish intake. Of the four studies identified that looked specifically at premenopausal breast cancer, three reported a nonsignificant weak positive association and one reported a nonsignificant weak negative association. Of three studies that looked at postmenopausal breast cancer, one reported no association, one reported a nonsignificant increased risk, and one reported a nonsignificant decreased risk of breast cancer with fish consumption. In summary, there was no conclusive evidence to support an association between fish intake and breast cancer based on evidence from cohort studies; the conclusions from the 2007 report remain [67].

13.10.3 Other Types of Cancer

The association between fish intake and pancreatic cancer has been investigated in several studies [68–70] and it was suggested that anti-inflammatory properties of long-chain PUFAs may reduce the risk of pancreatic cancer, which has been suggested to have an inflammatory pathogenesis [68]. WCRF/AICR concluded in their 2007 report [67] that the evidence for an association between fish and pancreatic cancer was limited and no conclusion could be drawn.

Also other studies and meta-analyses investigating the association with prostate, bladder, stomach, and ovaries cancer did not suggest that fish intake has a protective effect from these types of cancer.

13.11 Fish Intake in Early Childhood and Risk of Asthma and Atopic Conditions

A systematic review looking into early life fish exposure and risk of atopy identified 14 studies that looked at fish intake during infancy or childhood and atopic outcomes (including asthma and eczema). Nine of these studies observed a beneficial effect of fish intake during infancy/childhood on atopic outcomes (three were prospective cohort, two were case–control, and four were cross-sectional studies); two studies (one case control, one cross sectional) found a negative effect; and three prospective cohort studies observed no associations. The authors of the systematic review suggested that most studies that reported a protective effect of fish intake in infancy and childhood have found a risk reduction between 50% and 60% [71].

Data from around 5000 infants from Western Sweden showed the introduction of fish at months 3–5, and 6–8 was associated with a significantly reduced risk of eczema at 1 year of age (OR 0.7; 95% CI, 0.6–0.9; and OR 0.6; 95% CI, 0.5–0.7, respectively), compared with fish introduction at 9–12 months [72]. This is aligned with the view that there are critical windows during early development for establishing immune tolerance [73].

It appears, therefore, that fish intake during early childhood is associated with a decreased risk of atopic outcomes, but the findings have not been found very consistent.

13.12 Fish Intake and Cognitive Functions in Later Life

13.12.1 The Risk of Dementia and Alzheimer's Disease

Dementia develops generally in aging people. 6% of people >65 years of age are affected by dementia, including Alzheimer's disease (AD). There is increasing interest in identifying dietary factors that may influence risk of developing these conditions, including fish and long-chain *n*-3 PUFA consumption.

Cohort studies investigating the association between fish and/or dietary long-chain *n*-3 PUFA intake and risk of dementia in general and AD specifically have reported conflicting results, with some studies proposing a protective effect of dietary fish or DHA intakes or plasma DHA levels on risk of dementia and/or AD [74–76], whereas others reporting no association [77, 78].

In the sub-cohort (815 subjects) randomly selected of the Chicago Health and Aging Project [74], free of AD at baseline and followed for an average of 3.9 years, participants who consumed fish at least once a week had a 60% lower risk of developing AD compared with those who rarely or never ate fish at baseline (RR 0.4; 95% CI, 0.2–0.9), taking into account several potential confounders. A protective effect of DHA on risk of AD was also observed [RR in highest (median 100 mg/day) vs. lowest (median 30 mg/day) quintile: 0.3; 95% CI, 0.1–0.9], whereas EPA and ALA intakes were not associated with risk of AD.

In The Framingham Heart Study [76], 1921 subjects aged 55 years or above who were free of dementia were included in the study and were followed for an average of 9.1 years. Based on data from 899 men and women, the authors reported a significantly reduced incidence of dementia (including AD) in the highest quartile of plasma DHA levels (measured at baseline) compared with the lower three quartiles (RR 0.57; 95% CI, 0.33–0.97).

A cross-sectional analysis of a sub-cohort of the Rancho Bernardo Study [76] resulted in similar findings. Altogether, 266 men and women aged 67–100 years were examined for dementia and AD, and plasma DHA levels were assessed

(1991–1993). After adjusting for various potential confounding factors, those who were in the highest tertile of plasma DHA had a 65% lower odds of all-cause dementia (OR 0.35; 95% CI, 0.17–0.92), and a 60% lower odds of AD, although the findings for AD were not statistically significant (OR 0.40; 95% CI, 0.15–1.10). Dietary DHA intake in the highest tertile (mean 0.31 g/day, range 0.16–1.86 g/day) was associated with a 73% reduced odds of all-cause dementia (OR 0.27; 95% CI, 0.09–0.79) and a 72% reduced odds of AD (OR 0.28; 95% CI, 0.09–0.93).

While studies on US cohorts (as those illustrated above) showed a risk reduction for dementia in subjects who consumed fish, in European and Canadian cohort studies the results were negative and fish intake was not associated with a reduction of the risk.

One of these negative studies was a large cohort study conducted in the Netherlands, The Rotterdam Study [77], in which 5395 people 55 years of age or older, free from dementia at baseline, were followed for 9.6 years. Total fish intake didn't result to be associated with dementia risk. Compared with participants who typically ate no fish, those with a higher fish intake had a similar dementia risk (HR 0.95; 95% CI, 0.76–1.19) as did those who ate fatty fish compared with those who typically did not eat fish (HR 0.98; 95% CI, 0.77–1.24). Dietary intakes of long-chain *n*-3 PUFA were also not associated with dementia risk. When AD specifically was considered, the results were similar [77].

Another negative study was the Canadian Study of Health and Aging, a cohort study in which 1219 subjects free from dementia provided blood samples for analysis of fatty acid levels in blood erythrocyte membranes and were included at study baseline. After a median follow-up of 4.9 years, a study sample of 663 subjects was available for analysis. The study authors found no association between blood levels of total *n*-3 PUFA, EPA or DHA and risk of dementia and AD [78].

13.12.2 Fish Intake and the Risk of Cognitive Decline

Cognition is a combination of skills that include attention, learning, memory, language, visuospatial skills, and executive function such as decision-making, goal setting, planning, and judgment. Decline in cognition ranges from severe dementia, such as Alzheimer's disease, to mild cognitive impairment (MCI) and age-related cognitive decline (ARCD). Cognitive decline is multi-causal, and mild cognitive impairment does not always progress to dementia.

According to DSM-IV 1994, criteria for diagnosis of mild cognitive decline (MCI) or age-related cognitive decline (ARCD) include the objective decline in cognitive functioning associated with the aging process but within normal limits given the person's age.

Numerous studies have investigated association of single nutrients with MCI and ARCD, including fish intake.

Actually, fish intake has been associated with a slower decline of cognitive function with aging. However, also in this case, the results were uncertain, in that an association of fish with a slower mental decline was also observed, but with data not statistically significant.

The Chicago Health and Aging project looked at whether fish and long-chain ω-3 PUFA intakes were associated with slower cognitive decline. The authors found that fish intake was associated with a slower rate of cognitive decline over a follow-up period of 6 years, even after adjusting for several potential confounders. Compared with those who consumed fish less than weekly, the rate of cognitive decline was 10% slower among those who consumed one fish meal per week ($P = 0.03$), and 13% slower among those who consumed two or more fish meals per week ($P = 0.04$). However, the authors found no association between total *n*-3 PUFA, DHA or EPA intake and cognitive decline [79].

The Zutphen Elderly Study [80] also investigated the effect of fish intake on cognitive decline in 342 men aged 70 years or above over a period of 3 years. The authors found that fish consumption was inversely, but not significantly, associated with cognitive decline.

In an analysis of a sub-cohort of the French SU.VI.MAX study (3294 subjects), self-reported cognitive difficulties were less frequent among subjects who had higher intakes of total long-chain *n*-3 PUFA 13 years prior to cognitive assessment (OR highest vs. lowest quartile 0.68; 95% CI, 0.53–0.85), EPA (OR 0.69; 95% CI, 0.55–0.87) and DHA (OR 0.75; 95% CI, 0.60–0.95). There was no significant association between fish intake and self-reported cognitive difficulties. No association was found between intake of any of the fatty acids or fish and odds of poor score on cognitive tests [81].

13.13 Fish Intake and Bone Health

The optimization of bone health is crucial throughout life to reduce the burden of health issues associated with poor bone health, such as osteomalacia, which can lead to bone deformation, and osteoporosis in later life, which significantly increases the risk of fractures.

Calcium and vitamin D play critical roles in bone mineralization. Calcium is a main component of the skeleton and teeth, where the majority of total body calcium (99%) is found. Vitamin D is crucial for maximizing gut absorption of calcium via vitamin D-dependent calcium receptors, and also stimulates bone formation and maturation.

Calcium is present in a wide range of foods, although not all calcium is equally available for absorption in the gut. Dairy products are a major contributor to calcium intake, and the calcium from dairy products is generally well absorbed [82]. Fish is another good source of calcium. Pulses, wholegrain, nuts and seeds, dried fruit, and green vegetables also contain calcium usually at lower concentrations, but calcium from plant sources is generally less well absorbed [82].

Vitamin D is primarily made in the skin on exposure to sunlight, when skin is exposed to UV radiation. There are only a few natural dietary sources of vitamin D, with oil-rich fish being the richest source.

A role of PUFAs in bone metabolism has also been suggested, in particular long-chain *n*-3 PUFA and *n*-6 derivatives of PUFAs.

Several prospective cohort studies have investigated whether there is an association between fish consumption or long-chain n-3 PUFA intake and bone health in older adults. The Framingham Osteoporosis Study [83] followed 623 adults with a mean age of 75 years over a period of 4 years and looked at changes in hip bone mineral density (BMD) during this time. After adjusting for a variety of potential confounders, including vitamin D and calcium, the researchers found that high intakes (3 servings/week) of dark fish (oil-rich fish) and tuna in men, and of dark fish (excluding tuna) in women, relative to lower intakes, were associated with maintenance of or an increase in femoral neck BMD ($P < 0.05$). Cross-sectional analysis of baseline data found that both men and women with high fish intakes (3 servings/week) had a greater mean baseline femoral neck BMD than did those with moderate or low fish intakes, but the associations were not significant. However, no significant association between fish consumption or EPA and DHA intake and risk of hip fracture was found [83].

The Women's Health Initiative studies investigated the association between dietary fatty acids and risk of fracture in 137,486 postmenopausal women, who were 50–79 years of age at baseline. During an average follow-up of 7.8 years, 20,399 fractures, including 1638 hip fractures, were reported. In this cohort, high intake of saturated fatty acids was associated with a significant 31% increase in hip fractures (HR 1.31; 95% CI, 1.11–1.55), but not with total fracture risk. Total PUFA and total n-3 PUFA intake were not associated with total fracture risk. EPA and DHA intakes in the highest quartile of intake (mean intake of 0.09 g/day or 1.6% of energy) compared with the lowest quartile (mean intake of 0 g/day or 0.03% of energy) were associated with a nonsignificant decreased risk of hip fracture (HR 0.86; 95% CI, 0.72–1.01) [84].

A cross-sectional analysis in Chinese women aged 48–63 years ($n = 685$) found that intake of sea fish was significantly associated with BMD and bone mineral content (BMC) in the whole body, the spine and the hip. After adjusting for potential confounders, mean BMDs were 3.2–6.8% higher, and BMCs 5.1–9.4% higher in the top quintile of sea fish intake (average intake 65 g/day) compared with the bottom quintile (average intake 0.6 g/day) at the whole body and hip sites. Osteoporosis risk was also significantly lower in women in the highest intake quintile compared with the lowest for whole body (OR 0.23; 95% CI, 0.08–0.66), total hip (OR 0.12; 95% CI, 0.03–0.59) and the femur neck (OR 0.06; 95% CI, 0.01–0.44). [85].

In summary, there is some evidence from cohort and cross-sectional studies that fish intake may be associated with better bone health, but not all studies have found such an association.

13.14 Recommendations for Fish Intake

Recommendations for fish and long-chain n-3 PUFA intake have been published by a variety of organizations for both primary and secondary prevention of CHD.

The American Heart Association (AHA) recommends that adults eat two portions of fish per week, preferably oil-rich fish [86]. The AHA recommendation was confirmed to be in line with other findings (a benefit for heart health with intakes of EPA plus DHA of up to 500 mg), with 2 portions of oil-rich fish per week expected to equate to 400–500 mg EPA plus DHA per day [87]. For secondary prevention in people with established CHD, AHA recommends an intake of 1000 mg EPA plus DHA per day [86].

The recommendations of the National Institute of Health and Clinical Excellence (NICE) have been based on the findings of a single study (the GISSI trial) [88]. In the GISSI trial, patients with prior MI within 3 months of recruitment were included and a significant protective effect of long-chain *n*-3 PUFA supplementation was found. NICE also referred to another study [89] that failed to find a protective effect. NICE suggested that this outcome happened because patients who had suffered a MI more than 3 months prior to recruitment had been included, and that treatment with long-chain *n*-3 PUFA supplements may only be effective if it is started within 3 months of MI (based on the GISSI findings).

References

1. Serhan CN, Dalli J, Colas RA, Winkler JW, Chiang N. Protectins and maresins: new pro-resolving families of mediators in acute inflammation and resolution bioactive metabolome. Biochim Biophys Acta. 2015;1851:397–413.
2. Gao F, Taha AY, Ma K, Chang L, Kiesewetter D, Rapoport SI. Aging decreases rate of docosahexaenoic acid synthesis-secretion from circulating unesterified α-linolenic acid by rat liver. Age. 2012;35:597–608.
3. Bibus D, Lands B. Balancing proportions of competing omega-3 and omega-6 highly unsaturated fatty acids (HUFA) in tissue lipids. Prostaglandins Leukot Essent Fat Acids. 2015;99:19–23.
4. Lands WE. n-3 fatty acids as precursors for active metabolic substances: dissonance between expected and observed events. J Intern Med Suppl. 1989;731:11–20.
5. Smith WL. Nutritionally essential fatty acids and biologically indispensable cyclooxygenases. Trends Biochem Sci. 2008;33:27–37.
6. Wada M, Delong CJ, Hong YH, Rieke CJ, Song I, Sidhu RS, Yuan C, Warnock M, Schmaier AH, Yokoyama C, Smyth EM, Wilson SJ, FitzGerald GA, Garavito RM, Sui de X, Regan JW, Smith WL. Enzymes and receptors of prostaglandin pathways with arachidonic acid-derived versus eicosapentaenoic acid-derived substrates and products. J Biol Chem. 2007;282:22254–66.
7. Cleland LG, James MJ, Proudman SM. Fish oil: what the prescriber needs to know. Arthr Res Ther. 2006;8:202.
8. Mickleborough T. Dietary omega-3 polyunsaturated fatty acid supplementation and airway hyperresponsiveness in asthma. J Asthma. 2005;42:305–14.
9. Broughton KS, Johnson CS, Pace BK, Liebman M, Kleppinger KM. Reduced asthma symptoms with n-3 fatty acid ingestion are related to 5-series leukotriene production. Am J Clin Nutr. 1997;65:1011–7.
10. Lee HJ, Rao JS, Rapoport SI, Bazinet RP. Antimanic therapies target brain arachidonic acid signaling: lessons learned about the regulation of brain fatty acid metabolism. Prostaglandins Leukot Essent Fat Acids. 2007;77:239–46.
11. Morita M, Kuba K, Ichikawa A, Nakayama M, Katahira J, Iwamoto R, Imai Y. The lipid mediator protectin D1 inhibits influenza virus replication and improves severe influenza. Cell. 2013;153:112–25.
12. Merched AJ, Ko K, Gotlinger KH, Serhan CN, Chan L. Atherosclerosis: evidence for impairment of resolution of vascular inflammation governed by specific lipid mediators. FASEB J. 2008;22:3595–606.

13. Deng B, Wang CW, Arnardottir HH, Li Y, Cheng CY, Dalli J, Serhan CN. Maresin biosynthesis and identification of maresin 2, a new anti-inflammatory and pro-resolving mediator from human macrophages. PLoS One. 2014;9:e102362.
14. Oh DY, Talukdar S, Bae EJ, et al. GPR120 is an omega-3 fatty acid receptor mediating potent anti-inflammatory and insulin-sensitizing effects. Cell. 2010;142:687–98.
15. Hirasawa A, Tsumaya K, Awaji T, et al. Free fatty acids regulate gut incretin glucagonlike peptide-1 secretion through GPR120. Nat Med. 2005;11:90–4.
16. Burns RN, Moniri NH. Agonism with the omega-3 fatty acids a-linolenic acid and docosahexaenoic acid mediates phosphorylation of both the short and long isoforms of the human GPR120 receptor. Biochem Biophys Res Commun. 2010;396:1030–5.
17. Brown MD, Sacks DB. Protein scaffolds in MAP kinase signalling. Cell Signal. 2009;21:462–9.
18. Miller WE, Lefkowitz RJ. Expanding roles for b-arrestins as scaffolds and adapters in GPCR signaling and trafficking. Curr Opin Cell Biol. 2001;13:139–45.
19. Uozumi N, Kume K, Nagase T, et al. Role of cytosolic phospholipase A2 in allergic response and parturition. Nature. 1997;390:618–22.
20. Sapirstein A, Bonventre JV. Specific physiological roles of cytosolic phospholipase A2 as defined by gene knockouts. Biochim Biophys Acta. 2000;1488:139–48.
21. Fujishima H, Sanchez Mejia RO, Bingham CO 3rd, Lam BK, Sapirstein A, Bonventre JV, Austen KF, Arm JP. Cytosolic phospholipase A2 is essential for both the immediate and the delayed phases of eicosanoid generation in mouse bone marrow-derived mast cells. Proc Natl Acad Sci U S A. 1999;96:4803–7.
22. Pawliczak R, Logun C, Madara P, Lawrence M, Woszczek G, Ptasinska A, Kowalski ML, Wu T, Shelhamer JH. Cytosolic phospholipase A2 Group IVa but not secreted phospholipase A2 Group IIA, V, or X induces interleukin-8 and cyclooxygenase-2 gene and protein expression through peroxisome proliferator-activated receptors c1 and 2 in human lung cells. J Biol Chem. 2004;279:48550–61.
23. Clark JD, Lin LL, Kriz RW, Ramesha CS, Sultzman LA, Lin AY, Milona N, Knopf JL. A novel arachidonic acid-selective cytosolic PLA2 contains a Ca2 + -dependent translocation domain with homology to PKC and GAP. Cell. 1991;65:1043–51.
24. Lin LL, Wartmann M, Lin AY, Knopf JL, Seth A, Davis RJ. cPLA2 is phosphorylated and activated by MAP kinase. Cell. 1993;72:269–78.
25. Kramer RM, Roberts EF, Um SL, Borsch-Haubold AG, Watson SP, Fisher MJ, Jakubowski JA. p38 mitogen-activated protein kinase phosphorylates cytosolic phospholipase A2 (cPLA2) in thrombin-stimulated platelets. Evidence that proline-directed phosphorylation is not required for mobilization of arachidonic acid by cPLA2. J Biol Chem. 1996;271:27723–9.
26. Sharp JD, White DL, Chiou XG, et al. Molecular cloning and expression of human Ca2 + -sensitive cytosolic phospholipase A2. J Biol Chem. 1991;266:14850–3.
27. Funk CD. Prostaglandins and leukotrienes: advances in eicosanoid biology. Science. 2001;294:1871–5.
28. Giuliano F, Warner TD. Origins of prostaglandin E2: involvements of cyclooxygenase (COX)-1 and COX-2 in human and rat systems. J Pharmacol Exp Ther. 2002;303:1001–6.
29. Liu Y, Chen LY, Sokolowska M, Eberlein M, Alsaaty S, Martinez-Anton A, Logun C, Qi HY, Shelhamer JH. The fish oil ingredient, docosahexaenoic acid, activates cytosolic phospholipase A_2 via GPR120 receptor to produce prostaglandin E_2 and plays an anti-inflammatory role in macrophages. Immunology. 2014;143:81–95.
30. Dyerberg J, Bang HO. Haemostatic function and platelet polyunsaturated fatty acids in eskimos. Lancet. 1979;2:433–5.
31. Dyerberg J, Bang HO, Hjorne N. Fatty acid composition of the plasma lipids in Greenland eskimos. Am J Clin Nutr. 1975;28:958–66.
32. Dyerberg J, Bang HO, Stoffersen E, Moncada S, Vane JR. Eicosapentaenoic acid and prevention of thrombosis and atherosclerosis? Lancet. 1978;1:117–9.
33. Goodnight SH Jr, Harris WS, Connor WE. The effects of dietary omega 3 fatty acids on platelet composition and function in man: a prospective, controlled study. Blood. 1981;58:880–5.

34. Bays HE, Ballantyne CM, Kastelein JJ, Isaacsohn JL, Braeckman RA, Soni PN. Eicosapentaenoic acid ethyl ester (AMR101) therapy in patients with very high triglyceride levels (from the multi-center, plAcebo-controlled, randomized, double-blINd, 12-week study with an open-label extension [MARINE] trial). Am J Cardiol. 2011;108:682–90.
35. Jacobson TA, Ito MK, Maki KC, Orringer CE, Bays HE, Jones PH, McKenney JM, Grundy SM, Gill EA, Wild RA, et al. National Lipid Association recommendations for patient-centered management of dyslipidemia: part 1 - executive summary. J Clin Lipidol. 2014;8:473–88.
36. Miller M, Stone NJ, Ballantyne C, Bittner V, Criqui MH, Ginsberg HN, Goldberg AC, Howard WJ, Jacobson MS, Kris-Etherton PM, et al. Triglycerides and cardiovascular disease: a scientific statement from the American Heart Association. Circulation. 2011;123:2292–333.
37. Bays HE, Tighe AP, Sadovsky R, Davidson MH. Prescription omega-3 fatty acids and their lipid effects: physiologic mechanisms of action and clinical implications. Expert Rev Cardiovasc Ther. 2008;6:391–409.
38. Le Jossic-Corcos C, Gonthier C, Zaghini I, Logette E, Shechter I, Bournot P. Hepatic farnesyl diphosphate synthase expression is suppressed by polyunsaturated fatty acids. Biochem J. 2005;385:787–94.
39. Horton JD, Bashmakov Y, Shimomura I, Shimano H. Regulation of sterol regulatory element binding proteins in livers of fasted and refed mice. Proc Natl Acad Sci U S A. 1998;95:5987–92.
40. Harris WS, Bulchandani D. Why do omega-3 fatty acids lower serum triglycerides? Curr Opin Lipidol. 2006;17:387–93.
41. Park Y, Harris WS. Omega-3 fatty acid supplementation accelerates chylomicron triglyceride clearance. J Lipid Res. 2003;44:455–63.
42. Khan S, Minihane AM, Talmud PJ, Wright JW, Murphy MC, Williams CM, Griffin BA. Dietary long-chain n-3 PUFAs increase LPL gene expression in adipose tissue of subjects with an atherogenic lipoprotein phenotype. J Lipid Res. 2002;43:979–85.
43. Mason RP, Jacob RF. Eicosapntaenoic acid inhibits glucose-induced membrane cholesterol crystalline domain formation through a potent antioxidant mechanism. Biochim Biophis Acta. 2015;1848:502–9.
44. Willett WC, Stampfer MJ, Manson JE, Colditz GA, Speizer FE, Rosner BA, Sampson LA, Hennekens CH. Intake of trans fatty acids and risk of coronary heart disease among women. Lancet. 1993;341:581–5.
45. Oomen CM, Ocke MC, Feskens EJ, van Erp-Baart MA, Kok FJ, Kromhout D. Association between trans fatty acid intake and 10-year risk of coronary heart disease in the Zutphen elderly study: a prospective population-based study. Lancet. 2001;357:746–51.
46. Charnock JS. Dietary fats and cardiac arrhythmia in primates. Nutrition. 1994;10:161–9.
47. McLennan PL, Bridle TM, Abeywardena MY, et al. Dietary lipid modulation of ventricular fibrillation threshold in the marmoset monkey. Am Heart J. 1992;123:1555–61.
48. Lemaitre RN, King IB, Raghunathan TE, Pearce RM, Weinmann S, Knopp RH, Copass MK, Cobb LA, Siscovick DS. Cell membrane trans-fatty acids and the risk of primary cardiac arrest. Circulation. 2002;105:697–701.
49. McLennan PL, Abeywardena MY, Charnock JS. The influence of age and dietary fat in an animal model of sudden cardiac death. Aust NZ J Med. 1989;19:1–5.
50. Charnock JS, Abeywardena MY, Poletti VM, et al. Differences in fatty acid composition of various tissues of the marmoset monkey after different lipid supplemented diets. Comp Biochem Physiol Comp Physiol. 1992;101:387–93.
51. McLennan PL, Bridle TM, Abeywardena MY, Charnock JS. Comparative efficacy of n23 and n26 polyunsaturated fatty acids in modulating ventricular fibrillation threshold in marmoset monkeys. Am J Clin Nutr. 1993;58:666–9.
52. Billman GE, Hallaq H, Leaf A. Prevention of ischemia-induced ventricular fibrillation by n23 fatty acids. Proc Natl Acad Sci U S A. 1994;91:4427–30.
53. Siscovick DS, Raghunathan TE, King I, et al. Dietary intake and cell membrane levels of long-chain n-3 polyunsaturated fatty acids and the risk of primary cardiac arrest. JAMA. 1995;274:1363–7.

54. Leaf A. The electrophysiologic basis for the antiarrhythmic actions of polyunsaturated fatty acids. Eur Heart J. 2001;22:D98–D105.
55. Siscovick DS, Raghunathan T, King I, Weinmann S, Bovbjerg VE, Kushi L, Cobb LA, Copass MK, Psaty BM, Lemaitre R, Retzlaff B, Knopp RH. Dietary intake of long-chain n-3 polyunsaturated fatty acids and the risk of primary cardiac arrest. Am J Clin Nutr. 2000;71(1 Suppl):208S–12S.
56. Christensen JH. N-3 fatty acids and the risk of sudden cardiac death. Emphasis on heart rate variability. Dan Med Bull. 2003;50:347–67.
57. Albert CM, Campos H, Stampfer MJ, Ridker PM, Manson JE, Willett WC, Ma J. Blood levels of long-chain n-3 fatty acids and the risk of sudden death. N Engl J Med. 2002;346:1113–8.
58. Jouven X, Charles MA, Desnos M, Ducimetiere P. Circulating nonesterified fatty acid level as a predictive risk factor for sudden death in the population. Circulation. 2001;104:756–61.
59. Albert CM, Hennekens CH, O'Donnell CJ, et al. Fish consumption and risk of sudden cardiac death. JAMA. 1998;279:23–8.
60. Kang JX, Leaf A. Antiarrhythmic effects of polyunsaturated fatty acids: recent studies. Circulation. 1996;94:1774–80.
61. Billman GE, Kang JX, Leaf A. Prevention of ischemia-induced ventricular arrhythmias by dietary pure n-3 polyunsaturated fatty acids in dogs. Circulation. 1999;99:2452–7.
62. Mozaffarian D, Rimm E. Fish intake, contaminants, and human health. Evaluating the risks and the benefits. J Am Med Assoc. 2006;296:1885–99.
63. De Goede J, Geleijnse JM, Boer JMA, Kromhout D, Verschuren WMM. Marine (n-3) fatty acids, fish consumption and 10-year risk of fatal and nonfatal coronary heart disease in a large population of Dutch adults with a low fish intake. J Nutr. 2010;140:1023–8. https://doi.org/10.3945/jn.109.119271.
64. Skeaff C, Miller J. Dietary fat and coronary heart disease: summary of evidence from prospective cohort and randomised controlled trials. Annals of. Nutr Metab. 2009;55:173–201.
65. He K, Song Y, Daviglus MU, Liu K, Van Horn L, Dyer AR, Golbourt U, Greenland P. Fish consumption and incidence of stroke. A meta-analysis of cohort studies. Stroke. 2004;35:1538–42.
66. Chowdhury R, Stevens S, Gorman D, Pan A, Warnakula S, Chowdhury S, Ward H, Johnson L, Crowe F, Hu FB. Association between fish consumption, long chain omega 3 fatty acids, and risk of cerebrovascular disease: systematic review and meta-analysis. Br Med J. 2012;345:e6698.
67. WCRF & AICR (World Cancer Research Fund & American Institute for Cancer Research). Food, nutrition, physical activity and the prevention of cancer: a global perspective. Washington, DC: WCRF & AICR; 2007.
68. Farrow B, Evers B. Inflammation and the development of pancreatic cancer. Surg Oncol. 2002;10:153–69.
69. Qin B, Xun P, He K. Fish or long-chain (n-3) PUFA intake is not associated with pancreatic cancer risk in a meta-analysis and systematic review. J Nutr. 2012;142:1067–73.
70. Rohrmann S, Linseisen J, Nothlings U, Overvad K, Egeberg R, Tjønneland A, Boutron-Ruault MC, Clavel-Chapelon F, et al. Meat and fish consumption and risk of pancreatic cancer: results from the European prospective investigation into cancer and nutrition. Int J Cancer. 2012;132:617–24.
71. Kremmyda L-S, Vlachava M, Noakes P, Diaper ND, Miles EA, Calder PC. Atopy risk in infants and children in relation to early exposure to fish, oily fish, or long-chain omega-3 fatty acids: a systematic review. Clin Rev Allergy Immunol. 2011;41:36–66.
72. Alm B, Aberg N, Erdes L, Möllborg P, Pettersson R, Norvenius SG, Goksör E, Wennergren G. Early introduction of fish decreases the risk of eczema in infants. Arch Dis Child. 2009;94:11–5.
73. BNF (British Nutrition Foundation). Nutrition and Development. Short- and long-term consequences for health. Oxford, UK: Wiley Blackwell; 2013.
74. Morris M, Evans D, Bienias J, Tangney CC, Bennett DA, Wilson RS, Aggarwal N, Schneider J. Consumption of fish and n-3 fatty acids and risk of incident Alzheimer disease. Arch Neurol. 2003;60:940–6.

75. Schaefer E, Bongard V, Beiser A, Lamon-Fava S, Robins SJ, Au R, Tucker KL, Kyle DJ, Wilson PW, Wolf PA. Plasma phophatidylcholine docosahexaenoic acid content and risk of dementia and Alzheimer disease: the Framingham heart study. Arch Neurol. 2006;63:1545–50.
76. Lopez L, Kritz-Silverstein D, Barrett-Connor E. High dietary and plasma levels of the omega-3 fatty acid docosahexaenoic acid are associated with decreased dementia risk: the rancho Bernardo study. J Nutr Health Aging. 2011;15:25–31.
77. Devore E, Grodstein F, van Rooij F, Hofman A, Rosner B, Stampfer MJ, Witteman JC, Breteler MM. Dietary intake of fish and omega-3 fatty acids in relation to long-term dementia risk. Am J Clin Nutr. 2009;90:170–6.
78. Kroger E, Verreault R, Carmichael PH, Lindsay J, Julien P, Dewailly E, Ayotte P, Laurin D. Omega-3 fatty acids and risk of dementia: the Canadian study of health and aging. Am J Clin Nutr. 2009;90:184–92.
79. Morris M, Evans D, Tangney C, Bienias JL, Wilson RS. Fish consumption and cognitive decline with age in a large community study. Arch Neurol. 2005;62:1849–53.
80. Kalmijn S, Feskens E, Launer L, Kromhout D. Polyunsaturated fatty acids, antioxidants, and cognitive function in very old men. Am J Epidemiol. 1997;145:33–41.
81. Kesse-Guyot E, Péneau S, Ferry M, Jeandel C, Hercberg S, Galan P. SU.VI.MAX 2 Research Group. Thirteen-year prospective study between fish consumption, long-chain n-3 fatty acids intakes and cognitive function. J Nutr Health Aging. 2011;15:115–20.
82. Diet PF. Bone health. Nutr Bull. 2004;29:99–110.
83. Farina E, Kiel D, Roubenoff R, Schaefer EJ, Cupples LA, Tucker KL. Protective effects of fish intake and interactive effects of long-chain polyunsaturated fatty acid intakes on hip bone mineral density in older adults: the Framingham osteoporosis study. Am J Clin Nutr. 2011;93:1142–51.
84. Orchard T, Cauley J, Frank GC, Neuhouser ML, Robinson JG, Snetselaar L, Tylavsky F, Wactawski-Wende J, Young AM, Lu B, Jackson RD. Fatty acid consumption and risk of fracture in the Women's health initiative. Am J Clin Nutr. 2010;92(145):2–60.
85. Chen Y, Ho S, Lam S. Higher sea fish intake is associated with greater bone mass and lower osteoporosis risk in postmenopausal Chinese women. Osteoporos Int. 2010;21:939–46.
86. Kris-Etherton PM, Harris WS, Appel LJ. Omega-3 fatty acids and cardiovascular disease: new recommendations from the American Heart Association. Arterioscler Thromb Vasc Biol. 2003;23(2):151.
87. Harris WS, Kris-Etherton PM, Harris KA. Intakes of long-chain omega-3 fatty acid associated with reduced risk for death from coronary heart disease in healthy adults. Curr Atheroscler Rep. 2008;10:503–9.
88. GISSI-Prevenzione Investigators. Dietary supplementation with n-3 polyunsaturated fatty acids and vitamin E after myocardial infarction: results of the GISSI-Prevenzione trial. Lancet. 1999;354:447–55.
89. Burr M, Ashfield-Watt P, Dunstan F, Fehily AM, Breay P, Ashton T, Zotos PC, Haboubi NA, Elwood PC. Lack of benefit of dietary advice to men with angina: results of a controlled trial. Eur J Clin Nutr. 2003;57:193–200.
90. Clark JD, Schievella AR, Nalefski EA, Lin LL. Cytosolic phospholipase A2. J Lipid Mediat Cell Signal. 1995;12:83–117.
91. Marchioli R, Barzi F, Bomba E, Chieffo C, Di Gregorio D, Di Mascio R, et al. on behalf of the GISSI-Prevenzione Investigators. Early protection against sudden death by n-3 polyunsaturated fatty acids after myocardial infarction. Time course analysis of the results of the Gruppo Italiano per lo Studio della Sopravivenza nell'Infarto Miocardico (GISSI)-Prevenzione. Circulation. 2002;105:1897–903.

14 The Smells and Tastes of the Mediterranean Diet: Herbs

14.1 Premises

The herbs that grew in abundance in the Mediterranean area were used from the early years not only in foods to add flavor, but also in drinks to give taste, and in general to add "spice" to the everyday life of people. Herbs and their derivatives together with spices from trees and bushes were collected and used when in season or they were dried to be used as and when needed.

In recent years when the Mediterranean diet was formulated and depicted in the form of the Mediterranean diet pyramid, initially Mediterranean culinary herbs and spices have not taken the place they deserved. In a latter revision of the Mediterranean diet pyramid they were glamorously introduced and the Mediterranean diet pyramid was updated. Herbs and spices are in the "every-day-use" level and are used to form the basis of an everyday Mediterranean diet meal. Due to variety of the herbs and the degree of their use by the 16 Mediterranean countries and nations, herbs and spices contribute to the individuality, culinary tastes, and identity of the variations of the various Mediterranean cuisines.

The main reason that culinary herbs and spices were introduced in the Mediterranean diet pyramid was the fact that recent studies have identified their medicinal properties and effects on the health of the people following the Mediterranean diet. While the effects of olive oil and wine were very well known in the prevention of cardiovascular diseases, the antioxidant effects of culinary herbs and spices were "ignored" until recent studies have revealed them and thus they took the position that they deserve in the Mediterranean diet pyramid.

Culinary herbs and spices form a food group and as a food group they have been identified to have more medicinal properties and be as effective at preventing cardiovascular diseases as olive oil and wine. The reason behind this effectiveness is their antioxidant property. A recent study has revealed that out of top 50 antioxidant foods, five are spices and the leading antioxidant spice is Oregano, a spice that originates from the Mediterranean basin. It was found that Oregano has four times more antioxidant activity and benefits than blueberry.

A. Capurso et al., *Benefits of the Mediterranean Diet in the Elderly Patient*, Practical Issues in Geriatrics, https://doi.org/10.1007/978-3-319-78084-9_14

Also other Mediterranean spices and herbs have strong antioxidant effects and these are: parsley, basil, rosemary, sage, onion, and garlic. All these spices are part of the traditional Mediterranean cuisine and apart from helping in the fight against cardiovascular diseases they protect against cancer, Alzheimer's, and diabetes.

It is beyond question that due to the fact that the Mediterranean diet is a way of living and a diet which has resulted very healthy over the pass of the centuries, it has managed to balance and exploit all the properties and benefits of the plant and animal kingdom that used to grow and graze in the Mediterranean basin and has been transformed to probably the healthiest diet of the world.

14.2 Parsley

Parsley or garden parsley (*Petroselinum crispum*) is a species of flowering plant in the family Apiaceae, native to the central Mediterranean region (southern Italy, Greece, Portugal, Spain, Malta, Morocco, Algeria, and Tunisia), naturalized elsewhere in Europe, and widely cultivated as a herb, a spice, and a vegetable.

14.2.1 Culinary Use

The main use of parsley is culinary. Parsley is widely used in European, Middle Eastern, and American cooking. In central Europe, eastern Europe, and southern Europe, as well as in western Asia, many dishes are served with fresh green chopped parsley sprinkled on top. In southern and central Europe, parsley is part of *bouquet garni*, a bundle of fresh herbs used as an ingredient in stocks, soups, and sauces. Freshly chopped green parsley is used as a topping for soups such as chicken soup, green salads, or salads such as *salade Olivier*, and on open sandwiches with cold cuts or *pâtés.*

Parsley is also the main ingredient in Italian *salsa verde*, which is a mixed condiment of parsley, capers, anchovies, garlic, and sometimes bread soaked in vinegar. It is an Italian custom to serve it with *bollito misto* or fish. *Gremolata*, a mixture of parsley, garlic, and lemon zest, is a traditional accompaniment to the Italian veal stew, *ossobuco alla milanese*. In England, parsley sauce is a roux-based sauce, commonly served over fish or gammon.

Parsley, Fresh
Vitamins and mineral content per 100 g
Source: USDA Database

Energy	151 KJ (36 kcal)
Carbohydrates	6.33 g
Protein	2.97 g
Fat	0.79 g

Vitamin A equiv.	421 μg	(53% DV)
Beta-carotene	5054 μg	47% DV
Lutein-zeaxanthin	5561 μg	
Thiamine	0.086 mg	(7% DV)
Riboflavin	0.09 mg	(8% DV)
Niacin	1.313 mg	(9% DV)
Pantothenic acid	0.4 mg	(8% DV)
Vitamin B_6	0.09 mg	(7% DV)
Folate	152 μg	(38% DV)
Vitamin C	133 mg	(160% DV)
Vitamin E	0.75 mg	(5% DV)
Vitamin K	1640 μg	(1562% DV)

Calcium	136 mg	(14% DV)
Iron	6.2 mg	(48% DV)
Magnesium	50 mg	(14% DV)
Manganese	0.16 mg	(8% DV)
Phosphorus	58 mg	(8% DV)
Potassium	554 mg	(12% DV)
Sodium	56 mg	(4% DV)
Zinc	1.07 mg	(11% DV)

DV = Daily Value

14.2.2 Nutritional Content

Parsley (*Petroselinum crispum*) is a rich source of flavonoid and antioxidants, especially apigenin, luteolin, folic acid, vitamin K, vitamin C, and vitamin A. Half a tablespoon (a gram) of dried parsley contains about 6.0 μg of lycopene and 10.7 μg of alpha carotene as well as 82.9 μg of lutein + zeaxanthin and 80.7 μg of beta-carotene (see table "**Parsley, Fresh**").

Parsley has been shown to contain at least 85 compounds, with flavonoids being the dominant compounds [1]. The main parsley's flavonoids are apigenin, luteolin, quercetin, isorhamnetin, chrysoeriol, kaempferol, apiin (glycoside), cnidilin, diosmetin (glycoside), cosmosiin (glycoside) [1]. Parsley is particularly rich of the flavones apigenin and luteolin. Fresh parsley contains 216 mg/100 g while dried parsley contains 4523 mg/100 g of apigenin [1].

The flavone apigenin is primarily present in parsley as apiin, the 7-*O*-apioside of apigenin.

Seeds, roots, and leaves of parsley produce high amount of essential oil. Myristicin and apiol are the two main components of *Petroselinum crispum* essential oil which are responsible for its antioxidant activity. α-Pinene, sabinene, β-pinene, ρ-cymene, limonene, β-phellandrene, γ-terpinene, myristicin, elemicin, 1-allyl-2,3,4,5-tetramethoxy-benzene, carotol, eugenol, and apiol have been also identified in *Petroselinum crispum* seed essential oil [2, 3].

Parsley contains also coumarin products. Oxypeucedanin is the major furocoumarin of *Petroselinum crispum*. It doesn't act as anticoagulant but is responsible for contact photodermatitis that can be induced by the plant.

Also carotenoids, including B-carotene, lutein, violaxanthin, and neoxanthin, have been detected in *Petroselinum crispum.*

14.2.3 Ethnomedicinal and Modern Medicinal Use

In traditional and folklore medicines or oriental populations, parsley has been used as carminative, gastro tonic, diuretic, antiseptic of urinary tract, anti-urolithiasis, antidote, and anti-inflammatory and for the treatment of amenorrhea, dysmenorrhea, gastrointestinal disorder, hypertension, cardiac disease, urinary disease, otitis, sniffle, diabetes, and also various dermal disease.

In modern medicine, parsley has been found to have a wide range of pharmacological activities, including antioxidant, hepatoprotective, brain protective, antidiabetic, analgesic, spasmolytic, immunosuppressant, antiplatelet, gastroprotective, cytoprotective, laxative, estrogenic, diuretic, hypotensive, antibacterial, and antifungal activities.

14.2.4 Antioxidant Activity

Flavonoids of parsley (present in leaves, roots, and seeds) are potent antioxidants (see also antioxidants flavonoids Chap. 10, Sect. 10.10). Apigenin and myristicin are the main compounds responsible for this antioxidant activity in the essential oil from seeds and leaves [2]. Other extracts from *Petroselinum crispum* leaves and stems have shown antioxidant activity in in vitro models, as free radical scavenging [4–7]. In an in vitro study, dichloromethane extract of *Petroselinum crispum* DPPH showed potent radical scavenging properties and to exert a significant protection against DNA damage in normal cells [8].

Very interesting was a randomized crossover study in which the effect of intake of parsley (*Petroselinum crispum*), with high levels of the flavone apigenin, on the urinary excretion of flavones and on biomarkers of oxidative stress was evaluated in seven women [10]. The subjects received a strictly controlled diet low in flavones and other naturally occurring antioxidants during the 2 weeks of intervention. This basic diet was supplemented with parsley providing 3.73–4.49 mg apigenin/MJ in one of the intervention weeks. Urinary excretion of apigenin was 1.59–409.09 μg/MJ per 24 h during intervention with parsley and 0–112.27 μg/MJ per 24 h on the basic diet. Erythrocyte glutathione reductase and superoxide dismutase activities increased during intervention with parsley ($P < 0.005$) as compared with the levels on the basic diet. No significant changes were observed in plasma protein 2-adipic semialdehyde residues, a biomarker of plasma protein oxidation. Apigenin, therefore, was demonstrated to be actively absorbed from parsley and excreted in low amount (0.58% on average) with urine.

14.2.5 Antidiabetic Activity

Antidiabetic activity of parsley has been shown in studies on animals. *Petroselinum crispum* leaves have been shown to decrease blood glucose level and exert hepatoprotective effects in diabetic rats via antioxidant activity [11, 12]. This antihyperglycemic activity of *Petroselinum crispum* was not due to improvement and regeneration of secretory granules and β-cells of pancreas islets [13]. Furthermore, *Petroselinum crispum* improved hyperglycemia-induced heart and aorta oxidative damage via its antioxidant activity in the heart and aorta tissue [14].

14.2.6 Intestinal Activity

In experimental animals, analgesic and spasmolytic activity have been demonstrated. *Petroselinum crispum* seed hydroalcoholic extract has shown analgesic activity in mice [15]. It also reduced KCl- and $CaCl_2$-induced contractions on rat isolated ileum dose dependently via blocking voltage-gated calcium channels [16]. Different extracts from aerial parts demonstrated antispasmodic activity on spontaneous and acetylcholine-induced contractions of rat isolated ileum [17]. Aqueous extract from *Petroselinum hortense* seeds demonstrated also a laxative activity in rat by significant absorption of sodium and water and also enhancing $NaKCl_2$ transporter activity in the colon [18].

14.2.7 Genitourinary System

The methanolic extract from the aerial parts of *Petroselinum crispum* has shown to possess a potent estrogenic activity [19]. Several flavone glycosides and a new flavone glycoside, 6'-acetylapiin, with estrogenic activity have been isolated, together with a new monoterpene glucoside, petroside. The estrogenic activities of these flavones were nearly equal to those of the isoflavones daidzein and genistein. The methanolic extract of parsley, apiin, and apigenin restored the uterus weight in ovariectomized mice when orally administered for consecutive 7 days [19].

14.2.8 Hypotensive Effect and Antiplatelet Activity

Parsley leaves extracts decreased mean blood pressure in anesthetized rats. This effect was attenuated with muscarinic receptor antagonist. It also decreased the rate and amplitude of contraction on isolated rat atria. These data demonstrated that parsley has a hypotensive and negative inotropic and chronotropic activity [20].

Petroselinum crispum leaves have also a strong antiplatelet aggregation effect in rats and human [21, 22]. The effect of genins (aglycone flavonoids without sugar group) isolated from parsley leaves was investigated in vitro on human platelet aggregation and adhesion [22]. Genins inhibited dose dependently platelet aggregation induced by thrombin, ADP, and collagen. The strongest effect was observed in collagen-induced aggregation. The HPLC identification of genins compounds revealed the presence of aglycone flavonoids kaempferol, apigenin, and other not identified compounds. In addition, adhesion of human platelets to collagen was greatly decreased (over 75%) by genins [22].

14.2.9 Antimicrobial Activity

Petroselinum crispum leaves and steams have antibacterial activity on *B. subtilis* and *E. coli* [4]. Hot and cold water extract from *Petroselinum crispum* leaves have shown to exert antibacterial activity against *Pseudomonas aeruginosa*, *S. aureus* and *S. pyogenes* isolated from patient with burn infection [23]. Ethanol extract of parsley leaves inhibited the growth of *Lactobacillus plantarum* and *Leuconostoc mesenteroides* [24]. The furocoumarins isolated from parsley leaves showed inhibitory activity against *E. coli*, *L. monocytogenes*, *Erwinia carotovora*, and *Listeria innocua* [25].

14.2.10 Antiprostate Cancer Activity

Studies have shown that apigenin is an anticancer agent selectively toxic to cancer cells by inducing cycle arrest and apoptosis. These apigenin-mediated growth inhibitory responses have been demonstrated as due to inhibition of class I histone deacetylases (HDACs) (see side BOX) in prostate cancer cells [10, 26]. Apigenin-mediated HDAC inhibition resulted in global histone H3 and H4 acetylation, as well as localized hyperacetylation of histone H3 on the p21/waf1 promoter. The downstream events demonstrated cell cycle arrest and induction of apoptosis in cancer cells. Actually, numerous evidences suggest that in the pathophysiology of prostate cancer epigenetic modifications play a considerable role. HDACs have strong crosstalk with prostate cancer progression as they regulate various genes meant for tumor suppression. Histone deacetylase inhibitors (HDACi), the small molecules interfering HDACs may be propitious chemotherapeutic agents as they tune the altered acetylation homeostasis for attenuating disease signaling. More than 20 synthetic HDACi have entered into the clinical trials. Despite the therapeutic benefits, the synthetic HDACi cause detrimental side effects like atrial fibrillation, raising concerns regarding their applicability. Apigenin, a plant-derived HDAC inhibitor, has shown a promising role in prostate cancer therapy. Apigenin provokes apoptotic signaling by multiple mechanisms like restraining HDACs and declining the levels of antiapoptotic proteins. Apigenin also hampers NFκB signaling and down-modulates its regulated gene products for bringing therapeutic effect. Furthermore, apigenin has shown synergistic effect in combinatorial therapy inducing apoptosis even in prostate cancer models resistant to conventional therapeutic regimens.

The Role of Histone Deacetylases

Histone is a basic protein associated with the DNA in the chromatin of eukaryotes, implicated in the spatial organization of DNA. Histone tails are normally positively charged due to amine groups present on their lysine and arginine amino acids. These positive charges help the histone tails to interact with and bind to the negatively charged phosphate groups on the DNA backbone. Acetylation, which occurs normally in a cell, neutralizes the positive charges on the histone by changing amines into amides and decreases the ability of the histones to bind to DNA. This decreased binding allows chromatin expansion, permitting genetic transcription to take place. Histone deacetylases remove the acetyl groups, increasing the positive charge of histone tails and encouraging high-affinity binding between the histones and DNA backbone. The increased DNA binding condenses DNA structure, preventing transcription.

Gene transcription is "switched on" when histone protein is acetylated, and "switched off" when histone protein is deacetylated. These functional gene modifications, which do not imply any gene sequence modification, are reversible and are generally due to epigenetic phenomena, linked to variations in environmental factors, including diet (see also Chap. 7, Sect. 7.3.2)

14.3 Oregano

Oregano is a flowering plant in the mint family. It originated in temperate western and southwestern Eurasia and the Mediterranean region.

Oregano (*Origanum vulgare*) is the anglicized form of the Italian word *origano*, derived from the Classical Latin *origanum,* which probably referred specifically to *sweet marjoram,* and itself derived from Greek *origanon,* which simply referred to *"an acrid herb."*

14.3.1 The History

The Greek and Roman cultures first started the practice of using oregano as a flavoring agent in food. The rich aroma of oregano and its spicy flavor perfectly complemented the Italian and Greek food, and the herb soon gained popularity in other European countries. Being considered as a symbol of joy and happiness, oregano was used not only in Greek and Italian cuisines, but also as a symbol of celebrating. For instance, it was a common practice among Greeks and Romans to crown their brides and grooms with laurels of oregano during a marriage ceremony. The French started using oregano in their food during the Middle Ages. The herb became so popular among the French that it is still a very important component of Mediterranean cuisine. It took a while for oregano to enter the United States from Europe but when it did, the Americans could not ignore the flavor which had already captured the taste buds of people in Europe. It was the US soldiers serving in Europe during the

Second World War who introduced oregano to fellow Americans. Oregano was chiefly used as a seasoning in pizzas in Italy and therefore the aromatic herb became known as the "pizza herb" in the USA, a culinary concept that is still popular.

14.3.2 Chemical Components

Oregano is rich in polyphenols, particularly flavanones and flavones. Dried oregano contains 412 mg/100 g flavanones, and 1046 mg/100 g flavones [1].

The essential oil of oregano contains high concentration of monoterpenoids and monoterpenes with the relative concentration of each compound varying widely across geographic origin and other factors. Over 60 different compounds have been identified, with the primary ones being carvacrol and thymol ranging to over 80%, while lesser abundant compounds include p-cymene, γ-terpinene, caryophyllene, spathulenol, germacrene-D, β-fenchyl alcohol, and δ-terpineol.

Oregano, Dried

Vitamins and mineral content per 100 g

Source: USDA Database, Basic Report 02027

Energy	265 kcal
Carbohydrates	68.92 g
Protein	9.00 g
Fiber	42.5 g
Fat	4.28 g
Saturated	1.551 g
Monounsaturated	0.716
Polyunsaturated	1.369

Vitamin A RAE	85 μg
Vitamin A IU	1.701 μg
Thiamine	0.177 mg
Riboflavin	0.528 mg
Niacin	4.640 mg
Vitamin B_6	1.044 mg
Folate	237 μg
Vitamin C	2.3 mg
Vitamin E	18.26 mg
Vitamin K	621.7 μg

Calcium	1.597 mg
Iron	36.80 mg
Magnesium	270 mg
Phosphorus	148 mg
Potassium	1.260 mg
Sodium	25 mg
Zinc	2.69 mg

14.3.3 Culinary

Oregano is an important culinary herb, used for the flavor of its leaves, which can be more flavorful when dried than fresh. It has an aromatic, warm, and slightly bitter taste, which can vary in intensity. Factors such as climate, season, and soil composition may affect the aromatic oils present, and this effect may be greater than the differences between the various species of plants. Among the chemical compounds contributing to the flavor are carvacrol, thymol, limonene, pinene, ocimene, and caryophyllene.

Oregano's most prominent modern use is as the staple herb of Italian-American cuisine. Its popularity in the USA began when soldiers returning from World War II brought back with them a taste for the "pizza herb," which had probably been eaten in southern Italy for centuries. There, it is most frequently used with roasted, fried, or grilled vegetables, meat, and fish. Oregano combines well with spicy foods popular in southern Italy. It is less commonly used in the north of the country, as marjoram generally is preferred. The dried and ground leaves are most often used in Greece to add flavor to Greek salad, and is usually added to the lemon-olive oil sauce that accompanies fish or meat grills and casseroles.

14.3.4 Health Benefits

The flavonoids and terpenes from *Origanum vulgare* and *Origanum majorana* have been shown to have numerous beneficial effects.

14.3.4.1 Radical Scavenging Properties

The essential oil from O*riganum* species was found to contain 39 compounds. Thymol and trans-sabinene hydrate were the most prominent compounds, followed by gamma-terpinene, terpinen-4-ol, and alpha-terpinene. The total phenol content showed a high free radical scavenging activity, with some variability explained by the climate variables, the temperature being the most important climatic variable [27].

Origanum majorana essential oil was analyzed by gas chromatography-mass spectrometry (GC-MS) and evaluated for free radical scavenging and anti-acetylcholinesterase (AChE) activities [28]. GC-MS analysis revealed the presence of 4-terpineol (29.97%), γ-terpinene (15.40%), trans-sabinene hydrate (10.93), α-terpinene (6.86%), 3-cycolohexene-1-1 methanal,a,a4-trimethyl-,(*S*)-(CAS) (6.54%), and sabinene (3.91%) as main constituents. The essential oil exhibited a potent concentration-dependent inhibitory effects on hydroxyl radical, hydrogen peroxide, reducing power and lipid peroxidation. Interestingly, an important acetylcholine esterase (AChE) inhibitory activity was also demonstrated, leading to the conclusion that the *Origanum majorana* essential oil has a significant potential to be used as a natural antioxidant and anti-AChE [28].

14.3.4.2 Gastric Protection Activity

The ethanol extract of *Origanum majorana* showed an anti-ulcerogenic activity in experimentally induced gastric ulcers in rats. Marjoram at doses of 250 and 500 mg/kg of body weight significantly decreased the incidence of ulcers, basal gastric secretion, and acid output. Ulcer preventing potential was further confirmed by histopathological assessment. The phytochemical screening of aerial parts of marjoram revealed the presence of volatile oil, flavonoids, tannins, sterols, and/or triterpenes [29].

14.3.4.3 Antidiabetic Activity

In vitro studies have demonstrated significant inhibitory effects of methanolic extract of the leaves of *Origanum majorana* (*OM*) on the formation of advanced glycation end products. The advanced glycation end products (AGEs) are the final products of the nonenzymatic reaction between reducing sugars and amino groups in proteins, lipoproteins, and nucleic acids. AGEs accumulation in vivo has been considered to play a major role in the pathogenic process of diabetes and its complications, including neuropathy, nephropathy, retinopathy, and cataract.

The *OM* antiglycation activity was not only brought about by its antioxidant activities but also related to its abilities to scavenge reactive carbonyls species such as methylglyoxal, an intermediate reactive carbonyl of AGE formation. The data of a recent study [30] demonstrated that *OM* has significant effects on in vitro AGE formation, and the glycation inhibitory activity was demonstrated to be more effective than the effects obtained using as standard antiglycation agent aminoguanidine. The ability of *OM* to react with carbonyls appeared to be the major mechanism for protein glycation inhibition. Furthermore, *OM* alleviated oxidative stress under diabetic conditions through the inhibition of lipid peroxidation, so preventing and/or delaying the onset of renal damage. These results have suggested that *OM* might prevent or improve the AGE-associated chronic conditions. Therefore, *OM* could has been suggested as a candidate for use in studies looking at the effects of natural herbal complement in the prevention of diabetes complications, since it possesses both antioxidant and antiglycation activities. Finally, treatment of streptozotocin-diabetic mice with *Origanum majorana* and glibenclamide for 28 days had beneficial effects on renal metabolic abnormalities including glucose level and AGEs formation [30].

14.3.4.4 Anticancer Activity

Numerous papers have documented the antiproliferative anticancer activity of *Origanum majorana (OM)*.

Lymphoblastic leukemia [31]. The antiproliferative activity of plant extracts from *OM* was tested on human lymphoblastic leukemia cell line. At noncytotoxic concentrations, the viability of cells decreased with the increase of concentration of plant extract. The antiproliferative effect was found to be dose-dependent. Analysis via flow cytometry showed that marjoram extracts stimulated apoptosis. Induction of apoptosis was caused by an upregulation of p53 protein levels and downregulation of Bcl-2alpha. Marjoram exhibited also a strong scavenging activity. The data of this study suggested that marjoram extracts have antiproliferative effect and high antioxidant activity.

Hepatocellular carcinoma [32]. The antiproliferative activity of OM was demonstrated also on human hepatocellular carcinoma (HepG2) cell line, with aqueous and ethanol extracts of *Origanum majorana* leaf [32]. The effects of aqueous and ethanol extracts of *Origanum majorana L.* on HepG2 cell viability, nuclear factor kappa B (NF-kB) gene expression were examined. The results of the cell viability assays showed that aqueous and ethanol extracts exhibited a highly significant inhibitory effect on HepG2 cell proliferation which was evidenced by a reduction in viable cell count. The results were confirmed by microscopical examination of cell morphology. Furthermore, the *Origanum majorana L.* extracts suppressed the activity of NF-kB gene expression of HepG2 cells compared to the control. The conclusions from this study suggested that marjoram extracts have antiproliferative effect against hepatocellular carcinoma through suppressing the activity of NF-kB gene expression and high antioxidant activity.

Breast cancer. *Origanum majorana* has shown to be active also on human breast cancer. The effect of *OM* ethanolic extract on the survival of the highly proliferative and invasive triple-negative p53 mutant breast cancer cell line MDA-MB-231 was investigated [33]. It was found that *Origanum majorana* extract (OME) was able to inhibit the viability of the MDA-MB-231 cells in a time- and concentration-dependent manner. The effect of OME on cellular viability was further confirmed by the inhibition of colony growth. It was shown that, depending on the concentration used, OME elicited different effects on the MDA-MB 231 cells. Lower concentrations of OME (150 and 300 μg/mL) induced an accumulation of apoptotic-resistant population of cells arrested in mitosis and overexpressing the cyclin-dependent kinase inhibitor p21, and the inhibitor of apoptosis survivin. Higher concentrations of OME (450 and 600 μg/mL) triggered a massive apoptosis through the extrinsic pathway, including the activation of tumor necrosis factor-α (TNF-α), caspase 8, caspase 3, and cleavage of PARP, downregulation of survivin as well as depletion of the mutant p53 in MDA-MB-231 cells. Furthermore, OME induced also an upregulation of γ-H2AX, a marker of double strand DNA breaks and an overall histone H3 and H4 hyperacetylation. These data provided strong evidence that *Origanum majorana* may be a promising chemopreventive and therapeutic candidate against cancer especially for highly invasive triple negative p53 mutant breast cancer, thus validating its complementary and alternative medicinal use.

14.4 Basil

Basil (*Ocimum basilicum*) is a culinary herb of the family of Lamiaceae (mints). It is also called the "king of herbs" and the "royal herb." The name "basil" comes from Greek *basilikón phutón*, "royal plant." Basil is possibly native to India, and has been cultivated there for more than 5000 years. It was thoroughly familiar to the Greek authors Theophrastus and Dioscorides. It is a tender plant, best known as a culinary herb prominently featured in Italian cuisine, and also plays a major role in Southeast

Asian cuisines of Indonesia, Thailand, Malaysia, Vietnam, Cambodia, Laos, and Taiwan. There are many varieties of basil. The type used in Italian food is called sweet basil (or Genovese basil), as opposed to other type of basil (Thay basil, lemon basil, holy basil) used in Asia.

14.4.1 Culinary Use

Basil is most commonly used fresh in cooked recipes. In general, it is added at the last moment, as cooking quickly destroys the flavor. Basil is one of the main ingredients in *Pesto,* a green Italian oil-and-herb sauce. The Chinese also use fresh or dried basils in soups and other foods. In Taiwan, people add fresh basil leaves to thick soups. They also eat fried chicken with deep-fried basil leaves. Basil (most commonly Thai basil) is commonly steeped in cream or milk to create an interesting flavor in ice cream or chocolates (such as truffles). Thai basil is also a condiment in a Vietnamese noodle soup.

Basil (*Ocimum basilicum*)
Vitamins and mineral content per 100 g
Source: USDA Database, Basic Report 02044

Energy	23 kcal (94 kJ)
Carbohydrates	2.65 g
Protein	3.15 g
Fiber	1.6 g
Fat	0.64 g
Saturated (16:0)	0.041 g
Monounsaturated (18:1)	0.088 g
Polyunsaturated (18:3)	0.316 g

Vitamin A RAE	264 µg
Vitamin A IU	5275 IU
Lutein + zeaxanthin	5650 µg
Carotene, beta	3142 µg
Cryptoxanthin	46 µg
Thiamine	0.034 mg
Riboflavin	0.076 mg
Niacin	0.902 mg
Pantothenic acid	0.209 mg
Vitamin B_6	0.155 mg
Folate	68 µg
Vitamin C	18 mg
Vitamin E (a-tocopherol)	0.80 mg
Vitamin K	414.8 µg

Calcium	177 mg
Copper,	0.385 mg
Iron	3.17 mg
Magnesium	64 mg
Manganese	1.148 mg
Phosphorus	56 mg
Potassium	295 mg
Selenium	0.3 μg
Sodium	4 mg
Zinc	0.81 mg

14.4.2 Chemical Components [See Table "Basil (*Ocimum basilicum*)"]

Basil leaves contain essential oil at a percentage of 0.2–1%, with the main components being *linalool* and *estragole* (methyl chavicol), as well as *o-cymene, citral, alpha-pinene, camphene, beta-pinene, geraniol,* and *geranial.* The major components of basil oil vary extensively, depending on genetic factors, geographical origins, nutritional status, the extracted plant parts (stem, leaf, and flower), and the extraction methods. However, because of the variations of the plant and oil composition, several chemotypes have been described with the basic components of linalool, *eugenol, methyleugenol, methyl chavicol, methyl cinnamate,* and *bergamotene*, either alone or in the form of a mixture [34].

The strong clove scent of sweet basil is derived from eugenol. The citrus scent of lemon basil and lime basil reflects their higher portion of *citral*, which causes this effect in several plants including lemon mint, and of limonene, which gives actual lemon peel its scent.

In a comparative evaluation of North American commercially available *Ocimum* basil cultivars, 44 different cultivars have been listed. Many of the cultivars evaluated belonged to the "Sweet" basil group, with "Genovese," "Italian large leaf," "Mammoth," "Napoletano," and "Sweet" dominating the American fresh and dry culinary herb markets. By chemical analysis, basil plants showed a wide variety of oil compounds reflecting a diversity of available aromas and flavors. Many contained a combination of *linalool* and *methyl chavicol* and/or *1,8-cineole*, reflecting the traditional sweet basil aroma. Others had distinct aromas. The predominant aroma compound was *eugenol* (62%) in "East Indian" and "Tree" basil; *camphor* (61%) in "Camphor" basil; *thymol* in "Green" basil; *b-caryophyllene* in "Holy" and "Sacred" basil; and *methyl chavicol* in "New Guinea" and "Thai—Richters" basil. *Citral* was the predominant compound in all the lemon-scented basils.

In a study [35] with gas chromatography/mass spectrometry conducted to identify volatile compounds in *Ocimum* basil, four major constituents were identified: 3,7-dimethyl-1,6-octadien-3-ol (*linalool*; 3.94 mg/g), 1-methoxy-4-(2-propenyl) benzene (*estragole*; 2.03 mg/g), *methyl cinnamate* (1.28 mg/g), 4-allyl-2-methoxyphenol (*eugenol*; 0.896 mg/g), and *1,8-cineole* (0.288 mg/g). Twelve aroma constituents of basil were examined for their antioxidant activities using the aldehyde/carboxylic acid assay. *Eugenol, thymol, carvacrol,* and *4-allylphenol* showed stronger antioxidant activities than did the other components tested in the assay.

They all inhibited the oxidation of hexanal by almost 100% for a period of 30 days at a concentration of 5 μg/mL. Their antioxidant activities were comparable to those of the known antioxidants, α-tocopherol and butylated hydroxy toluene (BHT).

In another study [36], the basil essential oil components were linalool and naphthalene. The essential oil components of plants exhibited different profiles with respect to nitrogen applications. Average linalool content ranged from 57.93% to 61.10% in the control. The highest and lowest average naphthalene content were 13.87% and 11.58% 150 kg N ha^{-1} application, respectively.

14.4.3 Methyleugenol and Eugenol Biological Actions

Methyleugenol and *eugenol* are among the main components of basil essential oil. Studies have shown that *methyleugenol* derives from *eugenol* by a specific methylation involving an S-adenosylmethionine dependent O-methyltransferase.

Methyleugenol is the prevalent component (58.7%) of the herb, and belongs to the phenylpropanoid group, an important natural constituent of a large number of herbs, spices, and vegetables. *Methyleugenol* is an active pesticide ingredient and as such has been registered in the USA. *Methyleugenol* is also an insect parapheromone which is attractive to male fruit flies and is used in insect traps to attract certain species such as the oriental fruit flies. *Eugenol* is also an ingredient of various dental preparations and oral solutions owing to its antiseptic effects.

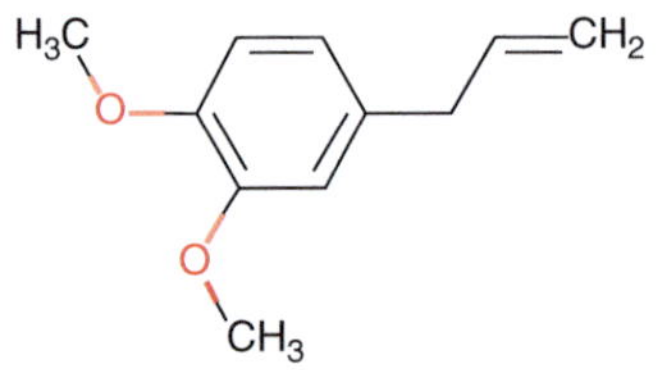

Methyleugenol

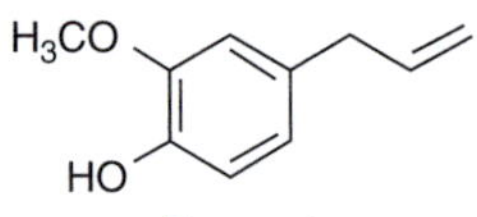

Eugenol

Although *methyleugenol* and *estragole* are approved for commercial use as a flavoring agent in food and as fragrance in perfumes, creams, and detergents, human exposure to these compounds is of some toxicological concern. It has been reported that *methyleugenol* and *estragole* are responsible for cytotoxic damage and carcerogenesis, and according to the Council of Europe, the former must not be detectable, and the latter must not exceed the limit of 0.05% mg/kg in food products.

No data are available on the ability of *methyleugenol* and *estragole* to induce DNA adducts, DNA strand breaks, mutations chromosomal effects, alteration in oncogenes or suppressor genes in tumors, or change in gene expression in humans. In animals, *methyleugenol* has been demonstrated to be mutagenic. In a 2-years study on mice given *methyleugenol* in 0.5% methylcellulose by gavage at variable doses for 105 weeks, *methyleugenol* caused significant dose-related increases in the incidence of hepatocellular adenoma, hepatocellular carcinoma, and hepatoblastoma [37]. In cultured human HepG2 hepatoma cells methyleugenol has induced DNA adducts [38].

The intake of *methyleugenol* with the human diet is usually very low. In US population the dietary intake of *methyleugenol* was estimated for a 60-kg body weight adult. The estimated dietary exposure was of 0.50–0.65 μg/kg/day, mainly derived from basil. The estimated dietary exposure from *methyleugenol* used as an added flavoring substance was 0.11 μg/kg body weight per day. Thus, the overall dietary exposure was estimated to be ~0.77 μg/kg body weight per day [39].

Ocimum basilicum, Genovese Gigante variety, is by far the most popular basil cultivar used in the production of the typical Italian sauce called "*Pesto.*" Pesto is traditionally prepared with basil that is 10–12 cm in height, when the percentage of *methyleugenol* in the essential oil is more that 40%. Considering that, at this stage of growth, the amount of essential oil in *Ocimum basilicum* (*Genovese Gigante*) corresponds to ~0.5% and that one portion of pesto contains ~10 g of basil, the resulting dietary exposure to *methyleugenol* could reach ~250 μg/kg body weight in adults. This *methyleugenol* intake could arise some concern about its potential carcinogenicity.

In a study [40], the basil cultivar used in the production of "*Pesto*" was found to have different aromatic composition at different growth stages. Plants from different areas of northwestern Italy were analyzed at 4 and 6 weeks after sowing and actually showed to have *methyleugenol* and *eugenol* as the main components. The content of these compounds, however, was shown to be correlated with plant height rather than plant age. In fact, the evaluation of *methyleugenol* and *eugenol* percentage in basil plants of various height, some of which were harvested at 4 weeks after sowing while others 2 weeks later, showed how different was the composition of essential oils based on the height of each plant. *Methyleugenol* was predominant in plants up to 10 cm in height, whereas *eugenol* was prevalent in taller plants. For this reason, "*Pesto*" sauce is at present prepared only with basil plants of over 10 cm height [40].

14.4.4 Antioxidant Activity

The antioxidant activity of basil extracts and essential oils has been evaluated in different cultivars of basil [41]. Five green basil cultivars and breeding lines including "Italian Large Leaf," "Sweet," "Cinnamon" (*Ocimum basilicum*), "Sweet Dani Lemon" (*O. citriodorum*), and "Holy" (*O. sanctum*), plus four purple basil cultivars, "Dark Opal," "Osmin Purple," "Purple Ruffles," and "Red Rubin" basil (*O. basilicum*) were evaluated. Basil ethanolic extracts and essential oils were tested for in vitro antioxidant activity. Total phenolics were higher in the purple basils than in the green cultivars. "Dark Opal" basil contained the highest concentration (126.2 mg phenolics/g dry weight). The green cultivars evaluated yielded significantly lower total phenols, varying from 35.6 mg in "Cinnamon" to 62.9 mg in "Italian Large Leaf." In all basils, the essential oil contribution to the total antioxidant activity was low, varying from 0.05% in "Purples Ruffles" to 5.9% in "Sweet" basil. These results suggested that the main antioxidant activity from different basil plants did not arise from their essential oils, but rather from other phenolics such as flavonoids in green basils and anthocyanins in purple basils. Given the high relative antioxidant activity of selected basils, these plants could be deemed a good source of antioxidant phenolics in the diet, providing 125 mg of gallic acid equivalents, 85–125 mg of Trolox, or 106–140 mg of ascorbic acid equivalents per gram of dry weight [41].

14.4.5 Antibacterial Activity

The basil essential oil has shown to have a powerful antibacterial activity, which has been attributed to its high content in *linalool* and *estragole*, whereas the antimicrobial spectrum is restricted to specific bacteria (*Staphylococcus* spp., *Enterococcus* spp., *E. coli*, *P. aeruginosa*, *A. baumannii*, *A. hydrophila*, *B. cereus*, *Bacillus subtilis*, *Enterobacter* spp., *Listeria* spp., *Proteus* spp., *Salmonella* spp., *Serratia marcescens*, and *Y. enterocolitica*) and fungi (*Candida* spp., *Rhodotorula* spp., and *Saccharomyces cerevisiae*) [42].

14.5 Rosemary

Rosmarinus officinalis, commonly known as rosemary, is a woody, perennial herb with fragrant, evergreen, needle-like leaves and white, pink, purple, or blue flowers, native to the Mediterranean region. It is a member of the mint family Lamiaceae, which includes many other herbs. The name "rosemary" derives from the Latin for "dew" (*ros*) and "sea" (*marinus*), or "dew of the sea."

According to myth, the Virgin Mary is said to have spread her blue cloak over a white-blossomed rosemary bush when she was resting, and the flowers turned blue. The shrub then became known as the "Rose of Mary." Rosemary was considered sacred to ancient Egyptians, Romans, and Greeks. In the Middle Ages, rosemary was associated with wedding ceremonies. The bride would wear a rosemary headpiece and the groom and wedding guests would all wear a sprig of rosemary. From this association with weddings, rosemary was thought to be a love charm.

14.5.1 Culinary Use

The leaves are used as a flavoring in foods such as stuffings and roast lamb, pork, chicken, and turkey. Fresh or dried leaves are frequently used in traditional Mediterranean cuisine. They have a bitter, astringent taste and a characteristic aroma which complements many cooked foods. When roasted with meats or vegetables, the leaves impart a mustard-like aroma with an additional fragrance of charred wood compatible with barbecued foods.

Rosemary extract has been shown to improve the shelf life and heat stability of omega 3-rich oils which are prone to rancidity

14.5.2 Chemical Components

Rosemary leaves contain certain phytochemical (plant-derived) compounds that are known to have disease preventing and health promoting properties. The herb parts, especially flower tops, include phenolic antioxidant rosmarinic acid as well as numerous health benefiting volatile essential oils such as *cineol, camphene, borneol, bornyl acetate,* and *α-pinene*. These compounds are known to have rubefacient (counterirritant), anti-inflammatory, anti-allergic, antifungal, and antiseptic properties.

The herb is exceptionally rich in many B-complex groups of vitamin, such as folic acid, pantothenic acid, pyridoxine, and riboflavin. It is one of the herbs containing high levels of folates, providing about 109 μg per 100 g (about 27% of RDA). Folates are essential to DNA synthesis and when given during the periconception period can help prevent neural tube defects in the newborns.

Rosemary herb carries also great amounts of vitamin A, 2924 IU per 100 g or about 97% of RDA. A few leaves a day in the diet would contribute enough of this vitamin. Vitamin A is known to have antioxidant properties and is essential for vision. It is also required for maintaining healthy mucosa and skin. Consumption of natural foods rich in vitamin A is known to help the body protect from lung and oral cavity cancers.

The rosemary oil, which is distilled from the flowering tops, contains volatile essential oil such as *camphene, cineol, borneol, bornyl acetate,* and other esters. These compounds are known to have tonic, astringent, diaphoretic, and stimulant properties. This oil has being used externally as a rubefacient to soothe painful ailments in gout, rheumatism, and neuralgic conditions. Rosemary herb extractions, when applied over the scalp, stimulate the hair-bulbs and help prevent premature baldness. It is said to be also an effectual remedy for the prevention of dandruff.

Rosemary Herb, Fresh Leaves

Vitamins and mineral content per 100 g

Source: USDA National nutrient Database

Energy	131 kcal
Carbohydrates	20.70 g
Protein	3.31 g
Fat	54.86 g
Fiber	14.10 g

Vitamin A	2924 IU	(97% DV)
Thiamine	0.036 mg	(3% DV)
Riboflavin	0.152 mg	(12% DV)
Niacin	0.912 mg	(6% DV)
Pantothenic acid	0.804 mg	(16% DV)
Vitamin B_6 (pyridoxine)	0.336 mg	(26% DV)
Folate	109 μg	(27% DV)
Vitamin C	21.8 mg	(36% DV)

Calcium	317 mg	(32% DV)
Iron	6.65 mg	(83% DV)
Magnesium	91 mg	(23% DV)
Manganese	0.960 mg	(42% DV)
Potassium	668 mg	(14% DV)
Sodium	26 mg	(2% DV)
Zinc	0.93 mg	(8.5% DV)

DV = Daily Value

14.5.3 Antioxidant Activity

Several studies have confirmed that leafy spices such as rosemary, sage, oregano, basil, parsley, and thyme have strong antioxidant activity [43]. Rosemary extracts contain a large number of phenolic compounds, including *carnosic acid, carnosol,* and *rosmarinic acid* [44]. It was reported that these phenolic compounds found in spice herb plants, including rosemary, are mainly responsible for the biological effects such as antioxidant potential [43]. These phenolic compounds exert their antioxidant activity through various mechanisms such as free-radical scavenging activity, transition-metal-chelating activity, and/or singlet-oxygen-quenching capacity [45]. The antioxidant activity has been demonstrated to retard or prevent lipid oxidation in a variety of foods.

In a study [46], methanol extracts from oregano and rosemary were demonstrated to retard oxidation of long-chain polyunsaturated fatty acids, docosahexaenoic acid C22:6 (DHA) and eicosapentaenoic acid C20:5 (EPA), in menhaden fish oil. The fish oils after mixing with the extracts at different concentrations were oxidized by heating at 150 °C for 30 min or incubating at 60 °C for 5 day. After heating at 150 °C, only 15.9% of DHA and 18.5% of EPA remained in the fish oil without extract, while 38.8–65.9% of DHA and 44.7–69.0% of EPA were retained in the fish oil mixed with 1–5% of oregano extract. The highest retained DHA (56.9%) and EPA (58.0%) in the fish oils mixed with rosemary extract were observed at 2.5% addition. After incubation at 60 °C for 5 day, the highest inhibition capability was also found at 2.5% of added rosemary extract, and the oil retained 88.2% DHA and 88.3% EPA. However, only 18.8% DHA and 23.6% EPA were retained in the fish oil mixed with 5% of oregano extract and no DHA and EPA were detected in the fish oil without extract after 5-day incubation at 60 °C. Thus, antioxidant activity of the rosemary extract results to be greater than that of oregano extract, but it is sensitive to heat. The rosemary extract also has shown higher DPPH free radical scavenging capability, which was approximately three times higher than oregano extract, although there was no significant difference in the total phenolic contents between both extracts.

14.5.4 Anticancer Activity

The main polyphenols found in rosemary extract (RE) include the diterpenes *carnosic acid* (CA) and *rosmarinic acid* (RA). Rosemary extract and its polyphenols CA and RA have recently been explored in vitro and found to exert potent anticancer effects [47–49]. RE, CA, and RA have been shown to have various potent and effective anticancer properties.

14.5.4.1 In Vitro Studies

Colon Cancer: Studies in vitro on colon cancer cell lines have demonstrated that RE decreases cell viability in a dose dependent way. Moreover, RE inhibits cell proliferation, induces cell cycle arrest, apoptosis, necrosis, cholesterol accumulation, and ROS accumulation [50–53].

Pancreatic Cancer: Exposure of pancreatic cancer cells PANC-1 and MIA-PaCa-2 to RE containing increasing concentrations of *carnosol* (CN) (1–3.8% *w*/*w*) and CA (10–30% *w*/*w*) resulted in significant inhibition of cell viability. The RE containing 25.66% *w*/*w* CA (sub-max) caused maximal inhibition compared to other RE's in PANC-1 cells, significantly inhibiting cell viability to approximately 60% at 40 μg/mL (48 h) [54].

Breast Cancer: Breast cancer is classified under three subtypes based on the sensitivity of the tumors to chemotherapeutic agents. The subtypes are (a) estrogen receptor positive (ER+), which express Erα and therefore respond to estrogens; (b) human epidermal growth factor receptor 2 positive (HER2+) which overexpress HER2 and can be either ER+ or ER−; and (c) triple negative (TN) which lack expression of ERα, progesterone receptor, and HER2. The effects of RE at 1–120 μg/mL (48 h) have been explored in all three breast cancer subtypes, ER+, HER2+, and TN, in vitro. RE caused dose-dependent inhibition of cell viability in all subtypes of breast cancer cells. Furthermore RE enhanced the effectiveness of the monoclonal antibody (mAb) trastuzumab and the chemotherapeutic drugs tamoxifen and paclitaxel, used in the treatment of breast cancer [55]. Taken together, these studies suggest a role for RE to inhibit pancreatic and breast cancer cell viability and proliferation, and induce apoptosis at concentrations in the 10–100 μg/mL range.

Prostate Cancer: Rosemary extract (RE) (6.25–50 μg/mL; 48 h) has shown to inhibit viability of DU145 and PC3 prostate cancer cells [56]. In agreement with these data, significant inhibition of LNCaP and 22RV1 prostate cancer cell proliferation and viability, and an induction of apoptosis has been observed with RE (50 μg/mL standardized to 40% CA; 24–48 h) [57]. RE was able to combat the enhanced prostate specific antigen (PSA) levels measured in cell culture media, indicative of prostate cancer, inhibiting levels to less than a fifth of what was seen in the control group. Correspondingly, levels of the androgen receptor, to which PSA binds, were significantly decreased by 50 μg/mL RE [57]. The inhibitory effects on both androgen sensitive and insensitive cell lines are important and suggest potential chemotherapeutic effects of RE in different prostate cancer subtypes.

Ovarian Cancer: Exposure of A2780 ovarian cancer cells to 0.08% (0.8 mg/mL; 48 h) RE containing media resulted in significant inhibition of proliferation and induction of apoptosis and cell cycle arrest. At 0.08% RE enhanced the sensitivity of A2780 and cisplatin-resistant A2780CP70 cell lines to growth inhibition by cisplatin treatment, suggesting that RE may be of use in combination with cisplatin or potentially other chemotherapeutic drugs in patients who have developed an acquired resistance [58]. Furthermore, in human ovarian cancer cells SK-OV3 and HO-8910 rosemary essential oil (0.0625%–1%) inhibited cell viability with an IC50 of 0.025% and 0.076% in each cell line, respectively [59]. This study noted that the rosemary essential oil was more potent than its individual components (*α-pinene, β-pinene, 1,8-cineole*) when tested alone at the same concentrations.

Lung Cancer: In lung cancer cells, RE has demonstrated to decrease viability of NCI-H82 small cell carcinoma cells (6.25–50 μg/mL; 48 h) [56] and decreased proliferation of A549 non-small cell carcinoma cells (2.5–200 μg/mL) [60] with an IC50 or 24.08 μg/mL and 15.9 μg/mL in each cell line, respectively.

Human Leukemia: A study examining the human leukemia HL-60 and K-562 cell lines and the murine RAW264.7, macrophage/monocyte cell line found significant inhibition of proliferation with an IC50 of 0.14% (1.4 mg/mL) and 0.25% (2.5 mg/mL) for the HL-60 and K-562 cells, respectively. In addition, 0.1% (1 mg/mL; 72 h) RE significantly increased differentiation of HL-60 cells [61]. RE inhibited viability at 50 μg/mL (48 h) in K-562 leukemia cells [56].

14.5.4.2 In Vivo Animal Studies

A limited number of studies have examined the effects of RE administration on tumor growth in animals in vivo.

Colon Cancer: Administration of RE (1 mg/mL) in the drinking water ad libitum for 32–35 days resulted in a significant decrease in tumor size in nude mice xenografted with SW620 colon cancer cells [54]. A similar study using HCT116 colon cancer xenografted athymic nude mice fed 100 mg/kg/day RE dissolved in olive oil (4 weeks) significantly decreased tumor size in treated animals compared to control [50]. Biochemical analysis of serum samples collected from Sprague Dawley rats with N-methylnitrosourea-induced colon cancer showed significant anticancer effects by both high (3333.3 mg/kg/day) and low (1666.6 mg/kg/day) dose RE after 4 months of treatment with significant alteration of gene and protein signaling and aggregation of lymphoid cells [62].

Liver Cancer: In a diethylnitrosamine (DEN)-induced liver cancer model in F344 rats, RE at 100 mg/kg/day (5 days) was administered intragastrically with an intraperitoneal (i.p.) injection of DEN on day 4. From this point, rats were fed a normal diet for 3 weeks until undergoing partial hepatectomy. Examination of liver tissue suggested RE may exert some protective antioxidant effects [63]. In accordance with this, use of Swiss mice exposed to 6 Grays (Gy) ionizing radiation (IR) in their liver once, followed by treatment with 1000 mg/kg RE fed orally daily for 5 days, suggested protective, antioxidant activity by RE. A delayed onset of IR-induced mortality and attenuated increases in glycogen and protein levels were seen in livers of mice exposed to IR and fed RE, compared to IR-exposed mice not fed RE [64]. Taken together, these studies suggest a role for RE inhibiting chemical- or IR-induced carcinogenesis, by exerting protective, antioxidant effects on healthy tissues. Thus, RE may display radioprotective effects, which would benefit healthy tissue during radiation treatment.

Myeloid Leukemia: In WEHI-3BD myeloid leukemia xenografted mice fed 1% *w/w* RE in their food ad libitum (29 days), investigators noted a significant decrease in both tumor volume and incidence. Furthermore, RE showed an additive effect when combined with vitamin D analogues (VDA) [65]. In WEHI-3BD xenografted mice administered RE (4% *w*/*w* in food) for up to 15 weeks combined with VDAs, median survival time was significantly increased and white blood cell count decreased to levels comparable to those seen in the control group of healthy mice [66].

14.5.4.3 Mechanism of Action: The Role of *carnosic* Acid and *rosmarinic* Acid

It was suggested that synergy between many components of the rosemary's extract plays a role in rosemary's anticancer effects [67]. Among different fractions of the RE, the fraction containing *carnosic acid* (CA) was found to be among the most active. Also the fraction containing *rosmarinic acid* (RE) showed an important role in anticancer activity.

The mechanisms involved in this anticancer activity are very complex. As an example, some mechanisms involved in colon cancer inhibition will be exposed.

Carnosic Acid (CA): Inhibition of cell proliferation and increased cell cycle arrest by CA in HT-29 colon cells was found to be orchestrated by the unfolded protein response and triggered by endoplasmic reticular stress which leads to apoptosis and thus destruction of cancerous cells [51]. Enhanced cholesterol and ROS accumulation in CA treated cancer cells was also shown to contribute to the inhibition of proliferation seen [51]. Similarly, activity of proapoptotic markers including p53, Bax, caspases, and PARP has be shown to be enhanced and anti-apoptotic markers MDM2, Bcl-2, and Bcl-xL to be decreased in HT-29, HCT116, and SW480 colon cells [68]. Levels of ROS and H_2O_2 are increased in vitro in the cell medium [52, 68] by CA which can trigger cellular stress and thus cancer cell death. The signaling molecules STAT3 and *survivin* have been shown to play a key role in regulating cell survival and CA inhibits activity of these molecules in colon cancer cells [68]. These studies provide strong evidence that CA at relatively low doses (1–100 μM) is capable of inhibiting colon cancer cell growth and survival by modulating expression of key signaling molecules and altering cell metabolism.

Rosmarinic Acid (RA): Treatment of HT29 colon cancer cells with RA (5–20 μM) has lead to a reduction in COX2 promoter activity and COX2 protein levels [69]. In HCT15 and CO115 colon cancer cells, RA (10–100 μM) has been demonstrated to induce apoptosis and to decrease levels of phosphorylated-ERK which regulates cell proliferation [70]. *Rosmarinic acid* (55–832.6 μM) decreases also ROS levels in association with a decreased migration and adhesion rates in Ls174-T colon cells [71]. Furthermore, treatment of CO115 cells with RA (50 μM) protects against BCNU-induced DNA damage, suggesting potential chemopreventive effects [72]. Treatment of MCF-7 and MDA-MB-231 breast cancer cells with RA (0–300 μM) has decreased cell viability [56, 73–75]. *Rosmarinic acid* has also shown to decrease methyltransferase activity, which inhibits hyper-methylation of DNA, associated with disease [74], and to sensitize a resistant cell line (MCF-7/Adr) to the chemotherapeutic agent Adriamycin [75].

14.5.4.4 Considerations on the Role of Rosemary in Anticancer Therapy

In recent years, focus has shifted towards establishing new targeted cancer treatments that can modulate specific pathways often mutated in cancer. RE and its polyphenols CA and RA may be used as chemicals to target specific pathways leading to induction of apoptosis and decreased cell survival. In addition, RE, CA, and RA may be used as neutraceuticals to enhance the anticancer effects of current chemotherapeutics. This could allow for lower doses of chemotherapeutics to be used and less toxicity induced in healthy surrounding tissue. Although studies examining signaling molecules and pathways targeted by RE, CA, and RA are limited, the existing studies provide supporting evidence for the use of these compounds both on their own and in combination with other cancer therapies. Overall, RE, CA, and RA have been shown to have various potent and effective anticancer properties.

14.6 Sage

The Sage (*Salvia officinalis*), also called common sage or culinary sage, is a perennial evergreen plant. It is a member of the mint family native of Mediterranean region, although it has naturalized in many places throughout the world. Actually, the *Salvia* genus comprises about 900 species, but *Salvia officinalis L* and *Salvia lavandulaefolia L* are probably the best known due to their long-standing reputation as traditional herbal remedies.

14.6.1 History

The sage has been used since ancient times for warding off evil, snakebites, increasing women's fertility, and more. Pliny the Elder said this plant was called *salvia* by the Romans, and used as a diuretic, a local anesthetic for the skin, a styptic, and for other uses. Charlemagne recommended the plant for cultivation in the early Middle Ages, and during the Carolingian Empire, it was cultivated in monastery gardens. The plant had a high reputation throughout the Middle Ages, with many sayings referring to its healing properties and value. It was sometimes called *S. salvatrix* (sage the savior), and was one of the ingredients of Four Thieves Vinegar, a blend of herbs which was supposed to ward off the plague. Pliny and Galen recommended sage as a diuretic, hemostatic, emmenagogue, and tonic. In past centuries it was also used for hair care, insect bites and wasp stings, nervous conditions, mental conditions, oral preparations for inflammation of the mouth, tongue and throat, and also to reduce fevers.

14.6.2 Chemical Components

Common sage is grown in parts of Europe for distillation of an essential oil. In fact, plants of the genus *Salvia* are rich in essential oils, with a large array of terpenoids including α and *β-thujone, camphor, 1,8-cineole, a-humulene, b-caryophyllene*, and *viridiflorol*. Moreover, they are rich sources of diterpenes and triterpenes such as *carnosic acid, ursolic acid, carnosol,* and *tanshinones.* Sage leaf contains *tannic acid, oleic acid, ursonic acid, ursolic acid, carnosol, carnosic acid, fumaric acid, chlorogenic acid, caffeic acid, niacin, nicotinamide, flavones, flavonoid glycosides*, and estrogenic substances.

The composition of the polyphenols and terpenoids can vary considerably across *Salvia* (S) species. For example, rosmarinic acid is high in *S. officinalis* but low in *S. hypoleuka*. Levels of thujone are also reported to be higher in *S. officinalis* compared with *S. lavandulaefolia*. Tanshinones are found in *S. miltiorrhiza*, and varying forms of *yunnaneic acids* and *salvianolic acids* differ across Salvia species.

14.6.3 Health Benefits

Salvia officinalis comes from the Latin word meaning "to heal" and is widely used in both culinary and medicinal preparations. Many species of *Salvia* are native to Mediterranean Europe and have been traditionally used for the treatment of a range of problems including digestive and circulation disturbances, bronchitis, coughs, asthma, memory problems, angina, mouth and throat inflammation, depression, and excessive sweating. *Salvia* plants are traditionally noted for their antioxidant effects and ability to enhance "head and brain" functions, improve memory, quicken the senses, and delay age-associated cognitive decline [76].

Sage Herb (*Salvia officinalis*) **Dried, Ground**
Vitamins and mineral content per 100 g
Source: USDA Database

Energy	315 kcal
Carbohydrates	60.73 g
Protein	10.63 g
Fiber	40.3 g
Fat	12.75 g

Vitamin A	5900 mg
Lutein zeaxanthin	1.895 μg
Carotene β	3.485 μg
Cryptoxanthin-β	109 μg
Thiamine	0.754 mg
Riboflavin	0.336 mg
Pyridoxine	2.690 mg
Niacin	5.720 mg
Folate	274 μg
Vitamin C	32.4 mg
Vitamin E	7.48 mg
Vitamin K	1.714 μg

Calcium	1652 mg
Copper,	0.757 mg
Iron	28.12 mg
Magnesium	428 mg
Manganese	3.133 mg
Zinc	4.70 mg

14.6.3.1 Antioxidant Effects

Salvia plants and their individual constituents possess strong antioxidant activity. In an analysis of 10 *Salvia* species, it was confirmed that all species exhibited significant antioxidant activity as measured by oxygen radical absorbance capacity, radical scavenging capacity and total phenolic content. The extent of antioxidant activity varied across species and extraction methods used, the ethanolic extract of *S. officinalis* exhibited the highest activity [77].

S. miltiorrhiza reduces the production of ROS by inhibiting oxidases, reducing the production of superoxide, inhibiting the oxidative modification of low-density lipoproteins and ameliorating mitochondrial oxidative stress. *S. miltiorrhiza* also increases the activities of catalase, manganese superoxide dismutase, glutathione peroxidase, and coupled endothelial nitric oxide synthase [78].

The majority of antioxidant effects are attributed to *Salvia* phenolic compounds such as *rosmarinic acid, salvianolic acid, sagecoumarin,* and *sagerinic acid* as they exhibit strong radical scavenging activity with approximately 90% of 2,2-diphenylpicrylhydrazyl (DPPH) scavenged under experimental conditions. Their effects are substantially greater than the sage flavonoids, *luteolin* and *apigenin* [79]. In an in vitro study, *salvianolic acid L* showed potent free radical scavenging activities for DPPH and superoxide anion radicals. It was identified as a significantly better scavenger of these free radicals than *trolox* (a water-soluble analogue of vitamin E), *caffeic acid* and *rosmarinic acid* [80]. The monoterpenes 1,8-cineole and a-pinene identified in *S. lavandulaefolia* essential oil were shown to be able to attenuate oxidative injury in astrocytes by inhibiting ROS production and increasing endogenous antioxidant compounds (e.g., glutathione, catalase, superoxide dismutase, heme oxygenase 1 activity and protein expression) [81]. *Carnosic acid* and *ursolic acid* are also powerful antioxidants [82, 83].

14.6.3.2 Anti-inflammatory Effects

Findings from in vitro and animal studies have demonstrated that *Salvia* species and their constituents have anti-inflammatory effects. An examination of the essential oils in *S. officinalis* (mainly comprising 1,8-cineole and camphor) revealed that it significantly inhibited nitric oxide production stimulated by LPS in mouse macrophages [84]. Acute inflammation induced with intraperitoneal administration of turpentine oil in mice was significantly reduced by *S. officinalis* tincture, demonstrated by reductions in total leukocyte and monocyte percentages, and the activation of circulating phagocytes [85]. Phenolic diterpenes (*carnosol and carnosic acid*) present in *S. officinalis* reduced nitric oxide and prostaglandin E2 (PGE2) production in

LPS-stimulated macrophages. They also significantly blunted gene expression levels of iNOS, cytokines/interleukins (IL-1a, IL-6) and chemokines including CCL5/RANTES and CXCL10/IP-10 [86].

A methalonic extract of *S. plebeian*, and several of its active components, significantly reduced inflammatory processes induced by the in vivo exposure of 12-O-tetradecanoylphorbol-12-acetate, and in vitro exposure to LPS-activated macrophages. *S. plebeian* decreased the release of nitric oxide, cyclooxygenase-2 (COX-2), PGE2 and the expression of iNOS [87]. Bioactive constituents contained in *S. miltiorrhiza* such as the *tanshinones* and *salvianolic acids* have also been shown to have anti-inflammatory mechanisms by influencing cytokine production and iNOS activity. They also inhibited COX-2, hypoxia-inducible factor-1a, and nuclear factor kB activity [88]. Moreover, in one study, *tanshinones* isolated from *S. miltiorrhiza* significantly inhibited the mRNA and protein expression of TNF-a, IL-1b, and IL-8 in LPS-stimulated macrophages [89]. Investigations into the constituents of *Salvia* plants have also confirmed that *caffeic acid, rosmarinic acid* [90], and *ursolic acid* [82] have strong anti-inflammatory properties.

14.6.3.3 Antidepressant and Anxiolytic Effects

Sage is known to have antidepressant and anxiolytic effects. However, these effects are more pronounced in other species, different from *S. officinalis*, particularly *S. elegans*, *S. verticillata*, *S. sclarea,* and *S. miltiorrhiza.*

The administration of hydroalcoholic extracts of *S. elegans* [91] and *S. verticillata* [92] has been shown to produce antidepressant and anxiolytic-like effects via animal models of depression and anxiety. The same has been observed following the administration of essential oils of *S. sclarea* [93, 94] and *S. miltiorrhiza* [95]. The effects of *S. sclarea* were more pronounced than those obtained from the administration of essential oils of *Anthemis nobilis* (chamomile), *Rosmarinus officinalis* (rosemary), and *Lavandula angustifolia* (lavender). The anti-stressor effect of *S. sclarea* was significantly blocked by pretreatment with dopamine receptor antagonists, indicating its influences via dopaminergic activity [94]. Several constituents from *S. officinalis* also influence benzodiazepine receptor activity, including the flavones, apigenin, hispidulin and cirsimaritin; and the diterpenes, 7-methoxyrosmanol and galdosol [96]. The phenolic acids *rosmarinic acid* and *caffeic acid* have also shown to possess antidepressant and anxiolytic-like activity. In a neuropharmacological analysis, neither of these substances affected either the uptake of monoamines to synaptosomes or mitochondrial monoamine oxidase activity in the mouse brain, suggesting that they produce their antidepressant effects via mechanisms other than the inhibition of monoamine transporters and monoamine oxidase [97, 98]. Moreover, *salvianolic acid B*, a compound from *S. miltiorrhiza* [99], and *salvinorin A* from *S. divinorum* [100] also exhibited antidepressant and anxiolytic effects in animals models.

14.6.3.4 Cognitive Effects

The *Salvia* genus comprises about 900 species, of which, *Salvia officinalis L* and *Salvia lavandulaefolia L* have a long-standing reputation as traditional herbal remedies having been used by ancient Greek and Roman, Ayurvedic, Native American and Chinese folk medicine. *Salvia officinalis L.* and *Salvia lavandulaefolia L.* have a long-standing use as traditional herbal remedies for enhancing memory and improving cognitive functions. In recent times, several studies have been done to evaluate the effects of *Salvia* plants on cognitive functions in normal individuals and in Alzheimer's disease (AD) patients.

Alzheimer's disease (AD) is a chronic progressive neurodegenerative disorder and is the most common cause for the development of progressive dementia in elderly. AD is characterized by the presence of amyloid plaques, neurofibrillary tangles and marked cholinergic degeneration clinically expressed through cognitive impairment. To explain the pathogenesis of AD, numerous processes have been involved, including free radical damage and inflammation. The *Salvia* plants have been demonstrated to have antioxidant, anti-inflammatory, anti-β-amyloid, and pro-cholinergic activities.

In a pilot, open-label study, 11 patients with probable Alzheimer's disease were administered capsules containing 50 μL of *S. lavandulaefolia* essential oil, administered 1–3 times/day over a 3-week period. There were statistically significant reductions in caregiver-rated neuropsychiatric symptoms, and improvements in attention over the 6-week period, although these findings were tempered by the open-label, no-placebo arm, and small sample size [101].

In a randomized, double-blind, placebo-controlled study, the efficacy of an ethanolic extract of *S. officinalis* was evaluated in patients with Alzheimer's disease. In this 4-month study, participants allocated to the active-drug condition (60 drops of *S. officinalis* daily) experienced significantly greater improvements in cognitive function as measured by the Alzheimer's Disease Assessment Scale, and the Clinical Dementia Rating Scale. *S. officinalis* administration was well tolerated with no differences in adverse effects across the active and placebo conditions [102].

The cognitive-enhancing effect of acute, single administration of different *Salvia* species has been investigated in six studies, five utilizing randomized, double-blind, placebo-controlled designs. In five studies, the efficacy of *Salvia* plants in healthy young adults was investigated, while one was conducted on healthy, older-age volunteers. Positive cognitive (e.g., secondary memory, attention, word recall, and speed of memory) and mood-enhancing (e.g., alertness, calmness, and contentedness) effects from the single administration of differing dosages of essential oil of *S. lavandulaefolia* in healthy adults was demonstrated [103–105]. Improvements in mood (e.g., alertness, contentedness, and calmness) and cognition were also demonstrated following the single administration of a *S. officinalis* extract to healthy young adults [106], and enhancement in memory and attention were revealed following the single administration of *S. officinalis* to healthy, older-age adults [107]. In a randomized, single-blinded design (participant-masked) positive cognitive and mood-enhancing effects from acute exposure to the aroma of *S. officinalis* and *S. lavandulaefolia* were also found [108].

However, it should be considered that herbal extracts may greatly vary in their biological actions, depending on several factors. Differences in the active constituents across each species are very likely to affect their influence on biological processes and therefore their therapeutic efficacy. Typical factors influencing the potency of herbal remedies include growing, harvesting, collection, drying, and extraction methods used. For example, an evaluation of antioxidant potential of ten *Salvia* species demonstrated that ethanol extracts possessed significantly higher antioxidant capacity and total phenolic content compared with aqueous and CO_2 extraction [77]. Ratios of amount-to-solvent, solvent temperature and duration of immersion also influence extract potency [109]. Even the season of *Salvia* plant collection is important as the highest content of rosmarinic acid in *S. officinalis* leaves was detected when collections occurred in May, July, and September [110].

14.6.3.5 Cognitive Effects: Sage Cholinergic Activity

Central cholinergic signaling has long been associated with features of memory, motivation, and mood. Acetylcholine (ACh), a neurotransmitter involved in cholinergic signaling, is believed to play an important role in several aspects of cognitive function and behavior, including attention, learning, memory, and motivation. Alterations in ACh signaling are involved in the pathophysiology of multiple neurodegenerative disorders including Alzheimer's disease [111]. Acetylcholine esterase (AChE) is an enzyme that catalyzes the breakdown of acetylcholine and there are several AChE inhibitor drugs available to increase overall ACh concentration. These drugs are based on the premise that increasing the availability of ACh at acetylcholine receptors in the brain enhances neuron-to-neuron transport and ultimately improves cognitive function [112].

In vitro and animal studies have shown that several *Salvia* species and their constituents are effective AChE inhibitors. An aqueous extract of *S. officinalis* lowered AChE activity in mice [113], and in vitro analyses revealed that ethanolic extracts of *S. officinalis* reduced AChE, with greater effects on butyrylcholinesterase [106, 107]. In mice subjected to β-amyloid (Aβ) peptide, pretreatment with *S. sahendica* significantly ameliorated reductions in AChE activity and memory performance [114]. The essential oil of *S. fruticosa* also showed inhibition of AChE [115], and similar findings were revealed from the essential oil of *S. lavandulaefolia*, although AChE inhibiting activity occurred exclusively via the monoterpenoids [103]. AChE inhibition has also been observed from the phenolic diterpenes, *7amethoxyrosmanol* and *isorosmanol*, isolated from *S. officinalis* [116]. The active constituents, *rosmarinic acid, carnosic acid,* and *qu6.1.ercetin*, found in several *Salvia* species can also inhibit AChE activity [116–118]. The tanshinones from *S. miltiorrhiza* also inhibit both AChE and butyrylcholinesterase activity [119, 120].

14.6.3.6 Cognitive Effects: Sage Effects on β-Amyloid

The accumulation of amyloid (Aβ peptide) is a characteristic of Alzheimer's disease and its deposition is considered partially responsible for the cognitive dysfunction seen in Alzheimer's disease. It is theorized that aggregated Aβ is accountable for the progressive nature of the disease, as the unregulated build-up of aggregates are neurotoxic, causing dysfunction to cholinergic neurons and calcium homeostasis, and promoting the formation of reactive oxygen species (ROS) and pro-inflammatory responses. Aβ is known to cause specific learning and memory impairment and its administration has been renowned for inducing memory loss in animal models [121].

Salvia miltiorrhiza has been shown to protect mice from Aβ-induced neurotoxicity by inhibiting increases in tumor necrosis factor-a (TNF-a), interleukin-6 (IL-6) levels, and acetylcholinesterase (AChE) activity [122]. Tanshinones from *S. miltiorrhiza* can also protect against Aβ-induced toxicity by ameliorating mRNA expression of inducible nitric oxide synthase (iNOS), matrix metalloproteinase 2, and nuclear transcription factor-j [9].

Animal studies have demonstrated that supplementation with *S. sahendica* attenuated memory deficits, modulated cAMP response element binding protein and its downstream molecules, and decreased apoptosis in Aβ-injected rats [123]. In mice exposed to an acute injection of Aβ, rosmarinic acid also prevented Aβ-induced nitration of proteins (an indirect indicator of peroxynitrite damage) in the hippocampus. Rosmarinic acid also prevented memory impairments induced by Aβ toxicity [124]. Protective effects from Aβ toxicity have also been observed following the administration of the *Salvia* constituents, *salvianolic acid* [125], *carnosic acid* [126], and *quercetin* [127].

14.6.3.7 Cognitive Effects: Sage Effects on Neurotrophins

Neurotrophins are a family of proteins that promote the survival, development, and function of neurons. They belong to a class of growth factors, secreted proteins that are capable of signaling particular cells to survive, differentiate, or grow.

Brain-derived neurotrophic factor (BDNF) is a neutrophin that has received particular attention in cognitive and neurological research due to its role in supporting the survival of existing neurons, stimulating the growth and differentiation of new neurons and synapses, and enhancing learning and memory [128]. Peripheral BDNF levels have been shown to be lower in patients with Alzheimer's disease and mild cognitive impairment [129]. In one study, the administration of *S. miltiorrhiza* to mice mitigated Aβ-induced reductions in BDNF [122].

Rosmarinic acid has been also shown to protect against memory deficits induced by cerebral artery occlusion in mice. One mechanism of the neuroprotective effects of rosmarinic acid was the increase in BDNF [130]. In rats exposed to chronic unpredictable stress, *rosmarinic acid* restored hippocampal BDNF. In vitro experiments showed that rosmarinic acid increased BDNF levels in cultured astrocytes [131].

Caffeic acid reduced immobility time of mice in the forced swim test and ameliorated stress-induced reductions in levels of BDNF mRNA in the frontal cortex. *Caffeic acid* did not modify the levels of BDNF in brain regions of naive mice, indicating that it primarily attenuates the downregulation of BDNF transcription during stressful conditions [132].

The flavonoid *luteolin* was identified to be highly active in inducing the synthesis and secretion of neurotrophic factors, including nerve growth factor, glial-derived neurotrophic factor, and BDNF in cultured astrocytes [133].

There have also been some reports that *quercetin* can increase BDNF levels in brain injury models [134]. The production of nerve growth factor, another neurotrophin important for the growth, maintenance, and survival of neurons, has also been shown to be enhanced *by carnosic acid, carnosol* [135], *tanshinones* [136], and *quercetin* [137].

14.6.3.8 Cognitive Effects: Conclusive Remarks

Salvia plants have historically been used for the treatment of several ailments, with traditional knowledge suggesting they have benefits for cognitive and neurological conditions. Findings from research confirm that many *Salvia* species and their individual active constituents influence several biological processes that may impact on neurological and cognitive function. In vitro, animal and preliminary human studies have supported the evidence of *Salvia* plants to enhance cognitive skills and guard against neurodegenerative disorders. At present, the majority of human studies have used *S. officinalis* and *S. lavandulaefolia* species, so the efficacy of other *Salvia* species is uncertain. Moreover, the extracts used have varied considerably across studies. Ethanolic, methanolic, and aqueous extracts have been used, along with the essential oils of *S. officinalis* and *S. lavandulaefolia*. The potency and pharmacodynamic effects of these different extracts are likely to vary considerably, potentially impacting on their therapeutic efficacy. It is important that standardized, replicable extracts be developed that include some measure of potency and purity.

14.6.3.9 Sage Anticancer Activity

Biological in vitro studies have shown that the essential oils of *Salvia* species have potential anticancer activity.

S. officinalis oil was able to inhibit the growth of renal cell adenocarcinoma with IC50 of 100.70 μg/mL. The oil was unable to react with human breast cancer cell (MCF-7) and hormone dependent prostate carcinoma cell (LNCaP) [138]. Additionally, the cytotoxicity of the essential oil on the squamous human cell carcinoma cell line of the oral cavity (UMSCC1) was also assessed with the XTT assay. It revealed that low concentrations of the essential oil increased vitality of the UMSCC1 cells. Beyond the concentration of the IC50 of 135 μg/mL, *S. officinalis* oil reduced UMSSC1 cells viability to a minimum [139].

The combination of the three bioactive compounds of *S. libanotica* essential oil, Linalyl acetate, Terpeniol, and Camphor was shown to cause significant growth suppression of HCT116 p53+/+ cells in PreG1 (64% at 48 h). In p53-/- cells, Linalyl acetate, Terpeniol and Camphor caused cell accumulation in PreG1 and G2/M phases. In response to the three components, 58% apoptosis occurred in p53+/+ cells and 38% in p53-/- cells [140].

The antiproliferative activity of *Salvia* oils on human cancer cell lines was also investigated. *S. leriifolia* exhibited a strong inhibitory activity on renal adenocarcinoma ACHN, large cell carcinoma COR-L23, amelanotic melanoma C32, and malignant melanoma A375 with IC50 values of 6.8, 7.5, 9.1, and 12.5 μg/mL, respectively. *S. acetabulosa* inhibited the viability of C32 and COR-L23 cell lines with IC50 values of 6.3 and 6.5 μg/mL. However, both *S. acetabulosa* and *S. leriifolia* couldn't exert antiproliferative activity against human skin fibroblast 142BR [141].

14.7 *"Allium"* Species: Onion and Garlic

Allium is a genus of flowering plants that includes hundreds of species, including the cultivated onion, garlic, scallion, and shallot. The generic name *Allium* is the Latin word for garlic, and the type species for the genus is *Allium sativum* which means "cultivated garlic."

Onion and garlic were not to be included in this chapter dedicated to the "Herbs," but they represent two basic ingredients to which many flavors and scents of Mediterranean diet are due. Moreover, they contribute their flavor to savory dishes without raising caloric content appreciably. For this reason we have included onion and garlic in this chapter.

14.7.1 Onion

The onion (*Allium cepa* L., from Latin *cepa* "onion"), also known as the bulb onion or common onion, is a vegetable and is the most widely cultivated species of the genus *Allium*. Its close relatives include the garlic, shallot, leek, and chive.

14.7.1.1 History

The onion plant has been grown and selectively bred in cultivation for at least 7000 years. Food uses of onions date back thousands of years in China, Egypt, and Persia. According to archaeologists, botanists, and food historians, onion probably originated in central Asia or Persia.

Traces of onions recovered from Bronze Age settlements in China suggest that onions were used as far back as 5000 BCE, not only for their flavor, but the bulb's durability to store and transport. Ancient Egyptians revered the onion bulb, viewing its spherical shape and concentric rings as symbols of eternal life. The Judeo-Christian Bible refers to the ancient Israelites consuming onions in Numbers 11:5 in a story of their Exodus: "*We remember the fish, which we did eat in Egypt freely, the cucumbers and the melons and the leeks and the onions and the garlic*." Dioscorides, a Greek physician of first century A.D., documented the medicinal uses of onions. Eating onions was a tradition to fortify athletes before the Olympic Games. Athletes consumed huge quantities of them, drink onion juice, and rubbed onions on their bodies.

Pliny the Elder wrote about the use of onions and cabbage in Pompeii. He documented Roman beliefs about the onion's ability to improve vision ailments, aid in sleep, and heal everything from mouth sores and toothaches, to dog bites, lumbago and even dysentery. Archeologists unearthing Pompeii long after it was buried in a volcanic explosion found gardens of Pliny's detailed narratives, where onions had grown. Apicius, the Roman gourmet and one of the first authors of a cookbook, used onions in many of his recipes.

Onions were taken by the first European settlers to North America, where the Native Americans were already eating wild onions raw or cooked in various foods. According to diaries kept by the colonists, bulb onions were one of the first crops planted by the Pilgrim fathers.

14.7.1.2 Nutrients and Chemical Components

Onions contain phytochemical compounds such as phenolics that are under basic research to determine their possible properties in humans. Considerable differences exist between onion varieties in polyphenol content, with shallots having the highest level, six times the amount found in Vidalia onions, the variety with the smallest amount. Yellow onions have the highest total flavonoid content, an amount 11 times higher than in white onions. Red onions have considerable content of anthocyanin pigments, with at least 25 different compounds identified representing 10% of total flavonoid content.

Raw Onion Bulbs

Vitamins and mineral content per 100 g
Source: USDA National nutrient Database

Energy	166 kJ (40 kcal)
Carbohydrates	9.34 g
Sugars	4.24 g
Protein	1.1 g
Fat	0.1 g
Fiber	1.7 g

Thiamine	0.046 mg	(4% DV)
Riboflavin	0.027 mg	(2% DV)
Niacin	0.116 mg	(1% DV)
Pantothenic acid	0.123 mg	(2% DV)
Vitamin B_6 (pyridoxine)	0.12 mg	(9% DV)
Folate	19 μg	(5% DV)
Vitamin C	7.4 mg	(9% DV)

Calcium	23 mg	(2% DV)
Iron	0.21 mg	(2% DV)
Magnesium	10 mg	(3% DV)
Manganese	0.129 mg	(6% DV)
Potassium	146 mg	(3% DV)
Fluoride	1.1 μg	(2% DV)
Zinc	0.17 mg	(2% DV)

DV = Daily Value

14.7.1.3 Eye Irritation

Freshly cut onions often cause a stinging sensation in the eyes of people nearby, and often uncontrollable tears. This is caused by the release of a volatile gas, *syn-propanethial-S-oxide*, which stimulates nerves in the eye creating a stinging sensation. This gas is produced by a chain of reactions which serve as a defense mechanism: chopping an onion causes damage to cells which releases enzymes called alliinases. These break down amino acid sulfoxides and generate sulfenic acids. A specific sulfenic acid, 1-propenesulfenic acid, is rapidly acted on by a second enzyme, the lacrimatory factor synthase, producing the syn-propanethial-S-oxide. This gas diffuses through the air and soon reaches the eyes, where it activates sensory neurons. Lacrimal glands produce tears to dilute and flush out the irritant.

Eye irritation can be avoided by cutting onions under running water or submerged in a basin of water. Leaving the root end intact also reduces irritation as the onion base has a higher concentration of sulfur compounds than the rest of the bulb. Refrigerating the onions before use reduces the enzyme reaction rate.

14.7.2 Garlic

Garlic (*Allium Sativum*) is a species in the onion genus "*Allium.*" Onion, shallot, leek, and Chinese onion are close relatives of garlic.

14.7.2.1 History

Garlic is believed to be originating in the mountainous Central Asia region and northeastern Iran, from where it spread all over the temperate and subtropical regions the world. It was known to Ancient Egyptians, and has been used both as a food flavoring and as a traditional medicine. It was consumed by ancient Greek and Roman soldiers, sailors, and rural classes and, according to Pliny the Elder, by the African peasantry. Galen eulogized it as the "rustic's theriac" (cure-all). Garlic was placed by the ancient Greeks on the piles of stones at crossroads, as a supper for Hecate. According to Pliny, garlic and onions were invoked as deities by the Egyptians at the taking of oaths. Pliny, in his *Natural History*, gives a list of scenarios in which garlic was considered beneficial. In the seventeenth century Dr. Thomas Sydenham valued it as an application in confluent smallpox.

Garlic was rare in traditional English cuisine (though it is said to have been grown in England before 1548) and has been a much more common ingredient in Mediterranean Europe. When the English came to America, they brought their anti-garlic attitude with them, and it took almost 300 years—likely because of continuing puritanism influence—for this viewpoint to diminish, though garlic was used as a folk medicine.

14.7.2.2 Nutrients and Chemical Components

In the typical serving size of 1–3 cloves (3–9 g), garlic provides no significant nutritional value, with the content of all essential nutrients below 10% of the Daily Value (DV). When expressed per 100 g, garlic contains several nutrients in rich amounts (20% or more of the DV), including vitamins B6 and C, and the dietary minerals, manganese and phosphorus. Per 100 g serving, garlic is also a moderate source (10–19% DV) of certain B vitamins, including thiamin and pantothenic acid, as well as the dietary minerals, calcium, iron, and zinc (see table "**Garlic, Raw**"). The composition of raw garlic is 59% water, 33% carbohydrates, 6% protein, 2% dietary fiber, and less than 1% fat.

Garlic, Raw

Vitamins and mineral content per 100 g

Source: USDA National nutrient Database

Energy	623 kJ (149 kcal)
Carbohydrates	33.06 g
Sugars	1 g
Protein	6.36 g
Fat	0.5 g
Fiber	2.1 g

Thiamine	0.2 mg	(17% DV)
Riboflavin	0.11 mg	(9% DV)
Niacin	0.7 mg	(5% DV)
Pantothenic acid	0.596 mg	(12% DV)
Vitamin B_6 (pyridoxine)	1.235 mg	(95% DV)
Folate	3 μg	(1% DV)
Vitamin C	31.2 mg	(38% DV)

Calcium	181 mg	(18% DV)
Iron	1.7 mg	(13% DV)
Magnesium	25 mg	(7% DV)
Manganese	1.672 mg	(80% DV)
Potassium	401 mg	(9% DV)
Fluoride	1.1 μg	(2% DV)
Selenium	14.2 μg	

DV = Daily Value

14.7.3 Health Effects of *"Allium"* Species

Onion (*Allium cepa* L.) and garlic (*Allium sativum* L) belong to the genus *Allium*. The National Cancer Institute ranked garlic at the top of the list of designer foods showing anticancer effects [142].

Generally, the biological activities of onion and garlic can be classified into two categories: cardiovascular disease prevention and cancer prevention. Activities in the former category include the inhibition of cholesterol synthesis, platelet aggregation, and arterial smooth muscle cell proliferation as well as anti-inflammatory, antioxidant, and hydrogen sulfide-mediated vasodilatory effects. The activities in the latter category include the effects on carcinogen metabolism (i.e., enhanced cellular glutathione synthesis that induces cell cycle arrest and apoptosis) and prevention of *Helicobacter pylori* infection, gastric cancer, and colorectal cancer [143–147]. However, an effective chronic disease prevention activity has been also described for numerous components of *Allium* species.

14.7.3.1 Onion (*Allium cepa*)

Constituents: The main chemical components of onion are: quercetin, fructose, quercetin-3-glucoside, isorhamnetin-4-glucoside, xylose, galactose, glucose, mannose, organosulfur compounds, allylsulfides, flavonoids, flavenols, S-alk(en)yl cysteine sulfoxides, cycloalliin, selenium, thiosulfinates, and sulfur and seleno compounds [148].

Antibiotic Effect: *Allium* plants, including Onion have been shown to exert antibiotic activity against Gram-positive and Gram-negative bacteria [149].

Anticancer Effect: Numerous in vitro, animal, and epidemiological studies indicate that onion or onion extract prevents cancer including gastrointestinal cancer, ovarian cancer, and skin cancer [150, 151]. The most common current theory is that the metabolites of organosulfur compounds, specifically S-alk(en)yl cysteine sulfoxide, found in these plants inhibit mutagenesis, induce phase II detoxification enzymes, influence cell arrest and apoptosis, scavenge free radicals, and inhibit DNA adduct formation [144, 150–152].

Antidiabetic Effect: Onion has been suggested to have antidiabetic activity. In a crossover comparative study [153] conducted in 20 cooperative diabetic outpatients the effects of a diet including onions or green beans on diabetic symptoms (hypercholesterolemia, serum glucose levels) was assessed. Ten of the patients consumed a specific diet (68% cal carbohydrate, 20% cal fat, 12% cal protein) plus 3 × 20 g fresh onion daily, or plus 3 × 200 g green beans daily in the first week, and the diet alone in the second week; the other half was assigned the other way around. The onion group had a significant decrease in blood sugar level (4.37 mg%, $p < 0.05$), but no blood lipid levels-changes occurred in these diets [153]. The effect of an aqueous extract of onion was studied on fasting blood sugar and experimentally induced hyperglycemia in man [154]. Graded doses of aqueous extract of onion used in the study, had no effect on fasting blood sugar levels, but reduced the rise in blood sugar in a dose-dependent manner, when administered along with glucose during oral glucose tolerance test. This effect was comparable to tolbutamide. The blood sugar lowering effect of raw and boiled onion extract was observed to be similar. Onion extract was also found to produce a reduction in blood sugar during intravenous glucose tolerance test and adrenaline induced hyperglycemia [154].

Anti-hypercholesterolemic Effect: Onion can help to prevent the rise of serum cholesterol. In a clinical study of alimentary hyperlipidemia, onion and onion essential oil prevented fat-induced increases in serum cholesterol and plasma fibrinogen and decreases in coagulation time and fibrinolytic activity [155]. The main active constituents were sulfur-containing compounds, mainly allyl propyl disulfide and diallyl disulfide.

Antihypertensive Effects: Antihypertensive effects of onion has been described. Twenty-four patients with arterial hypertension (WHO class I) received either four capsules of an onion-olive oil maceration product, essential ingredients of the Mediterranean diet, or placebo daily over a period of 1 week. The onion-olive oil maceration product led to a significant decrease in systolic blood pressure. There was also a trend towards a decrease in diastolic blood pressure. An improved blood fluidity resulting from a decrease in hematocrit was also described. All effects were observed immediately and after 1 week's administration [156].

Antithrombotic Effect: In pharmacologic and in vitro studies, onion and onion extract, alone and in combination with other products, have shown antithrombotic effects including inhibited platelet aggregation, reduced plasma viscosity, decreased hematocrit, and increased fibrinolytic activity [157–159]. In alimentary hyperlipidemia, onion also had a protective effect against increased plasma fibrinogen and it decreased coagulation time and fibrinolytic activity [155]. Onion's quercetin content is often hypothesized to stimulate these effects.

Anti-osteoclastic Effect: In animal studies, ingestion of onions has shown to inhibit bone resorption [160–162].

14.7.3.2 Garlic (*Allium sativum*)

Since time immemorial, garlic has been recognized as a prized herb in almost all the cultures for its medicinal properties as well as culinary uses. This herbal plant, grown for its underground root or bulb, contains numerous health promoting phytonutrients that has proven benefits against coronary artery diseases, infections, and cancers.

Garlic cloves contain many phytonutrients, minerals, vitamins, and antioxidants that have proven health benefits. Total measured antioxidant strength (ORAC value) is 5346 μmol TE/100 g.

The garlic bulbs contain important organic thiosulfinate compounds such as *diallyl disulfide, diallyl trisulfide,* and *allyl propyl disulfide*. Upon disruption of the bulb (while crushing, cutting, etc.), these compounds convert into allicin through an enzymatic reaction. Allicin, is responsible for the typical smell and taste of freshly cut or crushed garlic.

The garlic thiosulfinate compounds, particularly allicin, have been demonstrated to have numerous beneficial health effects. It clearly appears that these effects are very important in the context of Mediterranean diet, because they in part explain the positive health impact of this diet, in which numerous compounds synergize in a effective prevention of numerous acute and chronic disease.

Antimicrobial Activity: Reports about the targeted use of garlic as an antimicrobial agent go back to Louis Pasteur; in World War I, extracts of garlic were used in antibacterial and antiseptic therapeutics. Numerous scientific studies concerning the antibacterial potential of garlic have been published.

Allicin has been demonstrated to be the almost exclusively responsible for the antimicrobial activity of freshly crushed garlic. Allicin was shown to exert antibacterial, antibiotic-like activity against *Streptococcus* [161], *Staphylococcus aureus* [163], *Salmonella typhimurium* [164, 165]), *Escherichia coli* [166], *Pseudomonas syringae* [166], and *Vibrio cholera* [164]. As far as the mechanism of antibacterial action of allicin is concerned, it has been demonstrated that allicin, analogously to antibiotics, readily diffuses across the bacterial membrane, and once inside the bacteria it reacts with cysteine, as long as the –SH-group is freely available [167, 168].

Antifungal Activity: Beyond its well documented strong antibacterial properties allicin also shows toxic effects towards fungal cells and is able to inhibit spore germination and hyphal growth in vivo and in vitro [166]. Some efforts have been made to utilize this activity and develop allicin for application in medical therapy and agricultural plant protection.

It was claimed that allicin might be the basis of a strategy to treat aspergillosis in the lung, since allicin is highly volatile and thus can be delivered to the lung by inspiration [169]. It was also suggested that allicin can easily be applied topically to fungal infections of the skin and hence attempts were made to use allicin in the therapy of *Candida*-infections. Interestingly, allicin's activity was comparable to the frequently used antimycotic agent fluconazole [170]. There is an emerging interest in understanding the molecular basis of allicin's fungicidal properties.

Antioxidant Activity: Although allicin is chemically an oxidant, it acts in lower doses as *antioxidant* at the physiological level [171]. This observation is explained by the fact that mild oxidative conditions induce the expression of so-called phase II detoxifying enzymes, for instance by the activation of redox-sensitive transcription factors and build up protection against further and stronger oxidative insults. One example for the oxidation of a redox-sensitive transcription factor by allicin is the Nrf2/Keap1 system that regulates the expression of various anti-oxidative enzymes (among others of glutathione-biosynthesis). The fact that allicin can induce the Nrf2/Keap1 system has been shown in various studies [172, 173]. It is worth mentioning that the activation of Nrf2 by allicin is not only important in the context of cardiovascular diseases, but also for various other health-related events like neurodegenerative diseases. In that context it was shown that allicin attenuates age-related cognitive and memory deficits by activating the Nrf2-system [173].

Hypocholesterolemic Effect: Allicin has been shown to reduce serum cholesterol levels by reducing its synthesis. Different from statins that competitively inhibit the enzyme 3-hydroxy-3-methylglutaryl-coenzyme-A-reductase (HMG-CoA reductase), allicin suppresses cholesterol biosynthesis through inhibition of the squalene-monooxygenase and acetyl-CoA synthetase enzymes [167, 174, 175].

Antiplatelet Aggregation Activity: Platelet aggregation is a complex biochemical process. Its prerequisite is the activation of the GPIIb/IIIa receptor by thromboxane A2 which causes the binding, among others, of fibrinogen [176]. Classical platelet-aggregation-inhibitors like acetyl-salicylic acid (aspirin) inhibits endogenous thromboxane-biosynthesis and thus the GPIIb/IIIa receptor activation. Thiosulfinates like allicin are also potent platelet-aggregation inhibitors. While a final concentration of 0.4 mM allicin inhibits platelet aggregation to about 90%, a comparable concentration of 0.36 mM aspirin shows less than half this activity (~35% inhibition) [177].

Antihypertensive Activity: The antihypertensive effect of allicin is due to its reactivity. Since allicin decomposes rapidly to its degradation products, it has been shown that a complex reaction cascade with thiols (glutathione in particular) results in the release of hydrogen sulfide (H_2S) [178]. H_2S is a well known potent gaseous signaling molecule in regard to blood-pressure regulation [179]. H_2S lowers the blood pressure by relaxation of vessel smooth-muscle cells resulting in a lowering of blood pressure [178].

Immuno-modulatory Activity: Allicin stimulates lymphocytes by affecting $p21^{ras}$. Thioallylation, i.e., the binding of an allyl sulfenic acid to the thiol of cysteine^{118}, leads to an activation of $p21^{ras}$ and subsequently to stimulation of ERK1/2 phosphorylation [180, 181]. These processes are crucial for the activation of lymphocytes. Allicin, moreover, affects also the activity of the cytokine TNFα, through its action on macrophages that secrete TNFα. This effect inhibits the release of TNFα-dependent pro-inflammatory cytokines in intestinal epithelia [182]. Allicin also inhibits phosphatase-activity, so enhancing the phosphorylation of ERK1/2 [182], a central component of the signaling cascade that transfers extracellular signals into intracellular signaling cascades. Furthermore, allicin reduces the NO synthesis through inhibition of inducible nitric oxide synthase (iNOS) in LPS-stimulated macrophages [183, 184].

Anticancer Activity: In early studies in 1960, explants of mouse-tumors were incubated in allicin before implantation into healthy mice. In contrast to the control group (where the explants were not allicin-treated), mice with tumor explants incubated in allicin showed no further growth of the explant [185]. When the mechanisms were studied at molecular level, it became clear that the induction of apoptosis was crucial for the anticancer effect of allicin. Allicin also causes a redox-shift in human cell cultures [186]. This leads to the execution of cell death, both in a caspase-dependent [187] and caspase-independent manner [104]. Beside caspase activity, the apoptosis inducing factor (AIF), which contributes to the apoptotic DNA-laddering, is involved in allicin-induced cell death [188]. It was also shown that inNrf2 is involved in allicin-induced apoptosis [189, 190]. It should be noted that Nrf2 is generally described as an antiapoptotic factor regulating the expression of antiapoptotic proteins of the Bcl-2 family like Bcl-2 and Bcl-xL [191, 192]; however, under certain circumstances Nrf2 seems to have also a proapoptotic function [191, 192]. Also the ERK1/2 map kinases were shown to be influenced by allicin in immune cells; these kinases are also important for apoptosis induction by allicin [186–193].

The effects of allicin described above make allicin an attracting molecule for clinical use. However, its chemical instability has hampered its clinical application. Anyway, the potential for using garlic in a *nutriceutical* context, with health benefits not only for cancer prevention or therapy, but also for the other medical areas mentioned here, makes this molecule very attractive.

14.7.4 Conclusive Remarks

The many spice and herbs of the typical Mediterranean cuisine appear to give to this diet not only taste and smells but also a number of health protective effects, which derive from the rich set of their active components. It becomes clear that the health beneficial impact of Mediterranean diet is not the result of a single component but of a synergistic effect of its many extraordinary ingredients, from fresh vegetables (particularly cruciferous) to legumes and pulses, cereals, fish, fresh fruit, and on top, the extra virgin olive oil. All these components represent a rich source of active principles, from antioxidants to fibers, carbohydrates, mono- and polyunsaturated fatty acids and a rich set of vitamins. Spice and herbs complete this frame, adding to an extraordinary taste a potent antioxidant, anti-inflammatory, antidiabetic and anticancer activity.

References

1. Bhagwat S, Haytowits DB, Holden JM. USDA Database for the flavonoid content of selected foods. Nutrient Data Laboratory, Beltsville Human Nutrition Research Center Agricultural Research Service U.S. Departm Agricul. 2011:1–159.
2. Zhang H, Chen F, Wang X, Yao HY. Evaluation of antioxidant activity of parsley (Petroselinum crispum) essential oil and identification of its antioxidant constituents. Food Res Int. 2006;39:833–9.
3. Wagner H, Bladt S. Plant drug analysis. Berlin, Heidelberg: Springer; 1996. p. 154–75.
4. Wong PYY, Kitts DD. Studies on the dual antioxidant and antibacterial properties of parsley (Petroselinum crispum) and cilantro (Coriandrum sativum) extracts. Food Chem. 2006;97(3):505–15.
5. Popović M, Kaurinović B, Jakovljević V, Mimica-Dukic N, Bursać M. Effect of parsley (Petroselinum crispum (Mill.) Nym. ex A.W. Hill. Apiaceae) extracts on some biochemical parameters of oxidative stress in mice treated with CCl(4). Phytother Res. 2007;21:717–23.
6. Fejes SZ, Blázovics A, Lemberkovics E, Petri G, Szőke E, Kéry A. Free radical scavenging and membrane protective effects of methanol extracts from Anthriscus cerefolium L. (Hoffm.) and Petroselinum crispum (Mill.) nym. ex A.W. Hill. Phytother Res. 2000;14:362–5.
7. Vora SR, Patil RB, Pillai MM. Protective effects of Petroselinum crispum (Mill) Nyman ex A. W. Hill leaf extract on D-galactose-induced oxidative stress in mouse brain. Indian J Exp Biol. 2009;47:338–42.
8. Tang EL, Rajarajeswaran J, Fung S, Kanthimathi MS. Petroselinum crispum has antioxidant properties, protects against DNA damage and inhibits proliferation and migration of cancer cells. J Sci Food Agric. 2015;95:2763–71.
9. Jiang P, Li C, Xiang Z, Jiao B. Tanshinone IIA reduces the risk of Alzheimer's disease by inhibiting iNOS, MMP2 and NFkappaB p65 transcription and translation in the temporal lobes of rat models of Alzheimer's disease. Mol Med Rep. 2014;10:689–94.
10. Nielsen SE, Young JF, Daneshvar B, Lauridsen ST, Knuthsen P, Sandström B, Dragsted LO. Effect of parsley (Petroselinum crispum) intake on urinary apigenin excretion, blood antioxidant enzymes and biomarkers for oxidative stress in human subjects. Br J Nutr. 1999;81:447–55.
11. Bolkent S, Yanardag R, Ozsoy-Sacan O, Döger MM. Effects of parsley (Petroselinum crispum) on the liver of diabetic rats: a morphological and biochemical study. Phytother Res. 2004;18:996–9.
12. Ozsoy-Sacan O, Yanardag R, Orak H, Ozgey Y, Yarat A, Tunali T. Effects of parsley (Petroselinum crispum) extract versus glibornuride on the liver of streptozotocin-induced diabetic rats. J Ethnopharmacol. 2006;104:175–81.
13. Yanardağ R, Bolkent S, Tabakoğlu-Oğuz A, et al. Effects of Petroselinum crispum extract on pancreatic B cells and blood glucose of streptozotocin-induced diabetic rats. Biol Pharm Bull. 2003;26(8):1206–10.
14. Sener G, Saçan O, Yanardak R, Dülger GA. Effects of parsley (petroselinum crispum) on the aorta and heart of stz induced diabetic rats. Plant Food Hum Nutr. 2003;58:1–7.
15. Behtash N, Kargarzadeh F, Shafaroudi H. Analgesic effects of seed extract from Petroselinum crispum (Tagetes minuta) in animal models. Toxicol Lett. 2008;180(Suppl 5):S127–8.
16. Moazedi AA, Mirzaie DN, Seyyednejad SM, et al. Spasmolytic effect of Petroselinum crispum (Parsley) on rat's ileum at different calcium chloride concentrations. Pak J Biol Sci. 2007;10:4036–42.
17. Branković S, Kitić D, Radenković M, Ivetić V, Veljković S, Nesić M. Relaxant activity of aqueous and ethanol extracts of parsley (Petroselinum crispum (Mill) Nym. ex A. W Hill, Apiaceae) on isolated ileum of rat. Med Pregl. 2010;63:475–8.
18. Kreydiyyeh SI, Usta J, Kaouk I, Al-Sadi R. The mechanism underlying the laxative properties of parsley extract. Phytomedicine. 2001;8:382–8.

19. Yoshikawa M, Uemura T, Shimoda H, Kishi A, Kawahara Y, Matsuda H. Medicinal foodstuffs. XVIII. Phytoestrogens from the aerial part of Petroselinum crispum MIll. (Parsley) and structures of 6″-acetylapiin and a new monoterpene glycoside, petroside. Chem Pharm Bull. 2000;48(7):1039–44.
20. Brankovic S, Djosev S, Kitic D, Radenkovic M, Veljkovic S, Nesic M, Pavlovic D. Hypotensive and negative chronotropic and inotropic effects of the aqueous and ethanol extract from parsley leaves. J Clin Lipidol. 2008;2(Suppl 1):S191, S408.
21. Gadi D, Bnouham M, Aziz M, Ziyyat A, Legssyer A, Legrand C, Lafeve FF, Mekhfi H. Parsley extract inhibits in vitro and ex vivo platelet aggregation and prolongs bleeding time in rats. J Ethnopharmacol. 2009;125(1):170–4.
22. Gadi D, Bnouham M, Aziz M, Ziyyat A, Legssyer A, Bruel A, Berrabah M, Legrand C, Fauvel-Lafeve F, Mekhfi H. Flavonoids purified from parsley inhibit human blood platelet aggregation and adhesion to collagen under flow. J Complement Integr Med. 2012;9(1):19.
23. Aljanaby AAJJ. Antibacterial activity of an aqueous extract of Petroselinum crispum leaves against pathogenic bacteria isolated from patients with burns infections in Al-najaf Governorate, Iraq. Res Chem Intermed. 2013;39:3709–14.
24. Kim OM, Kim MK, Lee SO, Lee KR, Kim SD. Antimicrobial effect of ethanol extracts from spices against lactobacillus plantarum and Leuconostoc mesenteroides isolated from kimchi. Journal of the Korean Society of Food Science and. Nutrition. 1998;27:455–60.
25. Manderfield MM, Schafer HW, Davidson PM, Zottola EA. Isolation and identification of antimicrobial furocoumarins from parsley. J Food Prot. 1997;60:72–7.
26. Ganay SA. Plant-derived flavone Apigenin: the small-molecule with promising activity against therapeutically resistant prostate cancer. Biomed Pharmacother. 2017;85:47–56.
27. Dambolena JS, Zunino MP, Lucini EI, Olmedo R, Banchio E, Bima PJ, Zygadlo JA. Total phenolic content, radical scavenging properties, and essential oil composition of Origanum species from different populations. J Agric Food Chem. 2010;58:1115–20.
28. Mossa AT, Nawwar GA. Free radical scavenging and antiacetylcholinesterase activities of Origanum Majorana L. essential oil. Hum Exp Toxicol. 2011;30:1501–13.
29. Al-Howiriny T, Alsheikh A, Alqasoumi S, Al-Yahya M, El Tahir K, Rafatullah S. Protective effect of Origanum Majorana L. 'marjoram' on various models of gastric mucosal injury in rats. Am J Chin Med. 2009;37:531–45.
30. Perez Gutierrez RM. Inhibition of advanced glycation endproduct formation by Origanum Majorana L. in vitro and in streptozotocin-induced diabetic rats. Evid Based Complement Alternat Med. 2012;2012:598638.
31. Abdel-Massih RM, Fares R, Bazzi S, El-Chami N, Baydoun E, et al. The apoptotic and antiproliferative activity of Origanum Majorana extracts on human leukemic cell line. Leuk Res. 2010;34:1052–6.
32. Fathy SA, Emam MA, Abo Agwa SH, Abu Zahra FA, Youssef FS, Sami RM. The antiproliferative effect of Origanum Majorana on human hepatocarcinoma cell line: suppression of NF-κB. Cell Mol Biol. 2016;62(10):80–4.
33. Al Dhaheri Y, Eid A, AbuQamar S, Attoub S, Khasawneh M, Aiche G, Hisaindee S, Iratni R. Mitotic arrest and apoptosis in breast cancer cells induced by Origanum Majorana extract: upregulation of TNF-α and downregulation of survivin and mutant p53. PLoS One. 2013;8(2):e56649.
34. Zheljazkov VD, Callahan A, Cantrell CL. Yield and oil composition of 38 basil (Ocimum basilicum L.) accessions grown in Mississippi. J Agric Food Chem. 2008;56:241–5.
35. Lee SJ, Umano K, Shibamoto T, Lee KG. Identification of volatile components inbasil (Ocimum basilicum L.) and thyme leaves (Thymus vulgaris L), and their antioxidant properties. Food Chem. 2005;91:131–7.
36. Daneshian A, Gurbuz B, Cosge B, Ipek A. Chemical components od essential ols from basil (*Ocimum basilicum* L.) grown at different nitrogen levels. ResearchGate, January 2009.
37. Johnson JD, Ryan MJ, Toft JD II, Graves SW, Hejtmancik MR, Cunningham ML, Herbert R, Abdo KM. Two-year toxicity and carcinogenicity study of methyleugenol in F344/N rats and B6C3F(1) mice. J Agric Food Chem. 2000;48:3620–32.

38. Zhou GD, Moorthy B, Bi J, Donnelly KC, Randerath K. DNA adducts from alkoxyallylbenzene herb and spice constituents in cultured human (HepG2) cells. Environ Mol Mutagen. 2007;48:715–21.
39. Smith SB, Adams TB, Doull J, Feron VJ, Goodman JI, Marnett LJ, Portoghese PS, Waddell WJ, Wagner BM, Rogers AE, Caldwell J, Sipes IG. Safety assessment of allylalkoxybenzene derivatives used as flavouring substances – methyl eugenol and estragole. Food Chem Toxicol. 2002;40:851–70.
40. Miele M, Dondero R, Ciarallo G, Mazzei M. Methyleugenol in Ocimum basilicum L. Cv. genovese gigante. J Agric Food Sci. 2001;49:517–21.
41. Juliani HR, Simon JE. Antioxidant activity of basil. In: Janick J, Whipkey A, editors. Trends in new crops and new uses. Alexandria, VA: ASHS Press; 2002. p. 575–9.
42. Sakkas H, Papadopoulou C. Antimicrobial activity of basil, oregano, and thyme essential oils. J Microbiol Biothecnol. 2017;27:439–8.
43. Kähkönen MP, Hopia AI, Vuorela HJ, Rauha JP, Pihlaja K, Kujala TS, Heinonen M. Antioxidant activity of plant extracts containing phenolic compounds. J Agric Food Chem. 1999;47:3954–62.
44. Frankel EN, Huang S-W, Prior E, Aeschbach R. Evaluation of antioxidant activity of rosemary extracts, carnosol and carnosic acid in bulk vegetable oils and fish oil and their emulsion. Sci Food Agricol. 1996;72:201–8.
45. Shan B, Cai YZ, Sun M, Corke H. Antioxidant capacity of 26 spice extracts and characterization of their phenolic constituents. J Agric Food Chem. 2005;53:7749–77759.
46. Bhale SD, Xu Z, Prinyawiwatkul W, King JM, Godber JS. Oregano and rosemary extracts inhibit oxidation of long-chain n-3 fatty acids in menhaden oil. J Food Sci. 2007;72:C504–8.
47. González-Vallinas M, Reglero G, Ramírez de Molina A. Rosemary (Rosmarinus officinalis L.) extract as a potential complementary agent in anticancer therapy. Nutr Cancer. 2015;67:1221–9.
48. Petiwala SM, Puthenveetil AG, Johnson JJ. Polyphenols from the Mediterranean herb rosemary (Rosmarinus officinalis) for prostate cancer. Front Pharmacol. 2013;4:e1–4.
49. Petiwala SM, Johnson JJ. Diterpenes from rosemary (*Rosmarinus officinalis*): defining their potential for anti-cancer activity. Cancer Lett. 2015;367:93–102.
50. Yan M, Li G, Petiwala SM, Householter E, Johnson JJ. Standardized rosemary (*Rosmarinus officinalis*) extract induces Nrf2/sestrin-2 pathway in colon cancer cells. J Funct Foods. 2015;13:137–47.
51. Valdés A, Sullini G, Ibáñez E, Cifuentes A, García-Cañas V. Rosemary polyphenols induce unfolded protein response and changes in cholesterol metabolism in colon cancer cells. J Funct Foods. 2015;15:429–39.
52. Valdés A, García-Cañas V, Koçak E, Simó C, Cifuentes A. Foodomics study on the effects of extracellular production of hydrogen peroxide by rosemary polyphenols on the anti-proliferative activity of rosemary polyphenols against HT-29 cells. Electrophoresis. 2016;37:1795–804.
53. Valdés A, Artemenko KA, Bergquist J, García-Cañas V, Cifuentes A. Comprehensive proteomic study of the Antiproliferative activity of a polyphenol-enriched rosemary extract on colon cancer cells using Nanoliquid chromatography-Orbitrap MS/MS. J Proteome Res. 2016;15:1971–85.
54. González-Vallinas M, Molina S, Vicente G, Zarza V, Martín-Hernández R, García-Risco MR, Fornari T, Reglero G, de Molina AR. Expression of MicroRNA-15b and the glycosyltransferase GCNT3 correlates with antitumor efficacy of rosemary diterpenes in colon and Pancreatic cancer. PLoS One. 2014;9:e98556.
55. González-Vallinas M, Molina S, Vicente G, Sánchez-Martínez R, Vargas T, García-Risco MR, Fornari T, Reglero G, Ramírez de Molina A. Modulation of estrogen and epidermal growth factor receptors by rosemary extract in breast cancer cells. Electrophoresis. 2014;35:1719–27.
56. Yesil-Celiktas O, Sevimli C, Bedir E, Vardar-Sukan F. Inhibitory effects of rosemary extracts, carnosic acid and Rosmarinic acid on the growth of various human cancer cell lines. Plant Foods Hum Nutr. 2010;65:158–63.

57. Petiwala SM, Berhe S, Li G, Puthenveetil AG, Rahman O, Nonn L, Johnson JJ. Rosemary (*Rosmarinus officinalis*) extract modulates HOP/GADD153 to promote androgen receptor degradation and decreases Xenograft tumor growth. PLoS One. 2014;9:e89772.
58. Tai J, Cheung S, Wu M, Hasman D. Antiproliferation effect of rosemary (*Rosmarinus officinalis*) on human ovarian cancer cells in vitro. Phytomedicine. 2012;19:436–43.
59. Wang W, Li N, Luo M, Zu Y, Efferth T. Antibacterial activity and anticancer activity of *Rosmarinus officinalis* L. essential oil compared to that of its main components. Molecules. 2012;17:2704–13.
60. Moore J, Megaly M, MacNeil AJ, Klentrou P, Tsiani E. Rosemary extract reduces Akt/mTOR/p70S6K activation and inhibits proliferation and survival of A549 human lung cancer cells. Biomed Pharmacother. 2016;83:725–32.
61. Cheung S, Tai J. Anti-proliferative and antioxidant properties of rosemary *Rosmarinus officinalis*. Oncol Rep. 2007;17:1525–31.
62. Ahmad HH, Hamza AH, Hassan AZ, Sayed AH. Promising therapeutic role of *Rosmarinus officinalis* successive methanolic fraction against colorectal cancer. Int J Pharm Pharm Sci. 2013;5:164–70.
63. Kitano M, Wanibuchi H, Kikuzaki H, Nakatani N, Imaoka S, Funae Y, Hayashi S, Fukushima S. Chemopreventive effects of coumaperine from pepper on the initiation stage of chemical hepatocarcinogenesis in the rat. Jpn J Cancer Res Gann. 2000;91:674–80.
64. Soyal D, Jindal A, Singh I, Goyal PK. Modulation of radiation-induced biochemical alterations in mice by rosemary (*Rosemarinus officinalis*) extract. Phytomed Int J Phytothe Phytopharm. 2007;14:701–5.
65. Sharabani H, Izumchenko E, Wang Q, Kreinin R, Steiner M, Barvish Z, Kafka M, Sharoni Y, Levy J, Uskokovic M, et al. Cooperative antitumor effects of vitamin D3 derivatives and rosemary preparations in a mouse model of myeloid leukemia. Int J Cancer. 2006;118:3012–21.
66. Shabtay A, Sharabani H, Barvish Z, Kafka M, Amichay D, Levy J, Sharoni Y, Uskokovic MR, Studzinski GP, Danilenko M. Synergistic Antileukemic activity of Carnosic acid-rich rosemary extract and the 19-nor Gemini vitamin D analogue in a mouse model of systemic acute myeloid Leukemia. Oncology. 2008;75:203–14.
67. Borrás-Linares I, Pérez-Sánchez A, Lozano-Sánchez J, Barrajón-Catalán E, Arráez-Román D, Cifuentes A, Micol V, Carretero AS. A bioguided identification of the active compounds that contribute to the antiproliferative/cytotoxic effects of rosemary extract on colon cancer cells. Food Chem Toxicol Int J Publ Br Ind Biol Res Assoc. 2015;80:215–22.
68. Kim D-H, Park K-W, Chae IG, Kundu J, Kim E-H, Kundu JK, Chun K-S. Carnosic acid inhibits STAT3 signaling and induces apoptosis through generation of ROS in human colon cancer HCT116 cells. Mol Carcinog. 2016;55:1096–110.
69. Scheckel KA, Degner SC, Romagnolo DF. Rosmarinic acid antagonizes activator protein-1-dependent activation of cyclooxygenase-2 expression in human cancer and nonmalignant cell lines. J Nutr. 2008;138:2098–105.
70. Xavier CPR, Lima CF, Fernandes-Ferreira M, Pereira-Wilson C. Salvia fruticosa, Salvia officinalis, and rosmarinic acid induce apoptosis and inhibit proliferation of human colorectal cell lines: the role in MAPK/ERK pathway. Nutr Cancer. 2009;61:564–71.
71. Xu Y, Xu G, Liu L, Xu D, Liu J. Anti-invasion effect of rosmarinic acid via the extracellular signal-regulated kinase and oxidation-reduction pathway in Ls174-T cells. J Cell Biochem. 2010;111:370–9.
72. Ramos AA, Pedro D, Collins AR, Pereira-Wilson C. Protection by Salvia extracts against oxidative and alkylation damage to DNA in human HCT15 and CO115 cells. J Toxicol Environ Health A. 2012;75:765–75.
73. Moon DO, Kim MO, Lee JD, Choi YH, Kim GY. Rosmarinic acid sensitizes cell death through suppression of TNF-α-induced NF-κB activation and ROS generation in human leukemia U937 cells. Cancer Lett. 2010;288:183–91.
74. Paluszczak J, Krajka-Kuzniak V, Baer-Dubowska W. The effect of dietary polyphenols on the epigenetic regulation of gene expression in MCF7 breast cancer cells. Toxicol Lett. 2010;192:119–25.

75. Berdowska I, Zieliński B, Fecka I, Kulbacka J, Saczko J, Gamian A. Cytotoxic impact of phenolics from Lamiaceae species on human breast cancer cells. Food Chem. 2013;141:1313–21.
76. Perry EK, Pickering AT, Wang WW, Houghton PJ, Perry NS. Medicinal plants and Alzheimer's disease: from ethnobotany to phytotherapy. J Pharm Pharmacol. 1999;51:527–34.
77. Sulniute V, Ragazinskiene O, Venskutonis PR. Comprehensive evaluation of antioxidant potential of 10 salvia species using high pressure methods for the isolation of lipophilic and hydrophilic plant fractions. Plant Foods Hum Nutr. 2016;71:64–71.
78. Chang CC, Chang YC, Hu WL, Hung YC. Oxidative stress and salvia miltiorrhiza in aging-associated cardiovascular diseases. Oxidative Med Cell Longev. 2016;2016:4797102.
79. Lu Y, Foo Y. Antioxidant activities of polyphenols from sage (Salvia officinalis). Food Chem. 2001;75:197–202.
80. Lu Y, Foo Y. Salvianolic acid L, a potent phenolic antioxidant from Salvia officinalis. Tetrahedron Lett. 2001;42:8223–5.
81. Porres-Martinez M, Gonzalez-Burgos E, Carretero ME, Gomez-Serranillos MP. Major selected monoterpenes alpha-pinene and 1,8-cineole found in Salvia Lavandulifolia (Spanish sage) essential oil as regulators of cellular redox balance. Pharm Biol. 2015;53:921–9.
82. Kashyap D, Tuli HS, Sharma AK. Ursolic acid (UA): a metabolite with promising therapeutic potential. Life Sci. 2016;1:201–13.
83. Birtic S, Dussort P, Pierre FX, Bily AC, Roller M. Carnosic acid. Phytochemistry. 2015;115:9–19.
84. Abu-Darwish MS, Cabral C, Ferreira IV, Gonçalves MJ, Cavaleiro C, Cruz MT, Al-bdour TH, Salgueiro L. Essential oil of common sage (Salvia officinalis L.) from Jordan: assessment of safety in mammalian cells and its antifungal and anti-inflammatory potential. Biomed Res Int. 2013;2013:538940.
85. Oniga I, Parvu AE, Toiu A, Benedec D. Effects of Salvia officinalis L. extract on experimental acute inflammation. Rev Med Chir Soc Med Nat Iasi. 2007;111:290–4.
86. Schwager J, Richard N, Fowler A, Seifert N, Raederstorff D. Carnosol and related substances modulate chemokine and cytokine production in macrophages and chondrocytes. Molecules. 2016;21:465.
87. Akram M, Syed AS, Kim KA, Lee JS, Chang SY, Kim CY, et al. Heme oxygenase 1-mediated novel anti-inflammatory activities of Salvia Plebeia and its active components. J Ethnopharmacol. 2015;4:322–30.
88. Bonaccini L, Karioti A, Bergonzi MC, Bilia AR. Effects of salvia miltiorrhiza on CNS neuronal injury and degeneration: a plausible complementary role of tanshinones and depsides. Planta Med. 2015;81:1003–16.
89. Ma S, Zhang D, Lou H, Sun L, Ji J. Evaluation of the antiinflammatory activities of tanshinones isolated from salvia miltiorrhiza var. alba roots in THP-1 macrophages. J Ethnopharmacol. 2016;21:193–9.
90. Nabavi SF, Tenore GC, Daglia M, Tundis R, Loizzo MR, Nabavi SM. The cellular protective effects of rosmarinic acid: from bench to bedside. Curr Neurovasc Res. 2015;12:98–105.
91. Herrera-Ruiz M, Garcia-Beltran Y, Mora S, Diaz-Veliz G, Viana GS, Tortoriello J, Ramirez G. Antidepressant and anxiolytic effects of hydroalcoholic extract from Salvia elegans. J Ethnopharmacol. 2006;107:53–8.
92. Naderi N, Akhavan N, Aziz Ahari F, Zamani N, Kamalinejad M, Shokrzadeh M, Ahangar N, Motamedi F. Effects of hydroalcoholic extract from salvia verticillata on pharmacological models of seizure, anxiety and depression in mice. Iran J Pharm Res. 2011;10:535–45.
93. Gross M, Nesher E, Tikhonov T, Raz O, Pinhasov A. Chronic food administration of Salvia sclarea oil reduces animals' anxious and dominant behavior. J Med Food. 2013;16:216–22.
94. Seol GH, Shim HS, Kim PJ, Moon HK, Lee KH, Shim I, Suh SH, Min SS. Antidepressant-like effect of Salvia sclarea is explained by modulation of dopamine activities in rats. J Ethnopharmacol. 2010;130:187–90.
95. Liu AD, Cai GH, Wei YY, Yu JP, Chen J, Yang J, et al. Anxiolytic effect of essential oils of Salvia miltiorrhiza in rats. Int J Clin Exp Med. 2015;8:12756–64.

96. Kavvadias D, Monschein V, Sand P, Riederer P, Schreier P. Constituents of sage (Salvia officinalis) with in vitro affinity to human brain benzodiazepine receptor. Planta Med. 2003;69:113–7.
97. Takeda H, Tsuji M, Inazu M, Egashira T, Matsumiya T. Rosmarinic acid and caffeic acid produce antidepressive-like effect in the forced swimming test in mice. Eur J Pharmacol. 2002;449:261–7.
98. Pereira P, Tysca D, Oliveira P, da Silva Brum LF, Picada JN, Ardenghi P. Neurobehavioral and genotoxic aspects of rosmarinic acid. Pharmacol Res. 2005;52:199–203.
99. Feng Y, You Z, Yan S, He G, Chen Y, Gou X, Peng C. Antidepressant-like effects of salvianolic acid B in the mouse forced swim and tail suspension tests. Life Sci. 2012;90:1010–4.
100. Braida D, Capurro V, Zani A, Rubino T, Vigano D, Parolaro D, Sala M. Potential anxiolytic- and antidepressant-like effects of salvinorin A, the main active ingredient of Salvia divinorum, in rodents. Br J Pharmacol. 2009;157:844–53.
101. Perry NS, Bollen C, Perry EK, Ballard C. Salvia for dementia therapy: review of pharmacological activity and pilot tolerability clinical trial. Pharmacol Biochem Behav. 2003;75:651–9.
102. Akhondzadeh S, Noroozian M, Mohammadi M, Ohadinia S, Jamshidi AH, Khani M. Salvia officinalis extract in the treatment of patients with mild to moderate Alzheimer's disease: a double blind, randomized and placebo-controlled trial. J Clin Pharm Ther. 2003;28:53–9.
103. Kennedy DO, Dodd FL, Robertson BC, Okello EJ, Reay JL, Scholey AB, Haskell CF. Monoterpenoid extract of sage (Salvia lavandulaefolia) with cholinesterase inhibiting properties improves cognitive performance and mood in healthy adults. J Psychopharmacol. 2011;25:1088–100.
104. Tildesley NT, Kennedy DO, Perry EK, Ballard CG, Wesnes KA, Scholey AB. Positive modulation of mood and cognitive performance following administration of acute doses of Salvia lavandulaefolia essential oil to healthy young volunteers. Physiol Behav. 2005;83:699–709.
105. Tildesley NT, Kennedy DO, Perry EK, Ballard CG, Savelev S, Wesnes KA, Scholey AB. Salvia lavandulaefolia (Spanish sage) enhances memory in healthy young volunteers. Pharmacol Biochem Behav. 2003;75:669–74.
106. Kennedy DO, Pace S, Haskell C, Okello EJ, Milne A, Scholey AB. Effects of cholinesterase inhibiting sage (Salvia officinalis) on mood, anxiety and performance on a psychological stressor battery. Neuropsychopharmacology. 2006;31:845–52.
107. Scholey AB, Tildesley NT, Ballard CG, Wesnes KA, Tasker A, Perry EK, Kennedy DO. An extract of Salvia (sage) with anticholinesterase properties improves memory and attention in healthy older volunteers. Psychopharmacology. 2008;198:127–39.
108. Moss L, Rouse M, Wesnes KA, Moss M. Differential effects of the aromas of Salvia species on memory and mood. Hum Psychopharmacol. 2010;25:388–96.
109. Dent M, Dragovi-Uzelac V, Penic M, Brncic M, Bosiljkov T, Levaj B. The effect of extraction solvents, temperature and time on the composition and mass fraction of polyphenols in Dalmatian wild sage (Salvia officinalis L.) Extracts. Food Technol Biotechnol. 2013;51(1):84–91.
110. Gird CE, Nencu I, Costea T, Dutu LE, Popescu ML, Ciupitu N. Quantitative analysis of phenolic compounds from Salvia officinalis L. leaves. Farmacia. 2014;62:649–57.
111. Luchicchi A, Bloem B, Viana JN, Mansvelder HD, Role LW. Illuminating the role of cholinergic signaling in circuits ofattention and emotionally salient behaviors. Front Synaptic Neurosci. 2014;6:24.
112. Colovic MB, Krstic DZ, Lazarevic-Pasti TD, Bondzic AM, Vasic VM. Acetylcholinesterase inhibitors: pharmacology and toxicology. Curr Neuropharmacol. 2013;11:315–35.
113. Smach MA, Hafsa J, Charfeddine B, Dridi H, Limem K. Effects of sage extract on memory performance in mice and acetylcholinesterase activity. Ann Pharm Fr. 2015;73:281–8.
114. Foolad F, Khodagholi F. Dietary supplementation with Salvia sahendica attenuates acetylcholinesterase activity and increases mitochondrial transcription factor a and antioxidant proteins in the hippocampus of amyloid beta-injected rats. J Pharm Pharmacol. 2013;65:1555–62.
115. Senol FS, Orhan IE, Erdem SA, Kartal M, Sener B, Kan Y, Celep F, Karhaman A, Dogan M. Evaluation of cholinesterase inhibitory and antioxidant activities of wild and

cultivated samples of sage (Salvia fruticosa) by activity-guided fractionation. J Med Food. 2011;14:1476–83.
116. Sallam A, Mira A, Ashour A, Shimizu K. Acetylcholine esterase inhibitors and melanin synthesis inhibitors from Salvia officinalis. Phytomedicine. 2016;23:1005–11.
117. Merad M, Soufi W, Ghalem S, Boukli F, Baig MH, Ahmad K, Kamal MA. Molecular interaction of acetylcholinesterase with carnosic acid derivatives: a neuroinformatics study. CNS Neurol Disord Drug Targets. 2014;13:440–6.
118. Marcelo F, Dias C, Martins A, Madeira PJ, Jorge T, Florencio MH, Cañada FJ, Cabrita EJ, Jiménez-Barbero J, Rauter AP. Molecular recognition of rosmarinic acid from Salvia sclareoides extracts by acetylcholinesterase: a new binding site detected by NMR spectroscopy. Chemistry. 2013;19:6641–9.
119. Xu QQ, Xu YJ, Yang C, Tang Y, Li L, Cai HB, Hou BN, Chen HF, Wang Q, Shi XG, Zhang SJ. Sodium Tanshinone IIA sulfonate attenuates scopolamine-induced cognitive dysfunctions via improving cholinergic system. Biomed Res Int. 2016;2016:9852536.
120. Zhou Y, Li W, Xu L, Chen L. In Salvia miltiorrhiza, phenolic acids possess protective properties against amyloid beta-induced cytotoxicity, and tanshinones act as acetylcholinesterase inhibitors. Environ Toxicol Pharmacol. 2011;31:443–52.
121. More SV, Kumar H, Cho DY, Yun YS, Choi DK. Toxin-induced experimental models of learning and memory impairment. Int J Mol Sci. 2016;17:1447.
122. Teng Y, Zhang MQ, Wang W, Liu LT, Zhou LM, Miao SK, et al. Compound danshen tablet ameliorated a$\beta_{25\text{-}35}$-induced spatial memory impairment in mice via rescuing imbalance between cytokines and neurotrophins. BMC Complement Altern Med. 2014;14:23.
123. Khodagholi F, Ashabi G. Dietary supplementation with salvia sahendica attenuates memory deficits, modulates CREB and its down-stream molecules and decreases apoptosis in amyloid betainjected rats. Behav Brain Res. 2013;15:62–9.
124. Alkam T, Nitta A, Mizoguchi H, Itoh A, Nabeshima T. A natural scavenger of peroxynitrites, rosmarinic acid, protects against impairment of memory induced by Abeta(25-35). Behav Brain Res. 2007;180:139–45.
125. Lee YW, Kim DH, Jeon SJ, Park SJ, Kim JM, Jung JM, Lee HE, Bae SG, Oh HK, Son KH, Ryu JH. Neuroprotective effects of salvianolic acid B on an Aβ25-35 peptide-induced mouse model of Alzheimer's disease. Eur J Pharmacol. 2013;704(3):70–7.
126. Rasoolijazi H, Azad N, Joghataei MT, Kerdari M, Nikbakht F, Soleimani M. The protective role of carnosic acid against beta-amyloid toxicity in rats. Sci World J. 2013;2013:917082.
127. Patil CS, Singh VP, Satyanarayan PS, Jain NK, Singh A, Kulkarni SK. Protective effect of flavonoids against aging- and lipopolysaccharide-induced cognitive impairment in mice. Pharmacology. 2003;69:59–67.
128. Bowling H, Bhattacharya A, Klann E, Chao MV. Deconstructing brain-derived neurotrophic factor actions in adult brain circuits to bridge an existing informational gap in neuro-cell biology. Neural Regen Res. 2016;11:363–7.
129. Qin XY, Cao C, Cawley NX, Liu TT, Yuan J, Loh YP, Cheng Y. Decreased peripheral brain-derived neurotrophic factor levels in Alzheimer's disease: a meta-analysis study (N = 7277). Mol Psychiatry. 2017;22:312–20.
130. Fonteles AA, de Souza CM, de Sousa Neves JC, Menezes AP, Santos do Carmo MR, Fernandes FD, de Araújo PR, de Andrade GM. Rosmarinic acid prevents against memory deficits in ischemic mice. Behav Brain Res. 2016;15:91–103.
131. Jin X, Liu P, Yang F, Zhang YH, Miao D. Rosmarinic acid ameliorates depressive-like behaviors in a rat model of CUS and up-regulates BDNF levels in the hippocampus and hippocampalderived astrocytes. Neurochem Res. 2013;38:1828–37.
132. Takeda H, Tsuji M, Yamada T, Masuya J, Matsushita K, Tahara M, Iimori M, Matsumiya T. Caffeic acid attenuates the decrease in cortical BDNF mRNA expression induced by exposure to forced swimming stress in mice. Eur J Pharmacol. 2006;534:115–21.
133. Xu SL, Bi CW, Choi RC, Zhu KY, Miernisha A, Dong TT, Tsim KW. Flavonoids induce the synthesis and secretion of neurotrophic factors in cultured rat astrocytes: a signaling response mediated by estrogen receptor. Evid Based Complement Alternat Med. 2013;2013:127075.

134. Yao RQ, Qi DS, Yu HL, Liu J, Yang LH, Wu XX. Quercetin attenuates cell apoptosis in focal cerebral ischemia rat brain via activation of BDNF-TrkB-PI3K/Akt signaling pathway. Neurochem Res. 2012;37:2777–86.
135. Kosaka K, Yokoi T. Carnosic acid, a component of rosemary (Rosmarinus officinalis L.), promotes synthesis of nerve growth factor in T98G human glioblastoma cells. Biol Pharm Bull. 2003;26:1620–2.
136. Zhao Y, Xu P, Hu S, Du L, Xu Z, Zhang H, Cui W, Mak S, Xu D, Shen J, Han Y, Liu Y, Xue M. Tanshinone II A, a multiple target neuroprotectant, promotes caveolae-dependent neuronal differentiation. Eur J Pharmacol. 2015;765:437–46.
137. Wang W, Huang CY, Tsai FJ, Tsai CC, Yao CH, Chen YS. Growth-promoting effects of quercetin on peripheral nerves in rats. Int J Artif Organs. 2011;34:1095–105.
138. Loizzo MR, Tundis R, Menichini F, Saab AM, Statti GA, Menichini F. Cytotoxic activity of essential oils from Labiatae and Lauraceae families against in vitro human tumor models. Anticancer Res. 2007;27:3293–9.
139. Sertel S, Eichhorn T, Plinkert PK, Efferth T. Anticancer activity of Salvia officinalis essential oil against HNSCC cell line (UMSCC1). HNO. 2011;59:1203–8.
140. Itani WS, El-Banna SH, Hassan SB, Larsson RL, Bazarbachi A, Gali-Muhtasib HU. Anti colon cancer components from Lebanese sage (*Salvia libanotica*) essential oil. Cancer Biol Ther. 2008;7:1765–73.
141. Loizzo MR, Menichini F, Tundis R, Bonesi M, Nadjafi F, Saab AM, Frega NG, Menichini F. Comparative chemical composition and antiproliferative activity of aerial parts of Salvia leriifolia Benth and Salvia acetabulosa L. essential oils against human tumor cell in vitro models. J Med Food. 2010;13:62–9.
142. Theisen C. What ever happened to …? Looking back 10 years. J Natl Cancer Inst. 2001;93:1049–50.
143. Dewick PM. Medicinal natural products a biosynthetic approach. 2nd ed. London: Willey; 2002.
144. Rose P, Whiteman M, Moore PK, Zhu YZ. Bioactive S-alk(en)yl cysteine sulfoxide metabolites in the genus allium: the chemistry of potential therapeutic agents. Nat Prod Rep. 2005;22(3):351–68.
145. Amagase H. Clarifying the real bioactive constituents of garlic. J Nutr. 2006;136:716S–25S.
146. Corzo-Martinez M, Corzo N, Villamiel M. Biological properties of onions and garlic. Trends Food Sci Technol. 2007;18:609–25.
147. Smith S. In: Block E, editor. Garlic and Other *Alliums*: The Lore and Science. Cambridge: Royal Society of Chemistry; 2010. p. 100–223, 238–239.
148. Lanzotti V. The analysis of onion and garlic. J Chromatogr. 2006;1112:3–22.
149. Sivam GP. Protection against Helicobacter pylori and other bacterial infections by garlic. J Nutr. 2001;131(3S):1106S–8S.
150. Sengupta A, Ghosh S, Bhattacharjee S. Allium vegetables in cancer prevention: an overview. Asian Pac J Cancer Prev. 2004;5:237–45.
151. Fukushima S, Takada N, Hori T, Wanibuchi H. Cancer prevention by organosulfur compounds from garlic and onion. J Cell Biochem Suppl. 1997;27:100–5.
152. Wargovich MJ. New dietary anticarcinogens and prevention of gastrointestinal cancer. Dis Colon Rectum. 1988;31:72–5.
153. Tjokroprawiro A, Pikir BS, Budhiarta AA, Pranawa, Soewondo H, Donosepoetro M, Budhianto FX, Wibowo JA, Tanuwidjaja SJ, Pangemanan M, Widodo H, Surjadhana A. Metabolic effects of onion and green beans on diabetic patients. Tohoku J Exp Med. 1983;141(Suppl):671–6.
154. Sharma KK, Gupta RK, Gupta S, Samuel KC. Antihyperglycemic effect of onion: effect on fasting blood sugar and induced hyperglycemia in man. Indian J Med Res. 1977;65:422–9.
155. Bordia A, Bansal HC, Arora SK, Singh SV. Effect of the essential oils of garlic and onion on alimentary hyperlipemia. Atherosclerosis. 1975;21:15–9.
156. Mayer B, Kalus U, Grigorov A, Pindur G, Jung F, Radtke H, Bachmann K, Mrowietz C, Koscielny J, Wenzel E, Kiesewetter H. Effects of an onion-olive oil maceration product

containing essential ingredients of the Mediterranean diet on blood pressure and blood fluidity. Arzneimittelforschung. 2001;51:104–11.
157. Hubbard GP, Wolffram S, de Vos R, Bovy A, Gibbins JM, Lovegrove JA. Ingestion of onion soup high in quercetin inhibits platelet aggregation and essential components of the collagen-stimulated platelet activation pathway in man: a pilot study. Br J Nutr. 2006;96:482–8.
158. Kalus U, Pindur G, Jung F, Mayer B, Radtke H, Bachmann K, Mrowietz C, Koscielny J, Kiesewetter H. Influence of the onion as an essential ingredient of the Mediterranean diet on arterial blood pressure and blood fluidity. Arzneimittelforschung. 2000;50:795–801.
159. Agarwal RK, Dewar HA, Newell DJ, Das B. Controlled trial of the effect of cycloalliin on the fibrinolytic activity of venous blood. Atherosclerosis. 1977;27:347–51.
160. Muhlbauer RC, Lozano A, Reinli A. Onion and a mixture of vegetables, salads, and herbs affect bone resorption in the rat by a mechanism independent of their base excess. J Bone Miner Res. 2002;17:1230–6.
161. Small LD, Bailey JH, Cavallito CJ. Alkyl Thiosulfinates. J Am Chem Soc. 1947;69:1710–3.
162. Wetli HA, Brenneisen R, Tschudi I, Langos M, Bigler P, Sprang T, Schürch S, Mühlbauer RC. A gamma-glutamyl peptide isolated from onion (Allium cepa L.) by bioassay-guided fractionation inhibits resorption activity of osteoclasts. J Agric Food Chem. 2005;53:3408–14.
163. Cutler RR, Wilson P. Antibacterial activity of a new, stable, aqueous extract of allicin against methicillin-resistant Staphylococcus aureus. Br J Biomed Sci. 2004;61:71–4.
164. Cavallito C, Bailey J. Allicin, the antibacterial principle of *Allium sativum*. I. Isolation, physical properties and antibacterial action. J Am Chem Soc. 1944;66:1950–1.
165. Feldberg R, Chang S. In vitro mechanism of inhibition of bacterial cell growth by allicin. Antimicrob Agents Chemother. 1988;32:1763–8.
166. Curtis H, Noll U, Störmann J, Slusarenko AJ. Broad-spectrum activity of the volatile phytoanticipin allicin in extracts of garlic (*Allium sativum* L.) against plant pathogenic bacteria, fungi and Oomycetes. Physiol Mol Plant Pathol. 2004;65:79–89.
167. Focke M, Feld A, Lichtenthaler HK. Allicin, a naturally occurring antibiotic from garlic, specifically inhibits acetyl-CoA synthetase. FEBS Lett. 1990;261:106–8.
168. Rabinkov A, Miron T, Konstantinovski L, Wilchek M, Mirelman D, Weiner L. The mode of action of allicin: trapping of radicals and interaction with thiol containing proteins. Biochim Biophys Acta. 1998;1379:233–44.
169. Shadkchan Y, Shemesh E, Mirelman D, Miron T, Rabinkov A, Wilchek M, Osherov N. Efficacy of allicin, the reactive molecule of garlic, in inhibiting Aspergillus spp. in vitro, and in a murine model of disseminated aspergillosis. J Antimicrob Chemother. 2004;53:832–6.
170. Khodavandi A, Alizadeh F, Harmal NS, Sidik SM, Othman F, Sekawi Z, Jahromi MAF, Ng KP, Chong PP. Comparison between efficacy of allicin and fluconazole against Candida albicans in vitro and in a systemic candidiasis mouse model. FEMS Microbiol Lett. 2011;315:87–93.
171. Gruhlke MCH, Nwachukwu I, Arbach M, Anwar A, Noll U, Slusarenko AJ. Allicin from garlic, effective in controlling several plant diseases, ia a reactive sulfur species (RSS) that pushes cells into apoptosis. In: Modern Fungicides and Antifungal Compounds VI. Braunschweig, Gemany: DPG Publishers; 2011. p. 325–34.
172. Li XH, Li CY, Xiang ZG, Hu JJ, Lu JM, Tian RB, Jia W. Allicin ameliorates cardiac hypertrophy and fibrosis trought enhancing of Nrf2 antioxidant signaling pathways. Cardiovasc Drugs Ther. 2012;26:457–65.
173. Li XH, Li CY, Lu JM, Tian RB, Wei J. Allicin ameliorates cognitive deficits ageing-induced learning and memory deficits through enhancing of Nrf2 antioxidant signaling pathways. Neurosci Lett. 2012;514:46–50.
174. Gebhardt R, Beck H, Wagner KG. Inhibition of cholesterol biosynthesis by allicin and ajoene in rat hepatocytes and HepG2 cells. Biochim Biophys Acta. 1994;121:57–62.
175. Gupta N, Porter T. Garlic and garlic-derived compounds inhibit human squalene monooxygenase. J Nutr. 2001;131:1662–7.
176. Yip J, Shen Y, Berndt MC, Andrews RK. Primary platelet adhesion receptors. IUBMB Life. 2005;57:103–8.

177. Briggs WH, Xiao H, Parkin KL, Shen C, Goldman IL. Differential inhibition of human platelet aggregation by selected allium thiosulfinates. J Agric Food Chem. 2000;48:5731–5.
178. Benavides GA, Squadrito GL, Mills RW, Patel HD, Isbell TS, Patel RP, Darley-Usmar VM, Doeller JE, Kraus DW. Hydrogen sulfide mediates the vasoactivity of garlic. Proc Natl Acad Sci U S A. 2007;104:17977–82.
179. Zoccali C, Catalano C, Rastelli S. Blood pressure control: hydrogen sulfide, a new gasotransmitter, takes stage. Nephrol Dial Transplant. 2009;24:1394–6.
180. Tocque B, Delumeau I, Parker F, Maurier F, Multon MC, Schweighoffer F. Ras-GTPase activating protein (GAP): a putative effector for Ras. Cell Signal. 1997;9:153–8.
181. Patya M. Allicin stimulates lymphocytes and elicits an antitumor effect: a possible role of p21ras. Int Immunol. 2004;16:275–81.
182. Lang A, Lahav M, Sakhnini E, Barshack I, Fidder HH, Avidan B, Bardan E, Hershkoviz R, Bar-Meir S, Chowers Y. Allicin inhibits spontaneous and TNF-alpha induced secretion of proinflammatory cytokines and chemokines from intestinal epithelial cells. Clin Nutr. 2004;23:1199–208.
183. Haase H, Hieke N, Plum LM, Gruhlke MCH, Slusarenko AJ, Rink L. Impact of allicin on macrophage activity. Food Chem. 2012;134:141–8.
184. Dirsch VM, Kiemer AK, Wagner H, Vollmar AM. Effect of allicin and ajoene, two compounds of garlic, on inducible nitric oxide synthase. Atherosclerosis. 1998;139:333–9.
185. Dipaolo JA, Carruthers C. The effect of allicin from garlic on tumor growth. Cancer Res. 1960;20:431–4.
186. Miron T, Wilchek M, Sharp A, Nakagawa Y, Naoi M, Nozawa Y, Akao Y. Allicin inhibits cell growth and induces apoptosis through the mitochondrial pathway in HL60 and U937 cells. J Nutr Biochem. 2008;19:524–35.
187. Oommen S, Anto RJ, Srinivas G, Karunagaran D. Allicin (from garlic) induces caspase-mediated apoptosis in cancer cells. Eur J Pharmacol. 2004;485:97–103.
188. Park SY, Cho SJ, Kwon HC, Lee KR, Rhee DK, Pyo S. Caspase-independent cell death by allicin in human epithelial carcinoma cells: involvement of PKA. Cancer Lett. 2005;224:123–32.
189. Bat-Chen W, Golan T, Peri I, Ludmer Z, Schwartz B. Allicin purified from fresh garlic cloves induces apoptosis in colon cancer cells via Nrf2. Nutr Cancer. 2010;62:947–57.
190. Loboda A, Was H, Jozkowicz A, Dulak J. Janus face of Nrf2-HO-1 axis in cancer—Friend in chemoprevention, foe in anticancer therapy. Lung Cancer. 2008;60:1–3.
191. Niture SK, Jaiswal AK. Nrf2 protein up-regulates antiapoptotic protein Bcl-2 and prevents cellular apoptosis. J Biol Chem. 2012;287:9873–86.
192. Niture SK, Jaiswal AK. Nrf2-induced antiapoptotic Bcl-xL protein enhances cell survival and drug resistance. Free Radic Biol Med. 2013;57:119–31.
193. Cha JH, Choi YJ, Cha SH, Choi CH, Cho WH. Allicin inhibits cell growth and induces apoptosis in U87MG human glioblastoma cells through an ERK-dependent pathway. Oncol Rep. 2012;28:41–8.

Red and White Wines 15

15.1 Premises

In the context of the Mediterranean diet, wine has always covered a central role. In ancient times, Greek and Roman populations loved to conclude their banquets with wine libations, generally red wine diluted with water in a proportion of 1:3. In subsequent eras wine, which was always drunk in low to moderate amounts with meals, remained a fixed component in the diet of populations living to the north of the Mediterranean basin (As the southern Mediterranean population of north Africa and near East are Muslims, they do not drink alcohol or wine).

15.2 History

Wine can be considered the most ancient alcoholic beverage of mankind. In Valdarno Superiore, around Montevarchi (Tuscany, Italy), fossils of grapevines (*Vitis vinifera)* dating to 2 million years ago were found in lignite deposits. Several archaeological digs discovered that *Vitis vinifera* grew spontaneously already 300,000 years ago.

The earliest archaeological evidence of wine production was discovered at sites in Georgia (c. 6000 BC), Iran (c. 5000 BC), Greece (c. 4500 BC), and Armenia (c. 4100 BC). Wine production then spread to other sites in Greater Iran and Grecian Macedonia by c. 4500 BC.

In 1996, an American archaeological mission from the University of Pennsylvania found in the Neolithic village of *Hajji Firuz Tepe* in northern Iran, an earthenware jar capable of holding 9 L, containing a dry substance from grapes dating back to 5100 BC.

The oldest known winery was discovered in the "*Areni-1*" cave in *Vayots Dzor, Armenia*. Dating to c. 4100 BC, the site contained a wine press, fermentation vats, jars, and cups [1]. Archaeologists also found *Vitis vinifera* seeds and vines. The fact

A. Capurso et al., *Benefits of the Mediterranean Diet in the Elderly Patient*,
Practical Issues in Geriatrics, https://doi.org/10.1007/978-3-319-78084-9_15

that winemaking was already so well developed in 4000 BC presupposes that its technology dates to an even earlier time.

Wine played an important role in ceremonial life in ancient Egypt. Although it was predominantly red, residue from five clay amphorae in Tutankhamen's tomb revealed white wine, leading to the conclusion that the drink was made available to the Egyptians through trade.

The Phoenicians were instrumental in distributing wine, wine grapes, and winemaking technology throughout the Mediterranean region through their extensive trade network. Their use of amphorae for transporting wine was widely adopted and Phoenician-distributed grape varieties were crucial to the development of the wine industries of Rome and Greece.

Much of modern wine culture, however, has its roots in the practices of the ancient Greeks. Several ancient sources, such as the Roman *Pliny the Elder*, describe the ancient Greek method of using partly dehydrated *gypsum* (soft calcium sulfate dihydrate) before the grapes were fermented and some type of *lime* (a material containing inorganic calcium and carbonates) after they were fermented, in order to reduce the acidity of the wine. The Greek *Theophrastus* provided the oldest known description of this aspect of Greek winemaking.

The Roman Empire played a crucial role in the development of viticulture and oenology. Wine was an integral part of the Roman diet and winemaking became a regular business. Virtually all of today's major wine-producing regions of Western Europe were established during the Roman Imperial era. During the Roman Empire, social norms began to shift as the production of alcohol increased. Widespread drunkenness and true alcoholism among the Romans was already noted in the first century BC and reached its peak in the first century AD. Viniculture expanded so extensively that by c. 92 AD the emperor Domitian was forced to pass the first wine laws on record, banning the planting of any new vineyards in Italy and uprooting half of the vineyards in the provinces in order to increase the production of necessary but less profitable grains [2].

15.3 Wine Composition

Wine can be defined as a beverage made of the fermented juice of any of a variety of grapes, usually containing from 10% to 15% alcohol by volume. The main components of wine are water (850–900 g/L) and alcohol (100–150 g/L). Other components which are present in various quantities contribute to giving it its organoleptic characteristics, i.e., color, scent, flavor, and taste (sweet, sour, bitter, tannic, fructate) (see Table 15.1).

The chemical composition of grapes can be affected by many factors, including the grape variety or cultivar, environmental factors, seasonal variations, and viticultural management [3, 4].

The two principal types of wine, red and white wine, are processed in different ways. In fact, white wine is fermented without the skins while red wine is fermented with them. This means that red wines have more antioxidants and polyphenols,

Table 15.1 The major chemical components of wine

Constituent	g/L	% Volume
Water	850–900	80–90
Carbohydrates	1–10	
Glucose	0.5–5	
Fructose	0.5–5	
Acids	4.5–11	
Tartaric	1–6	0.17–0.45
Malic	0–8	0.0–0.44
Acetic	0.2–1.5	
Lactic	1–5	0.08–0.33
Alcohols		
Ethanol	80–150	8–16
Glycerol	3–14	0.32–1.19
Phenolics	Trace–5	
Simple phenolics	Trace–0.2	
Anthocyanins	Trace–0.5	
Inorganic	1.5–4	
Potassium	0.5–2	
Others	0.1–3 (sodium, calcium, iron, magnesium, phosphorus, zinc, copper, manganese, fluoride, selenium)	
Vitamins	Trace (thiamine, riboflavin, niacin, vitamins A, B, K, folate, choline, betaine, lutein, zeaxanthin)	

which are contained in the skin and seeds. White wines also contain some antioxidants, monophenols as well as catechins and stilbenes. Red wine, moreover, has about seven times more polyphenols than white wine.

Polyphenols, together with other minor compounds, are responsible for the bitterness, color, and astringency of wine, along with several important health benefits.

15.4 Is Drinking Wine Beneficial to Health?

Scientific data on wine drinking as well as that pertaining to other alcoholic beverages such as beer and liquors is often outlined together. This is due to the fact that most people normally do not drink wine exclusively, but also consume beer and/or liquors. In fact, studies regarding the effects of wine are often concerned with alcohol intake in general and they use "one drink" as the basic unit of measure of alcohol intake. According to many authors "one drink" corresponds to 100–150 mL of wine, 350–400 mL of beer, and 30–50 mL of liquor.

Numerous studies have shown that a moderate consumption of alcohol, particularly red wine, is beneficial to the health and in particular with regard to cardiovascular disease (CVD). The main health benefit of wine and other alcoholic beverages appears to be related to their effect on atherosclerosis.

The subjects appearing to benefit most from light to moderate alcohol drinking are middle-aged men and women, particularly those who are at increased risk of developing cardiovascular disease. These individuals have been shown to have about a 30% reduction in total mortality, an effect that is largely linked to the reduction in the risk of developing atherosclerosis disease.

Some observational studies on the beneficial effect of a low to moderate intake of wine or alcohol on health and cardiovascular disease are described below.

The Health Professional Follow-up Study [5] is an ongoing prospective cohort study on 51,529 US male health professionals, aged 40–75 years, that was begun in 1986. An article published in 2003 [5] refers to 38,077 subjects who at baseline were free from cardiovascular disease. The consumption of beer, red wine, white wine, and liquor and their relationship with cardiovascular mortality was assessed in these subjects. One drink was standardized as a 12-oz (355-mL) bottle or a can of beer, a 5-oz (148-mL) glass of wine, and 1.5 ounces (44 mL) of 80-proof distilled spirits. After a 12 year follow-up, study analysis showed the men who consumed alcohol 3–4 or 5–7 days/week had a significantly lower risk of having a myocardial infarction (MI) (multivariate relative risk, 0.68 and 0.63, respectively, equivalent to 32% and 37% risk reduction, respectively.

The Health Professional Health Follow-Up Study [6] monitored 1818 men who had survived a first MI between 1986 and 2006. Long-term average alcohol consumption was calculated beginning from the time period immediately before the first MI and updated every 4 years afterward. To determine the total grams of alcohol intake, the authors multiplied the frequency of each beverage type by the ethanol content in each portion (12.8 g for beer; 11.0 g for wine; 14.0 g for liquor). Compared with nondrinkers, the best reduction in the multivariable-adjusted hazard ratio (HR) for all-cause mortality and cardiovascular mortality (HR: 0.66 and 0.58, respectively) was observed in the moderate drinkers, i.e., those who drunk from 10.0 to 29.9 g/day alcohol. The study also showed a significant U-shaped association, with the greatest benefit observed in the moderate drinkers, and indicated that there was slight rise in mortality in the men who consumed more than 2 drinks/day post-MI.

The results of this last study were essentially in agreement with those of another study on survivors from myocardial infarction. The *US Physicians' Health Study* [7] showed that, compared with men who have rarely or never drank alcohol, those who consumed 1–4 drinks/month had a relative risk (RR) for total mortality of 0.85; for 2–4 drinks/week, the RR was 0.72; for 1 drink/day, the RR was 0.79. Finally, for 2 or more drinks/day, the RR was 0.84.

The data from studies on excessive drinking patterns were also interesting. In the *MI Onset Study* [8] the apparent benefit from light drinking after MI was entirely eliminated by episodes of binge drinking, confirming the U-shaped curve of alcohol amounts and morbidity-mortality rates.

The Copenhagen City Heart Study [9], a prospective cohort study on 13,329 eligible men and women between 45 and 84 years, was conducted to evaluate the relationships between alcohol consumption and the risk of ischemic stroke. The authors considered one bottle of beer to contain 12 g of alcohol, as well as the average alcohol content for the other types of drinks. After 16 year follow-up, a U-shaped relationship between alcohol intake and risk of stroke clearly emerged. The intakes of wine on a monthly, weekly, or daily basis were associated with a lower risk of stroke compared with no wine intake. The monthly relative risk (RR) was 0.83; the weekly RR was 0.59, and the daily RR was 0.70. No association between intake of beer or spirits and risk of stroke was found. These data indicated, in accordance with other studies, that the intake of a small amount of alcohol is very beneficial to the risk of stroke. This effect was strongest among the wine drinkers, as the subjects who drank wine had a lower risk of stroke than those who never drank wine. The risk of stroke among wine drinkers was not affected by the consumption of beer or spirits. High alcohol consumption, on the other hand, was associated with an increased risk of stroke, particularly hemorrhagic stroke, and there was evidence that at least some of these effects were mediated through the systolic blood pressure. The authors concluded that the differences in the effects of beer, wine, and spirits on the risk of stroke suggested that in addition to ethanol, other compounds of wine were responsible for the protective effect against stroke. These additional compounds in wine will be discussed later in this chapter.

15.5 What Are the Mechanisms in Wine and Alcohol That Help to Reduce Cardiovascular Risk?

The associations between moderate alcohol or wine consumption with lower risk and better prognosis of CVD seem to be linked to several biological mechanisms.

15.5.1 The Role of Alcohol

A large body of literature confirms the beneficial effects of moderate alcohol consumption on cardiovascular diseases and risk factors. Maximum cardiovascular benefit occurs at relatively low levels of consumption (i.e., 1–2 standard drinks a day in men (10–20 g alcohol) and up to one a day in women (10 g alcohol).

According to a large meta-analysis [10], a moderate alcohol consumption of 30 g/day was associated with a significant 4.0 mg/dL increase in HDL cholesterol. It should be emphasized that the level of HDL cholesterol normally expresses the ability of these particles to remove cholesterol from atherosclerotic plaques and transport it to the liver. This explains why the higher the HDL cholesterol, the greater the protection from atherosclerosis.

In addition to HDL's positive effects, moderate alcohol consumption has been also associated with improved insulin sensitivity [11], reduced fibrinogen levels [12], and levels of inflammatory markers [13] such as C-reactive protein and interleukin-6. A moderate alcohol consumption has been also significantly associated with less coronary calcification in asymptomatic subjects [14] as well as reduced progression of coronary atherosclerosis in serial angiographic measurements in MI survivors [15].

While some have postulated that the benefits of moderate alcohol consumption on CVD and mortality is entirely due to alcohol, others have hypothesized that additional benefits could be linked to other compounds present in wine. Wine in fact, particularly red wine, is rich in additional compounds, particularly polyphenols

Table 15.2 The phenolic compounds of wine

Flavonoids	Non-flavonoids
Anthocyanins	Stilbenoids (resveratrol)
Tannins	Phenolic acids (caffeic, benzoic, cinnamic acid)
Flavonols	Hydroxycinnamic acid
Proanthocyanidins (OPCs)	

(Table 15.2), which have been shown to be protective against atherosclerosis and many other diseases.

Up to 90% of red wine's phenolic content falls under the classification of flavonoids.

Anthocyanins and stilbenoids are largely present in the skin while phenolic acids in the pulp of grapes. Other phenols (catechins, proanthocyanidins, flavonols) are present in the skin and seeds. During the growth cycle of the grapevine, sunlight increases the concentration of phenolics in the grape berries, their development being an important component of canopy management. Red wines are richer in phenols, such as anthocyanin, proanthocyanidins, and flavonols, which are derived from the skin and seeds, while white wines mostly contain phenolic acids (caffeic acid) and lower quantities of catechins and stilbenes, which originate essentially from the pulp of berries.

Anthocyanins are responsible for the blue to red colors of red wines. Just as the sugars in the grape increase during ripening, so do the concentrations of anthocyanins. Likewise, anthocyanins are found in most grapes only in the outer cell layers of the skin, leaving the grape juice inside virtually colorless. Therefore, in order to provide wine with color pigmentation, during fermentation there must be contact with the grape skins in order for the anthocyanins to be extracted.

Tannins are a diverse family of chemical compounds in wine that can affect its color, aging ability and texture. They are perceived during wine tasting by the tactile drying sensation and sense of bitterness that they can leave in the mouth. Grape extracts are mainly rich in tannin monomers and small oligomers. The natural tannins found in grapes are known as proanthocyanidins, in view of their ability to release red anthocyanin pigments when they are heated in an acidic solution. Grape skin extracts contain four tannin monomers (catechin, epicatechin, gallocatechin, and epigallocatechin), as well as procyanidins and prodelphinidins oligomers.

15.5.2 The Role of Polyphenols: The Main Polyphenols in Red Wine

15.5.2.1 Resveratrol

Among the components in red wine, resveratrol is undoubtedly the most important and the best studied.

Resveratrol, a stilbenoid (3,5,4′-trihydroxy-trans-stilbene) with two phenolic rings, is contained in the skin of grape berries (*Vitis vinifera, Vitis labrusca*), but in lower amounts is also present in cranberries, blueberries, raspberry, and mulberries.

Plants produce resveratrol usually in response to mechanical injuries, ultraviolet radiation and as a defense against viral and fungal infections. Resveratrol is produced by grapes when they are stressed particularly by fungal pathogens, i.e., *Botrytis cinerea*. Grapes seem to use the resveratrol to increase their resistance to fungal growth and survive the stress it entails.

The resveratrol content in red wine is between 1.98 and 7.13 mg/L, depending upon the grape variety and the duration of the skin contact. White wine has much less resveratrol, between 0.05 and 1.80 mg/L, with respect to red wine which is fermented with the skins, allowing the wine to extract the resveratrol; white wine is fermented after the skin have been removed.

Here are some of resveratrol's numerous effects on health and diseases.

Cancer: Resveratrol has anticancer effects against several different tumor types at multiple stages of tumor initiation and proliferation. Specifically, resveratrol can induce cancer cell apoptosis by interfering with multiple signaling pathways activated in transformed cells [16]. Although resveratrol's anticancer action appears to be for tumors it can contact directly, such as cancer of the skin and the gastrointestinal tract, it has also been shown to prevent the development of mammary tumors in humans. According to a case–control study, women with high total intake of resveratrol had a lower risk of breast cancer compared with women with a low level of intake (OR: 0.39) [17]. More recently, a randomized, double-blind placebo-controlled trial reported that in women at an increased risk for breast cancer, twice daily resveratrol doses for a 12 week period was associated with a decrease in methylation of four cancer-related genes on posttreatment mammary tissue biopsies [18]. In cancer cell lines studied in vitro, resveratrol specifically killed cancer cells by a devastating increase in Ca^2 coupling between the greatly tethered endoplasmic reticulum and mitochondria [19]. Resveratrol moreover is active against bladder cancer. It has been demonstrated that resveratrol induces apoptosis and cell cycle arrest of human T24 bladder cancer cells in vitro and inhibits tumor growth in vivo [20]. In prostate cancer, resveratrol enhances prostate cancer cell response to ionizing radiation through a modulation of the AMPK, Akt, and mTOR pathways [21]. Finally, resveratrol has been demonstrated to inhibit human lung cancer cell proliferation and survival [22].

Antidiabetic Effects: Resveratrol acts as an agonist of PPARɣ, a nuclear receptor that is currently a pharmacological target of thiazolidinediones, also known as glitazones, for the treatment of type 2 diabetes mellitus [23].

Cognitive Effects: In aging free-living subjects with mild cognitive impairment, up to 1 drink/day of alcohol or wine has been found to decrease the rate of progression to dementia [24].

Cardioprotective Effects: Numerous studies have documented that a moderate intake of red wine is associated with a reduced risk of heart disease [25]. This effect has been attributed to alcohol and to other components of red wine, i.e., resveratrol. Resveratrol has been shown to inhibit platelet aggregation and to stimulate endothelial nitric oxide synthase (eNOS) leading to increased levels of NO [26, 27]. These specific effects of resveratrol should be considered additional to the heart benefits of alcohol.

Sirtuin Activation: The relationship between resveratrol and sirtuins is probably one of the most intriguing aspects linked to resveratrol. Sirtuins are hypothesized to play a key role in an organism's response to stresses (such as heat or starvation) and to be responsible for the life span-extending effects of calorie restriction. It has been found that resveratrol stimulates the activity of the sirtuin SIRT 1. (Sirtuin stands for "*silent mating type information regulation 2 homolog*") [1].

Seven sirtuin genes have been identified in mammals (SIRT 1–7). SIRT1 regulates processes such as glucose and insulin production, fat metabolism, and cell survival, leading to speculation that sirtuins might mediate the effects of caloric restriction in mammals [28].

SIRT 1, a NAD^+-dependent deacetylase, is a protein whose function in humans has not yet been elucidated, but its transgenic overexpression has been shown to prolong life span in yeast, *Caenorhabditis elegans*, *Saccharomyces cerevisiae*, and in flies, by activating the NAD^+-dependent histone deacetylase SIRT1. Yeast sirtuin proteins are known to regulate epigenetically gene silencing and suppress the recombination of rDNA. SIRT 1 has been also found to be downregulated in cells that have high insulin resistance. Inducing the expression of sirtuins in these cells increases insulin sensitivity, suggesting that these molecules, particularly SIRT-1, are associated with improved insulin sensitivity and glucose homeostasis in mice by stimulating the SIRT1-mediated deacetylation of the transcriptional coactivator PGC-1α [29].

Finally, SIRT1 stimulates autophagy by preventing the acetylation of proteins (via deacetylation) required for autophagy as demonstrated in cultured cells and embryonic and neonatal tissues [30]. Data obtained in *Caernorhabditis elegans* suggest that autophagy is required for the life span-extending effects of rapamycin as well as the increase in longevity promoted by caloric restriction and resveratrol [31]. Autophagy appears, therefore, to be the key mechanism that promotes life span extension and longevity in human and animal cells, worms and in flies. Autophagy is the target of caloric restriction and resveratrol. Resveratrol, therefore, appears to be involved in life span extension and longevity acting on autophagy through the same mechanisms of caloric restriction, that is through the SIRT-1-dependent induction of autophagy, the key mechanism of life span extension.

15.5.2.2 Anthocyanins

Anthocyanins are the second most represented antioxidant polyphenols in red wine. Anthocyanins and their downstream metabolites have been shown to have multiple metabolic effects. They alter signaling pathways involved in vascular inflammation, inhibit atherosclerosis development, improve endothelial function principally via improved blood flow, reduce NAD(P)H oxidase-dependent elimination of endothelial nitric oxide, and inhibit platelet function [32–36].

According to several short-term interventions, anthocyanins and flavanones led to a reduction in both systolic and diastolic blood pressure with favorable changes in arterial stiffness [37–42].

Anthocyanins have also been shown to exert beneficial effects on total and LDL cholesterol concentrations; some evidence has demonstrated that this effect is mediated by improvements in cholesterol efflux capacity [43, 44].

The findings of a recent trial have confirmed that anthocyanins have an anti-inflammatory effect in patients with hypercholesterolemia [45].

The relation between anthocyanin intake and coronary artery disease and stroke was also analyzed by the prospective *Health Professional Follow-up Study*. A multivariate analysis of data regarding a 24 year follow-up showed an inverse association between anthocyanins and nonfatal myocardial infarction (HR: 0.87). That study also showed that higher intakes of anthocyanins were associated with a lower risk of ischemic stroke (HR: 0.78) [32].

15.5.2.3 Proanthocyanidins (OPCs)

Proanthocyanidins are oligomeric flavonoids, essentially polymer chains of flavonoids such as catechins. They are also known as *OPCs* (*Oligomeric ProanthoCyanidins*), and are pycnogenol, leukocyanidin, and leucoanthocyanin. Found in grape seeds and skin, they are abundant in red wine, possibly the most abundant flavonoids according to some authors. It has been reported that *"Regions of the world with the greatest longevity also correspond to regions with the highest procyanidin flavonoids in their wines"* (*R. Corder—The red wine diet. Avery Publishing Group, Sept. 2007*).

The effects of proanthocyanidins include those of neutralizing oxidants and free radicals, depressing blood fat, and inhibiting the destruction of collagen, the most abundant protein in the body. These influences, along with other mechanisms, explain their beneficial effect with regard to venous and capillary disorders, including venous insufficiency, capillary fragility, diabetic retinopathy, and macular degeneration. The vascular benefits of red wine drinking have been reported to depend on the presence of oligomeric proanthocyanidins.

Some studies have shown that OPCs prevent cardiovascular disease by mitigating the negative effects of high cholesterol on the heart and blood vessels.

15.5.3 The Polyphenols in White Wine

15.5.3.1 Tyrosol

White wine is known to contain phenols, such as shikimic acid, caffeic acid, tyrosol, and hydroxy-tyrosol, that have antioxidant properties [46]. *n*-Tyrosol/2-(4-hydroxyphenyl) ethanol, a monophenol mostly contained in olive oil but also in white wine, is an active phenolic compound that has been shown in vitro to protect cells from oxidative stress. It was also shown that intravenous administration of *n*-tyrosol 10 min prior to coronary occlusion in an in vivo acute myocardial ischemia model of Wistar rats, significantly reduced the arrhythmic activity that occurs during myocardial ischemia and reperfusion [47].

It has been shown that the *n*-tyrosol/2-(4-hydroxyphenyl) ethanol of white wine provides cardioprotection against the ischemic stress induced by myocardial infarction in a rat in vivo LAD occlusion model. *n*-Tyrosol pretreatment significantly reduced the extent of the myocardial infarction and cardiomyocyte apoptosis followed by a decrease in ventricular remodeling as evidenced by a significant reduction in the collagenous fibrotic tissue. It also showed an improvement in left ventricular myocardial functions in conjunction with a significant increase in the levels of phosphorylated forms of Akt, eNOS, and FOXO3a along with an increased expression of nuclear SIRT1 in the *n*-tyrosol administered groups as compared to untreated controls [48].

15.5.3.2 Caffeic Acid

Caffeic acid is another monophenol contained in white wine with antioxidant properties. It has been reported to significantly reduce lipid peroxidation and diminish DNA damage in UVB-irradiated lymphocytes [49]. Furthermore, caffeic acid pretreatment significantly maintains antioxidant status and decreases UVB-induced cytotoxicity [49]. Moreover, it has also been shown that caffeic acid can reduce oxidative stress and inflammation induced by 12-*O*-tetradecanoyl-phorbol-13-acetate in vivo [50, 51].

At very low dosages, caffeic acid produces an effect that is similar to that observed after moderate white wine consumption. In fact, it exerts protective effects on human endothelial cell function by modulating NO release independently from eNOS expression and phosphorylation [52]. Caffeic acid-induced NO modulation has also been shown to limit cardiovascular and kidney disease progression associated with oxidative stress-mediated endothelial injury [52].

15.6 Melatonin in Wine

Recent studies have identified melatonin, an indoleamin (see BOX), in red and white wines (see also Chap. 10: Grapes).

Indolamines (or indoleamins) are a family of neurotransmitters that share a common molecular structure (namely, indolamine). Indolamines are a classification of monoamine neurotransmitters, along with catecholamines and melatonin. A common example of an indolamine is the tryptophan derivative serotonin, a neurotransmitter involved in mood and sleep. Another example of an indolamine is melatonin, which regulates the sleep-wake cycle (circadian rhythm) in humans.

Melatonin is synthesized during the winemaking process, specifically after the alcoholic fermentation of must by yeast. Indeed, melatonin is absent in grapes and musts and is formed during alcoholic fermentation. Melatonin, has been detected at 0.6, 0.5, and 0.4 ng mL^{-1} in Albana white, Sangiovese red, and Trebbiano white wines, respectively [53]. Other studies have reported melatonin also in Chardonnay, Malbec, and Cabernet Sauvignon wines, at 0.16, 0.24, and 0.32 ng mL^{-1}, respectively [54]. In Groppello and Merlot red wines, melatonin has been shown to vary between 5.2 and 8.1 ng mL^{-1}, depending on agrochemical treatments [55], while in rached wines higher concentration of melatonin have been found to range from 245 ng/mL (Merlot) to 423 ng/mL (Syrah) [56, 57].

The presence of melatonin in wines is a quite recent discovery. Melatonin was long believed to be a neurotransmitter secreted by the pineal gland only in vertebrates and humans, in whom it regulates sleep and circadian physiological functions through a receptor-mediated pathway. Receptor-independent processes have also been reported, mainly because of melatonin's powerful antioxidant activity. Melatonin can directly scavenge free radical species (both reactive oxygen and nitrogen species) and stimulate the activity of antioxidant enzymes; thus it is involved in immune responses and the pathogenesis of chronic-degenerative disorders.

The presence of melatonin in plants has been extensively described in the nineties also in a number of edible plants [58, 59]. So far, melatonin has been detected and quantified in roots, shoots, leaves, flowers, fruits, and seeds of a considerable variety of spermatophyte species, and its presence in plants has been confirmed [60].

The recently discovered melatonin in some relevant Mediterranean foods and in wines may represent a new factor contributing to the elucidation of the protective effects of diets rich in plant products. Therefore, in synergy with polyphenols and other bioactive phytochemicals (e.g., carotenoids and glucosinolates), melatonin may contribute to maximizing the benefits of a healthy dietary style such as the Mediterranean diet.

15.7 Concluding Remarks

Wine is probably the most ancient alcoholic beverage of mankind.

The maximum benefit from wine and alcohol occurs at relatively low levels of consumption (i.e., 1–2 standard drinks a day in men (10–20 g alcohol) and up to one a day in women (10 g alcohol)).

The most active compounds of wine are alcohol and phenolic compounds and the recently described presence of melatonin.

Alcohol, at low doses, is beneficial to lipoprotein metabolism reducing LDL cholesterol levels and increasing HDL cholesterol. It also improves insulin sensitivity, and it decreases fibrinogen and inflammatory markers [13] such as C-reactive protein and interleukin-6.

Resveratrol, the most active phenolic antioxidant of red wine, exerts beneficial effects with regard to the cardiovascular system, cancer, diabetes mellitus, age-related cognitive decline, and sirtuins involved in life-prolonging effects.

Anthocyanins, the second most active phenolic compounds in red wine, is beneficial in lowering LDL cholesterol, systolic and diastolic blood pressure, platelet aggregability, and the risk of myocardial infarction and ischemic stroke. Proanthocyanidins (OPCs) seem to be linked to longevity.

Thyrosol, a phenolic antioxidant of white wine, has cardioprotective effects against ischemic myocardial injuries.

Caffeic acid, the second most active phenolic antioxidant of white wine, protects endothelial functions and increases eNOS activity and NO production.

Melatonin, recently discovered in some relevant Mediterranean foods, may represent a new factor contributing to the elucidation of the protective effects of diets rich in plant products. In synergy with polyphenols and other bioactive phytochemicals (e.g., carotenoids and glucosinolates), melatonin may contribute to maximizing the benefits of Mediterranean diet, primarily linked to the prevention of numerous degenerative diseases and cancer.

References

1. Mark Berkowitz "World's Earliest Wine". Archaeology. Archaeological Institute of America, 1996; 49. Accessed 13 Jan 2011.
2. Jellinek EM. Drinkers and Alcoholics in Ancient Rome. Edited by Carole D. Yawney and Robert E. Popham. J Stud Alcohol. 1976;37:1718–40.
3. Cabras P, Martelli A. In: Chimica degli alimenti. Padova: Piccin Publisher; 2004. ISBN 88-299-1696-X.
4. Viticulture, volume 1—Resources, 2nd Edition, by Ed. Bryan Coombe and Peter Dry, 2004.
5. Mukamal KJ, Conigrave KM, Mittleman MA, Camargo CA, Stampfer MJ, Willet WC, Rimm EB. Roles of drinking pattern and type of alcohol consumed in coronary heart disease in men. New Engl J Med. 2003;348:109–18.
6. Pai JK, Mukamal KJ, Rimm EB. Long-term alcohol consumption in relation to all cause and cardiovascular mortality among survivors of myocardial infarction: the health professional follow-up study. Eur Heart J. 2012;33:1598–605.
7. Muntwyler J, Hennekens CH, Buring JE, Gaziano JM. Mortality and light to moderate alcohol consumption after myocardial infarction. Lancet. 1998;352:1882–5.
8. Mukamal KJ, Maclure M, Muller JE, Mittleman MA. Binge drinking and mortality after acute myocardial infarction. Circulation. 2005;112:3839–45.
9. Truelsen T, Grønbæk M, Schnohr P, Boysen G. Intake of beer, wine, and spirits and risk of stroke. The Copenhagen City Heart Study. Stroke. 1998;29:2467–72.
10. Rimm EB, Williams P, Fosher K, Criqui M, Stampfer MJ. Moderate alcohol intake and lower risk of coronary heart disease: meta-analysis of effects on lipids and haemostatic factors. BMJ. 1999;319:1523–8.
11. Kiechl S, Willeit J, Poewe W, Egger G, Oberhollenzer F, Muggeo M, Bonora E. Insulin sensitivity and regular alcohol consumption: large, prospective, cross sectional population study (Bruneck study). BMJ. 1996;313:1040–4.
12. Jensen T, Retterstol LJ, Sandset PM, Godal HC, Skjonsberg OH. A daily glass of red wine induces a prolonged reduction in plasma viscosity: a randomized controlled trial. Blood Coagul Fibrinolysis. 2006;17:471–6.
13. Pai JK, Hankinson SE, Thadhani R, Rifai N, Pischon T, Rimm EB. Moderate alcohol consumption and lower levels of inflammatory markers in US men and women. Atherosclerosis. 2006;186:113–20.
14. Vliegenthart R, Oei HH, van den Elzen AP, van Rooij FJ, Hofman A, Oudkerk M, Witteman JC. Alcohol consumption and coronary calcification in a general population. Arch Intern Med. 2004;164:2355–60.
15. Janszky I, Mukamal KJ, Orth-Gomer K, Romelsjo A, Schenck-Gustafsson K, Svane B, Kirkeeide RL, Mittleman MA. Alcohol consumption and coronary atherosclerosis progression—the Stockholm Female Coronary Risk Angiographic Study. Atherosclerosis. 2004;176:311–9.
16. Kotecha R, Takami A, Espinoza JL. Dietary phytochemicals and cancer chemoprevention: a review of the clinical evidence. Oncotarget. 2016;7:52517–29.
17. Levi F, Pasche C, Lucchini F, Ghidoni R, Ferraroni M, La Vecchia C. Resveratrol and breast cancer risk. Eur J Cancer Prev. 2005;14:139–42.
18. Medina-Aguilar R, Pérez-Plasencia C, Marchat LA, Gariglio P, García Mena J, Rodríguez Cuevas S, Ruíz-García E, Astudillo-de la Vega H, Hernández Juárez J, Flores-Pérez A, López-Camarillo C. Methylation landscape of human breast cancer cells in response to dietary compound resveratrol. PLoS One. 2016;11:e0157866.

19. Madreiter-Sokolowski CT, Gottschalk B, Parichatikanond W, Eroglu E, Klec C, Waldeck-Weiermair M, Malli R, Graier WF. Resveratrol specifically kills cancer cells by a devastating increase in the Ca^{2+} coupling between the greatly tethered endoplasmic reticulum and mitochondria. Cell Physiol Biochem. 2016;39:1404–20.
20. Bai Y, Mao QQ, Qin J, Zheng XY, Wang YB, Yang K, Shen HF, Xie LP. Resveratrol induces apoptosis and cell cycle arrest of human T24 bladder cancer cells in vitro and inhibits tumor growth in vivo. Cancer Sci. 2010;101:488–93.
21. Rashid A, Liu C, Sanli T, Tsiani E, Singh G, Bristow RG, Dayes I, Lukka H, Wright J, Tsakiridis T. Resveratrol enhances prostate cancer cell response to ionizing radiation. Modulation of the AMPK, Akt and mTOR pathways. Radiat Oncol. 2011;6:144.
22. Barron CC, Moore J, Tsakiridis T, Pickering G, Tsiani E. Inhibition of human lung cancer cell proliferation and survival by wine. Cancer Cell Int. 2014;14:6.
23. Wang L, Waltenberger B, Pferschy-Wenzig EM, Blunder M, Liu X, Malainer C, Blazevic T, Schwaiger S, Rollinger JM, Heiss EH, Schuster D, Kopp B, Bauer R, Stuppner H, Dirsch VM, Atanasov AG. Natural product agonists of peroxisome proliferator-activated receptor gamma (PPARγ): a review. Biochem Pharmacol. 2014;92:73–89.
24. Solfrizzi V, D'Introno A, Colacicco AM, Capurso C, Del Parigi A, Baldassarre Scapicchio P, Scafato E, Amodio M, Capurso A, Panza F, Italian Longitudinal Study on Aging Working Group. Alcohol consumption, mild cognitive impairment, and progression to dementia. Neurology. 2007;68:1790–9.
25. Szmitko PE, Verma S. Cardiology patient pages. Red wine and your heart. Circulation. 2005;111:e10–1.
26. Duffy SJ, Vita JA. Vita. Effects of phenolics on vascular endothelial function. Curr Opin Lipidol. 2003;14:21–7.
27. Olas B, Wachowicz B. Resveratrol, a phenolic antioxidant with effects on blood platelet functions. Platelets. 2005;16:251–60.
28. Guarente L, Picard F. Calorie restriction—the SIR2 connection. Cell. 2005;120:473–82.
29. Lagouge M, Argmann C, Gerhart-Hines Z, Meziane H, Lerin C, Daussin F, Messadeq N, Milne J, Lambert P, Elliott P, Geny B, Laakso M, Puigserver P, Auwerx J. Resveratrol improves mitochondrial function and protects against metabolic disease by activating SIRT1 and PGC-1alpha. Cell. 2006;127:1109–22.
30. Lee IH, Cao L, Mostoslavsky R, Lombard DB, Liu J, Bruns NE, Tsokos M, Alt FW, Finkel T. A role for the NAD-dependent deacetylase Sirt-1 in the regulation of autophagy. Proc Natl Acad Sci. 2008;105(9):3374.
31. Morselli E, Maiuri MC, Markaki M, Megalou E, Pasparaki A, Palikaras K, Criollo A, et al. Caloric restriction and resveratrol promote longevity through the Sirtuin-1 dependent induction of autophagy. Cell Death Dis. 2010;1:e10.
32. Cassidy A, Bertoia M, Chiuve S, Flint A, Forman J, Rimm EB. Habitual intake of anthocyanins and flavanones and risk of cardiovascular disease in men. Am J Clin Nutr. 2016;104:587–94.
33. Lamy S, Beaulieu E, Labbe D, Bedard V, Moghrabi A, Barrette S, Kissela BM, Kittner SJ, Lichtman JH, Lisabeth LD, et al. Delphinidin, a dietary anthocyanidin, inhibits platelet-derived growth factor ligand/receptor (PDGF/PDGFR) signaling. Carcinogenesis. 2008;29:1033–41.
34. Toufektsian MC, de Lorgeril M, Nagy N, Salen P, Donati MB, Giordano L, Mock HP, Peterek S, Matros A, Petroni K, et al. Chronic dietaryintake of plant-derived anthocyanins protects the rat heart against ischemiareperfusion injury. J Nutr. 2008;138:747–52.
35. Rizza S, Muniyappa R, Iantorno M, Kim JA, Chen H, Pullikotil P, Senese N, Tesauro M, Lauro D, Cardillo C, et al. Citrus polyphenol hesperidin stimulates production of nitric oxide in endothelial cells while improving endothelial function and reducing inflammatory markers in patients with metabolic syndrome. J Clin Endocrinol Metab. 2011;96:E782–92.
36. Jin YR, Han XH, Zhang YH, Lee JJ, Lim Y, Chung JH, Yun YP. Antiplatelet activity of hesperetin, a bioflavonoid, is mainly mediated by inhibition of PLC-gamma2 phosphorylation and cyclooxygenase-1 activity. Atherosclerosis. 2007;194:144–52.

37. Erlund I, Koli R, Alfthan G, Marniemi J, Puukka P, Mustonen P, Mattila P, Jula A. Favorable effects of berry consumption on platelet function, blood pressure, and HDL cholesterol. Am J Clin Nutr. 2008;87:323–31.
38. Basu A, Du M, Leyva MJ, Sanchez K, Betts NM, Wu M, Aston CE, Lyons TJ. Blueberries decrease cardiovascular risk factors in obese men and women with metabolic syndrome. J Nutr. 2010;140:1582–7.
39. Johnson SA, Figueroa A, Navaei N, Wong A, Kalfon R, Ormsbee LT, Feresin RG, Elam ML, Hooshmand S, Payton ME, et al. Daily blueberry consumption improves blood pressure and arterial stiffness in postmenopausal women with pre- and stage 1-hypertension: a randomized, double-blind, placebo-controlled clinical trial. J Acad Nutr Diet. 2015;115:369–77.
40. Dohadwala MM, Holbrook M, Hamburg NM, Shenouda SM, Chung WB, Titas M, Kluge MA, Wang N, Palmisano J, Milbury PE, et al. Effects of cranberry juice consumption on vascular function in patients with coronary artery disease. Am J Clin Nutr. 2011;93:934–40.
41. Habauzit V, Verny MA, Milenkovic D, Barber-Chamoux N, Mazur A, Dubray C, Morand C. Flavanones protect from arterial stiffness in postmenopausal women consuming grapefruit juice for 6 mo: a randomized, controlled, crossover trial. Am J Clin Nutr. 2015;102:66–74.
42. Morand C, Dubray C, Milenkovic D, Lioger D, Martin JF, Scalbert A, Mazur A. Hesperidin contributes to the vascular protective effects of orange juice: a randomized crossover study in healthy volunteers. Am J Clin Nutr. 2011;93:73–8.
43. Basu A, Betts NM, Nguyen A, Newman ED, Fu D, Lyons TJ. Freeze-dried strawberries lower serum cholesterol and lipid peroxidation in adults with abdominal adiposity and elevated serum lipids. J Nutr. 2014;144:830–7.
44. Zhu Y, Huang X, Zhang Y, Wang Y, Liu Y, Sun R, Xia M. Anthocyanin supplementation improves HDL-associated paraoxonase 1 activity and enhances cholesterol efflux capacity in subjects with hypercholesterolemia. J Clin Endocrinol Metab. 2014;99:561–9.
45. Zhu Y, Ling W, Guo H, Song F, Ye Q, Zou T, Li D, Zhang Y, Li G, Xiao Y, et al. Anti-inflammatory effect of purified dietary anthocyanin in adults with hypercholesterolemia: a randomized controlled trial. Nutr Metab Cardiovasc Dis. 2013;23(9):843.
46. Thirunavukkarasu M, Penumathsa SV, Samuel SM, Akita Y, Zhan L, Bertelli AAE, Das DK, Maulik N. White Wine induced Cardioprotection against ischemia-reperfusion injury is mediated by life extending Akt/FOXO3a/NFkappaB survival pathway. J Agric Food Chem. 2008;56:6733–9.
47. Chernyshova GA, Plotnikov MB, Smol'yakova VI, Golubeva IV, Aliev OI, Tolstikova TG, Krysin AP, Sorokina IV. Antiarrhythmic activity of n-tyrosol during acute myocardial ischemia and reperfusion. Bull Exp Biol Med. 2007;143:689–91.
48. Samuel SM, Thirunavukkarasu M, Penumathsa SV, Paul D, Maulik N. Akt/FOXO3a/SIRT1 mediated cardioprotection by n-tyrosol against ischemic stress in rat in vivo model of myocardial infarction: switching gears towards survival and longevity. J Agric Food Chem. 2008;56:9692–8.
49. Prasad NR, Jeyanthimala K. Ramachandran S. Caffeic acid modulates ultraviolet radiation-B induced oxidative damage in human blood lymphocytes. J Photochem Photobiol. B. 2009;95:196–203.
50. Khan AQ, Khan R, Qamar W, Lateef A, Ali F, et al. Caffeic acid attenuates 12-O-tetradecanoylphorbol-13-acetate (TPA)-induced NF-kB and COX-2 expression in mouse skin: abrogation of oxidative stress, inflammatory responses and proinflammatory cytokine production. Food Chem Toxicol. 2012;50:175–83.
51. Bertelli AA. Wine, research and cardiovascular disease: instructions for use. Atherosclerosis. 2007;195:242–7.
52. Migliori M, Cantaluppi V, Mannari C, Bertelli AAE, Medica D, Quercia AD, Navarro V, Scatena A, Giovannini L, Biancone L, Panichi V. Caffeic acid, a pieno found in white wine, modulates endothelial nitric oxide production and protects from oxidative stress-associated endothelial cell injury. PLoS One. 2015;10:e0117530.
53. Mercolini L, Mandrioli R, Raggi MA. Content of melatonin and other antioxidants in grape related foodstuffs: measurement using a MEPS-HPLC-F method. J Pineal Res. 2012;53:21–8.

54. Stege PW, Sombra LL, Messina G, Martinez LD, Silva MD. Determination of melatonin in wine and plant extracts by capillary electrochromatography with immobilized carboxylic multi-walled carbon nanotubes as stationary phase. Electrophoresis. 2010;31:2242–8.
55. Vitalini S, Gardana C, Zanzotto A, Fico G, Faoro F, Simonetti P, et al. From vineyard to glass: agrochemicals enhance the melatonin and total polyphenol contents and antiradical activity of red wines. J Pineal Res. 2011;51:278–85.
56. Rodriguez-Naranjo MI, Gil-Izquierdo A, Troncoso AM, Cantos E, Garcia-Parrilla MC. Melatonin: a new bioactive compound in wine. J Food Compos Anal. 2011;24:603–8.
57. Rodriguez-Naranjo MI, Gil-Izquierdo A, Troncoso AM, Cantos-Villar E, Garcia-Parrilla MC. Melatonin is synthesized by yeast during alcoholic fermentation in wines. Food Chem. 2011;126:1608–13.
58. Dubbels R, Reiter RJ, Klenke E, Goebel A, Schnakenberg E, Ehlers C, et al. Melatonin in edible plants identified by radioimmunoassay and by high performance liquid chromatography-mass spectrometry. J Pineal Res. 1995;18:28–31.
59. Hattori A, Migitaka H, Iigo M, Itoh M, Yamamoto K, Ohtani-Kaneko R, et al. Identification of melatonin in plants and its effects on plasma melatonin levels and binding to melatonin receptors in vertebrates. Biochem Mol Biol Int. 1995;35:627–34.
60. Paredes SD, Korkmaz A, Manchester LC, Tan D-X, Reiter RJ. Phytomelatonin: a review. J Exp Bot. 2009;60:57–69.

The Impact of the Mediterranean Diet on Aging, Frailty, and Longevity

16

16.1 Aging and Frailty

In the European Union, the number of people aged 65+ will almost double over the next 50 years, from 85 million in 2008 to 151 million in 2060 [1]. As reported by Clegg et al. [2], population aging is also accelerating rapidly worldwide. People older than 65 years increased from 461 million in 2004 to an estimated rate of 2 billion people by 2050 [3, 4]. This has profound implications for planning and provision of health and social care. The longer life does not go, however, perceived as a social and health problem. Indeed, it is an incredibly precious resource. It offers the opportunity to reconsider not only what older age might be, but how our whole life could unfold [5, 6]. For example, in high-income countries, there is evidence that many people are trying to spend these extra years of their advanced age in innovative ways, such as taking up a new career or continuing education; otherwise, they are pursuing a neglected passion [7]. However, the scope of opportunities that arise from these extra years of life are heavily dependent on the state of health and self-sufficiency of everyone. That is, if we live in good health the years of our old age, our ability to dedicate ourselves to our activities will be little different from that of a younger person. If these added years are dominated by the decline in the state of health and self-sufficiency and mental state, then the implications for older people and for society will be much more negative [6].

16.2 What Is Frailty

The probably most problematic expression of the aging population is the clinical condition of frailty. The frailty can be defined as a condition of the elderly characterized by a serious reduction of the functional reserve of organs and apparatuses, very close to the threshold of the clinical appearance of symptoms of organ decompensation. Frailty, therefore, is a state of the most vulnerables to poor resolution of homeostasis after a stress event, which increases the risk of negative outcomes,

A. Capurso et al., *Benefits of the Mediterranean Diet in the Elderly Patient*, Practical Issues in Geriatrics, https://doi.org/10.1007/978-3-319-78084-9_16

including falls, delirium, and disability [8–10]. Frail individuals are vulnerable and at high risk of adverse health outcomes. They have functional impairments, which often result in falls, immobility, and confusion. Frailty limits regular physical activity and its many health benefits, including the prevention of cognitive decline. People affected by frailty make the most use of community resources, hospitals, and long-term care institutions. The natural course of frailty is progressive, increasing the risk of comorbidity and disability over time [11]. It means that an apparently small insult (e.g., a new drug, minor infection, or minor surgery) results in a striking and disproportionate change in health state, i.e., from independent to dependent, mobile to immobile, postural stability to proneness to falling, or lucid to delirious [2]. Frailty develops because of age-related decline in many physiological systems, which altogether lead to a greater vulnerability to sudden changes in the state of health triggered by minor stress events. Between a quarter and half of people older than 85 years are estimated to be frail, and these people have a substantially increased risk of falls, disability, long-term care, and death [8, 12]. On the other hand, half of the three-quarters of people over 85 are estimated not to be frail, which raises several questions about how frailty develops, how it could be prevented, and how it can be reliably detected. Although most geriatricians intuitively recognize frailty, it is commonly neglected and confused with disability and various comorbidities [11].

Contrary to what one might think, frailty is not an inevitable consequence of aging, but has been recognized as an independent geriatric syndrome [8, 13–15]. It would therefore be more appropriate to define it as "*frailty syndrome,*" that is, the result of the interaction among various factors, including physiological alterations observed in aging, poly-pathology, nutritional deficiencies, negative impact of socio-environmental factors, and lifestyle (Fig. 16.1). Consequently, two goals are important for the clinician: first, identify the causes of frailty, hence its association

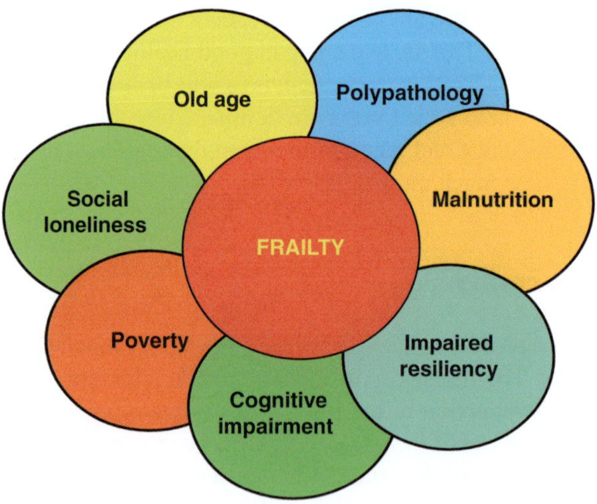

Fig. 16.1 The "rose of frailty"

with chronic inflammation and comorbidity; secondly, to develop an effective strategy for controlling the course and limiting disability.

16.3 Aging Is Not Synonymous with Frailty

Aging has been defined as the progressive loss of tissue and organ functionalities occurring throughout an individual's life [16]; it is due to the accumulation of senescent cells in the above tissues and organs. Cell senescence is regulated by a series of genes that are defined as pleiotropic antagonists [17] as they play an important role in anticancer protection, ultimately eliminating pre-neoplastic cells from the cell cycle, thus preventing malignant degeneration [18, 19]; the same genes are also implicated as responsible for aging and age-related diseases [20–22].

16.3.1 The Impact of Senescence on Human Health

Senescence causes a loss of tissue-repair capacity because of cell cycle arrest in progenitor cells. In addition, senescent cells produce pro-inflammatory and matrix-degrading molecules in what is known as the senescence-associated secretory phenotype (SASP). Persistent senescent cells in the adult are produced in two different contexts related to human health: healthy aging and age-related disease. In healthy aging, tissue and functional changes affect all individuals, while age-related diseases affect only a few. In aging individuals, the processes required for tissue homeostasis inevitably cause functional and structural degenerative alterations in the cells, resulting in senescence. These senescent cells can persist in the body due to defects in the immune system aged or because isolate senescent cells do not have sufficient signaling to attract resident immune cells. Similarly, senescent cells that are "acutely" generated by wound repair processes, tumor suppression processes, or other unknown processes can be completely disposed of by the aged immune system and survive in the body. Overall, senescent cells that arise from multiple mechanisms reduce the functional efficiency of the tissues and organs during aging. At the same time, they make tissues and organs more susceptible to further deterioration when attacked by other stressors [23].

In natural aging, senescence is probably induced by the combination of telomeric shortening, DNA oxidative damage, endoplasmic reticulum (ER) stress, and other degenerative factors responsible for macromolecular damage that slowly accumulate in cells [24–26]. The disease occurs when additional stress factors challenge the rich tissues of senescent cells, such as insulin-resistant fat, stressed by a high-fat diet [27–29]. Stress capable of causing disease may be unusual, such as DNA-damaging agents in cigarette smoke, or simply a more prolonged or more intense version of the same stresses operating in normal aging, such as telomere erosion following the repair of smoke-damaged lung epithelium [30]. When these results are taken together, a complex interaction between senescent cells and local and systemic environmental factors emerges.

Over time, these effects are added to cellular changes related to physiological aging, further reducing tissue function and decreasing stress resistance. That is, when stress persists in a tissue already affected by cellular senescence, it is more likely that a pathology condition develops [23].

16.4 Senescence, Diabetes, and Atherosclerosis

16.4.1 Senescence and Type 2 Diabetes Mellitus

In physiological conditions, circulating glucose triggers an insulin release from the pancreas, allowing insulin-susceptible peripheral tissues, such as fat and skeletal muscle, to take glucose for cellular respiration [31] (see also Chap. 4, this book). In obese, build-up of abdominal fat tissue, characterized by a chronic inflammatory state, and the excess of free circulating fatty acids, can cause a state of peripheral tissue insulin resistance [32, 33], which requires that the more insulin-producing pancreas maintain normal glucose levels. The proliferation of insulin-secreting beta-pancreatic cells is necessary to satisfy the demand. If insulin demand for peripheral tissue exceeds supply, it will develop Type-2 Diabetes Mellitus (T2DM). The increase in beta cells replication activity leads to senescence by telomeres attrition [34], thus limiting the adaptive response to insulin resistance and leading to the development of T2DM. The reduced ability to maintain glucose homeostasis in aging can lead to widespread glucose toxicity. This global stress can drive cellular senescence in various cell types such as fibroblasts, kidney tubular epithelial cells, endothelial cells, and mesenchymal stem cells [35–38]. This potential of glucose to drive cellular senescence globally may contribute to other important age-related pathologies, such as vascular diseases, kidney disease [38], and Alzheimer's disease.

16.4.2 Senescence and Atherosclerosis

In addition to causing T2DM, the stress of a high-fat diet can also drive atherosclerosis. Atherosclerosis is a disease of major arteries in which high levels of low-density lipoprotein (LDL) bearing oxidative modifications accumulate in vessel walls, attracting phagocytic immune cells to form plaques [39, 40]. During plaque formation and expansion, smooth-muscle proliferation and declining levels of endothelial nitric oxide synthase can lead to telomere shortening and oxidative stress, respectively [41, 42]. Because of the complex signaling between these cell types and immune cells recruited to plaques, these findings raise the possibility of a multistep role of senescent cells in atherogenesis. As in cancer prevention, senescence in atherosclerosis may serve an initial protective role by restricting proliferation within developing lesions and minimizing plaque-disrupting apoptosis. However, at some threshold of senescence burden, the pro-inflammatory, matrix-degrading SASP may exacerbate disease [23].

16.5 Diet, Metabolism, and Frailty

16.5.1 The Effects of Caloric Restriction

It is known that many metabolic changes, including modulation of mitochondrial function, decreases insulin sensitivity and alterations in substrate usage accompanies aging [43]. These changes can contribute to the aging of the phenotype and predisposes an individual to age-related conditions. In both experimental mouse models and humans, Caloric Restriction (CR) does have marked effects on weight and white adipose tissue (WAT) biology [44]. Although overall weight loss is common, a large fraction of the weight loss comes from the WAT and visceral fat stores [45, 46]. Interestingly, the common strains of laboratory rodents all experience extended life spans in response to CR, but this is not a universal effect. Indeed, certain inbred mice strains show only a modest effect or even a reductive effect on life span after CR [47]. Another bioenergetic effect of CR is a decreased reliance on carbohydrates and an increased utilization of fatty acid oxidation [48]. In fact, the degree of fat loss induced by food restriction is an important variable that seems to correlate with the beneficial effects of CR. In an analysis conducted on nearly 40 strains of mice, the beneficial longevity effects of CR were correlated with those mice that were best able to maintain fat stores, in the setting of a 40% CR regimen [49]. Moreover, results from a study conducted on progeroid mice models showed that a dietary restriction of 30% tripled the median and maximal remaining life spans of these mice. Mice undergoing dietary restriction retained 50% more neurons and maintained full motor function far beyond the life span of mice fed ad libitum.

Molecular analysis of gene expression suggested that dietary restriction increases resistance to DNA damage-induced stress, improves antioxidant defenses, and change insulin and other hormonal signaling pathways. Dietary restriction also changes mitochondrial function and apoptotic responses and induces a shift from pro- to anti-inflammatory cytokines [50]. It is well known, from randomized studies and subsequent meta-analysis, that aging is associated with a physiological reduction of appetite, resulting in reduced energy intake [51]. In addition, the results of some randomized human trials indicate that caloric restriction bolsters the body's ability to adapt to use whatever energy substrates are available, be those of glucose or fatty acids [52]. This adaptation is known as metabolic flexibility, a property that has long been linked to metabolic health and, increasingly, longevity [43]. There is also a strong link between CR and reduced inflammation, as shown in randomized data from nonhuman primates [53]. The exact molecular basis for these effects is unclear; however, it is of interest that a recent report has linked a rise in serum β-hydroxybutyrate, a ketone metabolite known to increase during fasting, to inhibition of the inflammasome [54]. Such metabolic-based inhibition of inflammasome activation may be at least one mechanism through which CR could suppress detrimental activation of the immune system. Other possibilities include a CR-induced delay in thymic involution, thus preserving T cell function [55], or a reduction in oxidative stress-induced inflammation [56].

16.5.2 Mitochondrial Activity and Aging

Numerous screens in model organisms involved nuclear-encoded mitochondrial proteins in the regulation of life span [57, 58]. Most of these genetic interventions have altered the expression of electron transport chain components that have compromised mitochondrial function and, however, have resulted in longer life expectancy [44]. This is difficult to conceptualize because human aging is generally associated with a decline in mitochondrial function [59]. Likewise, in mice models bearing significant mitochondrial genome mutations designed to significantly impair mitochondrial function, a phenotype characterized by accelerated aging was observed [60, 61]. The best explanation for these apparently contradictory observations is that they vary depending on the extent of the mitochondrial damage that has been achieved. For example, in experiments conducted on *C. elegans*, while a modest reduction in various components of mitochondrial electron transport leads to an increase in life expectancy, a significant reduction, i.e., a high mitochondrial damage, shorten the life span [62]. There is also genetic evidence in mammalian models that mild impairment of mitochondrial function might extend life span. This concept seems antithetical to the long-held belief that reactive oxygen species (ROS) fuels the aging process [63]. Although it is certainly clear that mithochondrial ROS can be harmful for the life span [64], there is also evidence that a small increase in mitochondrial ROS production may also trigger the activation of redox-sensitive pathways with long-lasting and prolonged protective effects.

The general concept that a little stress can protect against larger, subsequent stresses is often termed *hormesis*, and when specifically concerning the mitochondria, is termed as *mitohormesis* [65–67]. It is also apparent that ROS levels are not the only mediator of mitochondrial stress that can increase life span. Mitochondrial turnover—namely, the balance between the synthesis of new mitochondria (biogenesis) and the removal of old and damaged mitochondria (mitophagy)—represents an additional process that connects mitochondria to aging. Evidence suggests that interventions that increase longevity, such as CR, stimulate the mitochondrial-biogenesis through the induction of peroxisome proliferation-activated receptor gamma, and coactivator 1 alpha (PGC-1α) expression [68, 69]. Consequently, it is believed that a decline in the biogenesis both through the reduced activity of PGC-1a and through other routes contributes to various age-related diseases [70]. Mitochondrial quality control also requires the removal of mitochondria that are old and damaged. Aging seems to produce a gradual decline in autophagic activity [71], and it is presumed that the more specialized process of mitophagy follows a similar age-dependent decline. Indeed, in experimental models, the overexpression of gene products that appear to stimulate selectively mitochondria seems to prolong life expectancy [72].

16.6 The Mediterranean Diet

As already discussed above (see Chap. 1), the traditional Mediterranean Diet (MD) is characterized by a high intake of foods of plant origin (fruit, vegetables, breads, other cereals, potatoes, beans, nuts, and seeds) and fresh fruit as daily dessert [73].

Olive oil is the principal source of fats. Dairy products (mainly light cheese and yogurt), fish and poultry are consumed in low-to-moderate amounts, egg consumption is limited to a maximum of four per week, red meat is consumed in low amounts, sporadically, or no more than once a week. MD is low in saturated fats, which are no more than 8% of the total caloric intake. The caloric intake derived from fats does not exceed 30% of the total caloric intake [74]. Wine is consumed in low-to-moderate amounts, normally with meals [75]. From Ancel Keys' studies, which suggested beneficial health effects derived from the MD [76], the MD has been proposed as a healthy diet model, and has been associated with a lower risk of cardiovascular and metabolic diseases.

The traditional MD has also been proposed as an optimal weight-loss diet model. A population-based, prospective study conducted by Trichopoulou et al. [77] involving 22,043 Greek adults to assess the relation between adherence to the MD and total mortality, assessed by the Mediterranean Diet Score [78], showed that a two-point increment in the Mediterranean-diet score was associated with a 25% reduction in total mortality (adjusted HR = 0.75; 95%CI: 0.64–0.87; $P < 0.001$). Particularly, the adherence to the MD was associated to a 32% reduction of mortality from coronary heart disease (adjusted HR = 0.67; 95%CI: 0.47–0.94). Mortality from cancer was also reduced significantly (adjusted HR = 0.76; 95%CI: 0.59–0.98). This inverse association between the Mediterranean-diet score and total mortality was also evident after adjustment for age, sex, years of education, smoking status, body-mass index, waist-to-hip ratio, energy-expenditure score, and total energy intake. Importantly, the only measures that predicted total mortality were the intake of fruit and nuts and the relationship between monounsaturated lipids and saturated lipids.

This finding was later confirmed by the results of PREDIMED Study [79], which revealed that, among subjects at high cardiovascular risk, a MD supplemented with extra-virgin olive oil (EVOO), that is an intake of monounsaturated fatty acids and antioxidants, or nuts, this is a supply of n-3 polyunsaturated fatty acids, reduced the incidence of acute myocardial infarction, stroke, or death from any cardiovascular causes event (MD with EVOO: hazard ratio = 0.70, 95% CI: 0.53–0.91, $P = 0.009$; MD with nuts: hazard ratio = 0.70, 95% CI: 0.53–0.94, $P = 0.02$). Subsequently, [80] a large meta-analysis of prospective cohort studies which reviewed studies that analyzed prospectively the association between adherence to a MD pattern, mortality, and incidence of diseases, involving a total of 1,574,299 subjects followed for a time ranging from 3 to 18 years, established that a greater adherence to a MD is associated with a significant improvement in health status and with a reduced risk of mortality (RR = 0.91; 95%CI: 0.89–0.94; $P < 0.0001$). Particularly authors showed that a greater adherence to a MD pattern is associated with a significant reduction in mortality for cardiovascular diseases (RR = 0.91; 95%CI: 0.87–0.95; $P < 0.0001$) and for cancer (RR = 0.94; 95%CI: 0.92–0.96; $P < 0.0001$). A further meta-analysis conducted subsequently by the same authors on cohort prospective studies, involving 2,190,627 subjects [81], has confirmed the above findings, namely that a high adherence to the Mediterranean Diet model is associated to a better health status, better quality of life, and with a significant reduction of overall mortality (RR = 0.92; 95%CI: 0.90–0.94; $P < 0.0001$), cardiovascular incidence or

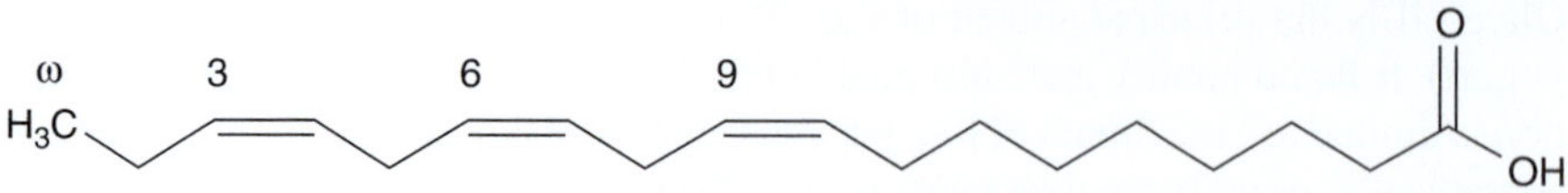

Fig. 16.2 Alpha-linolenic acid (ALA) formula

mortality (RR = 0.90; 95%CI: 0.87–0.93; $P < 0.0001$), cancer incidence or mortality (RR = 0.94; 95%CI: 0.92–0.96; $P < 0.0001$), and neurodegenerative diseases (RR = 0.87; 95%CI: 0.81–0.94; $P < 0.0001$), including mild cognitive impairment.

16.6.1 *n*-3 Polyunsaturated Fatty Acids

Concerning the dietary intake of *n*-3 polyunsaturated fatty acids, which is linked to a reduction in the incidence of aging-associated disease, including cardiovascular disease and stroke, an elegant study conducted by Qi et al. [82] showed that the treatment of *Caenorhabditis elegans* with α-linolenic acid (ALA) (Fig. 16.2), produced a dose-dependent increase in life span. The increased longevity of the GLP-1 mutant animals, which show an increased production of the ALA, is known to be dependent on both the NHR-49/PPARa and SKN-1/Nrf2 transcription factors. Authors found that ALA treatment increased the life span of wild-type worms and that these effects required both transcription factors. Specifically, NHR-49 was activated by ALA to promote the expression of genes involved in the b-oxidation of lipids, whereas SKN-1 is not directly activated by ALA, but instead, the exposure of ALA to air results in the oxidation of ALA to a group of compounds termed oxylipins. At least one of the oxylipins activates SKN-1 and enhances the increased longevity. Results of this study shows that *n*-3 fatty acids inhibit aging and that these effects could reflect the combined effects of the *n*-3 fatty acid and the oxylipin metabolites. The authors conclude by advancing the hypothesis that the benefits of *n*-3 fatty acid consumption on human health may similarly involve oxylipin production.

16.7 The Mediterranean Diet and Aging

16.7.1 The Mediterranean Diet, Mortality, and Life Span

It is well known that most of the interindividual variation in life span is explained by stochastic and environmental factors, including diet. It is also well known that dietary caloric restriction (CR, restriction in energy supply while ensuring adequate intake of all nutrients) can extend the life span in rodents and a similar effect has been demonstrated in several other model organisms including yeast, worms, flies, fish, and spiders [83]. The CR paradigm has been invaluable in elucidating the molecular pathways that modulate aging including the insulin-like growth factor-1/insulin signaling pathway, the sirtuin pathway, the AMP activated protein kinase pathway, and the mammalian target of rapamycin pathway, all of which interact [48, 84].

There is convincing evidence that CR and exercise prevent and defend from multiple forms of cellular and molecular damage associated with aging, which mediate intrinsic and progressive functional decline with aging. Conversely, excessive nutrition and physical inactivity increase the risk of disease and accelerate aging. CR and exercise enhance the resistance of an organism to challenges and maintain physiological function. However, in all conditions of compromised resilience, chronic illness, multimodality, disability, and frailty manifest themselves and compromise the health and longevity. In these cases, the CR has no beneficial effects; on the contrary, it can compromise the response to infections, as well as healing wounds and fractures, until it leads to a complete inability to recover. However, short-term refeeding may be able to undo these negative effects of CR [85] (Fig. 16.3).

Since 1995 Trichopoulou et al. [78] provided evidence that a nutritional pattern of the MD favorably affects life expectancy among elderly people. They showed that a high adherence to the MD, which was assessed with a validated extensive semiquantitative questionnaire on food intake, was associated with a significant 17% reduction in overall mortality. They also showed that a higher diet score was significantly associated with a sharply reduced risk of death, by 17% per one-unit increase and by more than 50% per four-unit increase. Subsequent evidence further confirmed the link between lifestyle and behavioral factors in the mid-life and their association with successful aging and the primary prevention or delay of disability, dementia, frailty, and noncommunicable chronic conditions, including cancer. The long-term impact of beneficial behavioral factors in middle to older age adults results in a greater chance of successful aging and in the primary prevention or delay of disability, dementia, frailty, and noncommunicable chronic conditions. Lafortune et al. [86] conducted a systematic review of 164 cohort and case-control

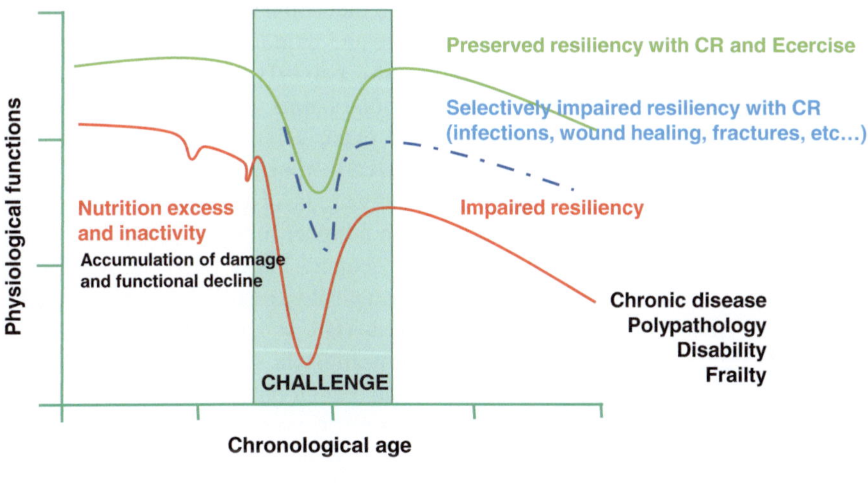

Fig. 16.3 Effect of Caloric Restriction on resiliency in healthy aging and in frailty. (Adapted from: Huffman DM [85])

studies. The authors have shown, with consistent evidence [87–89], that a healthy diet in mid-life is related to healthy and successful aging, where healthy and successful aging are defined as absence of major chronic diseases or major impairments in cognitive or physical function or mental health. A Mediterranean-type diet is associated to a more successful aging [89]. On the contrary, a Western dietary pattern (characterized by high intakes of fried and sweet food, processed food and red meat, refined grains, and high-fat dairy products) was associated with less successful aging. Doubtlessly, environment and lifestyle play a major role in human health and aging.

There is a consistent evidence that adherence to the Mediterranean dietary pattern is associated with reduced mortality risk, a benefit that appears to be independent of geography, as shown by the EPIC-elderly prospective cohort study [90], a multicenter, prospective cohort study, which examined whether adherence to the MD model was associated with greater life expectancy among older Europeans. Authors examined 74,607 men and women, aged 60 or more, from nine European countries (Denmark, France, Germany, Greece, Italy, the Netherlands, Spain, Sweden, and United Kingdom). They used a modified version of the Mediterranean Diet Score, where monounsaturated lipids were substituted with the sum of monounsaturated and polyunsaturated lipids in the numerator of the lipid ratio. This allowed the score to be applied to non-Mediterranean populations, in which intake of monounsaturated from olive oil is minimal. Authors showed that an increase in the modified Mediterranean Diet Score was associated with lower overall mortality; specifically, an increase of two units corresponded to a statistically significant reduction of 8% (95%CI 3–12%). In addition, the authors found no statistically significant evidence of heterogeneity among the countries in the association of overall mortality scores, although the association was stronger in Greece and Spain, probably because in these countries the modified Mediterranean diet was genuinely a MD and was followed uniformly by the entire population. In Italy, most deaths occurred in northern Italy, where the traditional diet could not be considered a MD.

Concerning the association between lifestyle and mortality, there are few studies among the oldest old in developing countries. Shi et al. [91] conducted an interesting study that examined the association between food habits, lifestyle factors, and all-cause mortality in people aged 80 years and older, using data from the Chinese Longitudinal Healthy Longevity Survey (CLHLS), from the baseline survey until 2011. 8959 participants aged 80 years and older were involved. Authors showed that daily fruit intake was inversely associated with a higher mortality risk (HR = 0.85; 95%CI: 0.77–0.92; $p < 0.01$), as also daily vegetables intake (HR = 0.74; 95%CI: 0.66–0.83; $p < 0.01$). On the contrary, there was a positive association between intake of salt-preserved vegetables and mortality risk (HR = 1.10; 95%CI: 1.03–1.18; $p < 0.001$). Authors also constructed a "healthy lifestyle score" that was based on three factors: daily intake of fruit, vegetable, and regular physical activity. A positive answer to each of the three-lifestyle factors was given a score of one. The maximum total score was three. Subjects who scored three, that means a healthy lifestyle score, had 2 years longer median survival, even if they had chronic diseases.

16.7.2 The Mediterranean Diet and Inflammation

There are now established evidence confirming that the MD significantly reduces mortality rates for various chronic diseases, including cardiovascular disease, neurodegenerative diseases, and cancer [92]. At the basis of this association there is the synergistic protective effect of the various components of the MD. In this regard, several intervention studies have investigated the potential role of MD in the prevention of cancer, obesity, and cardiovascular and neurodegenerative diseases. Serra-Majem and Estruch [93], in their systematic review of 35 experimental studies, confirmed that MD has favorable effects on lipoprotein levels, endothelium vasodilatation, insulin resistance, metabolic syndrome, antioxidant capacity, myocardial and cardiovascular mortality, and cancer incidence in obese patients and in those with previous myocardial infarction. In a subsequent systematic review of 11 randomized clinical trials for the Cochrane Collaboration involving 52,044 subjects, Rees and colleagues [94] have further concluded that MD positively affects cardiovascular risk factors, including reduction of total cholesterol and low-density lipoprotein (LDL) cholesterol. Sleiman et al. [95] conducted a systematic review on 24 studies (including cross-sectional, prospective, and controlled clinical trials) which showed that MD has some favorable effects on both glycemic control (particularly on fasting glucose and HbA1c) and cardiovascular disease.

In the Moli-sani study, a large prospective cohort study that recruited 24,325 men and women from the general population of the Molise Region, in Southern Italy, Bonaccio et al. showed that a MD pattern was significantly associated with lower values of glucose, lipids, CRP, and blood pressure and with reduction of 10-year cardiovascular risk, while the consumption of healthy foods with high content in antioxidant, vitamins, and phytochemicals was correlated with lower blood pressure and CRP plasma levels [96]. There is a consistent evidence that nutrition modulates multiple interconnected processes that play a major role in both carcinogenesis and inflammatory responses, including free radical production, NF-κB activation, expression of inflammatory cytokines, and the eicosanoids pathway [97]. MD may positively impact the so called "*inflammaging*" through either epigenetic mechanism (that include chromatin remodeling, DNA methylation and miRNAs) or preservation of gut microbiota homeostasis [92].

Concerning the relationship between dietary patterns and mental health [98] a healthy diet such as the Mediterranean-style diet including high consumption of vegetables, fruits, legumes, olive oil, fish, cereals, nuts, and seeds can provide a range of nutrients including B vitamins, omega-3 fatty acids, and antioxidants [99]. Antioxidants can protect the brain against oxidative damage to cellular membranes, which has been implicated in psychiatric disorders including depression [100] and in dementia. The omega-3 fatty acid docosahexaenoic acid is highly concentrated in the structure of the brain and is critical for brain development. Omega-3 fatty acids and vitamins also influence a variety of brain functions including production of neurotransmitters, neuronal cell growth and survival, and protection of the blood brain barrier [99].

16.8 The Mediterranean Diet and Frailty

16.8.1 Inflammation and Frailty

The state of chronic and low-grade inflammation in elderly people which has been defined as "*inflammaging*" [101] may be prodromal to the onset of cognitive disability [102] and multimorbidity [103]. All the chronic diseases with a high prevalence in the older population may in fact be linked with altered immune and inflammatory response [104]. Chronic activation of the inflammatory response also impacts survival, contributing with cognitive symptoms, depression, and poor physical performance to define a high-risk profile for mortality [105, 106]. The role of nutrition in these processes is of great importance. Chronic low-grade inflammation, resulting from comorbidity, is one of the determining factors of loss of appetite and reduced energy intake in the elderly, also known as "anorexia of aging," while acute inflammation may contribute to raising energy requirements, thus driving the onset of "disease-related malnutrition" [107]. The anabolic imbalance resulting from nutrition and nutritional needs has been associated with the onset of frailty, muscle mass loss, muscle strength reduction, and functional dependence that leads to disability. Diminished food intake and increased energy creates a vicious circle with unfavorable prognostic trajectory [108]. This catabolic state is greatest during critical illness conditions characterized by poor response to nutritional intervention [109].

In older individuals admitted to hospital for acute illness or chronic disease reactivation, inflammation degree has a greater influence on prognosis than nutritional status [110]. More importantly, the low-grade catabolic state present outside the acute phase is strongly related to inflammaging. This phenomenon, defined as "anabolic resistance," implies a nonoptimal protein synthesis of skeletal muscle in response to physiological stimuli and is one of the major determinants of sarcopenia [111].

16.8.2 Mediterranean Diet Patterns, Osteoporosis, and Sarcopenia

There are convincing evidences about the association of a healthy diet rich in vegetables, fruits, legumes, and omega-3 fish, or a diet based on the Mediterranean diet model, with a lower risk to developing osteoporosis and sarcopenia, in old individuals. An interesting cross-sectional study conducted on 2570 women aged 18–79 years from the UK [112] for evaluating the associations between the MD score and FFM% (fat-free mass/weight × 100), FFMI (fat–free mass/height^2), hand grip strength, and leg explosive power (LEP, watts/kg) showed that higher adherence to MD was positively associated with a significantly higher fat-free mass and LEP, with a significant difference of 1.7% for FFM% and 9.6% for LEP (P trend <0.001).

Concerning the risk of sarcopenia, a cross-sectional study conducted on 327 community-dwelling elderly people from northern Taiwan [113] showed that a high daily intake of protein, mostly vegetable proteins, confer a protection against depletion of the muscle mass. Participants in the lowest total protein quartile had a higher risk for depletion of the muscle mass than those in the highest quartile (OR = 3.03; 95%CI: 1.37–6.72). Similarly, participants in the lowest vegetable protein quartile had a higher risk for depletion of the muscle mass than those in the highest quartile (OR = 2.34, 95%CI: 1.14–4.83). Two different studies conducted on Dutch population, respectively, from the Maastricht Sarcopenia Study—MaSS [114] (227 subjects) and from the PROVIDE Study [115] (136 subjects), to investigate whether there were differences in the intake of nutrients and micronutrients and in the quality of life between sarcopenic and nonsarcopenics older adults, confirmed that sarcopenic older adults differed in certain nutritional intakes and biochemical nutrient status compared with nonsarcopenic older adults. Including dietary and supplement intakes, sarcopenic older adults from the MaSS Study had a lower intake of protein ($p = 0.048$) and n-3 fatty acids ($p = 0.022$), but a higher intake of ALA ($p = 0.018$), and a lower intake of folic acid ($p = 0.016$) and magnesium ($p = 0.024$). Also, sarcopenics subjects had a lower intake of vitamin B6 from dietary intake ($p = 0.005$); when dietary supplements were included in analysis, no significant differences were observed between sarcopenic and nonsarcopenic older adults (0.679). When considering the subjects from the PROVIDE Study, all the sarcopenics older adults had a lower practice of physical activity ($p < 0.001$) and a lower quality of life ($p < 0.001$). Compared to nonsarcopenics, the sarcopenic group had a lower intake of protein/kg ($p = 0.044$), vitamin D ($p = 0.007$), vitamin B-12 ($p = 0.011$), magnesium ($p = 0.015$), phosphorus ($p = 0.014$), and selenium ($p = 0.039$) (all $p < 0.05$).

16.8.3 Mediterranean Diet Patterns and Frailty

Several studies conducted on different populations around the world have shown that a healthy diet rich in vegetables, fruits, legumes, and fish omega-3 or a diet based on the Mediterranean-style model was associated with a lower risk to develop frailty, even in very oldest individuals. On the other hand, it is well known that nutrition plays a decisive role in the development of frailty. It is well established that nutritional supplements, in addition to high intensity resistance exercise training, is an effective way of counteracting muscle weakness and physical frailty in older people [116].

Bonnefoy et al. [117] in their narrative review summarizing the current corpus of knowledge on nutrition and frailty have reiterated that the MD is the best diet to maintain the health status. Even though there are many reports on the composition of such diet, most of the authors agree that the main components are each day several vegetables (especially raw vegetables), fruits (including nuts), which provide many vitamins, raw cereals (bringing antioxidant trace elements), and olive oil. This MD is poor in red meat and rich in fish, source of n-3 fatty acids. Also, many spices with antioxidant properties and garlic with antihypertensive properties are largely used [77] (see also Chap. 14, this book). The Mediterranean Diet can therefore be considered a key component of healthy aging and the best strategy to prevent age-related disability [83, 118].

It has been shown that adherence to a Mediterranean diet has positive effects on mobility, in a sample of 935 men and women aged 65 years and more from the InCHIANTI Study, after a follow-up of 9 years [119]. Authors showed that a high adherence to the MD was associated with a better lower body performance, which was measured using the Short Physical Performance Battery (SPPB), at baseline. Also, participants with higher adherence to the MD experienced less decline in SPPB score at 3, 6, and 9 years and a lower risk of developing mobility disability. In a subsequent study which evaluated dietary quality in 192 community-dwelling volunteers older than 75 years by using the MD Score, high adherence to the MD measured by the MD Score was associated to a lower risk of developing frailty (OR = 0.26; 95 CI: 0.07–0.98) [120]. Diets rich in *n*-6 PUFA and poor in *n*-3 PUFA eicosapentaenoic acid (EPA) and docosahexaenoic acid (DHA) may result in a pro-inflammatory environment that may be deleterious for muscle or other tissues. It is known that *n*-6 PUFA are a precursor of arachidonic acid that are a substrate of cyclooxygenase and lipoxygenase enzymes (see Chap. 13, Sect. 13.4.2, this book). Fish-oil supplementation enhanced the benefits of strength training for lower limb strength, in a randomized study in Brazilian women [121]. In the same study, a greater improvement for chair-rising performances was observed for the trained group supplemented with fish oil. In another interventional study, fish oil supplementation resulted in an improvement in walking speed in postmenopausal women [122]. On the contrary, a low intake of EPA or DHA is associated with poor functional mobility, according to the results of a cross-sectional study involving 417 Japanese elderly men [123]. The results of this study suggest that fish oil supplementation has a favorable effect particularly when is taken in addition to strength training and may represent a promising preventive therapeutic strategy in the cure of frail sarcopenics patients.

The abnormal synthesis of muscle protein in sarcopenic elderly may result from various factors such as lower response to insulin or impaired response to amino acids [124, 125]. Dietary strategies should be developed to compensate for this impairments and to help counteract muscle atrophy caused by immobilization periods that are frequently observed in the elderly [126]. However, in everyday life, the distribution of protein input seems to be very heterogeneous among different meals with less than 10 g of protein ingested during the breakfast in a population of frail and institutionalized elderly [127]. In nursing homes, this clearly implies a huge period of nearly 18 h between dinner and lunch without sufficient amounts of protein. Therefore, this could explain why anabolism could be compromised even if daily protein intake is apparently adequate in this population at risk of negative outcomes.

Still on frailty, the results of a longitudinal study on 690 community-living persons older than 65 years, from the InCHIANTI Study [128], have shown that a high adherence to MD was associated with a significant lower risk of developing frailty (OR = 0.30; 95%CI: 0.14–0.66). A higher adherence to a MD pattern was also associated with a lower risk of low physical activity (OR = 0.62; 95%CI: 0.40–0.96) and low walking speed (OR = 0.48; 95%CI: 0.27–0.86). Results from a subsequent prospective cohort study involving 1872 noninstitutionalized individuals older than 60 years from the Seniors-ENRICA cohort Study [129] showed that high adherence to a *Prudent Pattern,* characterized by a high consumption of olive oil, vegetables, potatoes, legumes, blue fish, pasta, and meat, was associated to a lower risk of developing frailty (OR = 0.40; 95%CI: 0.20–0.81; *P*-trend = 0.009), as compared to a *Westernized Pattern* (WP), characterized by a high consumption of refined bread, whole dairy products, and red and processed meat, as well as low intake of whole grains, fruit, low-fat dairy, and vegetables; high adherence to the WP was associated to a high risk of developing frailty (OR = 1.61; 95%CI: 0.85–3.03; *P*-trend = 0.14). Furthermore, with respect to Fried's criteria of the frailty [8], authors showed that a high adherence to a WP was associated to high risk of slow walking speed (OR = 1.85; 95%CI: 1.19–2.87; *P*-trend = 0.007) and weight loss (OR = 2.12; 95%CI: 1.22–3.70; *P*-trend = 0.007).

Another interesting study was conducted on a sample of 2724 Chinese community-dwelling, men and women, more than 65 years old, to examine the relationship of diet patterns with incident frailty [130]. A validated semiquantitative food frequency questionnaire (FFQ) [131, 132] was used to assess the dietary intake. The following quantitative scales were then used: the first, the Dietary Quality Index-International (DQI-I), which total score ranges from 0 to 94, was used to indicate the quality of the diet, where higher score indicate better diet quality [133, 134]; the second, the Mediterranean Diet Score (MDS) was used to assess the adherence to the MD [77, 135]. Authors showed that every 10-unit increase in DQI-I was associated with 41% reduced risk of frailty in the sex- and age-adjusted model (OR = 0.59; 95%CI: 0.42–0.85; $p = 0.004$). The association attenuated after adjusting for Body Mass Index (BMI), energy intake, physical activity, education level, smoking status, alcohol use, depression, cognitive impairment, living alone, and marital status at baseline (OR = 0.69; 95%CI: 0.47–1.02; $p = 0.056$). It is interesting to note that in the no association of MDS, with frailty was observed among Chinese older people.

A further confirmation of the protective role of the Mediterranean diet towards the onset of frailty came from two studies conducted on a French and US population, respectively.

In the first study [136] involved a sample of 560 subjects older than 75 years was selected from the participants of the Bordeaux Centre of the Three-City (3C) Study [137], a population-based prospective cohort study. Food habits were evaluated by a Qualified Research Assistant using a semiquantitative Food Frequency Questionnaire (FFQ), which estimated the weekly consumption of 12 food and food groups, including fats. Adherence to the MD was evaluated by the MDS [77]. Even in this case, a high adherence to the MD was associated with a low incidence of frailty ($p = 0.02$). Indeed, after adjusting for age, sex, marital status, education, BMI, diabetes, cardiovascular history, taking more than 5 drugs/day, hypertension, MMSE score depression state, subjects with the highest adherence to MD had a significantly 68% decreased risk of developing frailty over time (OR = 0.32; 95%CI 0.14–0.72, $p = 0.006$). Compared to the Fried's criteria of frailty [8], authors showed that a high adherence to MD was associated to low risk of poor muscle strength (OR = 0.44; 95%CI: 0.20–0.98, $p = 0.04$), slowness (OR = 0.45; 95%CI: 0.20–0.99, $p = 0.04$), and low physical activity (OR = 0.39, 95%CI: 0.18–0.82; $p = 0.01$).

The second study [138] investigated whether adherence to a MD pattern was associated with a lower incidence of frailty in a large cohort of US people. 4421 participants whose data were gathered from the Osteoarthritis Initiative (OAI) were studied [139, 140]. Participants' diet patterns were analyzed using the Block Brief 2000 food frequency (FFQ) questionnaire during the baseline appointment [141]. Adherence to a MD pattern was evaluated using the Mediterranean diet score (aMED) proposed by Panagiotakos et al. [142]. The score was calculated based on a food frequency questionnaire completed during the baseline OAI visit. After adjusting for 10 potential confounders (age, sex, race, body mass index, education, smoking habits, yearly income, physical activity level, Charlson comorbidity index, and daily energy intake), participants with the highest adherence to a MD pattern were found to have a significant reduction in incident frailty (HR = 0.71; 95%CI: 0.50–0.99, $p = 0.047$), compared to those in the lower category. Concerning individual components of the MD, low consumption of poultry was associated with higher risk of frailty (HR = 1.34; 95%CI: 1.07–1.67, $p = 0.009$).

16.9 Concluding Remarks on Sarcopenia

The association between nutrition and frailty becomes evident during the clinical course of frailty (Fig. 16.4). Aging is characterized by a decrease in lean body mass, bone mineral density, and to a lesser extent fat mass. The sarcopenia leads to

Predisposing causes	Clinical aspects of frailty	Consequences of frailty
1. Polypathology 2. Polypharmacy 3. Decline of psycho-physical functions 4. Decline of the functional reserve	**Symptoms** - Weakness - Fatigue - Anorexia - Malnutrition - Weight loss **Signs** - Reduced muscle strength - Reduced bone mass - Gait and balance compromises - Cardiovascular deconditioning	- Fractures - Wounds - Acute illness - Hospitalization - Disability - Addiction - Institutionalization - Death

Fig. 16.4 The clinical course of frailty

weakness and decreased physical activity. The progression of sarcopenia may be accelerated by inadequate protein intake, which also characterizes aging [143]. The "*anorexia of aging,*" namely the loss of appetite with the consequent reduction of energy supply in the elderly, contributes to inadequate protein intake. Moreover, older people avoid consuming animal protein because of age-related factors, mainly difficulty in chewing and changes in taste and smell. Moreover, even when protein intake is adequate there are many age-related factors (insulin resistance, impairments in protein digestion and amino acid absorption) that can inhibit muscle protein synthesis stimulation in older people [144].

Poor dietary intake may also produce micronutrient deficiencies that could contribute to the development of frailty. Vitamin D and calcium are of high interest, as they may affect bone health and, hence, mobility. Insufficient intakes of both calcium and vitamin D intakes have been observed in the elderly population and may accelerate bone resorption observed in the elderly. Additionally, social isolation resulting from depression or diminished health overall may reduce the chances for sunlight exposure, and thus vitamin production in the skin, or for physical exercise, that is the major stimuli for bone calcium retention.

Food components with antioxidant properties may also be involved in the development of frailty. A progressive, although slow, deterioration of antioxidant status has been observed in healthy free-living elderly [145] along with an increase in markers of oxidative stress [146]. This could be the result of decreased dietary intake [146, 147] or the aging process per se. Increased oxidative stress is strongly implicated in the pathophysiology of aging, but also in specific pathologies of frailty, including the decline in bone mass and strength [148], and muscle atrophy [149]. While our understanding of the relationship between frailty, nutrients, and antioxidants continues to grow in terms of molecular mechanisms, the most convincing evidence connecting the nutritional and antioxidant intake and the prevention of frailty is probably the association between adherence to the MD and frailty prevention that has been observed in many cross-sectional and prospective studies described above.

References

1. Available for public access at http://ec.europa.eu/eurostat/statistics-explained/index.php/Population_structure_and_ageing.
2. Clegg A. Frailty in elderly people. Lancet. 2013;381:752–62.
3. Kinsella K, Phillips DR. Global aging: the challenge of success. Population bulletin vol. 60, no. 1. Population Reference Bureau: Washington; 2005.
4. United Nations. The world at six billion. 12 October 1999. www.un.org/esa/population/publications/sixbillion/sixbilpart1.pdf.
5. Beard JR. The World report on ageing and health: a policy framework for healthy ageing. Lancet. 2016;387:2145–54.
6. Beard JR, Bloom DE. Towards a comprehensive public health response to population ageing. Lancet. 2015;385:658–61.
7. Age Wave, Sun America. Age Wave/Sun America Retirement Reset Study. Los Angeles, CA: Age Wave, Sun America; 2011.

8. Fried LP, Tangen CM, Walston J, et al. Frailty in older adults: evidence for a phenotype. J Gerontol A Biol Sci Med Sci. 2001;56:M146–56.
9. Walston J, Hadley EC, Ferrucci L, et al. Research agenda for frailty in older adults: toward a better understanding of physiology and aetiology: summary from the American Geriatrics Society/National Institute on Aging Research Conference on Frailty in Older Adults. J Am Geriatr Soc. 2006;54:991–1001.
10. Eeles EM, White SV, O'Mahony SM, et al. The impact of frailty and delirium on mortality in older inpatients. Age Ageing. 2012;41:412–6.
11. Strandberg TE, Pitkälä KH. Frailty in elderly people. Lancet. 2007;369:1328–9.
12. Song X, Mitnitski A, Rockwood K. Prevalence and 10-year outcomes of frailty in older adults in relation to deficit accumulation. J Am Geriatr Soc. 2010;58:681–7.
13. Fried LP, Ferrucci L, Darer J, et al. Untangling the concepts of disability, frailty, and comorbidity: implications for improved targeting and care. J Gerontol. 2004;59:255–63.
14. Bandeen-Roche K, Xue Q-L, Ferrucci L, et al. Phenotype of frailty: characterization in the women's health and aging studies. J Gerontol A Biol Sci Med Sci. 2006;61:262–6.
15. Morley JE, Haren MT, Rolland Y, Kim MJ. Frailty. Med Clin N Am. 2006;90:837–47.
16. Flatt T. A new definition of aging? Front Genet. 2012;3:148.
17. Giaimo S, d'Adda di Fagagna F. Is cellular senescence an example of antagonistic pleiotropy? Aging Cell. 2012;11:378–83.
18. Sharpless NE. Loss of p16Ink4a with retention of p19Arf predisposes mice to tumorigenesis. Nature. 2001;413:86–91.
19. Sager R. Senescence as a mode of tumor suppression. Environ Health Perspect. 1991;93:59–62.
20. Baker DJ. Clearance of p16Ink4a-positive senescent cells delays ageing-associated disorders. Nature. 2011;479:232–6.
21. Baker DJ. Opposing roles for p16Ink4a and p19Arf in senescence and ageing caused by BubR1 insufficiency. Nat Cell Biol. 2008;10:825–36.
22. Baker DJ. BubR1 insufficiency causes early onset of aging-associated phenotypes and infertility in mice. Nat Genet. 2004;36:744–9.
23. Childs BG, Durik M, Baker DJ, van Deursen JM. Cellular senescence in aging and age-related disease: from mechanisms to therapy. Nat Med. 2015;21(12):1424–35.
24. Kaszubowska L. Telomere shortening and ageing of the immune system. J Physiol Pharmacol. 2008;59(suppl. 9):169–86.
25. Titus S. Impairment of BRCA1-related DNA double-strand break repair leads to ovarian aging in mice and humans. Sci Transl Med. 2013;5:172ra121.
26. Brown MK, Naidoo N. The endoplasmic reticulum stress response in aging and age-related diseases. Front Physiol. 2012;3:263.
27. Shimizu I. p53-induced adipose tissue inflammation is critically involved in the development of insulin resistance in heart failure. Cell Metab. 2012;15:51–64.
28. Minamino T. A crucial role for adipose tissue p53 in the regulation of insulin resistance. Nat Med. 2009;15:1082–7.
29. Ryan AS. Insulin resistance with aging: effects of diet and exercise. Sports Med. 2000;30:327–46.
30. Walters MS. Smoking accelerates aging of the small airway epithelium. Respir Res. 2014;15:94.
31. Wilcox G. Insulin and insulin resistance. Clin Biochem Rev. 2005;26:19–39.
32. Xu H. Chronic inflammation in fat plays a crucial role in the development of obesity-related insulin resistance. J Clin Invest. 2003;112:1821–30.
33. Roden M. Mechanism of free fatty acid-induced insulin resistance in humans. J Clin Invest. 1996;97:2859–65.
34. Guo N. Short telomeres compromise beta-cell signaling and survival. PLoS One. 2011;6:e17858.
35. Yang TK. Davallialactone from mushroom reduced premature senescence and inflammation on glucose oxidative stress in human diploid fibroblast cells. J Agric Food Chem. 2013;61:7089–95.

36. Liu J. Receptor for advanced glycation end-products promotes premature senescence of proximal tubular epithelial cells via activation of endoplasmic reticulum stress-dependent p21 signaling. Cell Signal. 2014;26:110–21.
37. Mortuza R, Chen S, Feng B, Sen S, Chakrabarti S. High glucose induced alteration of SIRTs in endothelial cells causes rapid aging in a p300 and FOXO regulated pathway. PLoS One. 2013;8:e54514.
38. Kim YJ. miR-486–5p induces replicative senescence of human adipose tissue-derived mesenchymal stem cells and its expression is controlled by high glucose. Stem Cells Dev. 2012;21:1749–60.
39. Jialal I, Devaraj S. The role of oxidized low-density lipoprotein in atherogenesis. J Nutr. 1996;126:1053S–7S.
40. Ilhan F, Kalkanli ST. Atherosclerosis and the role of immune cells. World J Clin Cases. 2015;3:345–52.
41. Salpea KD, Humphries SE. Telomere length in atherosclerosis and diabetes. Atherosclerosis. 2010;209:35–8.
42. Kawashima S, Yokoyama M. Dysfunction of endothelial nitric oxide synthase and atherosclerosis. Arterioscler Thromb Vasc Biol. 2004;24:998–1005.
43. Riera CE, Dillin A. Tipping the metabolic scales towards increased longevity in mammals. Nat Cell Biol. 2015;17:196–203.
44. Finkel T. The metabolic regulation of aging. Nat Med. 2015;21(12):1416–23.
45. Bertrand HA, Lynd FT, Masoro EJ, Yu BP. Changes in adipose mass and cellularity through the adult life of rats fed ad libitum or a life-prolonging restricted diet. J Gerontol. 1980;35:827–35.
46. Barzilai N, Banerjee S, Hawkins M, Chen W, Rossetti L. Caloric restriction reverses hepatic insulin resistance in aging rats by decreasing visceral fat. J Clin Invest. 1998;101:1353–61.
47. Liao CY, Rikke BA, Johnson TE, Diaz V, Nelson JF. Genetic variation in the murine lifespan response to dietary restriction: from life extension to life shortening. Aging Cell. 2010;9:92–5.
48. Speakman JR, Mitchell SE. Caloric restriction. Mol Asp Med. 2011;32:159–221.
49. Liao CY. Fat maintenance is a predictor of the murine lifespan response to dietary restriction. Aging Cell. 2011;10:629–39.
50. Vermeij WP. Restricted diet delays accelerated ageing and genomic stress in DNA-repair-deficient mice. Nature. 2016;537:427–47.
51. Giezenaar C. Ageing is associated with decreases in appetite and energy intake—a meta-analysis in healthy adults. Forum Nutr. 2016;8:28. https://doi.org/10.3390/nu8010028.
52. Huffman KM. Caloric restriction alters the metabolic response to a mixed-meal: results from a randomized, controlled trial. PLoS One. 2012;7:e28190.
53. Willette AA. Interleukin-8 and interleukin-10, brain volume and microstructure, and the influence of calorie restriction in old rhesus macaques. Age (Dordr). 2013;35:2215–27.
54. Youm YH. The ketone metabolite β-hydroxybutyrate blocks NLRP3 inflammasome–mediated inflammatory disease. Nat Med. 2015;21:263–9.
55. Yang H, Youm YH, Dixit VD. Inhibition of thymic adipogenesis by caloric restriction is coupled with reduction in age-related thymic involution. J Immunol. 2009;183:3040–52.
56. Masoro EJ. Overview of caloric restriction and ageing. Mech Ageing Dev. 2005;126:913–22.
57. Dillin A. Rates of behavior and aging specified by mitochondrial function during development. Science. 2002;298:2398–401.
58. Lee SS. A systematic RNAi screen identifies a critical role for mitochondria in C. elegans longevity. Nat Genet. 2003;33:40–8.
59. Short KR. Decline in skeletal muscle mitochondrial function with aging in humans. Proc Natl Acad Sci U S A. 2005;102:5618–23.
60. Trifunovic A. Premature ageing in mice expressing defective mitochondrial DNA polymerase. Nature. 2004;429:417–23.
61. Kujoth GC. Mitochondrial DNA mutations, oxidative stress, and apoptosis in mammalian aging. Science. 2005;309:481–4.

62. Rea SL, Ventura N, Johnson TE. Relationship between mitochondrial electron transport chain dysfunction, development, and life extension in Caenorhabditis elegans. PLoS Biol. 2007;5:e259.
63. Harman D. Aging: a theory based on free radical and radiation chemistry. J Gerontol. 1956;11:298–300.
64. Barja G. The mitochondrial free radical theory of aging. Prog Mol Biol Transl Sci. 2014;127:1–27.
65. Yun J, Finkel T. Mitohormesis. Cell Metab. 2014;19:757–66.
66. Ristow M. Unraveling the truth about antioxidants: mitohormesis explains ROS-induced health benefits. Nat Med. 2014;20:709–11.
67. Ristow M, Schmeisser K. Mitohormesis: promoting health and lifespan by increased levels of reactive oxygen species (ROS). Dose-Response. 2014;12:288–341.
68. López-Lluch G. Calorie restriction induces mitochondrial biogenesis and bioenergetic efficiency. Proc Natl Acad Sci U S A. 2006;103:1768–73.
69. Finley LW. Skeletal muscle transcriptional coactivator PGC-1α mediates mitochondrial, but not metabolic, changes during calorie restriction. Proc Natl Acad Sci U S A. 2012;109:2931–6.
70. Gomes AP. Declining NAD+ induces a pseudohypoxic state disrupting nuclear-mitochondrial communication during aging. Cell. 2013;155:1624–38.
71. Cuervo AM. Autophagy and aging: the importance of maintaining "clean" cells. Autophagy. 2005;1:131–40.
72. Rana A, Rera M, Walker DW. Parkin overexpression during aging reduces proteotoxicity, alters mitochondrial dynamics, and extends lifespan. Proc Natl Acad Sci U S A. 2013;110:8638–43.
73. Capurso C, Vendemiale G. The mediterranean diet reduces the risk and mortality of the prostate cancer: a narrative review. Front Nutr. 2017;4:38. https://doi.org/10.3389/fnut.2017.00038.
74. Willett WC, Sacks F, Trichopoulou A, et al. Mediterranean diet pyramid: a cultural model for healthy eating. Am J Clin Nutr. 1995;61(Suppl 6):S1402–6.
75. Fundación Dieta Mediterránea. (2010). https://dietamediterranea.com.
76. Keys AB. Seven Countries: A multivariate analysis of death and coronary heart disease. Cambridge, MA: Harvard University Press; 1980. p. 381.
77. Trichopoulou A. Adherence to a mediterranean diet and survival in a greek population. N Engl J Med. 2003;348:2599–608.
78. Trichopoulou A. Diet and overall survival in the elderly. BMJ. 1995;311:1457–60.
79. Estruch R. Primary prevention of cardiovascular disease with a Mediterranean diet. N Engl J Med. 2013;368:1279–90.
80. Sofi F. Adherence to Mediterranean diet and health status: meta-analysis. BMJ. 2008;337:a1344. https://doi.org/10.1136/bmj.a1344.
81. Sofi F. Accruing evidence on benefits of adherence to the Mediterranean diet on health: an updated systematic review and meta-analysis. Am J Clin Nutr. 2010;92:1189–96.
82. Qi W. The ω-3 fatty acid α-linolenic acid extends Caenorhabditis elegans lifespan via NHR-49/PPARα and oxidation to oxylipins. Aging Cell. 2017;16(5):1125–35.
83. Mathers JC. Nutrition and ageing: knowledge, gaps and research priorities. Proc Nutr Soc. 2013;72(2):246–50.
84. Bishop NA, Lu T, Yankner BA. Neural mechanisms of ageing and cognitive decline. Nature. 2011;464:529–35.
85. Huffman DM. Energetic interventions for healthspan and resiliency with aging. Exp Gerontol. 2016;86:73–83.
86. Lafortune L. Behavioural risk factors in mid-life associated with successful ageing, disability, dementia and frailty in later life: a rapid systematic review. PLoS One. 2016;11(2):e0144405. https://doi.org/10.1371/journal.pone.0144405.
87. Britton A, Shipley M, Singh-Manoux A, Marmot MG. Successful aging: the contribution of early life and midlife risk factors. J Am Geriatr Soc. 2008;56:1098–105.
88. Akbaraly T, Sabia S, Hagger-Johnson G, et al. Does overall diet in midlife predict future aging phenotypes? A cohort study. Am J Med. 2013;126:411–9.

89. Samieri C. The association between dietary patterns at midlife and health in aging an observational study. Ann Intern Med. 2013;159:584–91.
90. Trichopoulou A. Modified Mediterranean diet and survival: EPIC-elderly prospective cohort study. BMJ. 2005;330(7498):991.
91. Shi Z. Food habits, lifestyle factors and mortality among oldest old Chinese: the Chinese longitudinal healthy longevity survey (CLHLS). Forum Nutr. 2015;7:7562–79.
92. Carruba G. Nutrition, aging and cancer: lessons from dietary intervention studies. Immun Ageing. 2016;13:13. https://doi.org/10.1186/s12979-016-0069-9.
93. Serra-Majem L, Roman B, Estruch R. Scientific evidence of interventions using the Mediterranean diet: a systematic review. Nutr Rev. 2006;64:S27–47.
94. Rees K. "Mediterranean" dietary pattern for the primary prevention of cardiovascular disease. Cochrane Database Syst Rev. 2013;8:CD009825. https://doi.org/10.1002/14651858.CD009825.pub2.
95. Sleiman D, Al-Badri MR, Azar ST. Effect of Mediterranean diet in diabetes control and cardiovascular risk modification: a systematic review. Front Public Health. 2015;3:69. https://doi.org/10.3389/fpubh.2015.00069.
96. Bonaccio M, Cerletti C, Iacoviello L, de Gaetano G. Mediterranean diet and low-grade subclinical inflammation: the moli-sani study. Endocr Metab Immune Disord Drug Targets. 2015;15:18–24.
97. Di Renzo L. Changes in LDL oxidative status and oxidative and inflammatory gene expression after red wine intake in healthy people: a randomized trial. Mediat Inflamm. 2015;2015:317348. https://doi.org/10.1155/2015/317348.
98. Milte CM, McNaughton SA. Dietary patterns and successful ageing: a systematic review. Eur J Nutr. 2016;55:423–50.
99. Parletta N, Milte CM, Meyer BJ. Nutritional modulation of cognitive function and mental health. J Nutr Biochem. 2013;24:725–43.
100. Smaga I. Oxidative stress as an etiological factor and a potential treatment target of psychiatric disorders. Part 2. Depression, anxiety, schizophrenia and autism. Pharmacol Rep. 2015;67:569–80.
101. Ticinesi A. Nutrition and inflammation in older individuals: focus on vitamin D, n-3 polyunsaturated fatty acids and whey proteins. Forum Nutr. 2016;8:186. https://doi.org/10.3390/nu8040186.
102. Giunta B. Inflammaging as a prodrome to Alzheimer's disease. J Neuroinflammation. 2008;5:51. https://doi.org/10.1186/1742-2094-5-51.
103. Stepanova M. Age-independent rise of inflammatory scores may contribute to accelerated aging in multimorbidity. Oncotarget. 2015;6:1414–21.
104. Ostan R. Inflammaging and cancer: a challenge for the mediterranean diet. Forum Nutr. 2015;7:2589–621.
105. Brown PJ. Inflammation, depression, and slow gait: a high mortality phenotype in later life. J Gerontol A Biol Sci Med Sci. 2016;71:221–7.
106. Giovannini S. Interleukin-6, C-reactive protein, and tumor necrosis factor-alpha as predictors of mortality in frail, community-living elderly individuals. J Am Geriatr Soc. 2011;59:1679–85.
107. Cederholm T. The role of malnutrition in older persons with mobility limitations. Curr Pharm Des. 2014;20:3173–7.
108. Jensen GL. Malnutrition and inflammation—"burning down the house": inflammation as an adaptive physiologic response versus self-destruction? J Parenter Enter Nutr. 2015;39:56–62.
109. Batt J, Dos Santos CC, Herridge MS. Muscle injury during critical illness. J Am Med Assoc. 2013;310:1569–70.
110. Nouvenne A. The prognostic value of high-sensitivity C-reactive protein and prealbumin for short-term mortality in acutely hospitalized multimorbid elderly patients: a prospective cohort study. J Nutr Health Aging. 2016;20:462–8.
111. Haran PH, Rivas DA, Fielding RA. Role and potential mechanisms of anabolic resistance in sarcopenia. J Cachexia Sarcopenia Muscle. 2012;3:157–62.

112. Kelaiditi E. Measurements of skeletal muscle mass and power are positively related to a Mediterranean dietary pattern in women. Osteoporos Int. 2016;27:3251–60.
113. Huang RY. The association between total protein and vegetable protein intake and low muscle mass among the community-dwelling elderly population in Northern Taiwan. Nutrients. 2016;8(6):E373. https://doi.org/10.3390/nu8060373.
114. Ter Borg S. Differences in nutrient intake and biochemical nutrient status between Sarcopenic and Nonsarcopenic older adults-results from the Maastricht sarcopenia study. J Am Med Dir Assoc. 2016;17(5):393–401.
115. Verlaan S. Nutritional status, body composition, and quality of life in community-dwelling sarcopenic and non-sarcopenic older adults: a case-control study. Clin Nutr. 2017;36(1):267–74.
116. Fiatarone MA. Exercise training and nutritional supplementation for physical frailty in very elderly people. N Engl J Med. 1994;330(25):1769–75.
117. Bonnefoy M. Frailty and nutrition: searching for evidence. J Nutr Health Aging. 2015;19(3):250–7.
118. Kiefte-de Jong JC, Mathers JC, Franco OH. Nutrition and healthy ageing: the key ingredients. Proc Nutr Soc. 2014;73(2):249–59.
119. Milaneschi Y, Bandinelli S, Corsi AM, et al. Mediterranean diet and mobility decline in older persons. Exp Gerontol. 2011;46(4):303–8.
120. Bollweinlu J, Diekmann R, Kaiser MJ, et al. Dietary quality is related to frailty in community-dwelling older adults. J Gerontol A Biol Sci Med Sci. 2013;68(4):483–9.
121. Rodacki CLN. Fish-oil supplementation enhances the effects of strength training in elderly women. Am J Clin Nutr. 2012;95(2):428–36.
122. Hutchins-Wiese HL. The impact of supplemental n-3 long chain polyunsaturated fatty acids and dietary antioxidants on physical performance in postmenopausal women. J Nutr Health Aging. 2013;17(1):76–80.
123. Takayama M. Association of marine-origin n-3 polyunsaturated fatty acids consumption and functional mobility in the community-dwelling oldest old. J Nutr Health Aging. 2013;17(1):82–9.
124. Biolo G. Short-term bed rest impairs amino acid-induced protein anabolism in humans. J Physiol Lond. 2004;558(Pt 2):381–8.
125. Volpi E, Mittendorfer B, Rasmussen BB, Wolfe RR. The response of muscle protein anabolism to combined hyperaminoacidemia and glucose-induced hyperinsulinemia is impaired in the elderly. J Clin Endocrinol Metab. 2000;85:4481–90.
126. Magne H, Savary-Auzeloux I, Rémond D, Dardevet D. Nutritional strategies to counteract muscle atrophy caused by disuse and to improve recovery. Nutr Res Rev. 2013;26(2):149–65.
127. Tieland M, Borgonjen-Van den Berg KJ, van Loon LJC, de Groot LCPGM. Dietary protein intake in community-dwelling, frail, and institutionalized elderly people: scope for improvement. Eur J Nutr. 2012;51(2):173–9.
128. Talegawkar SA. Development of frailty in community-dwelling elderly men and women. J Nutr. 2012;142:2161–6.
129. Luz M, León-Muñoz LM. Major dietary patterns and risk of frailty in older adults: a prospective cohort study. BMC Med. 2015;13:11. https://doi.org/10.1186/s12916-014-0255-6.
130. Chan R, Leung J, Woo J. Dietary patterns and risk of frailty in Chinese community-dwelling older people in Hong Kong: a prospective cohort study. Forum Nutr. 2015;7:7070–84.
131. Woo J, Leung SSF, Ho SC, Lam TH, Janus ED. A food frequency questionnaire for use in the Chinese population in Hong Kong: description and examination of validity. Nutr Res. 1997;17:1633–41.
132. Chan R, Chan D, Woo J. Associations between dietary patterns and demographics, lifestyle, anthropometry and blood pressure in Chinese community-dwelling older men and women. J Nutr Sci. 2012;1:e20. https://doi.org/10.1017/jns.2012.19. eCollection 2012.
133. Kim S, Haines PS, Siega-Riz AM, Popkin BM. The diet quality index-international (DQI-I) provides an effective tool for cross-national comparison of diet quality as illustrated by China and the United States. J Nutr. 2003;133:3476–84.

134. Woo J, Cheung B, Ho S, Sham A, Lam TH. Influence of dietary pattern on the development of overweight in a Chinese population. Eur J Clin Nutr. 2008;62:480–7.
135. Chan R, Chan D, Woo J. The association of a priori and a posterior dietary pattern with the risk of incident stroke in Chinese older people in Hong Kong. J Nutr Health Aging. 2013;17:866–74.
136. Rahi B, Ajana S, Tabue-Teguo M, Dartigues JF, Peres K, Feart C. High adherence to a Mediterranean diet and lower risk of frailty among French older adults community-dwellers: Results from the Three-City-Bordeaux Study. Clin Nutr. 2017. https://doi.org/10.1016/j.clnu.2017.05.020.
137. The Three City Study Group. Vascular factors and risk of dementia: design of the Three-City Study and baseline characteristics of the study population. Neuroepidemiology. 2003;22:316–25.
138. Veronese N, Stubbs B, Noale M, et al. Adherence to a Mediterranean diet is associated with lower incidence of frailty: a longitudinal cohort study. Clin Nutr. 2017. https://doi.org/10.1016/j.clnu.2017.08.028.
139. Felson DT, Nevitt MC. Epidemiologic studies for osteoarthritis: new versus conventional study design approaches. Rheum Dis Clin N Am. 2004;30:783–97.
140. Available for public access at http://www.oai.ucsf.edu.
141. Block G, Hartman AM, Naughton D. A reduced dietary questionnaire: development and validation. Epidemiology. 1990;1:58–64.
142. Panagiotakos DB, Pitsavos C, Stefanadis C. Dietary patterns: a Mediterranean diet score and its relation to clinical and biological markers of cardiovascular disease risk. Nutr Metab Cardiovasc Dis. 2006;16:559–68.
143. Yannakoulia M, Ntanasi E, Anastasiou CA, Scarmeas N. Frailty and nutrition: from epidemiological and clinical evidence to potential mechanisms. Metabolism. 2017;68:64–76.
144. Burd NA, Gorissen SH, van Loon LJ. Anabolic resistance of muscle protein synthesis with aging. Exerc Sport Sci Rev. 2013;41:169–73.
145. Andriollo-Sanchez M. Age-related oxidative stress and antioxidant parameters in middle-aged and older European subjects: the ZENITH study. Eur J Clin Nutr. 2005;59(Suppl. 2):S58–62.
146. Junqueira VB. Aging and oxidative stress. Mol Asp Med. 2004;25:5–16.
147. Zujko ME, Witkowska AM, Waskiewicz A, Mironczuk-Chodakowska I. Dietary antioxidant and flavonoid intakes are reduced in the elderly. Oxidative Med Cell Longev. 2015;2015:843173.
148. Manolagas SC. From estrogen-centric to aging and oxidative stress: a revised perspective of the pathogenesis of osteoporosis. Endocr Rev. 2010;31:266–300.
149. Meng SJ, YLJ O. Stress, molecular inflammation and sarcopenia. Int J Mol Sci. 2010;11:1509–26.

MIX
Papier aus verantwortungsvollen Quellen
Paper from responsible sources
FSC® C105338

If you have any concerns about our products,
you can contact us on
ProductSafety@springernature.com

In case Publisher is established outside the EU,
the EU authorized representative is:
Springer Nature Customer Service Center GmbH
Europaplatz 3, 69115 Heidelberg, Germany

Printed by Libri Plureos GmbH
in Hamburg, Germany